Echocardiographic Anatomy

Understanding Normal and Abnormal Echocardiograms

Ivan A. D'Cruz, M.D., F. R. C. P. (Lond & Edin)
Professor of Medicine, University of Tennessee
Director, Echocardiography Laboratories of Memphis VA Medical Center
Director, University of Tennessee Bowld Hospital
Memphis, Tennessee

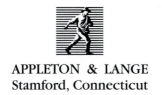

APPLETON & LANGE
Stamford, Connecticut

96 97 98 99 / 10 9 8 7 6 5 4 3 2 1

Prentice Hall International (UK) Limited, *London*
Prentice Hall of Australia Pty. Limited, *Sydney*
Prentice Hall Canada, Inc., *Toronto*
Prentice Hall Hispanoamericana, S.A., *Mexico*
Prentice Hall of India Private Limited, *New Delhi*
Prentice Hall of Japan, Inc., *Tokyo*
Simon & Schuster Asia Pte. Ltd., *Singapore*
Editora Prentice Hall do Brasil Ltda., *Rio de Janeiro*
Prentice Hall, *Englewood Cliffs, New Jersey*

Library of Congress Cataloging-in-Publication Data
D'Cruz, Ivan A.
    Echocardiographic anatomy: understanding normal and abnormal
    echocardiograms / Ivan D'Cruz.
        p.   cm.
    Includes index.
    ISBN 0-8385-2037-5 (case)
    1. Echocardiography. 2. Heart—Anatomy   I. Title
    [DNLM: 1. Echocardiography—methods.   2. Heart Diseases
    —diagnosis.   3. Heart—anatomy & histology.   WG 141.5.E2 D277ea
    1995]
    RC683.5.U5D379   1995
    616.1'207543—dc20
    DNLM/DLC
    for Library of Congress   95-14256
                                                                       CIP

Acquisitions Editor: Jane Licht
Production Service: Editorial Services of New England
Designer: Libby Schmitz

PRINTED IN THE UNITED STATES OF AMERICA

ISBN 0-8385-2037-5

*Dedicated to the eighty
cardiac fellows who have read
echocardiograms with me over
the past twenty years,
in Chicago, Augusta, and Memphis*

Acknowledgments

I am very grateful to the following persons, most of whom were at the Augusta, Georgia VA Medical Center during the period when this book was written:

• Ms. Carol Brown, for excellent word processing, exercising great patience, and deciphering my wayward handwriting.

• Mr. Russ Baltesar (Augusta) and Ms. Sibyl Waring (Chicago) for improving on my freehand drawings of diagrams.

• Ms. Karen McBride for high expertise in photography.

• Ms. Pat Orander for making the labels for the illustrations.

• Ms. Mary Walden, Lelia Childers, Renee Herron, and Janice Cook for recording most of the echocardiograms illustrated.

• Drs. Leo Horan, Charles Gross, M. Sridharan, and Ernest Madu whose collegial friendship and encouragement elevated the practice of echocardiography from an arduous duty to a pleasant and stimulating experience.

• Ms. Jane Licht of Appleton & Lange, whose unremitting help, advice, and cooperation facilitated progress of this book at every stage from inception to completion.

Contents

Preface

It has been my consistent experience over a 20-year period of running an echocardiography laboratory that the majority of cardiologists and cardiologists in training are unaware of most details of cardiac anatomy. Until about 20 years ago, clinical cardiologists could function adequately with no more knowledge of cardiac anatomy than that the heart possessed four chambers and four valves, as well as the knowledge of which structures represent the various bulges of the cardiac silhouette on the chest x-ray. Cardiologists who performed angiocardiography did become better acquainted with the shape, size, and location of cardiac chambers and vessels—but only to the extent of recognizing contours of shadows cast on cine films by opacified blood.

Recent noninvasive imaging techniques including echocardiography, magnetic resonance imaging (MRI), and computed tomography (CT) reveal cardiac and mediastinal anatomy in fuller detail and in a multiplicity of planes as never before. The versatile electronic retinas of such probes can detect spatial relationships, distinguish textures and densities, and even capture (by echo Doppler technology) rapid sequences of motion and flow within the heart and great vessels. To understand the imagery displayed on videoscreens by these newer devices, and to fulfill the richer and more realistic promises of three-dimensional echocardiography, requires a much greater knowledge of anatomy than in earlier, less-sophisticated decades.

Typical medical students have brief encounters with thoracic anatomy in their freshman year. This scant store of knowledge further dwindles until they start their cardiology fellowship six or more years later.

Sonographers trained at a good center may have had the benefit of instruction in cardiac anatomy and in ultrasound technique. But a good grasp of the relevance and application of the former to the latter is often lacking. The recent wide usage of transesophageal echocardiography has made it necessary for echocardiographers to acquire orientation with respect to a whole new series of posterior acoustic windows in addition to the several transthoracic windows already in use.

In order for echocardiographers to develop a sense of topography that can adjust to any acoustic cardiac window and recognize both normal variants as well as cardiac pathology, a thorough, comprehensive foundation of cardiac and mediastinal anatomy is essential—hence, this book.

Several excellent textbooks on echocardiography of the traditional, classic type have been published, including recent ones of vast scope and monumental size. This volume is not a textbook in the usual sense. It endeavors, instead, to provide a basis on which to build echocardiographic expertise and interpretive skills for those who have recently embarked on the discipline of cardiac ultrasound. Others, who have already been performing or reading echocardiograms empirically, may find their work more interesting and rewarding, the deeper and sounder knowledge they have of the cardiac structures they study on the videoscreen. They might find it better and safer to set sail on charted, rather than uncharted, seas.

Some of the greatest pioneers of cardiology (Harvey, Corvisart, Laennec, Osler—to mention a few) were outstanding anatomists as well as physicians. For various reasons, modern cardiologists seldom have the opportunity to view or section normal or abnormal human hearts. However, in another sense, they are more privileged than those illustrious predecessors; with the all-seeing electronic eye of the ultrasound probe, they can study the beating heart as the ancients never could. But in order to understand the moving anatomy that videoscreens reveal, students must first be instructed in what there is to see. Echocardiographic images make full sense only when the configurations they represent have already been imprinted on the trained mind. Not only normal cardiac anatomy, but also important aspects of pathological anatomy are depicted here. I have included those aspects of abnormal cardiac anatomy essential to the comprehension of the imaging of common cardiac entities.

The diagrams have been made as uncluttered as possible so that the reader is presented with easily comprehended, clear, simple images rather than elaborate works of art. The echocardiograms chosen are those that depict normal anatomy or illustrate common abnormalities. It is hoped that these illustrations as well as the text of this book will help bridge the gap between cardiac anatomy and gross pathology on the one hand, and echocardiographic interpretation and diagnosis on the other.

Except for the first three and the last two chapters, the sequence of chapters follows the path of circulating blood, from Systemic Great Veins (Chapter 4) to Aorta (Chapter 20).

In deciding which anatomic or echocardiographic information to include, I have been guided by what, in my experience, is helpful in understanding echocardiographic appearances: what data might be of practical use to the clinician, what information might prevent potential pitfalls in interpretation, and what instruction might fill in common lacunae in the knowledge of students or practitioners of cardiac ultrasound. I was often tempted to lengthen the text or include more figures, to make an extra point here or illustrate an additional variant or abnormality there, but my criteria for inclusion were practical usefulness and relevance to echocardiography. Also, I have aimed for readability, conciseness, and ease of comprehension. As Leonardo da Vinci, who dissected the heart nearly five centuries ago, wrote: "How in words can you describe this heart without filling a whole book? Yet the more detail you write concerning it, the more you will confuse the mind of the hearer." Cardiac anatomy has not changed since then, nor has the dilemma of how best to teach it.

Foreword

It gives me great pleasure to write this foreword for Dr. Ivan D'Cruz's book *Echocardiographic Anatomy: Understanding Normal and Abnormal Echocardiograms*. Dr. Ivan D'Cruz has been in the forefront of echocardiography for the past several years and has done pioneering work in relation to echocardiographic assessment of mitral annular calcification and pericardial effusion and cardiac tamponade. Because of his background and tremendous experience in echocardiography, he is very well suited to write a book of this type. With rapid advances occurring in echocardiography and other non-invasive modalities, it is essential to have a comprehensive knowledge of cardiac anatomy and a thorough understanding of the complex spatial interrelationships of various cardiac structures; this becomes even more important when one deals with the emerging, exciting technique of three- and four-dimensional echocardiography. Dr. D'Cruz's book superbly fulfills these needs: it consists of 22 chapters which cover all aspects of echocardiographic anatomy. In addition, it is amply illustrated with high quality line drawings and graphic displays. There is no question in my mind that this book would be of great value to both cardiac sonographers and physician echocardiographers. It will not only help build a sound basis for enhancing technical and interpretive skills of echocardiographers by relating anatomic features to echocardiographic findings but also help them recognize and avoid pitfalls. I commend Dr. Ivan D'Cruz for doing a super job.

Navin C. Nanda, M.D.
Professor of Medicine and
Director, Heart Station and
Echocardiography Laboratories
University of Alabama at Birmingham
Birmingham, Alabama

Abbreviations

AAO, AS AO	Ascending aorta	**OBL SIN**	Oblique sinus
AI	Aortic incompetence	**PA**	Pseudoaneurysm
AML	Anterior mitral leaflet	**PDA**	Patent ductus arteriosus
ANEU	Aneurysm	**PER**	Pericardium
AO, AOR	Aorta	**PER EFF**	Pericardial effusion
AOA, AO AR	Aortic arch	**PL**	Pacemaker lead
ARC	Arch of aorta	**PLE EFF**	Pleural effusion
AR	Aortic root	**PM**	Papillary muscle
AS, ASC	Ascites or atrial septum	**PML**	Posterior mitral leaflet
ATL	Anterior tricuspid leaflet	**PS**	Pulmonary stenosis
AV	Aortic valve	**PT**	Pulmonary trunk
AZV	Azygos vein	**PULM**	Pulmonary
CS, COR SIN	Coronary sinus	**PV**	Pulmonary valve or vein
CSV	Crista supraventricularis	**RA**	Right atrium
CT	Chordae tendineae	**RPA**	Right pulmonary artery
DA, DAO, DE AO	Descending aorta	**RPV**	Right pulmonary vein
ECG	Electrocardiogram	**RV**	Right ventricle
EFF	Effusion	**RV INFL**	Right ventricular inflow
EPSS	Mitral e-point septal separation	**RVO, RVOT**	Right ventricular outflow tract
HV	Hepatic vein	**SAM**	Systolic anterior motion (mitral)
IVC	Inferior vena cava	**SEP**	Septum (ventricular)
LA	Left atrium	**SI**	Superior-inferior
LAPW	Left atrial posterior wall	**SMC**	Submitral calcification
LAA	Left atrial appendage	**ST**	Stomach
LIG ART	Ligamentum arteriosum	**STL**	Septal tricuspid leaflet
LIV	Liver	**SVC**	Superior vena cava
LPA	Left pulmonary artery	**TDA**	Thoracic descending aorta
LPV	Left pulmonary vein	**THR**	Thrombus
LSVC	Left superior vena cava	**TR**	Tricuspid regugitation
LV	Left ventricle	**TR SIN**	Transverse sinus (pericardial)
LVOT	Left ventricular outflow tract	**TUM**	Tumor
LVPW, LVW	Left ventricular posterior wall	**TV**	Tricuspid valve
LYMP	Lymphoma	**VAL**	Valve
MA, MAS	Mass	**VEG**	Vegetation
MR,	Mitral regurgitation	**VERT**	Vertebra
MV	Mitral valve	**VSD**	Ventricular septal defect

Two-Dimensional Echocardiographic Views

ECHO "WINDOWS"

The heart and great vessels are surrounded by the air-filled lungs on either side as well as to a large extent anteriorly, and ultrasound cannot penetrate these areas. There are only a few anatomic locations uncovered by lung through which an ultrasound probe might succeed in depicting cardiac structures.

On the anterior chest wall these "windows" include the left parasternal region, the cardiac apex, and any point in between. These views sometimes may be obtained with the patient lying flat supine, but they are commonly of better quality with the patient lying in a partial left-lateral position, which allows the ventricles to "fall" nearer to the left anterior chest wall. The parasternal window exists because the anterior lower edge of the left lung (unlike the right) does not extend all the way to the sternum but exposes a small "bare" area of the heart to view, with only pericardium and chest wall interposed between it and the ultrasound probe.

Other echo windows routinely used include the *subcostal* (formerly called *subxiphoid*); the ultrasound probe is placed on the upper epigastric area and directed upward toward the cardiac chambers or posteriorly toward the inferior vena cava and abdominal aorta. Another conventional window is the *suprasternal,* which permits the echocardiographer to look downward behind the manubrium sternum at the aortic arch and other mediastinal structures. The *right parasternal* window probably has been underutilized; it is particularly revealing when the ascending aorta is dilated. Large *pleural effusions* may

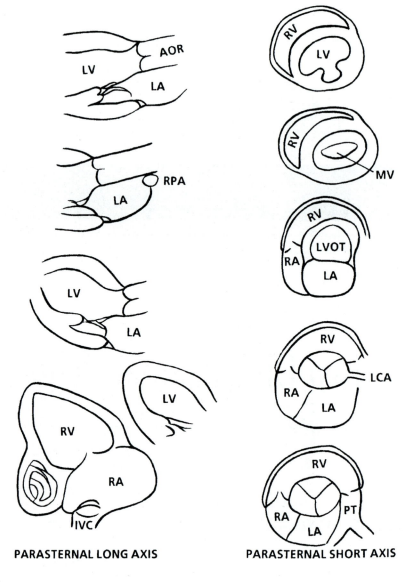

Figure 1–1. (Left) The upper four diagrams are variants of the parasternal long-axis view. The difference between them lies in whether the sector image is closer to the base or to the apex of the heart. The lowest diagram on the left represents the parasternal right heart inflow view, obtained by angling the transducer toward the right hip instead of perpendicular to the chest wall. (Right) Parasternal short-axis view, progressing from the papillary muscle level (top) through LV-mitral, LV outflow–LA, aortic valve–RV outflow, and finally aorta–pulmonary arteries views.

PARASTERNAL LONG AXIS   **PARASTERNAL SHORT AXIS**

provide lateral thoracic windows to the heart, since fluid is a good transmitter of ultrasound and the collapsed underlying lung is not a major echocardiographic obstacle.

No posterior thoracic echo windows are available because the vertebral column and paraspinal muscles are impenetrable to ultrasound. However, the esophagus has proven an excellent window to posterior mediastinal as well as cardiac structures. *Transesophageal echocardiography (TEE)* has shown rapid technological development in recent years so that it now provides the echocardiographer with a new panorama of imaging planes (discussed later in this book).

The heart, a three-dimensional (3D) object, can be viewed from multiple windows in a large number (theoretically infinite) of possible planes by varying transducer tilt and rotation. Each view, such as the parasternal, apical, and subcostal views, should not be regarded as a single fixed standard plane (analogous to an ECG chest lead) but rather as a family or range of planes. The echocardiographer can (and should) endeavor to adjust the tilt of the two-dimensional (2D) echo probe, as well as its rotation around its long axis, to best study the cardiac chamber or structure that is the focus of clinical or echocardiographic interest.

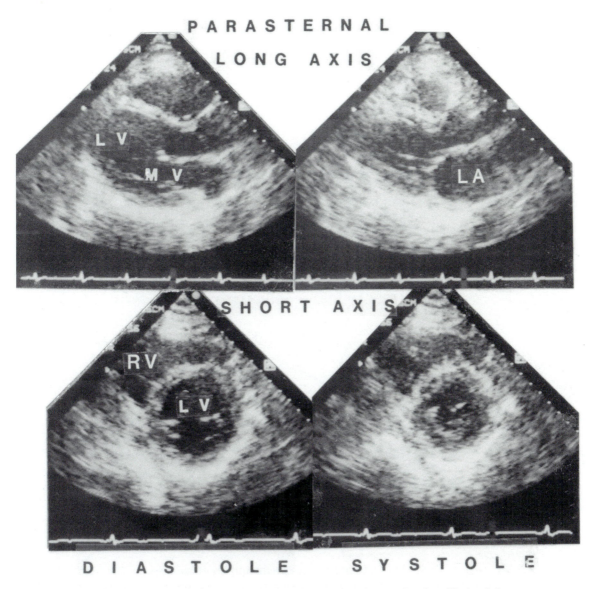

Figure 1–2. Parasternal long-axis view (above) and short-axis view (below) in a normal man. Left frames in diastole, right frames in systole. Long-axis view shows the mitral valve open in diastole and closed in systole.

PARASTERNAL LONG AXIS VIEW (Figures 1–1 to 1–3)

With the transducer near the mid-left sternal border, the plane interrogated is that of the left ventricular (LV) long axis. Good visualization is attained of the aortic and mitral valves as well as the basal LV and lower left atrial (LA) chambers. It may be possible to so manipulate the probe as to obtain a higher view of the base of the heart, including a greater length of ascending aorta (see Figure 1-1), as well as the whole length of the left atrium and even a cross section of the right pulmonary artery as it runs along the roof of the left atrium. At the other end of the parasternal long-axis range, it may be possible to visualize the LV chamber at and below the papillary muscle level; the contour and motion of the anteroseptal LV wall is particularly well seen in this view.

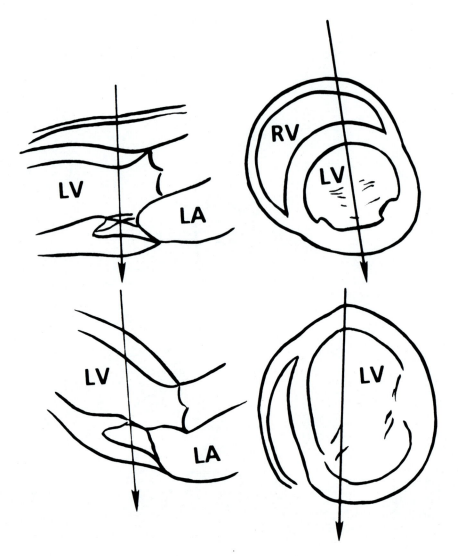

Figure 1–3. Diagram of parasternal long-axis and short-axis views. The long arrows indicate the proper cursor position for M-mode recordings of the LV chamber, at chordae level, bisecting the circular LV in short-axis view. Unsatisfactory 2D images for M-mode derivation are shown below. At the left, the LV long-axis is not perpendicular to the ultrasound beam; at the right, the LV cut is oblique, oval rather than circular cross section, and the cursor is not central.

PARASTERNAL SHORT-AXIS VIEW (Figures 1–1 to 1–3)

The LV chamber is roughly circular in this view, at right angles to the long-axis view. Within it can be seen the anterior mitral leaflet alone, both mitral leaflets, the chordae tendineae, and the papillary muscles as one proceeds from the LV base to the apex.

Above the mitral valve level, the aortic root and valve occupy the center of the image, with the tricuspid valve to the right, the right ventricle anterior to the aorta, the pulmonary valve to the left, and the left main coronary artery and left atrial appendage from front to back. The LA chamber is directly posterior to the aorta, and the right atrial (RA) chamber is right-posterior. In an even higher parasternal short-axis plane, the pulmonary trunk (main pulmonary artery) is seen in full length, as well as its bifurcation into right and left pulmonary arteries.

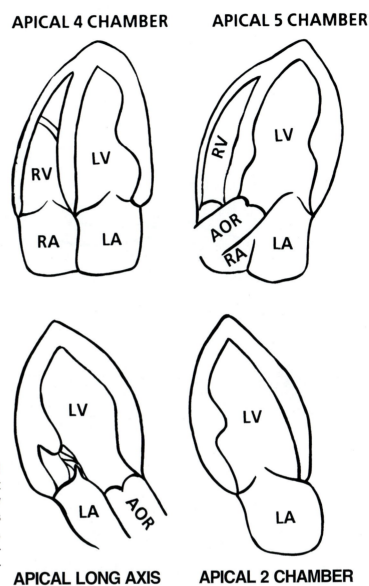

APICAL 4 CHAMBER   **APICAL 5 CHAMBER**

APICAL LONG AXIS   **APICAL 2 CHAMBER**

Figure 1–4. Diagram showing standard apical views. Of the two upper views, the one on the left is in a more posterior plane (ventricular inflow plane) than the one on the right, which includes the aortic valve and root. Of the two lower views, the aortic valve and root are imaged in the long-axis view but excluded in the apical two-chamber view.

PARASTERNAL RIGHT VENTRICULAR INFLOW VIEW (see Figure 1–1)

This view is obtained by angling the transducer downward and rightward from the standard parasternal view. The tricuspid valve is well seen; the roughly triangular right ventricular (RV) chamber above it and the roughly hemispherical RA chamber below it are seen in their greatest widths. The entry of the inferior vena cava (IVC) into the lower RA chamber, with the eustachian valve at its rim, is a feature of this scene.

APICAL VIEWS (Figures 1–4 to 1–9)

The standard apical four-chamber view depicts the mitral and tricuspid valves separating the inflow planes of both ventricles above from both atria below. In a (slightly anterior) variant of this view, the aortic valve and root are included (so-called five-chamber view).

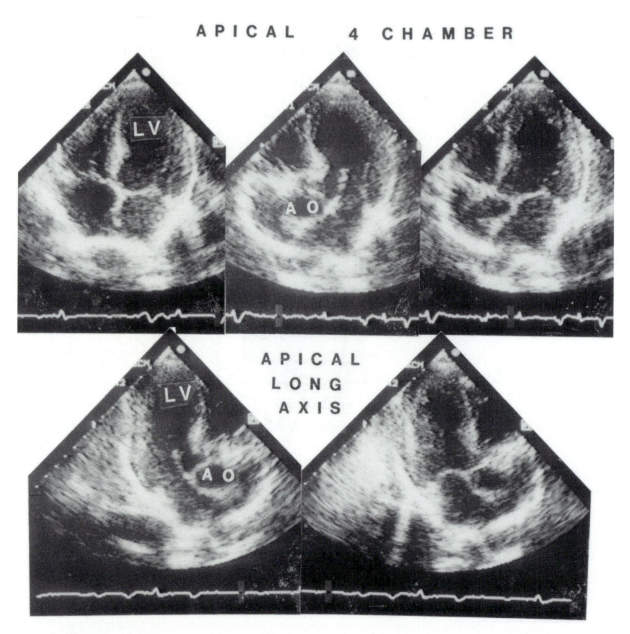

Figure 1–5. (Above, left) Apical four-chamber view, which is more posterior than the next (above, center), which includes the aortic valve and root. (Above, right) This shows the latter view in systole. The lower frames in apical long-axis view are in diastole (left) and systole (right).

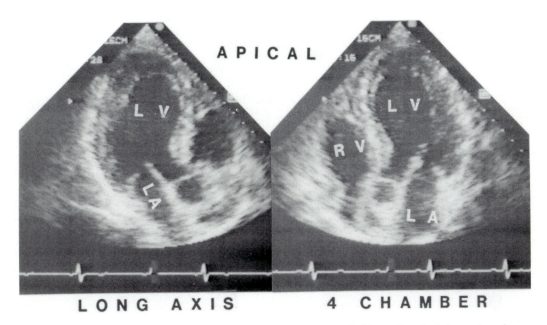

Figure 1–6. Normal 2D echo in apical long-axis view (left) and apical four-chamber view (right).

In other variations of this apical view obtained by appropriate angulation and rotation of the probe, the LA or RA chamber is partly or even entirely "cut off" from the imaging plane while the contralateral atrial and ventricular chamber are still in view.

In the apical view orthogonal to the standard four-chamber view, only the LV and LA chambers are imaged (two-chamber view). If the aortic valve and root are included, it is called the *apical long-axis view.* This is, in general, the most informative 2D echo view of all, providing a good idea not only of LV and LA size, shape, and wall motion but also of mitral and aortic valve motion and regurgitation. It has the additional advantage of being similar to the usual (RAO) angiocardiographic projection for studying LV contour and contraction.

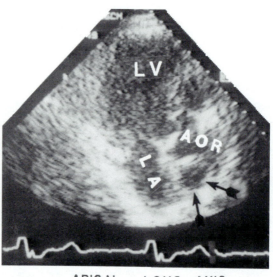

APICAL   LONG AXIS

Figure 1–7. Apical long-axis view. The round sonolucency adjacent to the superior pole of the left atrium (LA) and posterior to the aorta (AOR) is the right pulmonary artery (arrows) in cross section.

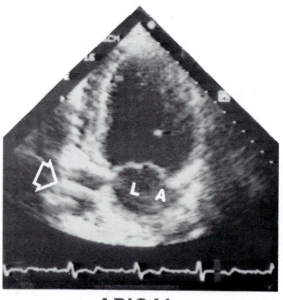

APICAL

Figure 1–8. Apical view intermediate between the four-chamber view and the two-chamber view; the LV and LA chambers are well seen, but only a narrow posterior part of the RV and RA chambers is included. The thick transverse-band echo in the RA represents the eustachian valve.

APICAL   4   CHAMBER

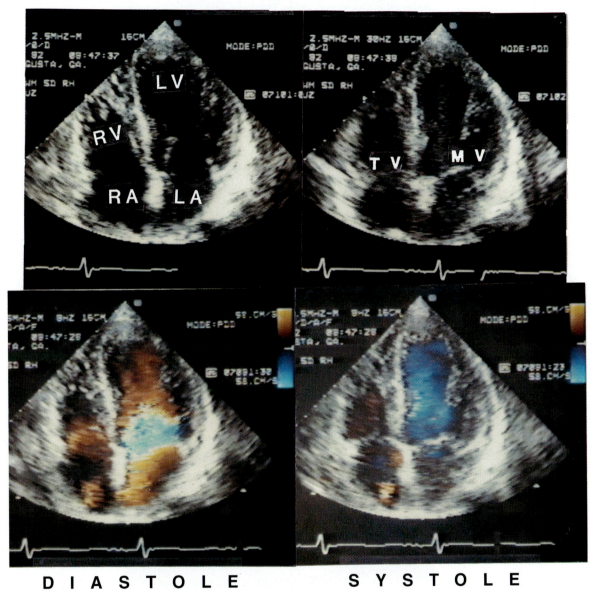

DIASTOLE   SYSTOLE

Figure 1–9. Apical four-chamber view in diastole (left) and systole (right). Colorflow Doppler shows a broad diastolic inflow stream toward the apex (below, left) and away from the apex (below, right).

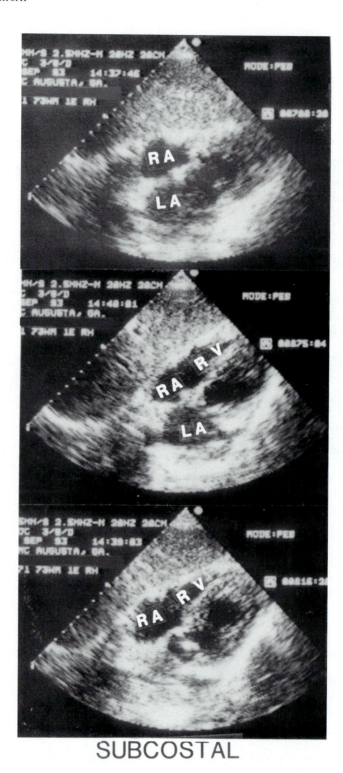

SUBCOSTAL

Figure 1–10. Subcostal four-chamber view in successively more anterior planes. The RV is imaged in the center but not top frame. The aortic valve is seen in the bottom but not the other planes.

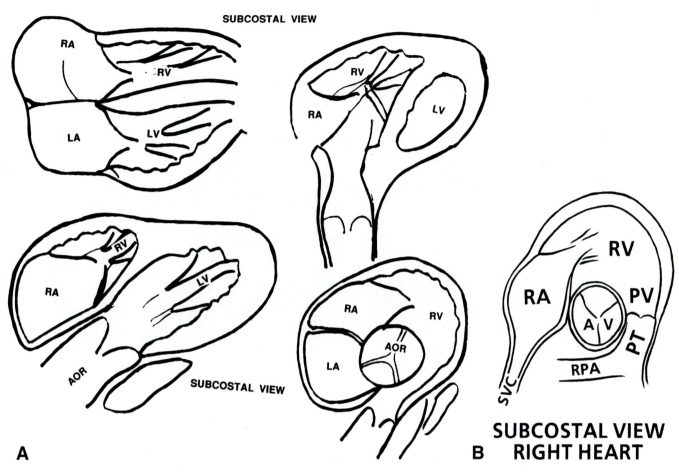

Figure 1–11. (A) Diagram showing four commonly used subcostal views. (B) Diagram showing a subcostal view in a plane transecting the superior vena cava (SVC), right atrium (RA), right ventricle (RV), pulmonic valve (PV), pulmonary trunk (PT), and right pulmonary artery (RPA). The right-sided heart chambers are situated circumferentially around the aortic root and valve (AV).

SUBCOSTAL VIEWS (Figures 1–10 to 1–17)

In the subcostal four-chamber view, the RV and RA are "anterior," i.e., closer to the transducer than the LA and LV (see Figure 1–10), though the imaging plane is as close or closer to the coronal plane than the true horizontal anatomic plane. The atrial and ventricular septa are perpendicular to the ultrasound beam and are therefore well suited to 2D echo and Doppler interrogation. Unlike the apical four-chamber view, the subcostal view does not show the LV apex.

SUBCOSTAL

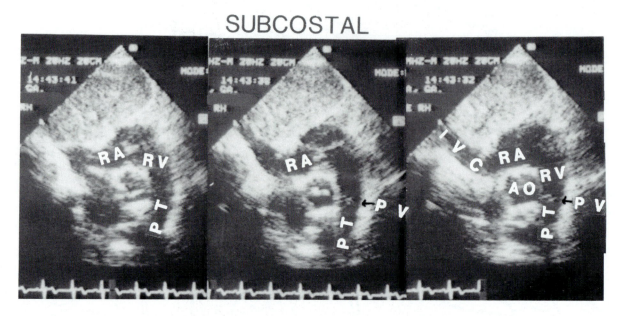

Figure 1–12. Subcostal view in slightly varying planes, showing IVC, RA, RV, PV, and pulmonary trunk in continuity, as in Figure 1–11.

Subcostal short-axis views can be obtained in several planes (see Figures 1-11 to 1-15), and when optimally displayed, they can demonstrate most or all of right-sided heart anatomy: the aortic root with valve in the field's center, with the RA chamber, tricuspid valve, entire RV length, pulmonic valve, pulmonary trunk, and the latter's bifurcation surrounding the aortic root.

Another useful subcostal plane is a sagittal or near-sagittal one that displays the IVC and hepatic veins entering it (see Figure 1-16) and the upper abdominal aorta in a slightly more posterior and leftward plane. The superior vena cava (SVC) entering the RA also can be visualized when the appropriate plane is attained (see Figure 1-17); in fact, the SVC, RA, and IVC often can be imaged in sonolucent continuity (see Figure 1-14).

SUBCOSTAL

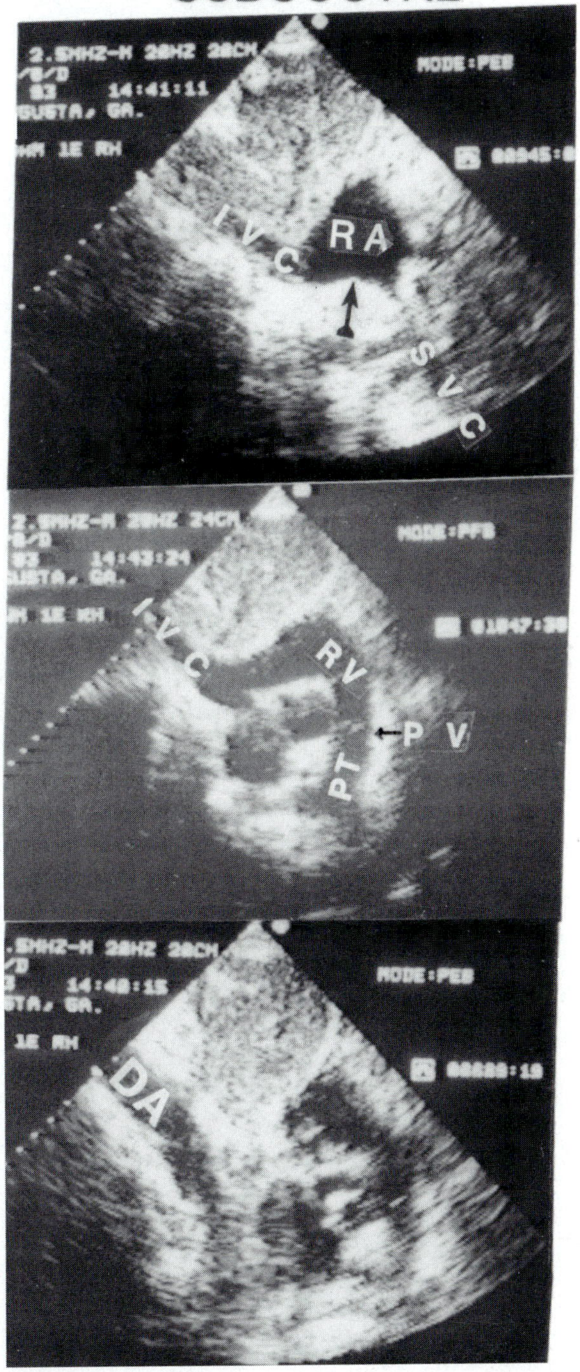

Figure 1–13. Three different planes, all subcostal, in the same patient. The top frame shows the IVC and SVC entering the RA. The bulge into RA is tuber of lower of anatomists (arrow). The center frame shows, in continuity, the IVC, RA, RV, and PV and PT. The bottom shows the abdominal aorta and its continuity with the descending thoracic aorta. The heart is seen anterior to it and superior to the liver.

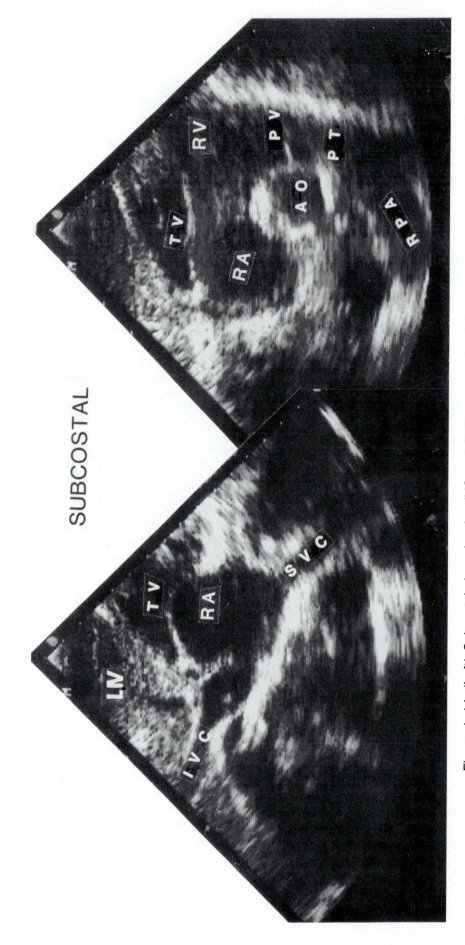

SUBCOSTAL

Figure 1–14. (Left) Subcostal view showing IVC and SVC entering the right atrium. The eustachian valve and tricuspid valve are also seen. (Right) The RA, RV, PT, and right pulmonary artery are seen winding around the aortic (Ao) hub.

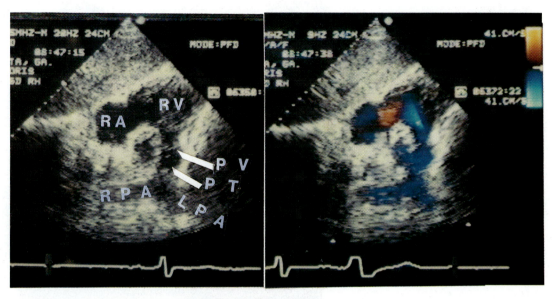

SUBCOSTAL

Figure 1–15. Subcostal view to show right atrium (RA), right ventricle (RV), pulmonic valve (PV), pulmonary trunk (PT), and its bifurcation into right and left pulmonary arteries (RPA and LPA).

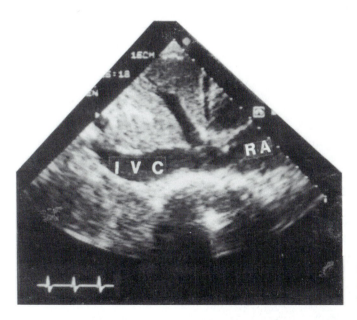

Figure 1–16. Subcostal view in the sagittal plane showing the IVC entering the RA after it receives a hepatic vein.

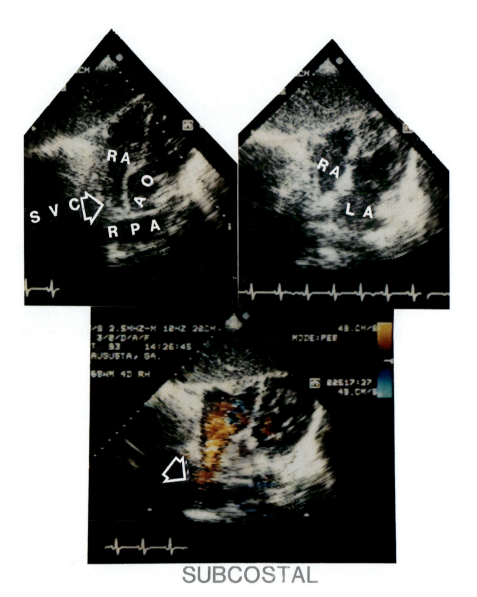

Figure 1–17. Subcostal views to show SVC (arrows). In the left upper frame, the aortic root (Ao) and right pulmonary artery (RPA) are imaged. In a more posterior plane, the left atrium comes into view. Mild atrial septal hypertrophy (lipomatous) separates the LA from the RA. Colorflow Doppler shows inflow into the RA through the SVC (below).

SUPRASTERNAL-SUPRACLAVICULAR VIEWS

Similar echographic appearances are obtained with the ultrasound probe in the midline suprasternal notch and above the medial end of the right clavicle (between the sternal and clavicular heads of the sternocleidomastoid muscle). In both cases, the ultrasound beam is directed almost directly inferiorly behind the bony landmark (manubrium sternum or clavicle).

In adults, this window is used mainly to visualize the aortic arch in its long axis. The ascending and descending aorta also can be imaged by suitable transducer manipulation. Dilated aortas are much easier to record. The ascending aorta can be differentiated easily from the descending aorta by colorflow Doppler: red for ascending and blue for descending aorta (toward and away from probe, respectively).

The three large arteries arising from the convexity of the aortic arch, the innominate, left common carotid, and left subclavian arteries, are well seen in the supraclavicular view and also serve as anatomic landmarks. The right pulmonary artery appears as a sonolucent space just below the arotic arch; below that, a large sonolucency represents the left atrium.

In the suprasternal aortic arch short-axis plane, the aortic arch appears as a circular or oval sonolucency. The right pulmonary artery and left atrium are seen below it.

SPATIAL ORIENTATION IN 2D ECHO IMAGING

Some echocardiographers, including some pediatric cardiologists and European proponents depict 2D echo images with right-left reversal, superior-inferior reversal, or both. The convention used in this book is that followed by the vast majority of American echocardiographers, including the textbooks of Feigenbaum and others and the journals of cardiology and echocardiography.

RIGHT PARASTERNAL VIEW (See also Chapter 20.)

The right parasternal window, at the second to fourth right intercostal spaces near the right sternal border, is particularly suitable for visualization of an immediately subjacent dilated ascending aorta.[1] Whereas the anterior edge of the right lung normally intervenes between the aorta and the chest wall, a dilated aortic root usually pushes the lung aside and approaches the chest wall at the right parasternal location. Moreover, the dilated ascending aorta itself may provide a window that permits visualization of other mediastinal structures, including the aortic arch, the descending aorta, the SVC, and the right pulmonary artery.

Marcella and Johnson[2] have shown recently that even in the absence of aortic dilatation, right parasternal scanning (in the right lateral position) can reveal several cardiac structures, in effect using the right atrium as a window to right-sided heart structures. It may be possible to obtain a plane that can image the SVC, right atrium, and IVC in continuity. A considerable extent of the right coronary artery may be imaged in approximately the plane of the tricuspid annulus.[2] The atrial septum and atrial septal defects also can be interrogated from the right parasternal view in some cases, as described earlier by Tei et al.[3] and Minagoe et al.[4]

REFERENCES

1. D'Cruz IA, Jain DP, Hirsch L, et al. Echocardiographic diagnosis of dilatation of the ascending aorta using right parasternal scanning. Radiology 1978;129:465.
2. Marcella CP, Johnson LE. Right parasternal imaging: An underutilized echocardiographic technique. J Am Soc Echocardiogr 1993;6:453.
3. Tei C, Tanaka H, Kashima T, et al. Real-time cross-sectional echocardiography of the interatrial septum by right atrium interatrial septum–left atrium direction of ultrasound beam. Circulation 1979;60:539.
4. Minagoe S, Tei C, Kisanuki A, et al. Noninvasive pulsed Doppler echocardiographic detection of the direction of shunt flow in patients with atrial septal defect: Usefulness of the right parasternal approach. Circulation 1985;71:745.

2

The Pericardium

The pericardium occupies a central position in the thorax, with pleura-encased lung on either side, the narrow anterior mediastinum in front, and the posterior mediastinum (containing mainly the esophagus and descending aorta) behind. The pericardial sac consists of (1) a strong fibrous outer membrane, the parietal pericardium, that is anchored firmly to the sternum anteriorly and to the central tendon of the diaphragm inferiorly (Figure 2-1) and (2) a delicate serous mesothelial layer, the visceral pericardium, that lines the inner aspect of the parietal pericardium and is continuous with a similar layer covering most of the cardiac surface. Some use the term *epicardium* as a synonym for *visceral pericardium*; for others, the word *epicardium* signifies the connective tissue deep to the visceral pericardium lining the heart, which contains fat, coronary arteries and veins, nerves, and lymphatics.

Pericardial fat is more abundant in obese and elderly individuals. Commonly restricted mainly to a fat pad on the right ventricular anterior wall, on occasion it may constitute a thick adipose envelope of ventricles up to 2 cm or more in maximum thickness.[1-3] On echocardiography, pericardial fat may be echogenic or appear sonolucent depending on the gain setting. On computed tomography (CT), a reliable differentiation can be made between pericardial fat, fluid, and thickening.

Visceral pericardium covers both ventricles entirely, almost all of the right atrium, and most of the left atrium. However, a "bare" area exists between the anterior left atrial wall and the aortic root; the absence of pericardium at this site may render it vulnerable to the spread of infection, and it is a common site of abscess formation in aortic or mitral

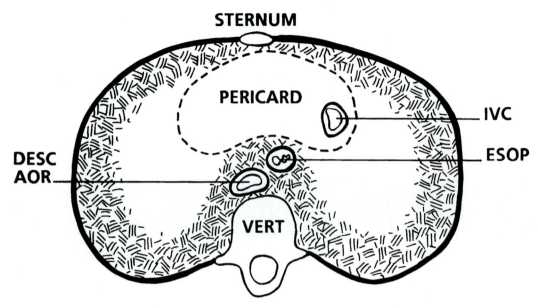

DIAPHRAGM: Viewed from above

Figure 2–1. Diagram showing the diaphragm as seen from above. The dotted line indicates the attachment of the pericardial sac to the central tendon of the diaphragm. The sites where the inferior vena cava (IVC), esophagus (ESOP), and the descending aorta (DESC AOR) pass through the diaphragm are shown (VERT, vertebra).

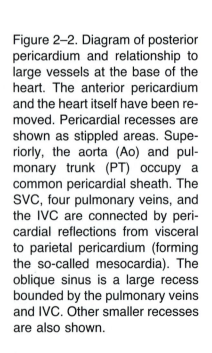

Figure 2–2. Diagram of posterior pericardium and relationship to large vessels at the base of the heart. The anterior pericardium and the heart itself have been removed. Pericardial recesses are shown as stippled areas. Superiorly, the aorta (Ao) and pulmonary trunk (PT) occupy a common pericardial sheath. The SVC, four pulmonary veins, and the IVC are connected by pericardial reflections from visceral to parietal pericardium (forming the so-called mesocardia). The oblique sinus is a large recess bounded by the pulmonary veins and IVC. Other smaller recesses are also shown.

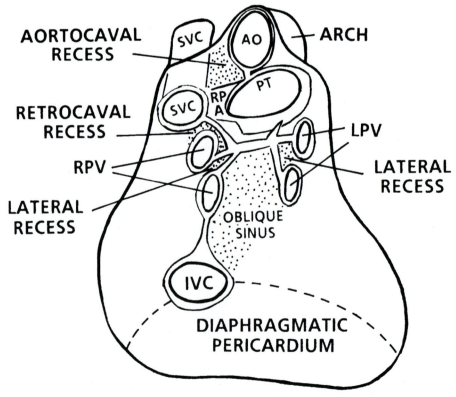

PERICARDIAL SAC AND RECESSES
(HEART AND ANTERIOR PERICARDIUM REMOVED)

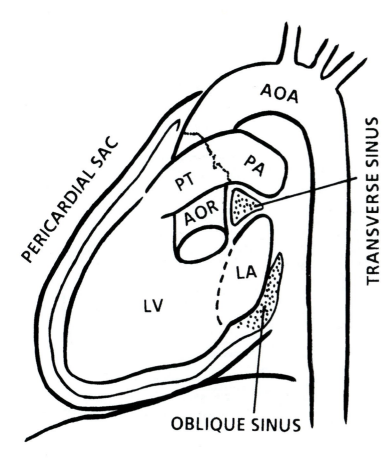

Figure 2–3. Diagram showing heart with pericardial sac in sagittal plane, including two pericardial recesses. The transverse sinus is located above and anterior to the upper pole of the left atrium (LA) and posterior to the ascending aorta (AOR). The oblique sinus extends upward posterior to the left atrium (AOA, aortic arch).

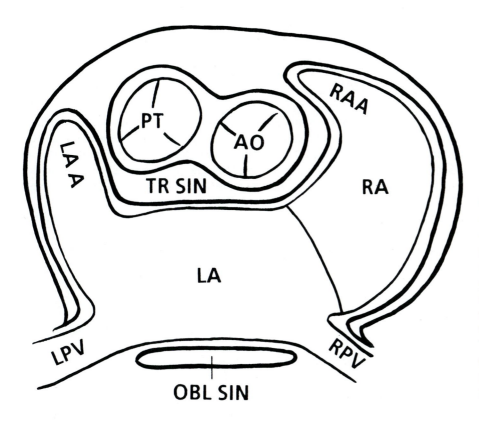

Figure 2–4. Diagram of horizontal section through the heart, looked at from above, to show extent of pericardial space and location of pericardial recesses. The pulmonary trunk (PT) and aortic root (Ao) occupy a common sheath of visceral pericardium anterior to the transverse sinus (TR SIN). The oblique sinus is posterior to the left atrium (LA) (LVP and RPV, left and right pulmonary veins; LAA, left atrial appendage).

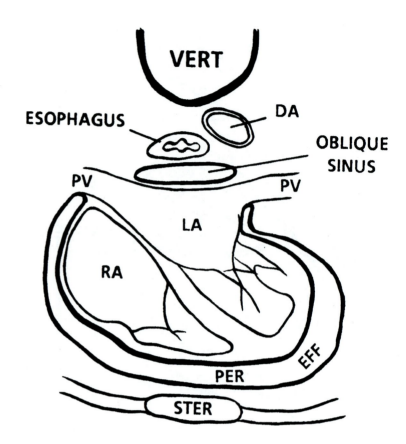

Figure 2–5. Transverse section through the thorax at the left atrial (LA) level to show the relationship of the oblique pericardial sinus to the left atrium anteriorly and to the esophagus and descending aorta (DA) posteriorly.

valve endocarditis. The visceral pericardium extends as short "sleeves" over the proximal few centimeters of great vessels emerging from or entering the heart: the aortic root, pulmonary trunk, both vena cavae, and the four pulmonary veins (Figures 2-2 and 2-3).

PERICARDIAL RECESSES (Figures 2–4 to 2–6)

The main serous pericardial space is bounded by the parietal pericardium on the one hand and the ventricles with right atrium on the other. Normally, this is essentially a "potential" space containing only a few milliliters of fluid (15 to 20 ml; an upper normal limit of 50 ml is widely quoted). However, the reflection of visceral pericardium from the cardiac chambers and the great vessels to the parietal pericardium is such that many small angular or pouchlike recesses are formed that open into the main pericardial sac.

The visceral pericardium covering the large vessels emerging from or entering the heart can be thought of as forming two tubes: (1) one ensheathing the ascending aorta and pulmonary trunk, and (2) the other containing the superior and inferior vena cavae as well as the four pulmonary veins. The visceral pericardium spanning the space between these large veins has been called the *venous mesocardium,* which forms a blind pouch opening inferiorly (the oblique pericardial sinus). The transverse sinus is that part of the visceral pericardial space lying between the two tubes.

During recent years, the availability of CT and magnetic resonance imaging (MRI) of the mediastinum has prompted a new interest in the anatomy of these recesses, and this has resulted in several excellent studies, all in radiology journals.[4-7]

To the echocardiographer, not all these pericardial recesses are important. The largest and most relevant recess is the *oblique sinus.* This is a cul-de-sac posterior to the left

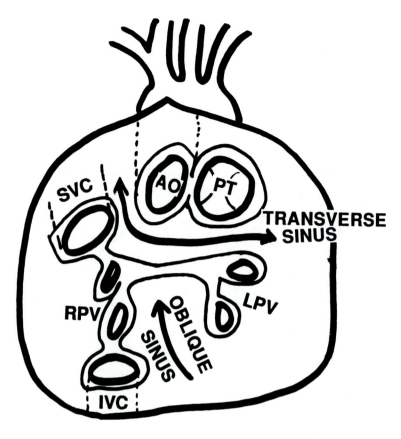

Figure 2–6. Diagram showing the interior of the pericardial sac after removal of the heart to show the anatomy of pericardial reflection from visceral to parietal pericardium. The upper reflection is as a pericardial sheath enclosing the aorta and pulmonary trunk. The lower reflection (mesocardium) encloses the SVC, IVC, and four pulmonary veins. Locations of transverse and oblique sinuses are shown by arrows.

atrium (Figure 2-4), limited on the left by the upper and lower pulmonary veins and on the right by the pulmonary veins and entry of the inferior vena cava into the right atrium. Superiorly, the oblique sinus ends blindly as the visceral pericardium is reflected onto posterior mediastinal structures. Inferiorly, the oblique sinus opens into the main pericardial space.

Another pericardial recess of note is the *transverse sinus* (Figure 2-6), posterior to the ascending aorta and pulmonary trunk, superior to the upper border of the left atrium, and anteroinferior to the right pulmonary artery as the latter crosses the midline horizontally to enter the hilum of the right lung. Yet another recess is a small nook between the left pulmonary artery and left superior pulmonary vein, behind the left atrial appendage.

PERICARDIAL EFFUSIONS

Normally, there is no appreciable separation between the parietal pericardium and the ventricles. Fluid accumulation in excess of 50 ml manifests on ultrasound as a sonolucent space, wider in systole than in diastole and commonly wider posterior than anterior to the ventricles, presumably because of the effect of gravity in the recumbent patient. Pericardial fluid is more uniformly distributed around the heart in the sitting position.

The very small film of normal pericardial fluid "holds" the atrial walls firmly to the parietal pericardium. This effect no longer prevails when a pericardial effusion (even a small effusion) is present so that atrial contraction increases the amplitude of atrial wall motion, which should not be mistaken for "atrial collapse" suggestive of tamponade. The

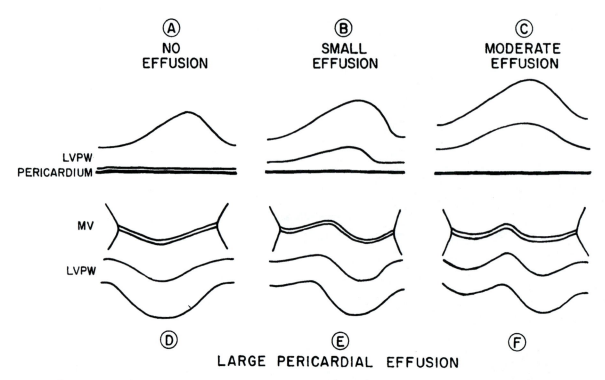

Figure 2–7. Diagram showing M-mode appearance with regard to LV posterior wall (LVPW) motion in (A) normal, (B) small pericardial effusion, and (C) moderate effusion. The pericardial space posterior to the LV wall appears in (B) and increases in (C); the LV wall motion amplitude increases but is in the normal direction. (D–F) Patterns of abnormal LV wall motion seen in large circumcardiac effusions with cardiac "swinging"; the mitral valve (MV) systolic echo participates in this LV motion and can simulate prolapse (pseudoprolapse).

shape of the sonolucent pericardial space in circumcardiac pericardial effusions conforms on its inner aspect to that of the ventricles and on its outer (parietal) aspect to that of the parietal pericardium. Thus the pericardial space is annular, or in smaller effusions crescentic, in the short-axis view. In apical or subcostal views, pericardial effusions appear as a sonolucent band behind the left ventricle with a narrower sonolucent rim anteriorly. Large pericardial effusions are characterized by preferential fluid accumulation in the lateral portions of the pericardial sac.[8,9] The typical contours of the pericardial space in the respective two-dimensional (2D) echo views serve to distinguish pericardial effusions from other sonolucent spaces adjacent to the heart, such as pleural effusions, ascites, LV pseudoaneurysms, or mediastinal cysts.

The width of the sonolucent pericardial space (separation between ventricles and parietal pericardium) is a rough measure of the size of the effusion (Figure 2-7). Another manifestation of moderate to large pericardial effusions is abnormal mobility of the ventricles.[10]

Such pendular, or "swinging," ventricular motion occurs because the ventricles lie completely free in a fluid-filled pericardial sac, whereas the base of the heart is attached to the mediastinum by a complex, partly flexible pedicle consisting of the aorta, the pulmonary artery, the vena cavae, and the pulmonary veins (Figure 2-8). The larger the pericardial effusion, the greater is the oscillatory swinging ventricular motion (Figure 2-9).

Electrical alternans (alteration in QRS voltage from beat to beat) has long been known to occur in some patients with large pericardial effusions. In such circumstances, echocar-

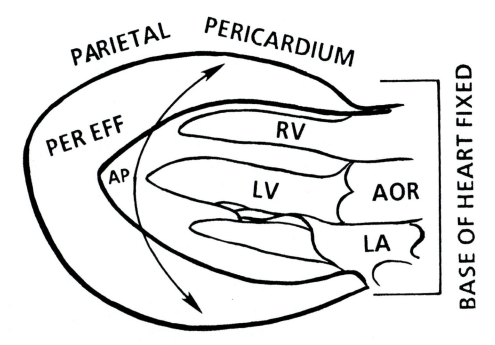

Figure 2–8. Diagram showing how the heart is fixed at its base by a pedicle of large vessels, whereas the ventricles lie free within a large pericardial effusion (PER EFF). The curved line with arrowheads at each end indicates the arc of ventricular "swinging" or oscillation.

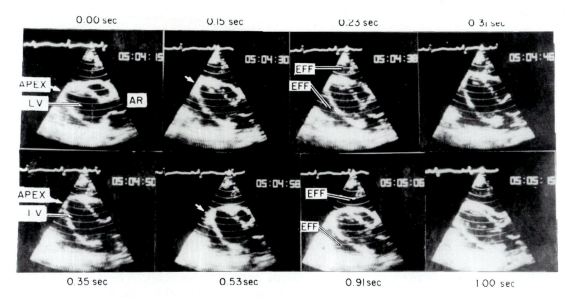

Figure 2–9. Eight serial frames in long-axis view over a 1-second period in a patient with a large pericardial effusion and "swinging" heart. The much exaggerated antero-posterior motion of the cardiac apex with the cardiac cycle is evident.

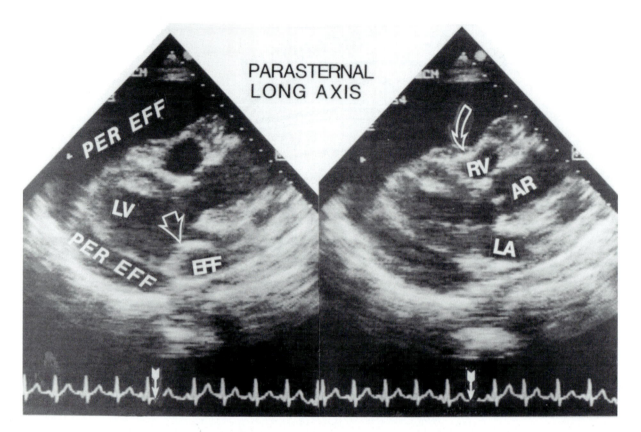

Figure 2–10. Parasternal long-axis views in a patient with a large pericardial effusion with tamponade. Left atrial collapse (arrow) is seen at left, and right ventricular in-curving (dimpling) is seen at right.

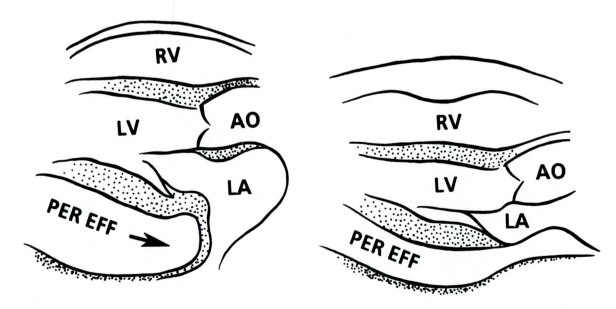

Figure 2–11. Diagram showing the parasternal long-axis view. (Left) A large loculated posterior pericardial effusion (regional tamponade) with conspicuous distension of the oblique pericardial sinus (arrow) distorting left atrial (LA) shape. This finding is not present in tamponade due to circumcardiac pericardial effusion (right).

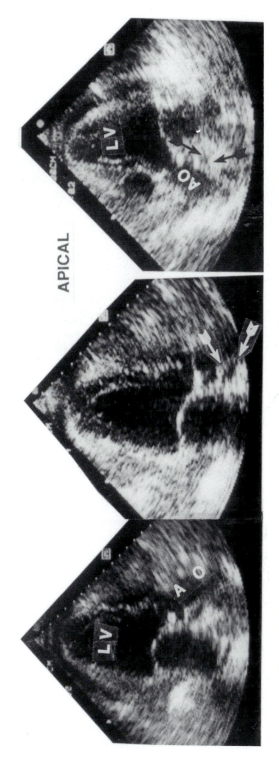

Figure 2–12. Apical long-axis views (left and center) and four-chamber view (right) showing effusion in transverse sinus manifesting as a small space (arrows) between the left atrium and ascending aorta.

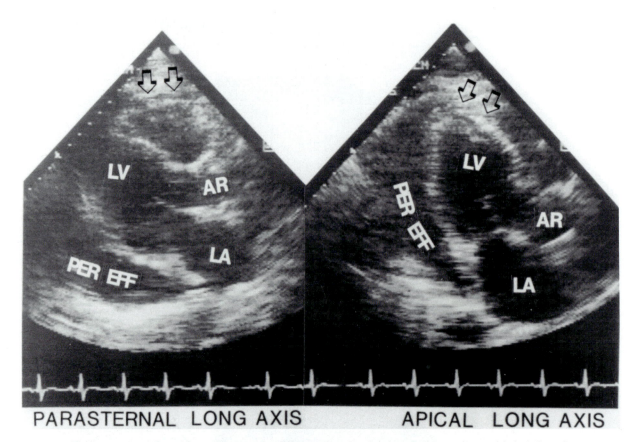

PARASTERNAL LONG AXIS   APICAL LONG AXIS

Figure 2–13. 2D echocardiogram in different long-axis views of a patient with loculated posterior pericardial effusion (PER EFF). No sonolucent space is seen anteriorly because of pericardial adhesions.

diography demonstrates *alternation in ventricular position.*[11,12] Tamponade is usually present. Why exactly alteration of cardiac position (and of ECG voltage) occurs in some patients with large effusions but not in others has not been explained.

Retroatrial extension of pericardial fluid was not recognized during the early years of echocardiography. In fact, the erroneous teaching at that time was that fluid behind the left atrium was typical of pleural effusions but not pericardial effusions. However, it was demonstrated on M-mode and subsequently on 2D echocardiography that pericardial fluid often does extend into the oblique pericardial sinus in large pericardial effusions.[13] In fact, patients with tamponade may show transient phasic inward dipping motion of the left atrial wall during atrial contraction, sometimes called *left atrial collapse* (Figure 2-10). A more remarkable type of oblique sinus distension (Figure 2-11) has been reported in patients with large loculated posterior pericardial effusions under high pressure; the left atrium is compressed and deformed, becoming concave toward the oblique pericardial sinus.[14,15]

Other pericardial recesses do not show any remarkable or diagnostic appearances in patients with pericardial effusions, but occasionally fluid in these recesses (Figure 2-12) can register as small unusual sonolucencies that may be confused with other abnormalities. Thus a small pocket of pericardial fluid in the left pulmonary recess, posterior to the pulmonary trunk and lateral to the aortic root, could be mistaken for an aneurysm of the left main coronary artery.

Figure 2–14. (Facing Page) Apical four-chamber views of patient with loculated pericardial effusions ▶ compressing both atria. There is little fluid around the ventricles because of adhesions.

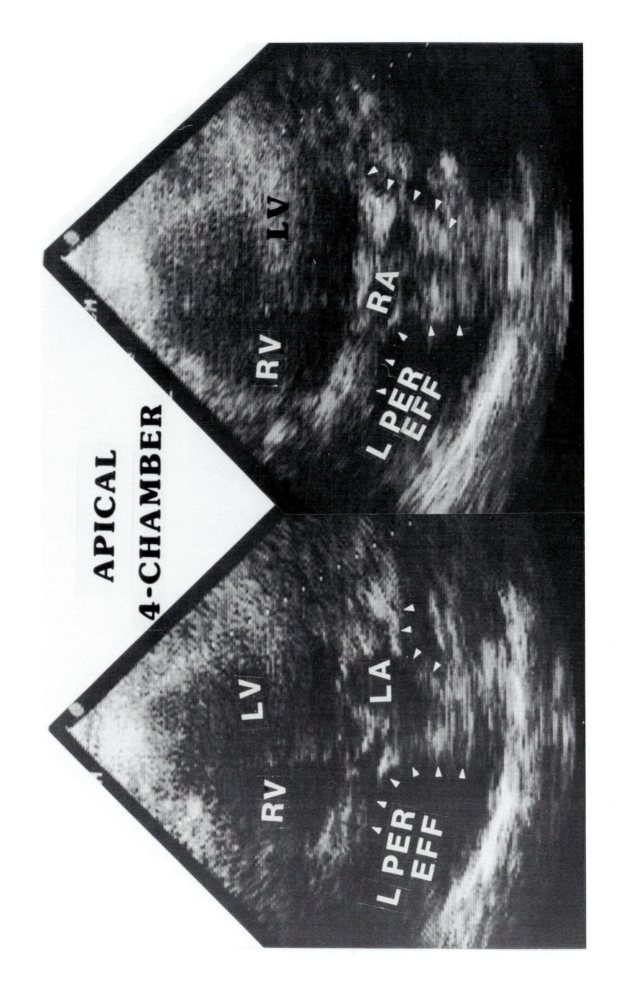

APICAL 4-CHAMBER

29

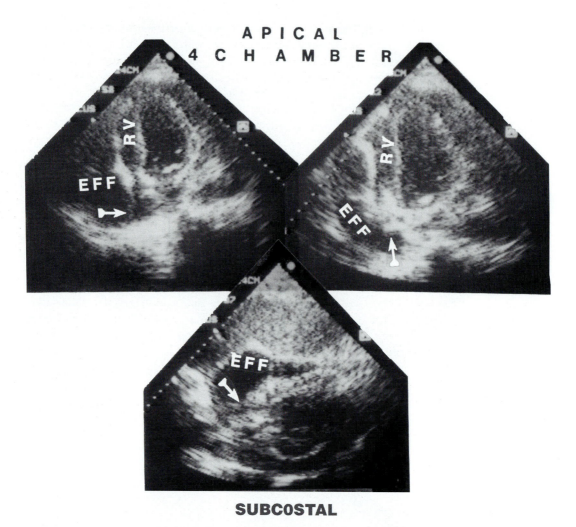

Figure 2–15. Apical four-chamber view (above) and subcostal view (below) showing a loculated pericardial effusion (EFF) compressing the right atrium (arrows) and the right ventricle (RV).

Loculated Pericardial Effusions (Figures 2–13 to 2–15)

Effusions that fill the whole pericardial sac are sometimes called *circumcardiac,* to distinguish them from effusions restricted to one portion or "pocket" of the pericardial space by intrapericardial adhesions.[16] The most common cause for such loculation is recent cardiac surgery, but certain other subacute forms of pericarditis are possible etiologies.[17] The size and location of loculated effusions can vary, but if they are large enough and under high tension, not only can they compress the subjacent chamber, but they can also cause overall cardiac tamponade.

Abnormal Structures Within Pericardial Effusions

Various "solid" objects may be noted within the pericardial sonolucency: (1) "Soft" fibrinous material resulting from pericardial inflammation may form an ill-defined layer on the parietal pericardium or mobile bands or ribbons undulating in the effusion with every heart beat. (2) Sharper, dense, and less mobile bands may bridge the pericardial space and anchor the ventricles to the parietal pericardium.[16] These intrapericardial adhesions are frequent in tuberculous and other subacute pericardial processes. (3) Rarely, metastases from malignant neoplasms elsewhere (Figure 2–16) are detected as solid intrapericardial masses.[18] (4) Thrombi or organizing hematomas following chest trauma or pericardial paracentesis have been reported.[19] (5) Immediately after egress of blood from a cardiac chamber into the pericardial sac, as a complication of perforation of the right atrial or ventricular wall by attempted paracentesis or by an intracardiac wire or catheter, the static but still fluid pericardial blood presents as a homogeneous echogenic "mass." (6) Spontaneous mobile, swirling or oscillating "dynamic echoes," resembling microbubble contrast material (Figure 2–17), have been reported in bloody pericardial effusions[20] or in pericardial infection by gas-producing organisms.[21,22] Echocardiographers need to be aware of the 2D echo appearances of these diverse intrapericardial abnormalities; they are of interest not only in themselves but also as clues to the nature and etiology of pericardial effusions.

Pericardial Shape and Volume

When the unopened external pericardium is viewed at surgery or autopsy, with the lungs retracted, the pericardial sac is somewhat flask-shaped, with its wide bottom resting on the diaphragm and a narrower neck above, through which the aorta, pulmonary artery, and superior vena cava emerge. However, when the serous pericardial sac is visualized by echocardiography or MRI, it approximates an ellipsoidal shape. This is true whether a pericardial effusion is present or not.

The volume of an ellipse of rotation can be estimated by the formula volume = $\frac{4}{3}\pi \cdot L/2 \cdot D_1/2 \cdot D_2/2$, where L is the length, or long axis, and D_1 and D_2 are two minor axes, perpendicular to each other. L and D_1 are measured in the apical four-chamber view; D_2 is measured in the parasternal short-axis view (see Figure 2–18). In the apical four-chamber view, the heart also is roughly ellipsoidal in shape, and its volume can be estimated by the same formula. In patients with large pericardial effusions, the volume of pericardial fluid can then be estimated as the difference between pericardial and cardiac volumes (Figure 2–18). The amount of pericardial effusion thus estimated correlated well with the actual quantity of fluid drained in a series of 13 patients with large pericardial effusions

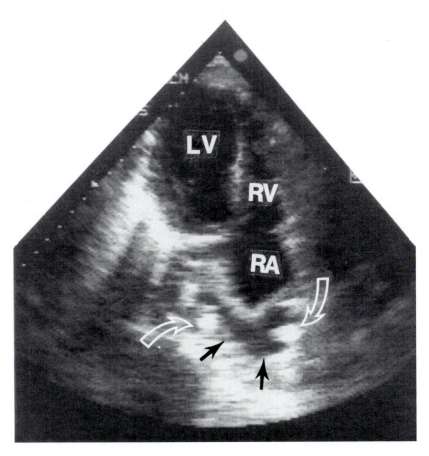

Figure 2–16. Apical view showing a loculated pericardial effusion (black arrows) adjacent to the right atrium containing solid nodules, (white arrows) which were metastases from a testicular seminoma. The effusion and nodules regressed after chemotherapy.

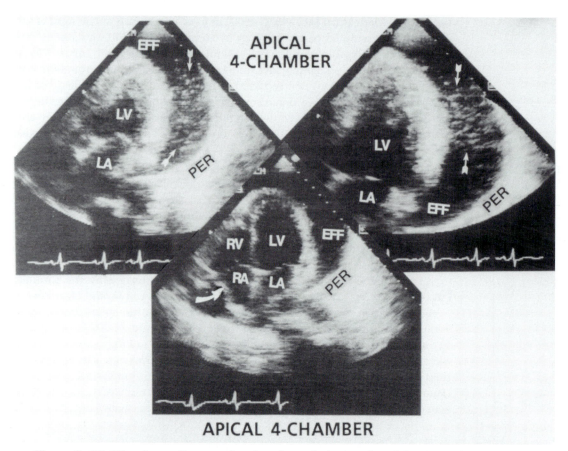

Figure 2–17. 2D echocardiogram showing dynamic intrapericardial echoes (arrows) in a large pericardial effusion in the upper frames. The lower frame shows right atrial wall indentation (arrow). (*Reproduced with permission from D'Cruz IA, Holman MS, Childers LS. Spontaneous Mobile Contrast-echoes in Pericardial effusion. Am. Heart J 1990;120:1472.*)

and tamponade.[23] Studying the same patients for pericardial shape, we found that the fluid-filled pericardial sac causing tamponade tended to be more spherical (Figure 2-19) than the same sac after fluid drainage; this shape alteration was caused by an increase in the transverse axes D_1 and D_2 with no significant change in length L.

The amount of pericardial effusion that compresses the cardiac chambers sufficiently to cause tamponade (significant rise of intracardiac diastolic pressures and eventual fall in cardiac output and arterial blood pressure) is variable and depends on three main factors: (1) the *time taken for fluid to accumulate* (this may be minutes to hours in "surgical tamponade" following penetrating chest wounds or immediately after cardiac surgery but many days to weeks in "medical tamponade" due to pericarditis of various etiologies), (2) the *rigidity and thickness of the pericardium* (intrapericardial pressure will rise more rapidly in a noncompliant than in a distensible pericardial sac), and (3) the *thickness of the ventricular walls* (inordinately high intrapericardial pressures exert their deleterious action on cardiac filling by transmitting this high pressure transmurally to the ventricles). The normal pericardium, though thin, is inelastic, since it consists of collagen but few elastic fibers.[24] It therefore has a steep pressure-volume curve; i.e., in acute experiments, increments in the amount of pericardial effusion produce substantial progressive rises in intrapericardial pressure, which in turn result in increasing tamponade.[24] On the other hand, chronic or subacute pericardial effusions that have acumulated over weeks or months do stretch the parietal pericardium so that 1 to 2 liters of effusion may sometimes be encountered with only mild tamponade. If the left or right ventricle has abnormally hypertrophied walls, the latter may "resist" the high pericardial pressure and "protect" that ventricle from transmission of elevated pericardial pressure.

2D - APICAL 4 - CHAMBER VIEW
PERICARDIUM

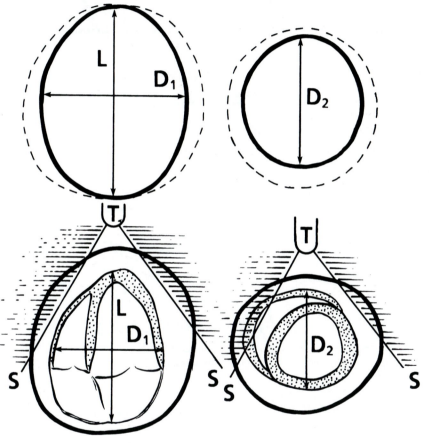

$$\text{VOLUME (Ellipse)} = \frac{4}{3} \cdot \pi \cdot \frac{L}{2} \cdot \frac{D_1}{2} \cdot \frac{D_2}{2}$$

$$= 0.523 \cdot L \cdot D_1 \cdot D_2$$

Figure 2–18. Diagram showing how the volume of a pericardial effusion can be estimated from the apical four-chamber view (left) and parasternal short-axis view (right). The pericardial sac and heart are presumed to be of ellipsoid shape, and the volume of each is calculated by the formula stated below. Then pericardial fluid volume = volume of pericardial sac *minus* cardiac volume. Note that the entire pericardial sac does not have to be visualized for this purpose.

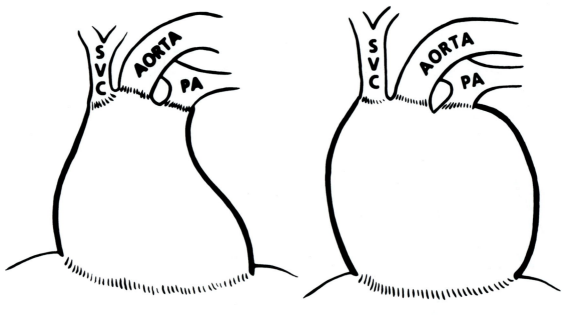

NORMAL PERICARDIUM

**LARGE
PERICARDIAL EFFUSION**

Figure 2–19. (Left) Diagram showing the flasklike shape of the normal pericardium. (Right) The pericardial sac is nearly globular in shape because it is distended by a large effusion.

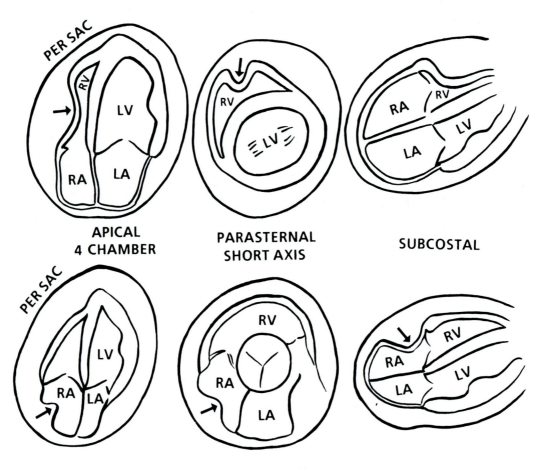

**APICAL
4 CHAMBER**

**PARASTERNAL
SHORT AXIS**

SUBCOSTAL

Figure 2–20. Diagram showing right ventricular collapse (above) and right atrial collapse (below) in apical four-chamber, parasternal short-axis, and subcostal views.

NORMAL

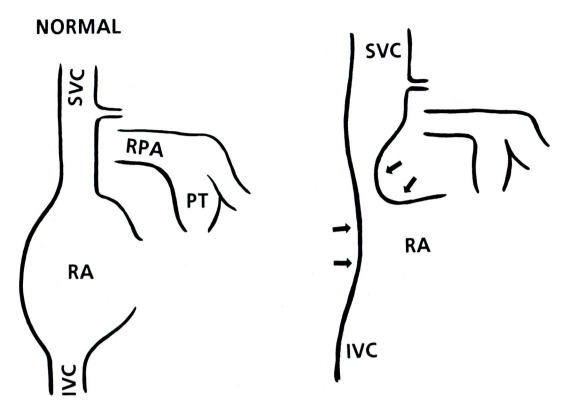

Figure 2–21. (Left) Diagram showing normal contour of SVC and right atrium. (Right) In tamponade due to a large pericardial effusion, the right atrial wall becomes flat or concave (arrows). The intrapericardial part of the SVC becomes compressed and narrowed below the level of the right pulmonary artery.

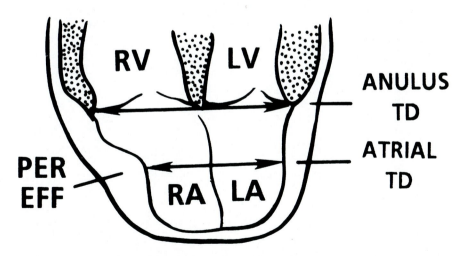

Figure 2–22. Diagram of apical four-chamber view in a patient with a large pericardial effusion and tamponade showing how the transverse dimension at the annulus level (Anulus TD) and the transverse dimension at the midatrial level (atrial TD) are measured. End-diastolic atrial TD/anulus TD is less than 0.85 in tamponade but greater than 0.85 after tamponade is relieved.

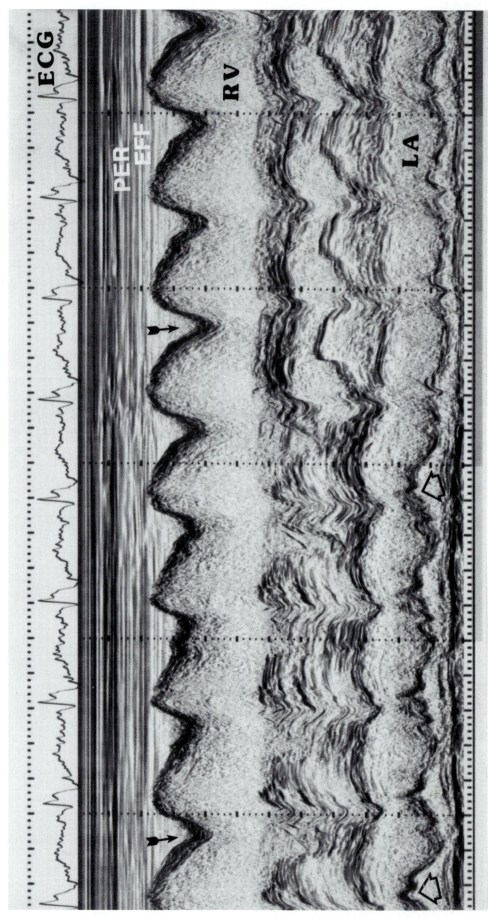

Figure 2–23. M-mode echocardiogram showing early diastolic collapse of the right ventricular wall (RVAW) and late diastolic–early systolic collapse of the left atrial posterior wall in a patient with tamponade.

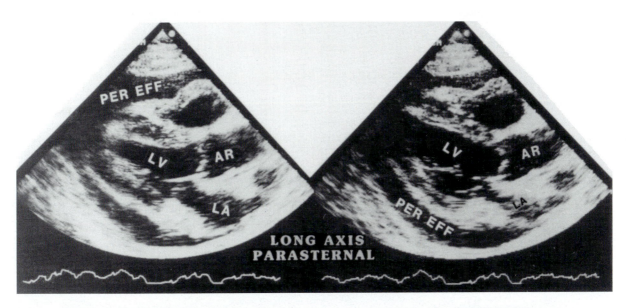

Figure 2–24. Parasternal long-axis view of a patient with a moderate to large circum-cardiac pericardial effusion. Mild "dimpling" of the RV anterior wall (left) and left atrial "collapse" (right) suggest the possibility of tamponade.

The pathophysiology of tamponade, a complex and extensively studied topic, is beyond the scope of this book. Although tamponade is a pathophysiologic state best diagnosed by intracardiac pressure recordings, its echocardiographic diagnosis is based on phasic anatomic changes, mainly *"collapse" of the right atrial or right ventricular wall* (Figures 2–20 to 2–25). Indentation or local infolding of the right atrial wall is noted in late diastole, concomitant with atrial contraction, with return to normal contour in early systole.[25] An inward curving or dimpling of the right ventricular wall in early diastole is typical of tamponade.[26] Common to RA and RV "collapse," as described above, is that the transient inward motion of the wall occurs at the phase of the cardiac cycle when pressure within that chamber is lowest so that intrapericardial pressure briefly overcomes it,

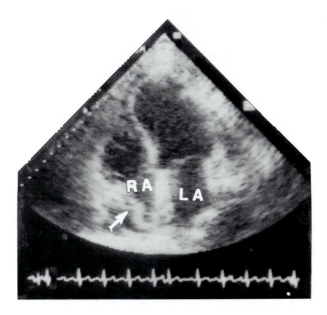

Figure 2–25. 2D echocardiogram in an apical four-chamber view showing indentation of the right atrial (RA) wall. The pericardial effusion is of a small size, and clinically, no tamponade was present.

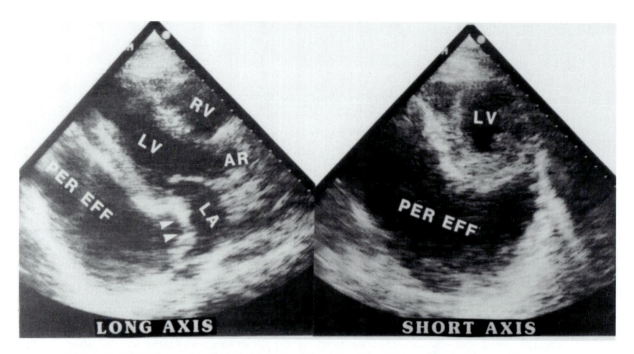

Figure 2–26. Long-axis view (left) and short-axis view (right) in a patient with a large loculated posterior pericardial effusion 7 weeks after coronary bypass surgery. Right-sided heart catheterization revealed typical signs of tamponade. Note distension of the oblique pericardial sinus (arrows).

pushing the RA and RV wall inward. The lower (intrapericardial) SVC may be compressed and narrowed, but not the upper (extrapericardial) SVC.

The left ventricle, because of its thicker wall, does not "collapse" in circumcardiac tamponade. The left atrial chamber does "collapse," i.e., decrease in volume at end-diastole as much as the right atrium.[27] However, conspicuous infolding of the left atrial wall is not visualized as it is with the right atrial wall. The reason for this may be anatomic rather than physiologic: The left atrial wall is firmly anchored by the four pulmonary veins, whereas the right atrium is fixed or tethered only at superior and inferior poles by the venae cavae, the rest of its anterior and lateral surface being free of attachments and covered by visceral pericardium. The RA wall is therefore capable of a greater amplitude of motion.

Large loculated pericardial effusions under high pressure can compress and distort the subjacent cardiac chamber or chambers, even causing hemodynamic and clinical changes like those of tamponade due to circumcardiac effusions. Distension of the oblique sinus and flattening of posterior LV wall by large loculated post-cardiac surgery pericardial effusions are not excessively rare (Figures 2-26 to 2-28).

Loculated pericardial effusions of sufficient size and tension (intrapericardial pressure) can cause selective tamponade of one or more cardiac chambers (Figures 2-29 and 2-30). That chamber or chambers may bear the main effect of compression, or the whole heart may suffer hemodynamic changes similar to generalized (circumcardiac) tamponade. Examples of regional tamponade have been imaged by echocardiography and reported with respect to each of the four cardiac chambers.[28-37]

Most instances of regional tamponade have occurred days to weeks after cardiac surgery, particularly in patients on anticoagulant therapy. Chest trauma and subacute pericarditis of various etiologies account for the remainder. Posterior loculated effusions compressing the left ventricle are the most common, causing distortion and perhaps paradoxical motion of the LV posteroinferior wall.[28,29] Distension of the oblique sinus is an

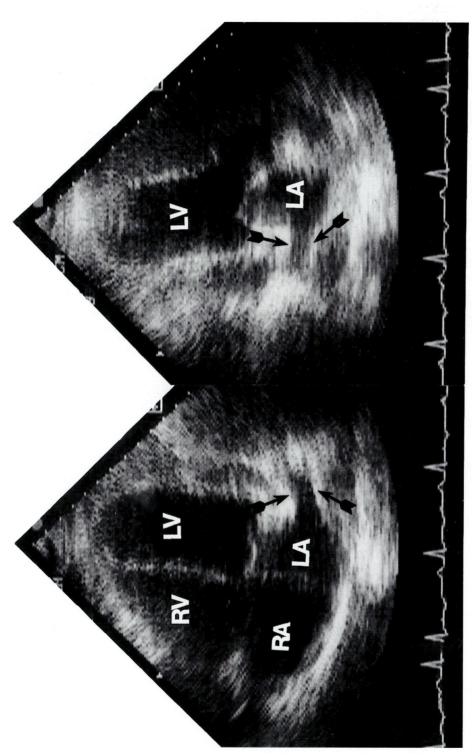

APICAL 4 - CHAMBER   APICAL LONG - AXIS

Figure 2–27. 2D echocardiogram shows prominent stretched pulmonary vein (arrows) in apical four-chamber view (left) and apical long-axis view (right) in a patient with loculated posterolateral pericardial effusion.

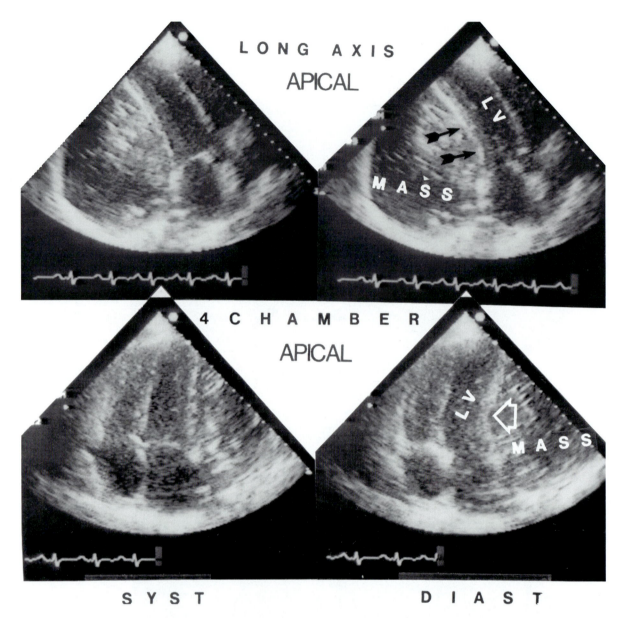

Figure 2–28. Apical long-axis view (above) and apical four-chamber view (below) show-ing a huge posterior intrapericardial mass (MASS) compressing the LV, more evident in diastole (DIAST) as in the two right frames than in systole (SYST) as in the two left frames. The LV posterior and posterolateral wall contour appears flat in systole, con-cave in diastole.

uncommon but diagnostically valuable 2D echo sign.[14,15] Many case reports of isolated right atrial or combined right atrial–tricuspid annulus–right ventricular compression have appeared. Isolated left atrial tamponade is the rarest form of regional tamponade. Transesophageal echocardiography (TEE) has proved most useful in visualizing loculated juxtaatrial pericardial effusions that may have been missed by transthorocic echocardiog-raphy (TTE) because of poor resolution and long distance from the transducer in apical or subcostal views.[2-10]

Exudative (Inflammatory) versus Transudative Effusions

Pericardial effusions can be either transudates or exudates. The former, also known as *hy-dropericardium,* result from passive noninflammatory flow of fluid as part of a general

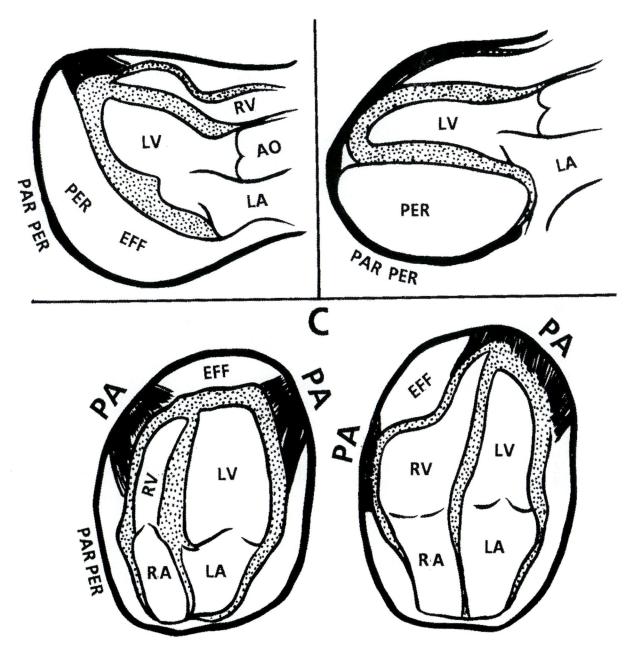

Figure 2–29. Diagram of long-axis views (above) and apical four-chamber views (below) in different patients, all of whom had tamponade and intrapericardial adhesions with fluid loculation. The untethered segments of ventricular wall are distorted and compressed by the high intrapericardial pressure. PAR PER, parietal pericardium. PA, pericardial adhesion.

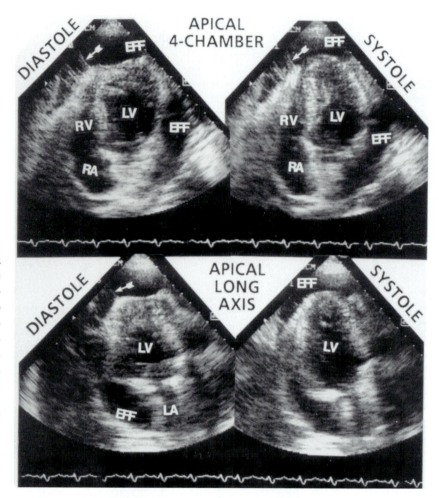

Figure 2–30. 2D echocardiogram of a patient with a large pericardial effusion and tamponade. Intrapericardial adhesions (arrows) tether some areas of the ventricular wall to the parietal pericardium; untethered areas of ventricular wall tend to become flat or even concave in diastole, resulting in bizarre ventricular contours. (*Reproduced with permission from D'Cruz IA, Jarrett J, Gross CM, Rogers W. Modification of the echocardiographic features of tamponade by intrapericardial adhesions. Am. J. Noninvasive Cardiology 1992; 6:69.*)

fluid retention and is usually accompanied by leg edema, pleural effusions, or ascites. The pericardial effusion is usually small but occasionally can be moderate in size.

Exudative pericardial effusions result from pericardial inflammation. Symptoms (chest pain) and ECG changes of pericarditis are common in varying degrees and may even be present without detectable pericardial effusion on echocardiography ("dry pericarditis"). Echocardiographically, an inflammatory pericardial process manifests with pericardial thickening, a finding best appreciated on the M-mode tracing; the visceral and parietal pericardia are detectable as definite layers, which in subacute and chronic pericarditis can be quite dense, more so than the myocardium of the ventricular wall. In hydropericardium, the pericardium is not thick.

The list of possible causes of pericarditis with effusion is very long and includes many viruses and bacteria, autoimmune processes, radiation, neoplastic invasion, and chemical irritation. In general, an effusion containing clear fluid is quite sonolucent, whereas an exudative pericardial effusion containing organizing exudate may manifest with turbidity or an amorphous, ill-defined layer (of fibrinous material) lying on the parietal pericardium. Certain bacterial forms of pericarditis, such as tuberculosis, have a strong tendency to form intrapericardial adhesions and fluid loculation.

PERICARDIAL THICKNESS

The parietal pericardium is normally about 2 mm thick, as measured on CT or MRI. The thickness of normal pericardium cannot be ascertained precisely by echocardiography,

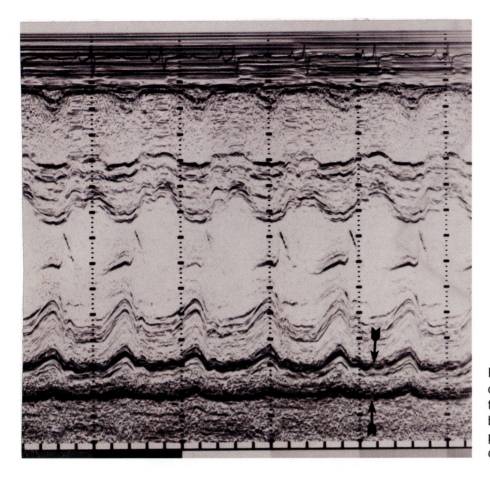

Figure 2–31. M-mode echocardiogram showing thickening of the posterior pericardium (small black arrows), visceral as well as parietal, which is more echodense than the LV posterior wall.

the ventricular-pericardial-pleural-lung interface appearing as a strong but ill-defined linear echo. Thickened pericardium, however, manifests on an M-mode echogram as a well-defined layer several millimeters in thickness[38] (Figures 2–31 and 2–32).

The entire circumference of the pericardium cannot be visualized by 2D echocardiography because of the wedge- or fan-shaped sector image; CT and MRI provide a more complete depiction of the entire pericardial perimeter. Both echocardiography and CT are useful in conveying an impression of the degree of thickening and of sclerosis and/or calcification of the pericardium, the density or "brightness" of the pericardial image being in proportion to the degree of sclerocalcific change (Figure 2–33). On the other hand, calcification does not register on the MRI and may in fact manifest as empty spaces. MRI pericardial images are most prominent when there is inflammatory change, i.e., in active subacute or chronic pericarditis.

CONSTRICTIVE PERICARDITIS

Only a small percentage of patients with pericardial thickening have hemodynamically significant pericardial constriction (Figure 2–34). However, the probability of constriction becomes higher if pericardial thickening is extensive and severe and approaches certainty if a circular or C-shaped dense calcific pericardial rim is evident on chest x-ray and CT.

The distribution of pericardial sclerocalcification is important. The ventricles are usually entirely encased in a thick pericardial sheath, and calcification is often most conspicuous in the atrioventricular (A-V) groove. The atria, however, are never constricted hemodynamically, although small calcific plaques or bands may sometimes adhere to the

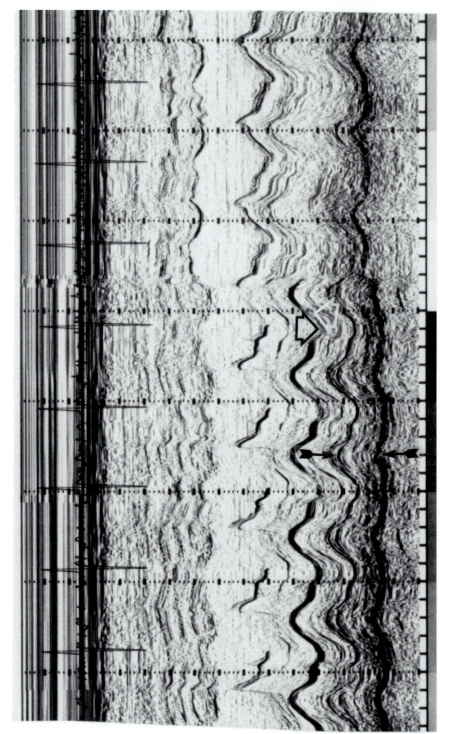

Figure 2–32. M-mode echocardiogram of a patient with pericardial thickening (small black arrows), which is more echodense than the LV posterior wall (open arrow).

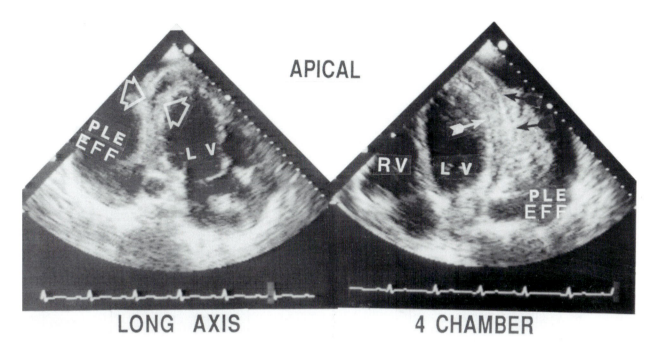

APICAL

LONG AXIS   4 CHAMBER

Figure 2–33. Apical views of a patient with left pleural effusion (PLE EFF) and pericarditis showing thickened pericardium (between arrows). A small pericardial effusion is seen in apical long-axis view.

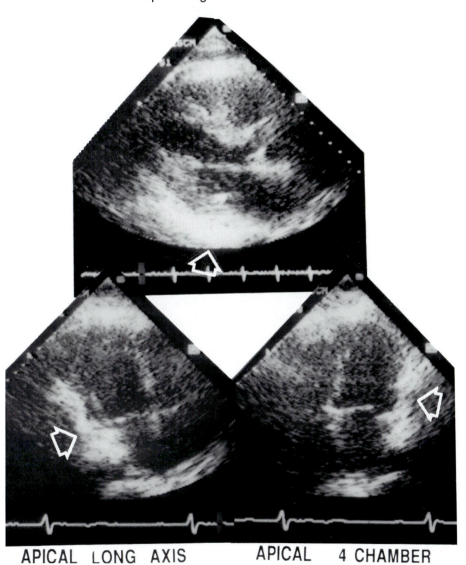

APICAL LONG AXIS   APICAL 4 CHAMBER

Figure 2–34. Parasternal long-axis view (above) and apical views (below) of a patient with conspicuous thickening of part of the pericardium (arrows). There were no signs of pericardial constriction.

45

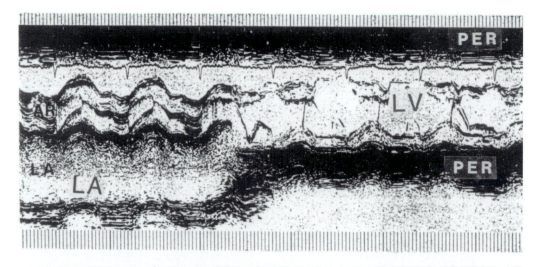

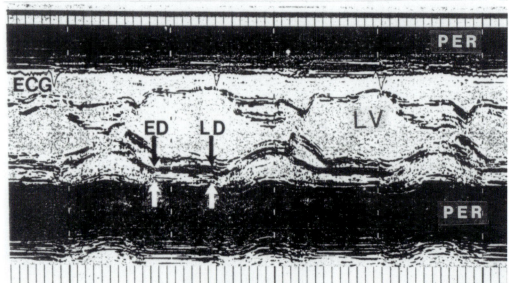

Figure 2–35. (Above) M-mode echocardiogram in a patient with constrictive pericarditis and heavy calcification of the pericardium (PER). Note that the posterior left atrial wall is at a much more posterior level than the posterior left ventricular wall because only the ventricles are constricted but the atria are not. (Below) M-mode echocardiogram in the same patient showing the so-called straight-line contour of LV posterior wall motion, i.e., failure of normal gradual ventricular expansion during middiastole (ED, early diastole; LD, late diastole).

atrial wall. The result of this is that imaging techniques including echocardiography show the ventricles to be of normal to small size, but both atria are always dilated. Very rare instances of localized pericardial constriction have been described, restricted to the left A-V groove causing *external mitral stenosis* or to the right ventricular outflow causing *external pulmonic stenosis.*

Echocardiography of Constrictive Pericarditis[39–45]

The features of constrictive pericarditis can be divided into four categories:

1. *Pericardial thickening,* often with dense sclerosis or calcification (Figure 2-35), the severity of which is extremely variable. The distribution of pericardial thickening

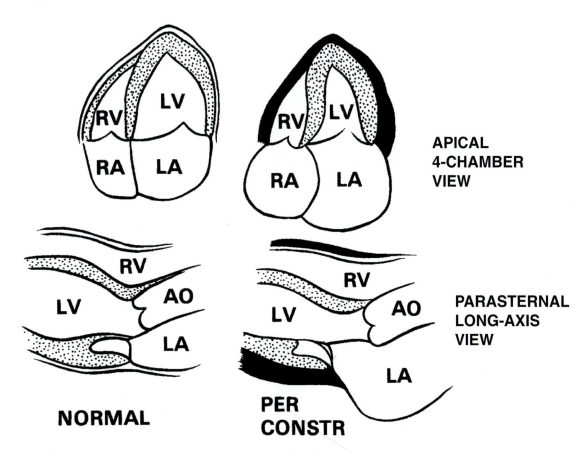

Figure 2–36. Diagram comparing normal 2D echocardiographic appearances with those of pericardial constriction. In the latter, the ventricles tend to be small, whereas the atria are dilated. In the parasternal long-axis view (below), the left atrial posterior wall is displaced posteriorly with respect to the left ventricular posterior wall, forming an abnormally small angle with it. (*Reproduced with permission D'Cruz IA. The noninvasive diagnosis of constrictive pericarditis. Am J Noninvas Cardiol 1990;4:65.*)

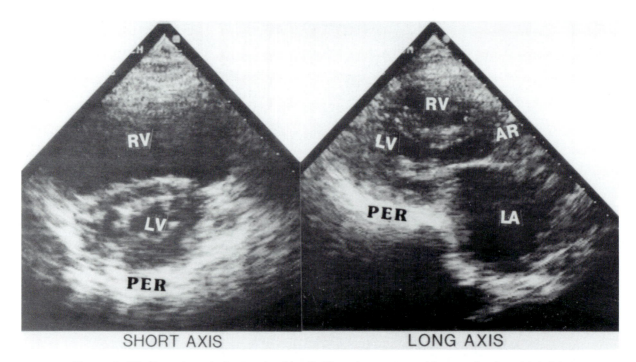

Figure 2–37. Parasternal short-axis view (left) and parasternal long-axis view (right) in a patient with pericardial constriction. The pericardium is thickened and densely sclerotic. The LA posterior wall is on a much more posterior plane than the LV posterior wall and forms almost a right angle with it at the LV-LA posterior junction.

around the ventricular perimeter is appreciated on 2D echo, but the precise thickness and "texture" of the posterior pericardium is more suitably defined by the higher resolution of M-mode.

2. *Abnormalities of ventricular septal motion,* which presumably reflect LV-RV pressure differences at various phases of the cycle and partly result from altered spatial motion and rotation of the heart secondary to adherent pericardium. Both these factors are not fully understood. The most useful M-mode signs are a very early diastolic anterior motion ("notch" on the M-mode tracing) and so-called flat motion of the LV posterior wall (absence of normal gradual posterior wall motion during the slow phase of ventricular filling). On the 2D echo, convexity or bowing of the ventricular and atrial septa toward the left-sided heart chambers were described by Lewis[42] and remain a useful sign in the absence of any other cause for RV overload.

3. *Abnormal chamber size and contour* (Figure 2-36). If the ventricles are not both normal to small in size and the atria not both dilated, the diagnosis of pericardial constriction remains in doubt. The atria are never constricted. In the parasternal long-axis view, this causes an unusual posterior cardiac contour (Figures 2-37 and 2-38): The left atrial posterior wall is in a plane 2 cm or more posterior to that of the left ventricle, and the LA-LV angle is abnormally small, less than 150 degrees.[43] This finding is seen in some patients with constrictive pericarditis, in my experience especially in those with conspicuous posterior pericardial thickening.

In constrictive pericarditis, the pericardium is densely thickened, fibrotic, and unyielding. The visceral and parietal layers are adherent. This final stage of pericardial scarring was presumably preceded by an acute exudative pericarditis, followed by a subacute stage of fibroblastic proliferation and organization during which the pericardial space becomes obliterated. Calcification varies from absent or minimal, to a thick, massive shell thicker than the ventricular wall. On the other hand, constricting pericardium sometimes can be hemodynamically important with leather-like toughness, even if its thickness is unimpressive and noncalcific.

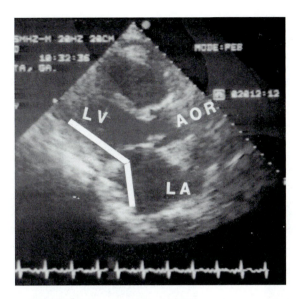

Figure 2–38. Parasternal long-axis view of a patient with pericardial constriction with an abnormally small posterior LV-LA angle.

4. *Abnormal motion resulting from hemodynamic abnormalities* of constriction. These include (a) premature opening of the pulmonic valve,[44] (b) a peculiar, even unique, brisk early diastolic rightward motion of the ventricular septum called the *septal bounce*,[45] and (c) *IVC dilatation and plethora* (absence of normal inspiratory IVC narrowing).[45]

Tuberculosis was the dominant etiology of constrictive pericarditis until the 1950s and is still so in developing countries. Prominent calcification is common. A dwindling prevalence of tuberculous pericarditis might explain the decreasing frequency of pericardial calcification in hemodynamically proved pericardial constriction during recent years.

Categorizing constrictive pericarditis by etiology, the largest group is idiopathic; i.e., the original cause of pericardial inflammation is unknown. Common varieties include (1) after radiation to the thorax for Hodgkin's lymphoma or breast cancer, (2) pyogenic pericarditis, (3) tumor encasement by neoplastic pericardial infiltration, (4) uremic pericarditis in patients on hemodialysis, (5) after hemopericardium following chest trauma, and (6) after cardiac surgery. The latter is rapidly growing in importance, and published data indicate that calcification or massive pericardial thickening is the exception in this situation.

Pericardial constriction exerts its deleterious effects by restricting diastolic filling of the ventricles. Rapid early diastolic filling is abruptly halted when intraventricular volume reaches the rigid limit imposed by the stiff, unyielding pericardium. A pericardial "knock" is often heard (and recorded by phonocardiography) at this point in the cardiac cycle.

The right and left ventricular chambers are of normal size or even reduced in size as a result of fibrotic scarring confining the ventricular dimensions. Their systolic function is normal. In long-standing instances, the myocardium may be superficially encroached on by the sclerotic pericardial process; some degree of myocardial atrophy may be present, perhaps accounting for the cardiac failure symptoms that follow pericardial resection in a small minority of cases.

Effusive-Constrictive Pericarditis

This is a subacute pericardial syndrome combining features of thickened constricting pericardium with some fluid pericardial contents (serous fluid, pus, or caseating material).[46] Thus the clinical presentation is that of constrictive pericarditis, but sonolucent pericar-

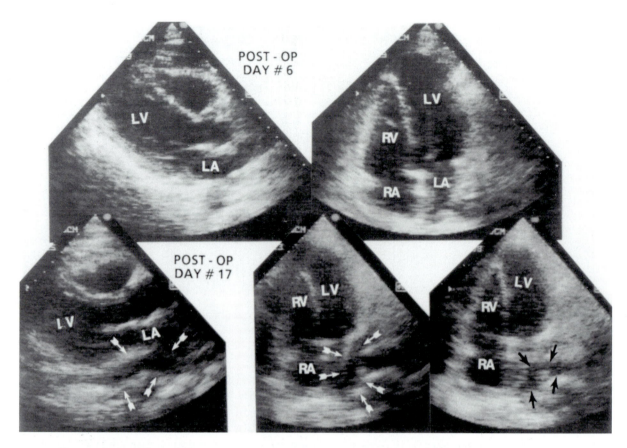

Figure 2–39. (Above) Parasternal long-axis and apical four-chamber views 6 days after cardiac surgery. (Below) Eleven days later a loculated pericardial effusion is seen adjacent to the left atrium. Catheterization showed typical findings of constrictive pericarditis. Surgical exploration revealed pus under pressure. *Diagnosis:* effusive-constrictive pericarditis.

dial spaces are detected on 2D echo, usually loculated by adhesions, and pockets of fluid or pus are found by surgical exploration (Figures 2-39 and 2-40). Another mode of presentation is that of persistence of signs of "tamponade" after paracentesis; this suggests unyielding epicardium rather than parietal pericardium as the constricting mechanism in such cases.

SEROUS EFFUSIONS ADJACENT TO THE HEART

The anatomic relationships of sonolucent spaces abutting the heart are well known to radiologists familiar with CT, MRI, or B-scan ultrasound imaging, but cardiologists interpreting echocardiograms are often ignorant to some degree of this topic. The subject is important, however, because such serous effusions could be mistaken for large loculated pericardial effusions. These include left pleural effusion, right pleural effusion, ascites, and pericardial or other mediastinal cysts.

Left Pleural Effusion

Other than pericardial effusions, a left pleural effusion is by far the most common sonolucent space seen on echocardiogram. The left pleura is extensively related to the posterior

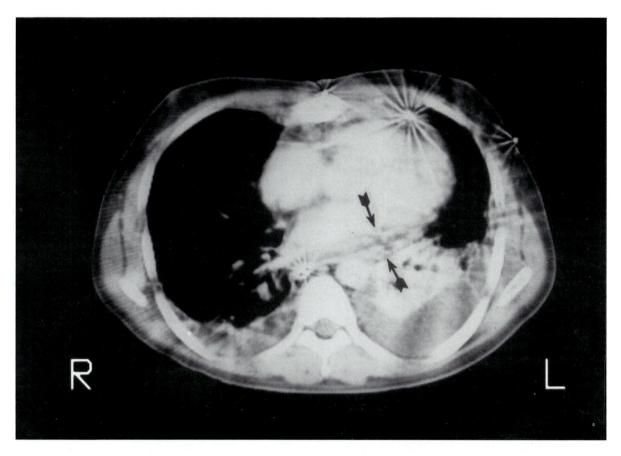

Figure 2–40. CT in same patient, showing the zone of loculated pus (arrows) and pneumonia of the left lower lobe.

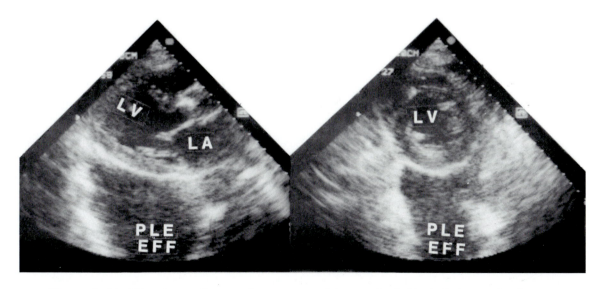

Figure 2–41. 2D echocardiogram in parasternal long-axis (left) and short-axis views (right) showing a sonolucent space posterior to the left ventricle (LV) representing a left pleural effusion (PLE EFF).

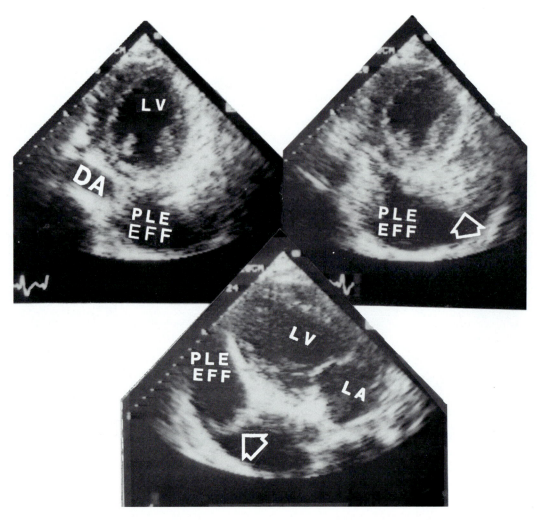

Figure 2–42. 2D echocardiogram in parasternal short-axis (above) and long-axis views (below). The collapsed lung appears as an opacity (arrows) within the left pleural effusion (PLE EFF).

and lateral aspects of the heart and pericardium. In patients with cardiorespiratory symptoms, the differential diagnosis between a left pleural effusion and a large loculated posterior pericardial effusion may be an important one.

One distinguishing feature is the shape of the sonolucent space (Figures 2-41 to 2-43). In the parasternal short-axis view, pericardial effusions follow the circular outline of the ventricles and therefore tend to be annular or crescentic in shape. On the other hand, a left pleural effusion is broad and band- or wedge-shaped.

Another very useful differentiating point is the relationship of the sonolucent space to the descending thoracic aorta (Figure 2-44). Pericardial effusions occupy a plane anterior to the round sonolucent space representing the descending aorta, whereas pleural effusions are posterior to the plane of the descending aorta.[47]

A large left pleural effusion is also important to the echocardiographer in another way. In patients who have poor anterior acoustic echo windows because of pulmonary emphysema or other reasons, the left pleural effusion can provide a good window to visualize the left ventricle and pericardium when the transducer is placed over the lateral or posterolateral left chest wall (Figure 2-45).

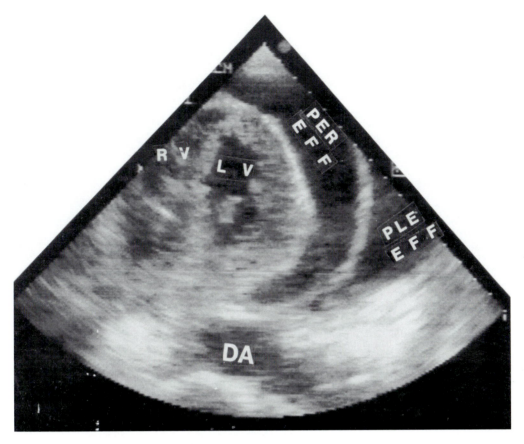

Figure 2–43. Apical view showing pericardial effusion as well as left pleural effusion. The pericardial-pleural interface appears as a curved linear echo between the sonolucencies of the two serous effusions.

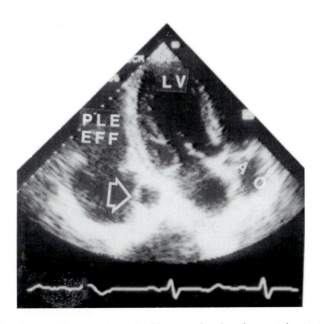

Figure 2–44. 2D echocardiogram in apical long-axis view in a patient with a left pleural effusion (PLE EFF) presenting as a large sonolucent space posterior to the heart. The pleural effusion is posterior to the plane of the descending thoracic aorta (open arrow).

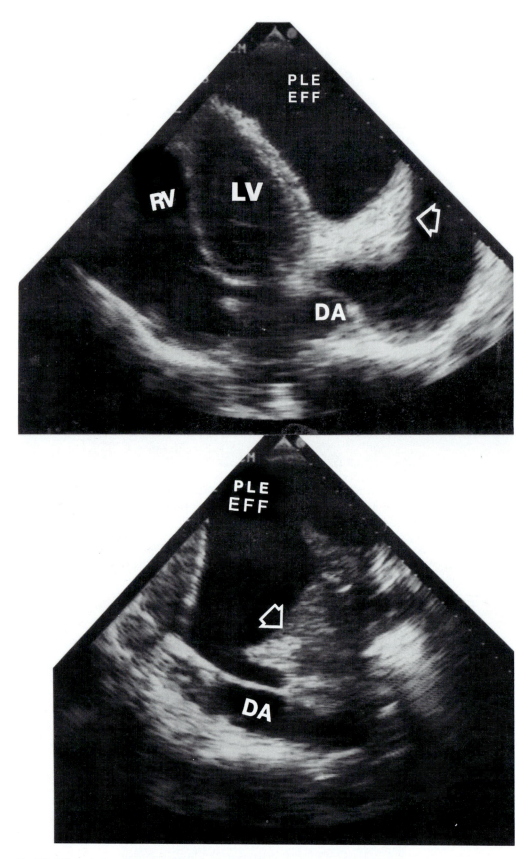

Figure 2–45. The left pleural effusion is itself used as an ultrasound window to image the effusion and beyond it the heart (above). The collapsed left lung appears as a bright opacity (arrow) within the effusion. In the lower frame the thoracic descending aorta is well seen in its long axis, posterior to the pleural effusion.

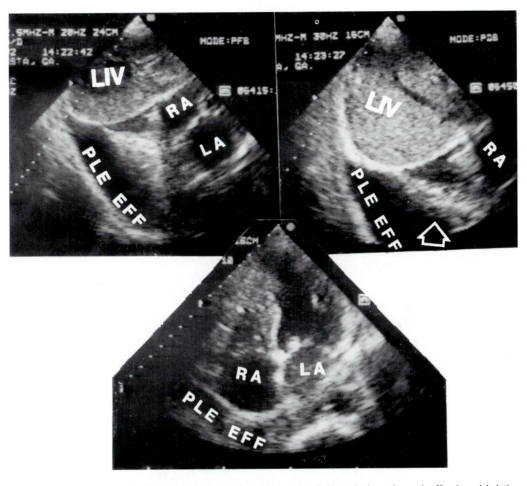

Figure 2–46. 2D echocardiogram in subcostal view (above) the pleural effusion (right) presenting as a sonolucent space bounded by the liver (LIV) inferiorly, chest wall posteriorly, and atria anteriorly and to the right. The collapsed lung (arrow) is seen within the pleural effusion. The effusion is seen adjacent to the right atrium in the apical four-chamber view (below).

Right Pleural Effusion (Figures 2–46 to 2–49)

The right pleura is contiguous with only one cardiac chamber—the right atrium (except for a very small corner of right ventricle). Right pleural effusions cannot be visualized from the conventional parasternal view and only indistinctly from the apical view, but they may be well seen in the subcostal view as a large sonolucent space adjacent to the right atrium and (intrathoracic) inferior vena cava.[48] In a sagittal or parasagittal subcostal plane, a right pleural effusion manifests as a triangular sonolucent space bounded inferiorly by the large, rounded, solid liver mass subjacent to the linear echo representing the right dome of the diaphragm, posteriorly by the posterior thoracic wall, and anteriorly by the right atrium and inferior vena cava.[48] Bilateral pleural effusions cause multiple sonolucent paracardiac spaces that need to be correctly identified (Figures 2-48 and 2-49).

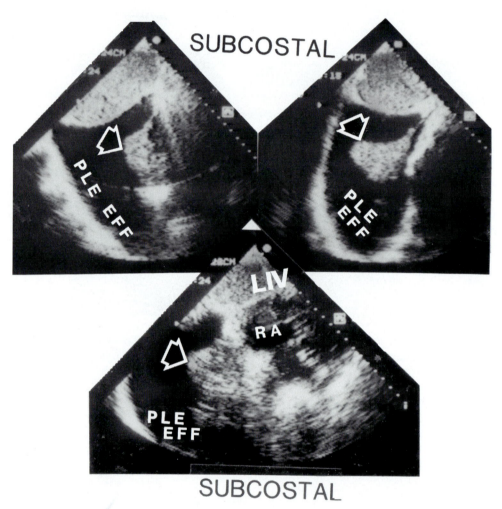

Figure 2–47. Subcostal view of a right pleural effusion showing that the effusion, with collapsed right lung within it (arrow), occupies the entire right hemithorax (above). In a different subcostal view (below), the bulky mass projecting into the effusion represents a malignant neoplasm within the collapsed right lung.

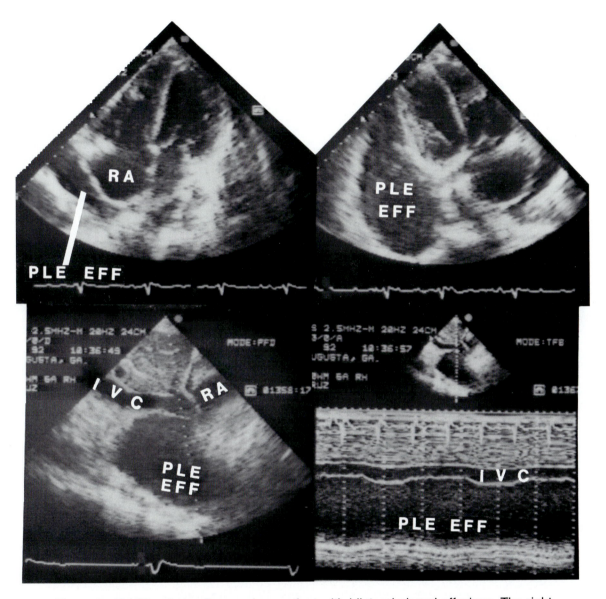

Figure 2–48. 2D echocardiogram in a patient with bilateral pleural effusions. The right effusion (above, left) appears as a sonolucent space adjacent to the right atrium (RA). The left effusion is represented by a larger sonolucent space posterior to the heart (above, right). The right pleural effusion is seen on 2D echo (below, left) and M-mode (below, right) as a large sonolucent space posterior to the plane of the inferior vena cava (IVC) and right atrium (RA) in the subcostal view.

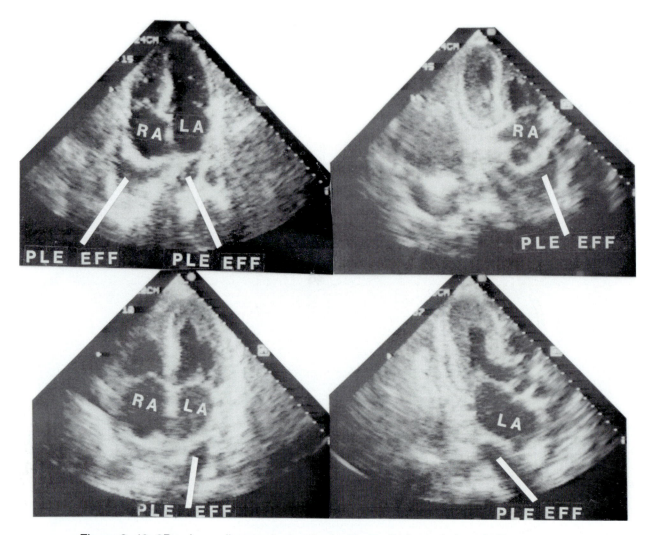

Figure 2–49. 2D echocardiogram in a patient with small bilateral pleural effusions (PLE EFF) which appear as sonolucent spaces posterior to the right and left atrium, respectively, in apical four-chamber views (left) and other apical views (right).

Ascites (Figure 2–50)

Ascites produces a large infradiaphragmatic sonolucent space in which various abdominal organs can be easily identified. Its importance to the echocardiographer can arise in two ways: First, in the subcostal view, with the transducer directed upward and backward from the epigastrium, a tense ascites can manifest as a sonolucent space "anterior" to the right ventricle (Figures 2-51 and 2-52). It could therefore be mistaken for a loculated anterior pericardial effusion or pericardial cyst.[49] Typically, this sonolucent space representing the most anterosuperior portion of the peritoneal cavity is bisected by a sharp, well-defined linear echo representing the ligamentum falciparum.[49] This falciform ligament is a normal triangular fold of peritoneum that is attached to the abdominal wall and anterior diaphragm on its convex border and to the convexity of the right lobe of the liver on its concave border. Exceptionally, the stomach can present as a similar "anterior" space (Figure 2-53). Second, in parasternal views, ascitic fluid just under the diaphragm can appear as a sonolucent "posterior" space (Figure 2-54) "behind" the left ventricle, though it is actually inferior to the heart in an anatomic sense.[39] An enlarged spleen (common in patients with tense ascites secondary to cirrhosis) can appear as a dense, solid echo "posterior" to the sonolucent fluid space, adding to the illusion of a posterior pericardial effusion.

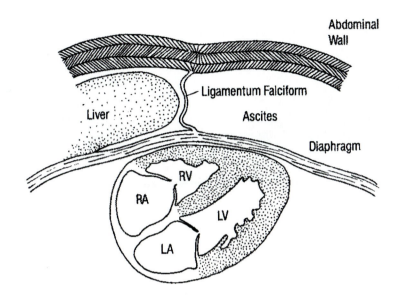

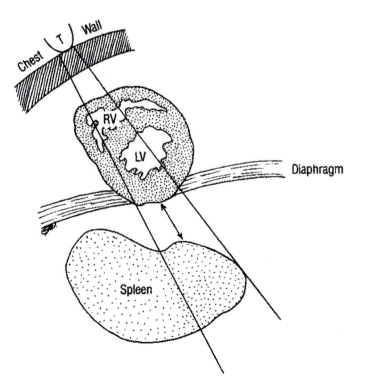

Figure 2–50. Ascites can simulate pericardial effusions. In the subcostal view (above), a sonolucent space representing ascites appears to be "anterior" to the heart and could be mistaken for a loculated anterior pericardial effusion. Ascites is identified by visualization of the left hepatic lobe and of the ligamentum falciform. In the parasternal view (below), ascitic fluid manifesting as a "posterior" sonolucent space (arrow) between the left ventricle and an enlarged spleen can simulate a loculated posterior pericardial effusion (T, transducer).

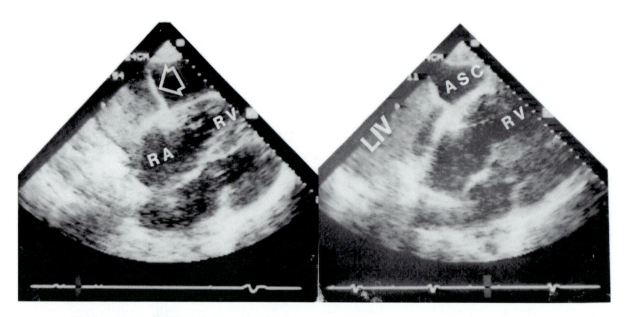

Figure 2–51. Subcostal four-chamber view showing a sonolucent space "anterior" to the right side of the heart representing ascites (ASC). A well-defined linear echo (arrow) within the ascites represents the falciform ligament. The solid mass of the liver (LIV) is seen adjacent to the ascites.

MEDIASTINAL CYSTS

Cystic masses of diverse origins, histology, size, and location can occur in the anterior mediastinum. Since they manifest as sonolucent spaces on echocardiography,[50-53] they could be mistaken for loculated anterior pericardial effusions. The list of such masses includes cystic thymomas, cystic hygromas, dermoid cysts, and cystic chondromas. However, the most common are pericardial cysts, which have a lining similar to pericardium or pleura and are thin-walled, containing clear, watery fluid. Although they may occur anywhere in the mediastinum, the most frequent site is in the angle between the right atrium and the diaphragm. In this location they may be visualized in the subcostal view.[52,53] The differential diagnosis of a sonolucent space adjacent to the right atrium and diaphragm includes a loculated pericardial effusion and a right pleural effusion. CT imaging demonstrates the lesion well.

CONGENITAL ABSENCE OF THE PERICARDIUM

This is a rare congenital anomaly affecting part (or more often all) of the left pericardium. Deficient right pericardium or total absence of pericardium is known but extremely rare. In 75% of cases there is also a large deficiency in the left parietal pleura so that the left lung may herniate through into the pericardial sac, thus becoming intimately contiguous with the base of the heart. Conversely, if the pericardial hiatus is of suitable size and location, herniation of the left atrial appendage or neighboring structures through it (incarceration) can cause arrhythmias, angina, syncope, or even sudden death.

The chest x-ray usually shows leftward cardiac shift with a straight left cardiac silhouette and long pulmonary trunk contour. Echocardiography shows right ventricular enlargement and perhaps abnormal septal motion.[54] Severe tricuspid regurgitation has been reported recently. The absent portions of pericardium cannot be visualized as such on echocardiography but have been identified on CT and MRI.[55,56]

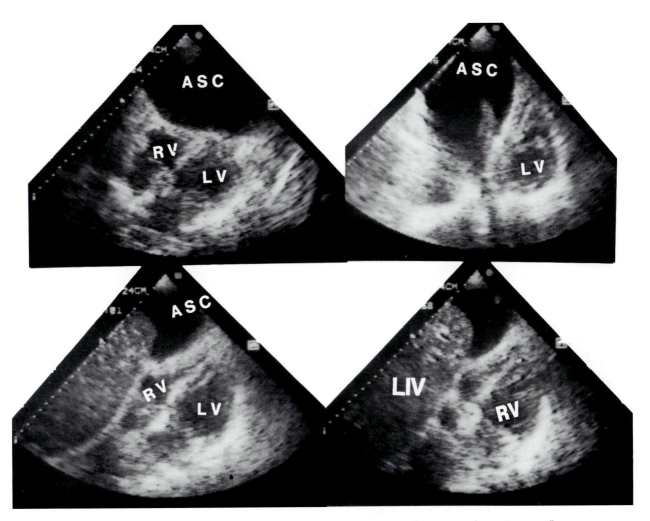

Figure 2–52. Subcostal views in different planes showing a large sonolucent space "anterior" to the heart which represents the uppermost part of a tense ascites (ASC). The liver (LIV) can be identified adjacent to the ascitic space in the lower frames.

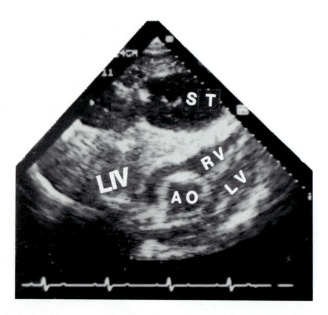

Figure 2–53. Subcostal view showing a sonolucent space "anterior" to the heart. In this patient it represents fluid within the stomach, which was displaced anteriorly by a large pancreatic pseudocyst.

DIAPHRAGMATIC HERNIA

The diaphragm, a large, dome-shaped musculofibrous sheet between the thorax and the abdomen, allows passage of certain important structures: the inferior vena cava, the esophagus, and the descending aorta. The gap, or hiatus, through which the esophagus passes sometimes becomes lax so that a variable extent of stomach slides up into the thorax. Such a *hiatus hernia* is quite common and often causes symptoms closely resembling ischemic cardiac pain. Hiatus hernias, especially when large, are of importance to the echocardiographer because they intrude into the posterior mediastinum and may encroach on the left atrium, simulating various extracardiac or intraatrial masses. Rare congenital defects in the posterolateral part of the diaphragm (foramen of Bochdalek) or in the most anterior part of the diaphragm just behind the sternum (foramen of Morgagni) give rise to abnormal thoracic radiographic and CT appearances but are of little relevance to the echocardiographer.

Rare instances of pericardiophrenic hernia have been reported—28 cases in total in a review published in 1985.[57] The defect was presumed to be congenital in most of these. (It also can be iatrogenic, as a complication of a subxiphoid window for pericardial fluid drainage.) Abdominal organs herniating into the pericardium in such a hernia are the omentum, stomach, colon, and liver in decreasing order of frequency. The clinical importance of this uncommon situation is that pericardial ingress of abdominal viscera, especially distended stomach or gut, can cause tamponade.[57]

Another form of acquired diaphragmatic perforation is caused by rupture of an amebic abscess of the left lobe of the liver—commonly into the right lung or pleura but sometimes into the pericardium. This grave complication occurs in tropical countries where amebiasis (*Entamoeba histolytica*) is rife; the clinical presentation can mimic acute myocardial infarction, with severe chest pain, hypotension, ST-segment changes on ECG (of pericarditis), and fatal outcome.[58]

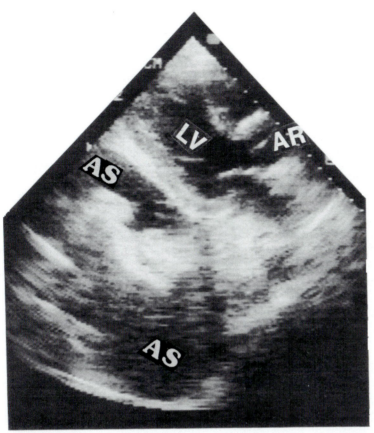

NEAR - APICAL LONG AXIS

Figure 2–54. Long-axis view showing sonolucent space posteroinferior to left ventricle (LV), which is ascites (AS) in this case secondary to hepatic cirrhosis. A pericardial effusion is simulated.

REFERENCES

1. Wada T, Honda M, Maysuyama S. Extra echo spaces: Ultrasonography and computerised tomography correlations. Br Heart J 1982;47:430.
2. Rifkin RD, Isner JM, Carter BL, et al. Combined posteroanterior subepicardial fat simulating the echocardiographic diagnosis of pericardial effusion. J Am Coll Cardiol 1984;3:1333.
3. Isner JM, Carter BL, Roberts WC, et al. Subepicardial adipose tissue producing echocardiographic appearance of pericardial effusion. Am J Cardiol 1983;51:565.
4. Levy-Ravetch M, Auh YH, Rubenstein WA, et al. CT of the pericardial recesses. AJR 1985;144:707.
5. Choe YH, Im J, Park JH, et al. The anatomy of the pericardial space: A study in cadavers and patients. AJR 1987;149:693.
6. Gale ME, Kiwak MG, Gale DR. Pericardial fluid distribution: CT analysis. Radiology 1987;162:171.
7. Miller SW. Imaging pericardial disease. Radiol Clin North Am 1989;27:1113.
8. Soulen R, Lapayowker MS, Cortes FM. Distribution of pericardial fluid: Dynamic and static influences. AJR 1968;103:583.
9. Byrk D, Kroope IG, Budow J. The effect of heart size, cardiac tamponade and phase of the cardiac cycle on the distribution of pericardial fluid. Radiology 1969;93:273.
10. Feginbaum H, Zaky A, Grabhorn LL. Cardiac motion in patients with pericardial effusion. Circulation 1966;34:611.
11. Gabor GE, Winsberg F, Bloom HS, Electrical and Mechanical Alternation in Pericardial Effusion. Chest 1971; 59:341.
12. Usher BW, Popp RL. Electrical alternans: Mechanism in pericardial effusion. Am Heart J 1972;83:459.

13. Lemire F, Tajik AJ, Giuliani ER, et al. Further echocardiographic observations in pericardial effusion. Mayo Clin Proc 1976;51:13.
14. D'Cruz IA, Kensey K, Campbell C, et al. Two-dimensional echocardiography in cardiac tamponade occurring after cardiac surgery. J Am Coll Cardiol 1985;5:1250.
15. D'Cruz IA, Macander PJ, Gross CM, et al. Distension of the oblique pericardial sinus in tamponade due to loculated posterior pericardial effusion. Am J Cardiol 1990;65:1520.
16. Martin RP, Bowen R, Fily K, et al. Intrapericardial abnormalities in patients with pericardial effusion. Circulation 1980;61:568.
17. Lam D, Rapaport E. Two-dimensional echocardiographic demonstration of intrapericardial fibrinous strands in rheumatoid pericarditis. Am Heart J 1987;114:442.
18. Chandaratna PAN, Aronow WS. Detection of pericardial metastases by cross-sectional echocardiography. Circulation 1981;63:197.
19. Schuster AH, Nanda NC. Pericardiocentesis-induced intrapericardial thrombus. Am Heart J 1982;104:308.
20. D'Cruz IA, Holman MS, Childers LS. Spontaneous mobile contrast echoes in pericardial effusion. Am Heart J 1990;120:1472.
21. Ku CS, Hsiung MC, Hsu TL, et al. Spontaneous contrast in the pericardial sac caused by gas-forming organisms. J Am Soc Echocardiogr 1991;4:67.
22. Manjana A, Marvric Z, Vukas D, et al. Spontaneous contrast echoes in pericardial effusion. Am Heart J 1992;124:521.
23. D'Cruz IA, Hoffman PK. A new cross-sectional echocardiographic method for estimating the volume of large pericardial effusions. Br Heart J 1991;66:448.
24. Holt JP. The normal pericardium. Am J Cardiol 1970;26:455.
25. Gillam LD, Guyer DE, Gibson TC, et al. Hydrodynamic compression of the right atrium: A new echocardiographic sign of cardiac tamponade. Circulation 1983;68:294.
26. Armstrong WF, Schilt BF, Helper DJ, et al. Diastolic collapse of the right ventricle with tamponade. Circulation 1982;65:1491.
27. Kronzon I, Cohen ML, Winer HE. Diastolic atrial compression: A sensitive echocardiographic sign of cardiac tamponade. J Am Coll Cardiol 1983;2:770.
28. D'Cruz IA, Kensey K, Campbell C, et al. Two-dimensional echocardiography in cardiac tamponade occurring after cardiac surgery. J Am Coll Cardiol 1985;5:1250.
29. Chuttani K, Pandian NG, Mohanty PK, et al. Left ventricular diastolic collapse: An echocardiographic sign of regional cardiac tamponade. Circulation 1991;83:1999.
30. Kronzon I, Cohen ML, Winer HE. Cardiac tamponade by loculated pericardial hematoma. J Am Coll Cardiol 1983;1:913.
31. Kochar GS, Jacobs LE, Kotler MN. Right atrial compression in postoperative cardiac patients. J Am Coll Cardiol 1990;16:511.
32. Fyke FE, Tancredi RG, Shub C. Detection of intrapericardial hematoma after open heart surgery. J Am Coll Cardiol 1985;5:1496.
33. Gheorghiade M, Cheek BH, Chakko SC. Isolated right heart tamponade following mediastinal irradiation. Am Heart J 1986;112:167.
34. Simpson IA, Munsch C, Smith EEJ, et al. Pericardial hemorrhage causing right atrial compression after cardiac surgery. Br Med J 1991;65:355.
35. Torelli J, Marwick TH, Salcedo EE. Left atrial tamponade. J Am Soc Echocardiogr 1991;4:413.
36. Safford RE, Blackshear JL, Kapples EJ. Clinical utility of transesophageal echocardiography. South Med J 1991;84:611.
37. Golub RJ, McNulty CM, McClellan JR, et al. Usefulness of transesophageal Doppler echocardiography in the surgical drainage of a loculated purulent pericardial effusion. Am Heart J 1993;126:724.
38. Schnittger I, Bowden RE, Abrams J, et al. Echocardiography: Pericardial thickening and constrictive pericarditis. Am J Cardiol 1978;42:388.
39. Pool PE, Seagren SC, Abbasi AL, et al. Echocardiographic manifestations of constrictive pericarditis. Chest 1975;68:684.
40. Voelkel AG, Pietro DA, Folland ED, et al. Echocardiographic features of constrictive pericarditis. Circulation 1978;58:871.
41. D'Cruz IA, Levinsky R, Anagnostopoulos C, et al. Echocardiographic diagnosis of partial pericardial constriction of the left ventricle. Radiology 1978;127:755.
42. Lewis BS. Real-time two-dimensional echocardiography in constrictive pericarditis. Am J Cardiol 1982;49:1789.

43. D'Cruz IA, Dick A, Gross CM, et al. Abnormal left ventricular–left atrial posterior wall contour: A new two-dimensional echocardiographic sign in constrictive pericarditis. Am Heart J 1989;118:128.
44. Wann LS, Weyman AE, Dillon JC, et al. Premature pulmonary valve opening. Circulation 1977;55:128.
45. Himelman RB, Lee E, Schiller NB. Septal bounce, vena cava plethora and pericardial adhesion: Informative two-dimensional echocardiographic signs in the diagnosis of pericardial constriction. J Am Soc Echocardiogr 1988;1:333.
46. Hancock EW. Subacute effusive-constrictive pericarditis. Circulation 1971;43:183.
47. Haaz WS, Mintz GS, Kotler MN, et al. Two-dimensional echocardiographic recognition of the descending thoracic aorta: Value in differentiating pericardial from pleural effusions. Am J Cardiol 1980;46:739.
48. D'Cruz IA. Echocardiographic simulation of pericardial fluid accumulation by right pleural effusion. Chest 1984;86:451.
49. D'Cruz IA. Echocardiographic simulation of pericardial effusion by ascites. Chest 1983;85:93.
50. Schloss M, Kronzon I, Geller PM, et al. Cystic hygroma simulating constrictive pericarditis. J Thorac Cardiovasc Surg 1975;70:143.
51. Koch PC, Kronzon I, Winer HE, et al. Displacement of the heart by a giant mediastinal cyst. Am J Cardiol 1977;40:445.
52. Felner JM, Fleming WH, Franch RH. Echocardiographic identification of a pericardial cyst. Chest 1975;68:386.
53. Hynes JK, Tajik AJ, Osborn MG, et al. Two-dimensional echocardiographic diagnosis of pericardial cyst. Proc Mayo Clin 1983;56:60.
54. Payvandi MN, Kerber RE. Echocardiography in congenital and acquired absence of pericardium. Circulation 1976;53:86.
55. Baim RS, MacDonald IL, Wise DJ, et al. Computed tomography of absent left pericardium. Radiology 1980;135:127.
56. Schiavone WA, O'Donnell JK. Congenital absence of the left portion of parietal pericardium demonstrated by nuclear magnetic resonance imaging. Am J Cardiol 1985;55:1439.
57. Nelson RM, Wilson RF, Huang CL, et al. Cardiac tamponade due to an iatrogenic pericardial diaphragmatic hernia. Crit Care Med 1985;13:607.
58. D'Cruz IA, Ramamoorthy K. Amebic pericarditis. J Ind Med Assoc 1967;49:342.

3

The Mediastinum

The heart is centrally situated in the mediastinum and is surrounded by important viscera and blood vessels, as well as smaller structures such as nerves, lymph nodes, fatty tissue, etc. The heart itself constitutes an echocardiographic window through which some parts of the mediastinum may be visualized. Conversely, anterior mediastinal masses might provide an ultrasound window through which superior mediastinal or right mediastinal structures, which are normally "hidden" by intervening lung tissues, can be imaged.

ANATOMIC TERMS (Figure 3–1)

The pericardium and its cardiac contents constitute the *middle mediastinum;* the *anterior mediastinum* lies between the anterior chest wall and the pericardium. The *posterior mediastinum* lies between the heart (or pericardium) and the vertebral column and paraspinal ligaments and muscles posteriorly. The diaphragm forms the inferior boundary of the anterior as well as posterior mediastinum. The upper boundary of these anatomic spaces is the plane of the sternal angle (of Louis) at the level of the second costal cartilage. The superior mediastinum is the mediastinal region between the thoracic inlet above (spine, first ribs, and upper border of manubrium sternum) and the plane of the angle of Louis inferiorly.

From the clinician's viewpoint, a distinction must be made between different degrees of cardiac "involvement" by mediastinal masses:

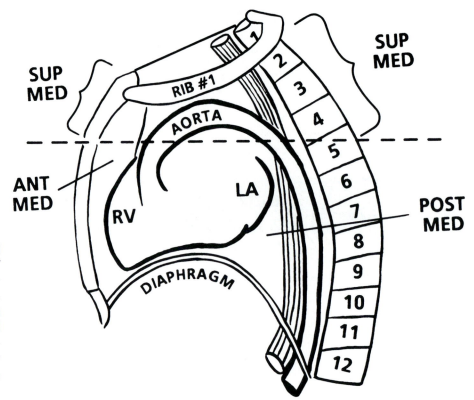

Figure 3–1. Diagram showing the demarcation of the superior mediastinum (SUP MED), anterior mediastinum (ANT MED), and posterior mediastinum (POST MED). The horizontal broken line runs through the sternal angle (of Louis) anteriorly and the lower border of the fourth dorsal vertebra posteriorly.

1. *Proximity.* The abnormal mass is contiguous or adjacent to the heart and recognizable in one or more of the two-dimensional (2D) echographic views but does not actually deform or indent cardiac chambers.

2. *Encroachment.* The mediastinal mass encroaches on one or more heart chambers, narrowing or otherwise distorting it, but does not cause adverse hemodynamic effects. (However, the patient may be symptomatic from pressure effects of the mass on the esophagus, trachea, or other noncardiac structures.) According to *Webster's Dictionary,* the meanings of *encroach* are (a) to trespass or intrude upon and (b) to advance beyond the proper, original, or customary limits.

3. *Compression.* The mediastinal mass is large and rigid or, if cystic, under high pressure and so located as to compress the heart, producing hemodynamic effects and symptoms akin to tamponade. The mediastinum can be considered to be a "box" with compliant lateral walls (pleura and lung on either side) but unyielding walls anteriorly (sternum and costal cartilages) and posteriorly (vertebral column). The latter renders it possible for a large, firm mass or a high-tension fluid accumulation or aortic aneurysm to seriously impair cardiac filling, in effect like tamponade.

Before discussing specific mediastinal viscera or structures giving origin to mediastinal masses, it is worth mentioning two types of tissue that pervade all mediastinal compartments: fat and lymph nodes.

Adipose Tissue

The distribution of fat within the thorax has been studied.[1] The major sites of fat accumulation are (1) retrosternally in the anterior mediastinum, extending downward into each cardiophrenic angle, (2) at the base of the heart between the ascending aorta and pulmonary trunk and around the base of the latter, (3) in the coronary groove around the coronary arteries and extending along the coronary branches, (4) in the posterior interatrial sulcus, where it becomes continuous with fat in the interatrial septum (lipomatous hypertrophy), a common finding in the elderly, (5) subepicardial fat, sometimes referred

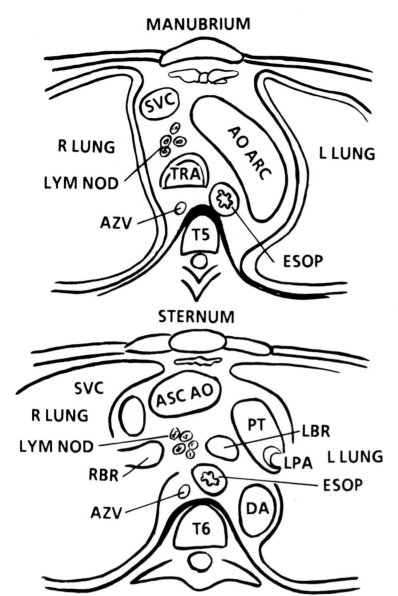

MANUBRIUM

SVC

R LUNG

AO ARC

L LUNG

LYM NOD

TRA

AZV

T5

ESOP

STERNUM

SVC

R LUNG

ASC AO

LYM NOD

PT

LBR

RBR

LPA   L LUNG

AZV

ESOP

DA

T6

Figure 3–2. Transverse sections (viewed from below) of the thorax at the levels of fifth and sixth thoracic vertebrae (T5 and T6) (SVC, superior vena cava; Ao ARCH, aortic arch; TRA, trachea; ESOP, esophagus; AZV, azygos vein; LYM NOD, lymph nodes; ASC AO, ascending aorta; PT, pulmonary trunk, RBR, right bronchus; LBR, left bronchus; DA, descending aorta).

to as *fat pads* (occasionally these exceed 1.5 or even 2 cm in thickness; large epicardial fat accumulations may occur anterior to the right ventricle and in the cardiophrenic angle, the right more frequently than the left[2,3]; in the cardiophrenic location, such a "mass" needs to be distinguished from a pericardial cyst, diaphragmatic hernia through the foramen of Morgagni, thymolipoma, and non-Hodgkin's lymphoma[4]), and (6) in the posterior mediastinum, anterior to the spine, between it and the descending thoracic aorta, usually more prominent on the left than right prevertebral region.

Pericardial fat sometimes may be mistaken for a small pericardial effusion on M-mode or 2D echocardiography. On the other hand, on CT, epicardial fat can be useful in outlining pericardial fluid and/or pericardial thickening. Mediastinal fat in general is more abundant in obese than in thin individuals.[1] However, there is much variation from person to person, and considerable local fat deposits can occur in certain locations in nonobese persons.

Impressive mediastinal fat accumulation is frequent in Cushing's syndrome and in patients on prolonged high-dose corticosteriod therapy (sometimes referred to as *mediastinal lipomatosis*).

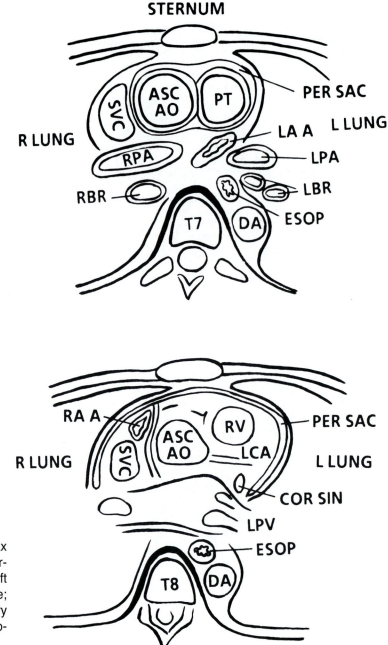

Figure 3–3. Transverse sections of the thorax at the levels of seventh and eighth thoracic vertebrae (RPA, right pulmonary artery; LPA, left pulmonary artery; LAA, left atrial appendage; LCA, left coronary artery; COR SIN, coronary sinus; RV, right ventricle; RAA, right atrial appendage; PER SAC, pericardial sac).

Lymph Nodes

The average number of lymph nodes in the mediastinum is 64, of which 50 are paratracheal or around the tracheal bifurcation.[6] A fair number are paraesophageal in location; the few remaining ones are scattered elsewhere in anterior or posterior mediastinal territory. Normal lymph nodes are usually less than 1.5 cm in size, rarely exceeding 2 cm. Lymph nodes can enlarge to a huge size due to lymphomatous or metastatic spread from lung, esophageal, or breast neoplasms, in which case they may compress adjacent viscera or veins and manifest as a mass on chest x-ray as well as echocardiography, CT, or MRI.

A convenient way to become familiar with mediastinal anatomy is by studying serial transverse sections at each of six vertebral levels (Figures 3–2 to 3–4). Figure 3–5 depicts the inferior aspect of the diaphragm to show the openings for passage of the inferior vena

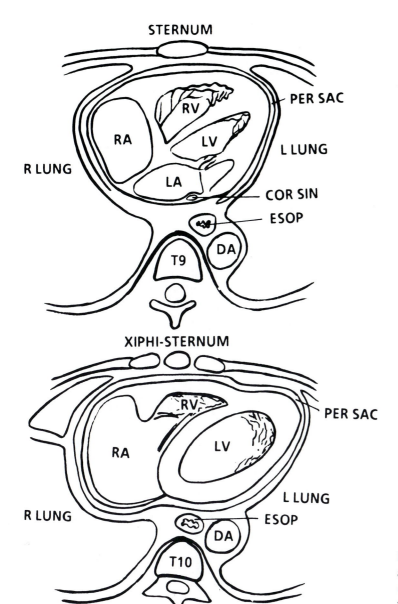

Figure 3–4. Transverse sections of the thorax at the levels of ninth and tenth thoracic vertebrae (RA, right atrium; RV, right ventricle; LV, left ventricle).

cava (IVC), esophagus, and descending aorta. The superior aspect was shown in Figure 2-1. The right aspect of the mediastinum (after removal of right lung and pleura) is shown in Figure 3-6. Figure 3-7 shows the heart as viewed from directly above, as well as from the left and above (after removal of the great vessels near their cardiac attachments). Figure 3-8 represents a coronal section through the mediastinum showing the anatomic relationships of some great vessels to each other and the heart.

Thymus

Other than adipose and lymphatic tissue, the only other *normal* structure in the anterior mediastinum (or anterior part of superior mediastinum) is the thymus gland. It weighs about 15 g at birth and grows to reach a maximum size at 12 to 19 years (average 35 g at puberty); then it regresses after age 20 so that at age 60 it is half of what it was at age 20.[7] However, the ratio of thymic to mediastinal size decreases during childhood so that on the chest x-ray or CT the thymus appears larger and more conspicuous in infancy than later. To pediatric echocardiographers this is fortunate because it helps provide a "win-

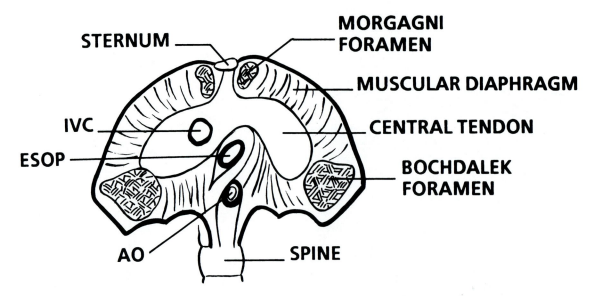

STERNUM

MORGAGNI
FORAMEN

MUSCULAR DIAPHRAGM

IVC

CENTRAL TENDON

ESOP

BOCHDALEK
FORAMEN

AO

SPINE

Figure 3–5. Diagram of diaphragm, viewed from below, showing the sites of orifices for passage of inferior vena cava (IVC), esophagus (ESOP), and descending aorta (AO). The central clear area represents the central tendon of the diaphragm. The sites of congenital diaphragmatic hernias of Morgagni (anteriorly) and of Bochdalek (postero-laterally) are also shown.

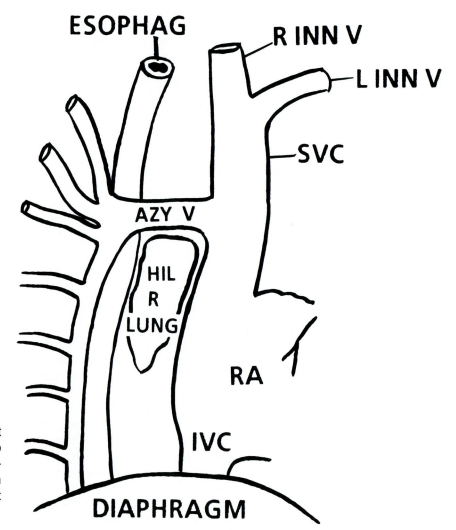

ESOPHAG

R INN V

L INN V

SVC

AZY V

HIL R LUNG

RA

IVC

DIAPHRAGM

Figure 3–6. Diagram of right aspect of mediastinum to show relationship of azygos vein (AZT V), SVC, innominate veins (INN V), right atrium (RA), and IVC to hilum (HIL) of right lung.

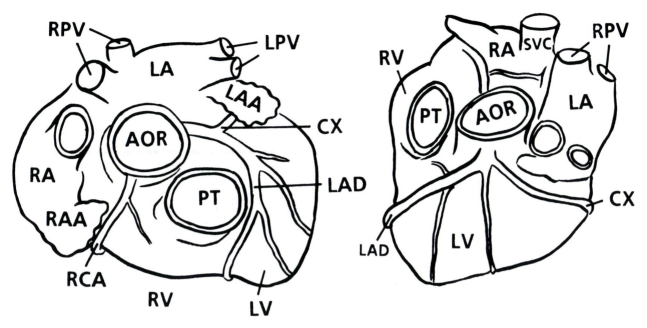

Figure 3–7. Diagram showing external anatomy of the excised heart, as viewed from directly above (left) and from the left and above (right). The aorta (AOR) and pulmonary trunk (PT) occupy a central position, the former somewhat posterior to the former. The left atrium (LA) is a posterior chamber; the right atrium (RA) is to the right and anterior. The locations of the right and left atrial appendages (RAA and LAA) are shown. Soon after emerging from the left aspect of the aortic root, the left main coronary artery divides into the left anterior descending (LAD) anteriorly and the circumflex (CX) posteriorly. The right coronary artery (RCA) courses anteriorly in the groove between right atrium and ventricle.

dow" to the upper mediastinum, often permitting visualization of large arteries and veins in infants and small children that is no longer available in teenagers because of obscuration by intervening lung.

Thymomas are the most common neoplasm encountered in the upper anterior mediastinum, 80% of which are located at the base of the heart. Thymomas have a strong association with myasthenia gravis and less commonly certain immunologic disorders. Thymic enlargement could represent (1) normal large thymus, (2) thymic hyperplasia, or (3) neoplastic thymic change; ultrasound and other imaging methods may not distinguish between them. Hodgkin's lymphoma is the main differential diagnosis of thymic mass on the chest x-ray; both present with "mediastinal widening," and both can be partly cystic sometimes and grow to considerable size.

Other anterior mediastinal masses include

1. *Teratomas,* also known as *dermoid tumors,* which may contain hair, teeth, or cartilage; a common location is anterior to the base of the heart.
2. *Anterior mediastinal hematoma,* resulting from chest trauma or diagnostic sternal bone marrow puncture; spontaneous hematoma following internal mammary vein rupture is known, especially in patients on chronic hemodialysis.
3. *Anterior mediastinal infection,* complicating sternum-splitting cardiac surgery.
4. *Paragangliomas,* more common in the posterior mediastinum, can also occur anterior to pulmonary trunk or aortic arch.

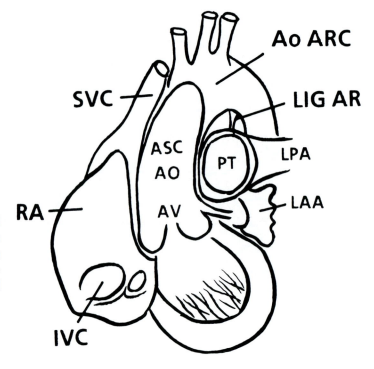

Figure 3–8. Coronal section through the heart and great vessels to show relationship of the right atrium (RA), ascending aorta (ASC Ao), aortic arch (AoARC), ligamentum arteriosum (LIG ART), pulmonary trunk (PT), left pulmonary artery (LPA), and left atrial appendage (LAA).

CORONAL SECTION THROUGH HEART

Aortic-Pulmonary Window

This refers to the mediastinal region just below the concavity of the aortic arch and must not be confused with the uncommon congenital shunt defect between the two great vessels. Parkinson and Bedford[8] called attention to this anatomic area limited by the aortic arch above and the left atrium below. Heitzman et al.[9] also studied the topic but considered the left pulmonary artery its lower boundary. The aortic-pulmonary window is bounded laterally by the mediastinal pleura, medially by the trachea and left bronchus, and posteriorly by esophagus and descending aorta. This aortic-pulmonary space contains lymph nodes, the left recurrent laryngeal nerve, the ligamentum arteriosum, the left bronchial arteries, and fat.

The relevance of this window to echocardiographers is that it can be visualized under the sonolucency of the aortic arch from the suprasternal window. Transesophageal echocardiography (TEE) can provide an even more detailed view of diagnostic value in masses in this location. These masses include (1) lymph nodes inferior to the tracheal bifurcation (subcarinal), most commonly from bronchogenic carcinoma spread, which form a solid lobulated mass, (2) bronchogenic cyst, also commonly subcarinal, which is a smooth, spherical or oval, fluid-containing benign structure, and (3) large intrapericardial space-occupying lesions, including giant left atrial dilatation and large posterior loculated pericardial effusions, which are discussed elsewhere.

POSTERIOR MEDIASTINAL MASSES

The posterior mediastinum is bounded anteriorly by the pericardium below and the trachea above, laterally by the right and left mediastinal pleura, and posteriorly by the vertebral column and adjacent ribs, the latter covered anteriorly by prespinal ligaments and muscles.

The main contents of the posterior mediastinum are two vertical tubes, the esophagus and descending thoracic aorta (DTA). Neural components of this space are the sympathetic trunk with ganglia and intercostal nerves. Prespinal fatty tissue and lymph nodes (mostly paraesophageal) are other normal components.

Abnormal posterior mediastinal masses include *aneurysmal dilatation of the descending thoracic aorta* and *traumatic rupture of the descending thoracic aorta*. Aneurysmal dilatation of the DTA usually results from aortic dissection and is discussed in Chapter 20. Large saccular aortic aneurysms due to syphilitic aortitis were common decades ago but are now rare. Because of aortic-esophageal proximity all through the thorax, TEE provides exquisite visualization of DTA pathology, especially of an intimal flap, and colorflow Doppler depicts true and false lumen flow in aortic dissection.

Traumatic rupture of the DTA is an important fatal complication of traffic accidents. In 95% of cases, the site of rupture is the junction of the aortic arch and the DTA, presumably due to whipping motion of the more mobile anterior aortic arch placing inordinate stress on the aorta where it joins the more fixed DTA. Complete aortic rupture results, of course, in immediate death, as do most instances of partial rupture, but 10% to 20% are said to survive more than 1 hour, i.e., long enough to receive clinical or radiologic evaluation, and thus may be examined by the echocardiographer in such emergent circumstances. A large posterior mediastinal hematoma (pseudoaneurysm) surrounds the ruptured DTA and may even be associated with longer survival if the tear is quite small. In a very small percentage, a traumatic aortic aneurysm is the eventual sequel.

Spontaneous rupture of the esophagus (Boerhaave's syndrome) is another emergency associated with a posterior mediastinal mass. It follows violent retching and vomiting.

Neurogenic tumors are the most common form of neoplastic masses in the posterior thorax. They arise from spinal nerve roots, intercostal nerves, or the sympathetic chain of ganglia. Histologically, the tumors are neurofibromas, neurilemmomas, ganglioneuromas, or more undifferentiated "blast" varieties of these neoplasms. They are round or oval in shape.

Other paraspinal masses include lymphomas, metastatic carcinoma, abscesses tracking downward from cervical or vertebral sources, mediastinal varices, dilated azygos or hemiazygos veins, and extramedullary hematopoietic tissue. The latter is associated with certain hemolytic anemias or bone diseases preventing normal bone marrow erythropoiesis.

All the various types of posterior mediastinal masses mentioned above have been well documented in the radiologic and CT literature but not in the echocardiographic literature (except for dissecting aneurysms). However, there remains one group of posterior mediastinal masses that are important to echocardiographers because they encroach on the left atrium posteriorly.[10] They include (1) esophageal neoplasms, (2) diaphragmatic hernias through the esophageal hiatus (such hiatus hernias involve migration of part of the stomach into the lower thorax), (3) surgical anastomosis of the stomach to the esophageal stump after resection of esophageal cancer, producing another variety of intrathoracic stomach, and (4) megaesophagus due to achalasia of the cardiac sphincter.

RECOGNITION OF MEDIASTINAL MASSES BY 2D ECHOCARDIOGRAPHY

A few studies have surveyed the ability of 2D echocardiography (2D echo) to recognize the presence of mediastinal masses in relatively large series of patients. Mancuso et al.[11] compared the sensitivity and specificity of transthoracic echocardiography (TTE) with that of chest radiography in 50 patients, 33 of whom showed mediastinal masses on CT. They found similar specificity (94%), but TTE had higher specificity (91% versus 61%) than chest x-ray.

In another more recent Italian study, Faletra et al.[12] compared the TTE with transesophageal echocardiography (TEE) in 30 patients with mediastinal masses; the diagnosis was confirmed by surgery, histology, and CT in virtually all cases. TEE was found to be more accurate than TTE in detecting the mediastinal mass (90% versus 73%). TEE was superior to TTE also in identifying the structure of the mass, i.e., solid versus cystic (100% versus 90%), and the relationship of the mass to contiguous structures (89% versus 81%). These authors pointed out an important advantage of 2D echo over CT: Motion or slight spatial displacement of the mass with reference to contiguous structures, due to cardiac pulsations or respiratory fluctuation, is usually detectable on careful scrutiny of the 2D echocardiogram. Faletra et al.[12] found that such mobility of the mediastinal mass in relation to neighboring structures was always absent if an invasive neoplastic mass had infiltrated these adjacent structures.

The Mayo Clinic group[13] reported their TEE experience in 83 patients with "cardiac mass lesions," either intra- or extracardiac. In 12 patients the mass was extracardiac; in 6 of them the mass was clearly detected by TTE. Five of the 12 patients appear to have had encroachment or compression of cardiac structures by the solid mediastinal mass; in one it encircled the left upper pulmonary vein and descending aorta, in another the left upper pulmonary vein and right pulmonary artery, in a third the left atrium, in the fourth there was extreme compression of the superior vena cava and right atrium.

These three reports[11-13] have provided valuable data for cardiologists and radiologists interested in the practice of noninvasive mediastinal imaging. However, with very few exceptions, hemodynamic or clinical evidence of actual cardiac compression was not reported.

On the basis of anatomic location and cardiac structure compressed, these mediastinal masses can be conveniently classified into the following groups:

1. *Anterior mediastinal,* compressing right-sided heart chambers
2. *Posterior mediastinal,* compressing left atrium and/or left ventricle
3. *Masses compressing large veins,* such as superior mediastinal ones compressing the superior vena cava or juxtahilar ones compressing pulmonary veins entering the left atrium
4. *Combinations* of the first three varieties or of one of them with a large pericardial effusion and tamponade.

ANTERIOR CARDIAC COMPRESSION (Figures 3–9 and 3–10)

In the M-mode era of the 1970s, several case reports appeared in which a large space was detected on echocardiography between the right ventricle and chest wall[14-18] that was either sonolucent (cystic space) or suggestive of a solid tumor mass. In some the mediastinal cyst was so large that not only cardiac compression but gross cardiac displacement rightward was produced.[17,18] In the case of Schloss et al.,[18] the cyst was of thymic origin. The large anterior mediastinal mass in the patient of Gottdiener and Maron[15] was lymphomatous and manifested as a separation between the chest wall and the right ventricular wall of over 5 cm. In the patient of Canedo et al.,[14] a large thymoma produced a tamponade-like presentation. Chandaratna et al.[16] described the M-mode echocardiographic findings of 5 patients with extrinsic cardiac masses. His patient 3 had cardiac compression by a large chest wall sarcoma. In patient 4, a large cystic hematoma complicating anticoagulant therapy compressed the right ventricle and was visualized echocardiographically as a sonolucent anterior space; cardiac catheterization showed elevated diastolic pressures in both the left and right sides of the heart.

Compression of the anterior aspect of the heart by large anterior mediastinal masses was visualized by 2D echo in many instances.[9-22] In the patient of Hsuing et al.,[20] a systolic pressure gradient of 28 mmHg across the right ventricular tract was demonstrated. The tumor was excised and found to be a teratoma. In the patient of Engle et al.,[19] the

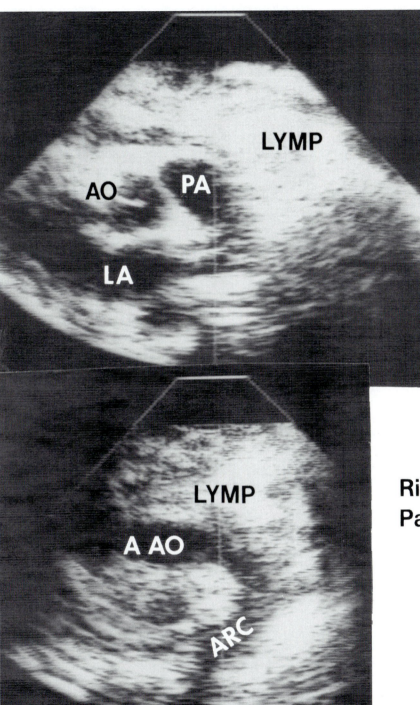

Parasternal
Short-Axis

Right
Parasternal

Figure 3–9. 2D echocardiogram in parasternal short-axis and right parasternal views in a patient with a large anterior mediastinal lymphoma. The lymphoma provides an ultrasound window to depict the ascending aorta and aortic arch.

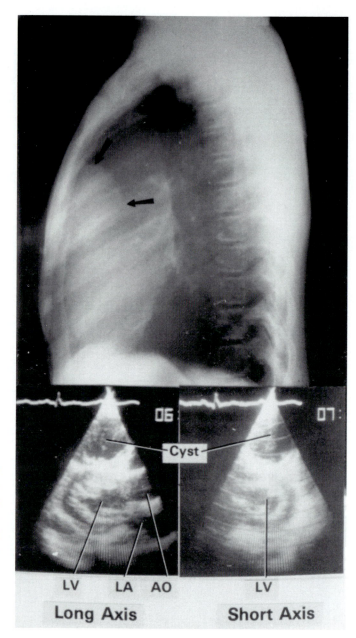

Figure 3–10. (Below) Parasternal long-axis (left) and short-axis views (right) showing a cystic sonolucent mass compressing the RV outflow tract. The lateral chest x-ray (above) shows the round anterior mediastinal mass, which was surgically removed and proved to be a cystic chondroma arising from the fourth left costal cartilage.

right ventricular cavity was almost obliterated by a pericardial cyst containing 400 g of altered blood; decompression of the cyst resulted in a fall in central venous pressure from 19 to 7 mmHg and relief of symptoms (edema, ascites, fatigability) and of hepatomegaly. In the patients of Chopra et al.[21] and Nishimura et al.,[22] the anterior mediastinal mass may not in itself have compressed the heart sufficiently to produce a tamponade-like state. However, in the former case, the mass (a large pericardial cyst) eroded the right ventricular wall myocardium; in the latter case, an invasive thymic tumor not only deformed the right ventricle and pulmonary trunk but invaded the wall and lumen of the latter vessel. Somewhat similar was the case of D'Cruz and Chiemmongkoltip,[23] in which right ventricular outflow was compressed by a rigid cystic chondroma arising from the fourth left costal cartilage.

POSTERIOR CARDIAC COMPRESSION

A few case reports have appeared of a huge posterior mediastinal space-occupying lesion compressing the left atrium or left ventricle or both. The heart as a whole may be compressed between the large posterior mass and the anterior chest wall so that the cardiac catheterization findings may be very similar to circumcardiac tamponade even though the heart is compressed only on its posterior aspect.

Solid posterior mediastinal tumors having such an effect have included a malignant lymphoma reported by Iwase et al.,[24] a liposarcoma reported by Chow et al.,[25] an anaplastic small cell carcinoma reported by Chandaratna et al.,[16] and mediastinal retrocardiac spread of bronchogenic carcinoma described by D'Cruz et al.[26] (Figure 3-11).

Another type of posterior cardiac compression manifesting as "atypical" tamponade is a large posterior high-tension loculated pericardial effusion following cardiac surgery (see Figures 2-26 and 2-28). Although such patients usually present a few weeks after surgery,[27] the effusion occasionally may be chronic. An example of this is patient 1 of Breall et al.,[28] who had hemodynamic signs of tamponade 2 years after coronary bypass surgery that were relieved by drainage of the "pericardial cyst." Dunlap et al.[29] described a somewhat similar situation in a young man who had suffered blunt chest trauma 4 years previously. 2D echo showed a large space posterior and lateral to the left ventricle; cardiac catheterization demonstrated elevated diastolic pressures in both the right and left sides of the heart; at surgery, an 8×10 cm partly organized hematoma was found.

Breall et al.[28] described a very unusual case where an enormous aneurysm of the descending thoracic aorta (15 cm in diameter) caused severe cardiac compression against the anterior chest wall with a tamponade-like situation. Lesser degrees of descending aorta dilatation are common, and sometimes such tortuous ectatic aortas encroach on the posterior aspect of the left atrium, but Doppler observations do not reveal any obstruction to the transit of blood through the atrium.[30]

Yoshikawa et al.[31] were one of the first groups to use 2D echocardiography in the diagnosis of mediastinal masses. They described the ultrasound visualization of a large posterior mediastinal neoplasm (esophageal carcinoma) and pointed out an important feature distinguishing extrinsic from intrinsic left atrial masses: The former may simulate intra-atrial masses when they invaginate the atrial wall but are immobile on real-time viewing, whereas intracardiac masses exhibit phasic motion with every cardiac cycle.

Kinney et al.[32] reported an instance of a posterior mediastinal lymphoma that compressed the left atrium so much that pulsed-wave Doppler of flow within this chamber showed abnormally high velocity (90 cm/s; normal 45 to 63 cm/s).

COMPRESSION OF VENOUS INFLOW TO THE HEART (SVC AND PULMONARY VEINS)

SVC

In adults, the superior vena cava (SVC) and the pulmonary veins are difficult, if not impossible, to visualize by conventional TTE. The SVC can sometimes be imaged from the suprasternal or right supraclavicular window, but even so, the quality of image resolution has been unsatisfactory because of the long distance of this structure from the transducer and beam-width artefact allowing echoes from adjacent structures to partly obscure the SVC lumen. TEE has been successful in obtaining good images not only of the SVC but also of other large venous channels in the mediastinum such as the innominate and azygos veins.[33]

Dawkins et al.[34] used TEE to image SVC compression by a malignant superior mediastinal mass. TEE also demonstrated tumor encasement of the ascending aorta, aortic arch, and right main pulmonary artery in this patient. Colorflow Doppler helped in diagnosing SVC obstruction by showing rapid turbulent flow in the compressed SVC.

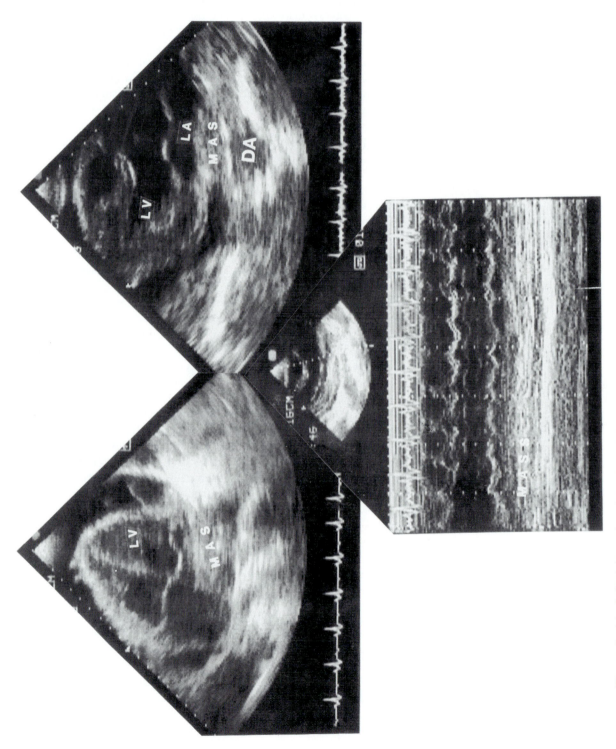

Figure 3–11. Apical four-chamber view (left) and M-mode echo (below) show an apparent left atrial mass. In the parasternal long-axis view (right), the mass is located between left atrium (LA) and descending aorta (DA). The mass (MAS) represented spread from bronchogenic carcinoma.

Pulmonary Veins

The openings of the right upper pulmonary vein and the left pulmonary veins into the left atrium often can be visualized in the apical four-chamber view. However, the veins themselves cannot be imaged adequately by conventional TTE. It has been shown by Pinherio et al.[35] that TEE in the colorflow Doppler mode can achieve excellent imaging of all four pulmonary veins.

Ren et al.[36] recently used TEE to demonstrate compression of the right upper pulmonary vein by neoplastic mediastinal masses in four patients. Obstruction of the pulmonary vein was diagnosed on the basis of (1) reduction in caliber of the vein as compared with normal values and (2) Doppler manifestations, such as increased velocity of flow in the vein by pulsed-wave Doppler. The latter velocities fell from (mean) 95 to 46 cm/s (systole) and from 62 to 39 cm/s (diastole) after chemotherapy or radiotherapy. In contrast, Doppler velocities in the unobstructed left upper pulmonary vein remained unchanged before and after therapy.

GASTROESOPHAGEAL MEDIASTINAL "MASSES" (Figures 3–12 to 3–18)

Although quite common, posterior mediastinal masses associated with abnormal intrathoracic migration of the stomach (or more rarely other abdominal contents) or with esophageal neoplasms or dilatation have received little attention in the cardiology or echocardiography literature.

The Mayo Clinic group[37] in 1985 reported 5 patients with hiatus hernia in whom the retrocardiac stomach impinged on the left atrium and simulated a left atrial mass when this chamber was imaged in a posterior atrial plane. Subsequently, only a very few additional reports have appeared.[38,39] The 2D echo features (see Figures 3–12 to 3–14) include a large, ill-defined mass posterior to the left atrium in long-axis views. Sometimes this mass, representing the diaphragmatic hernia, extends behind the left atrioventricular junction or even the basal left ventricular posterior wall. In the apical four-chamber view, the mass is seen lateral to the left atrium, encroaching on it to a variable degree when the posterior left atrium is imaged, but not in an anterior left atrial plane. Occasionally, the mass encroaches also on the right atrium posteriorly.[37,39] The mass sometimes appears "fixed"; its lack of mobility or participation in atrial wall motion helps to distinguish it from intraatrial masses such as myxomas or thrombi. If the patient ingests fluids, especially bubble-forming "pop" drinks, a swirling motion of the stomach contents may be observed within the posterior mediastinal mass.

I have encountered over a score of patients with the preceding echocardiographic findings over the last 3 years;[39a] the hiatus hernia, of sliding type, had been documented by upper gastrointestinal contrast studies (see Figure 3–15). In one case the diaphragmatic hernia was paraesophageal rather than sliding; in this variety, the contents of the intrathoracic hernial sac can include intraperitoneal structures such as bowel, omentum, and spleen. In this patient, the presence of a retrocardiac spleen could be demonstrated by a typical notched contour of a solid structure within the diaphragmatic hernia in the CT image and also identification of splenic tissue by radionuclide uptake study.[39] Rarely, the hiatus hernia may be huge, impinging on the entire length of the left atrium and ventricle posterolaterally (see Figure 3–4).

Another form of retrocardiac esophageal mass is carcinoma of the lower esophagus. On 2D echo such a neoplasm appears as a solid mass posterior to and often encroaching on the left atrium; its location is very typical (see Figure 3–16), between the sonolucencies of the left atrial chamber and the descending thoracic aorta.[40]

In contrast to hiatus hernia, the esophageal mass is sharply defined and relatively small (less than 5 cm in diameter) (see Figure 3–17). However, if the malignancy has been invasive enough to spread beyond the esophageal wall into the surrounding posterior mediastinum, the mass may be larger, not sharply demarcated from adjacent structures, and associated with pleural or pericardial effusions.

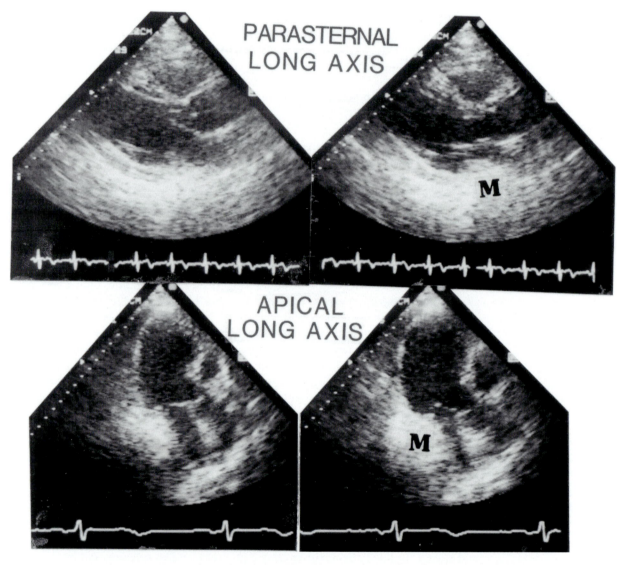

Figure 3–12. Parasternal long-axis view (above) and apical long-axis view (below) showing an ill-defined mass (M) posterior to the left atrioventricular junction. The degree to which the hiatal hernia mass encroaches on the left atrium varies phasically with respiration (more in the right than in the left frame).

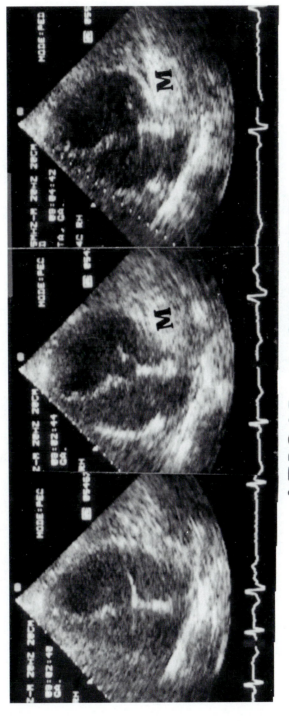

APICAL 4-CHAMBER

Figure 3–13. Apical four-chamber view in successively posterior planes showing normal appearance in an anterior plane (left); then an ill-defined mass (M) "appears" in the lateral left atrium (center) and seems to fill the chamber completely in the posterior plane (right). The mass was extrinsic to the heart, due to a hiatus hernia.

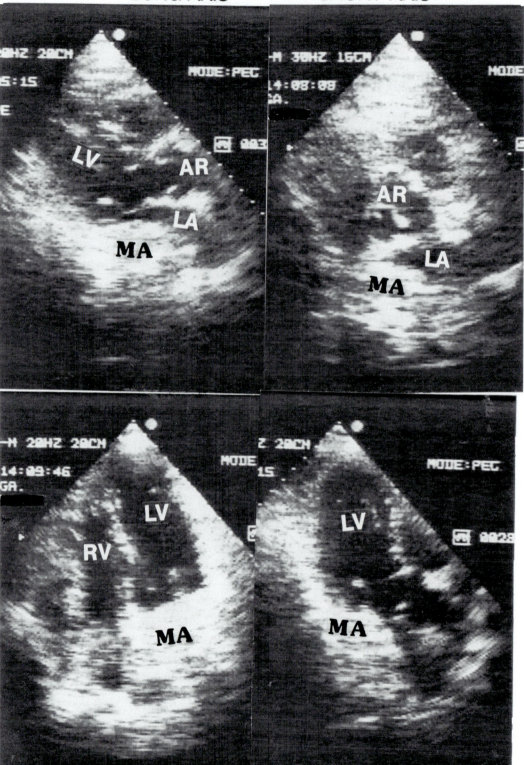

APICAL

Figure 3–14. Parasternal long and short-axis views (above) and apical four-chamber and long-axis views (below) in a patient with echodense-mass (MA) caused by hiatus hernia which encroaches not only on LA but also basal LV.

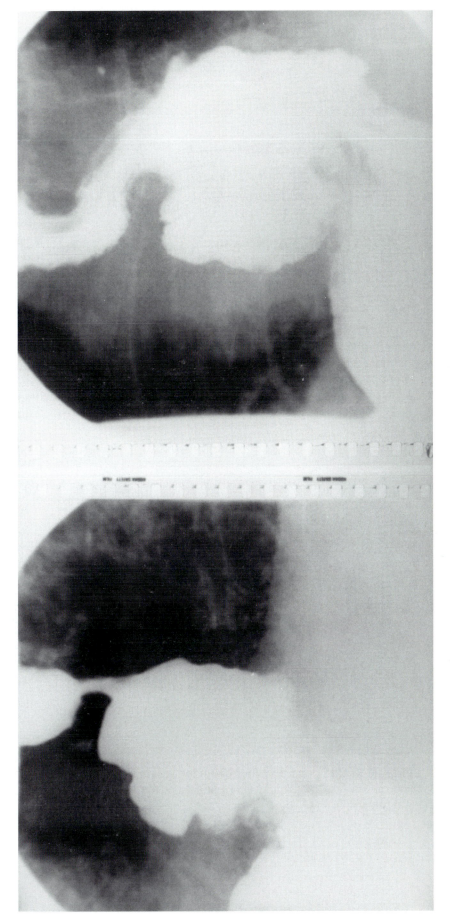

Figure 3–15. Barium opacification of the esophagus and stomach in a patient with hiatus hernia showing that the stomach is partly in the thorax behind the heart.

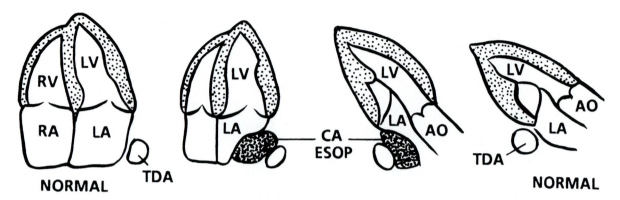

Figure 3–16. Diagram of apical four-chamber view in normals (extreme left) and in patient with esophageal carcinoma (center, left); apical long-axis view in normals (extreme right) and in patient with esophageal carcinoma (center, right). The esophageal mass (dark shading) manifests as a dense solid echo mass (CA-ESOP) intervening between the left atrium and descending aorta.

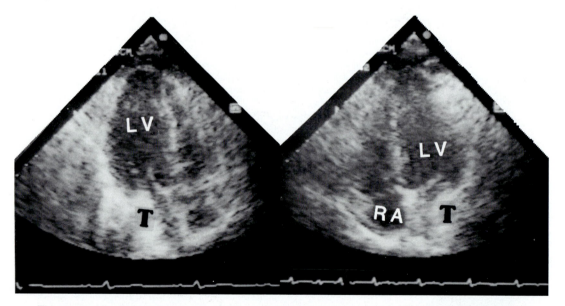

Figure 3–17. Apical long-axis (left) and four-chamber views (right) showing a solid mass encroaching on the posterior and lateral aspects of the left atrium. It proved to be an esophageal tumor (T).

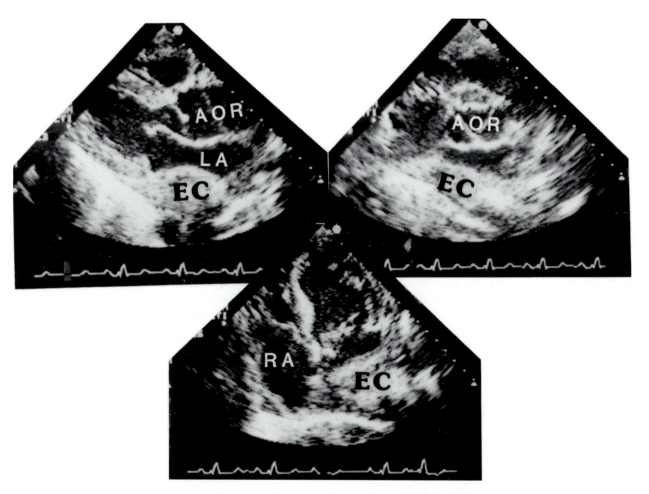

Figure 3–18. Parasternal long-axis and short-axis views (above) and apical four-chamber view (below) showing esophageal carcinoma (EC) as a solid mass posterior to the left atrium (above). In the apical four-chamber view the esophageal mass encroaches conspicuously on the LA, severely distorting the latter.

An isolated case report of massive esophageal dilatation due to achalasia of the cardiac sphincter has appeared.[41] Yet another type of intrathoracic gastric "mass" is that produced by the surgeon when the stomach is pulled up into the thorax to anastomose to the esophageal stump after resection of esophageal cancer. The echocardiographic appearances resemble those of a hiatus hernia, and like the latter, a large retrocardiac fluid level may be visible on the chest x-ray.

Although these retrocardiac gastroesophageal "masses" are often large, they rarely cause symptoms. I have encountered an exceptional patient who had syncopal episodes and another in whom dilatation of the intrathoracic stomach was associated with respiratory distress, but even then a causal relationship between the gastric mass and possible hemodynamic effects of cardiac compression was not conclusive.

REFERENCES

1. Genereux GP. The posterior pleural reflections. AJR 1983;141:141.
2. Holt JF. Epipericardial fat shadows in differential diagnosis. Radiology 1947;48:472.
3. Cohen SL. The right pericardial fat pad. Radiology 1953;60:391.

4. Rogers JV, Leigh TF. Differential diagnosis of right cardiophrenic angle masses. Radiology 1953;61:871.

5. Torrance DJ. Demonstration of subepicardial fat as an aid in diagnosis of pericardial effusion or thickening. AJR 1955;74:850.

6. Beck E, Beattie EJ. The lymph nodes in the mediastinum. J Int Coll Surg 1958;29:247.

7. Baven RL, Lee JKT, Sagel SS, et al. Computed tomography of the normal thymus. Radiology 1982;142:121.

8. Parkinson J, Bedford DE. The aortic triangle—A radiological landmark in the left oblique projection. Lancet 1936;2:909.

9. Heitzman ER, Lane EJ, Hammack DB, et al. Radiological evaluation of the aortic-pulmonary window. Radiology 1975;116:513.

10. D'Cruz IA, Feghali N, Gross CM. Echocardiographic manifestations of mediastinal masses compressing or encroaching on the heart. Echocardiography 1994;11:523.

11. Mancuso L, Pitrolo F, Bondi F, et al. Echocardiographic recognition of mediastinal masses. Chest 1988;93:144.

12. Faletra F, Ravini M, Moreo A, et al. Transesophageal echocardiography in the evaluation of mediastinal masses. J Am Soc Echocardiogr 1992;5:178.

13. Reeder GS, Khanderia BK, Seward JB, et al. Transesophageal echocardiography and cardiac masses. Mayo Clin Proc 1991;66:1101.

14. Canedo MI, Otken L, Stefadouros MA. Echocardiographic features of cardiac compression by a thymoma simulating cardiac tamponade and obstruction of the superior vena cava. Br Heart J 1977;39:1038.

15. Gottdiener JS, Maron BJ. Posterior cardiac displacement by anterior mediastinal tumor. Chest 1980;77:784.

16. Chandaratna PAN, Littman BB, Serafini A, et al. Echocardiographic evaluation of extracardiac masses. Br Heart J 1978;40:741.

17. Koch PC, Kronzon I, Winer HE, et al. Displacement of the heart by a giant mediastinal cyst. Am J Cardiol 1977;40:445.

18. Schloss M, Kronzon I, Geller PM, et al. Cystic thymoma simulating constrictive pericarditis. J Thorac Cardiovasc Surg 1975;70:143.

19. Engle DE, Tresch DD, Bonchek LI, et al. Misdiagnosis of pericardial cyst by echocardiography and computed tomography scanning. Arch Intern Med 1983;143:351.

20. Hsiung MC, Chen CC, Wang DJ, et al. Two-dimensional echocardiographic diagnosis of acquired right ventricular outflow obstruction due to external cardiac compression. Am J Cardiol 1984;53:973.

21. Chopra DS, Duke DJ, Pellet JR, et al. Pericardial cyst with partial erosion of the right ventricular wall. Ann Thorac Surg 1991;51:840.

22. Nishimura T, Kondo M, Miyazaki S, et al. Two-dimensional echocardiographic findings of cardiovascular involvement by invasive thymoma. Chest 1982;81:752.

23. D'Cruz IA, Chiemmongkoltip P. Echocardiographic diagnosis of an unusual anterior mediastinal mass. Clin Cardiol 1982;5:464.

24. Iwase M, Nagura E, Miyahara T, et al. Malignant lymphoma compressing the heart and causing acute left-sided heart failure. Am Heart J 1990;199:968.

25. Chow W-H, Chow T-C, Cheung H, et al. Mediastinal liposarcoma causing left ventricular inflow tract obstruction. Echocardiography 1993;10:141.

26. D'Cruz IA, Hoffman PK, Ewald FW. Echocardiography of posterior mediastinal masses encroaching on the left atrium. Echocardiography 1989;6:485.

27. D'Cruz IA, Kensey K, Campbell C, et al. Two-dimensional echocardiography in cardiac tamponade occurring after cardiac surgery. J Am Coll Cardiol 1985;5:1250.

28. Breall JA, Goldberger AL, Warren SE, et al. Posterior mediastinal masses: Rare causes of cardiac compression. Am Heart J 1992;126:523.

29. Dunlap TE, Sorkin RP, Mori KW, et al. Massive organized intrapericardial hematoma mimicking constrictive pericarditis. Am Heart J 1982;104:1373.

30. D'Cruz IA, Callaghan WE. Imaging of the aorta: II. Doppler and two-dimensional echocardiography of descending thoracic aortic abnormalities. Am J Cardiac Imaging 1987;1:331.

31. Yoshikawa J, Sabah I, Yanagihara K, et al. Cross-sectional echocardiographic diagnosis of large left atrium tumor and extracardiac tumor compressing the left atrium. Am J Cardiol 1978;42:853.

32. Kinney EC, Cotler RP, Sequeira RF, et al. Detection of posterior mediastinal lymphoma by pulsed Doppler echocardiography. Am Heart J 1984;108:365.

33. Nanda NC, Pinheiro L, Sanyal R, et al. Transesophageal echocardiographic of left sided superior vena cava and azygos and hemiazygos veins. Echocardiography 1991;8:731.

34. Dawkins PR, Stoddard MF, Liddell NE, et al. Utility of transesophageal echocardiography in the assessment of mediastinal masses and superior vena caval obstruction. Am Heart J 1991;122:1469.

35. Pinheiro L, Nanda NC, Jain H, et al. Transesophageal echocardiographic imaging of the pulmonary veins. Echocardiography 1991;8:741.

36. Ren WD, Nicholisi GL, Lestuzzi C, et al. Role of transesophageal echocardiography in evaluation of pulmonary venous obstruction by paracardiac neoplastic masses. Am J Cardiol 1992;70:1362.

37. Nishimura RA, Tajik AJ, Schattenberg TT, et al. Diaphragmatic hernia mimicking an atrial mass: A two-dimensional echocardiographic pitfall. J Am Coll Cardiol 1985;5:992.

38. Baerman JM, Hogan L, Swiryn S. Diaphragmatic hernia producing symptoms and signs of a left atrial mass. Am Heart J 1988;116:198.

39. Battu P, D'Cruz IA, Holman M, et al. Noninvasive imaging of a retrograde spleen: Unusual component of paraesophageal diaphragmatic hernia. Chest 1992;101:1159.

39a. D'Cruz IA, Hancock HL. Echocardiographic charactertics of diaphragmatic hiatus hernia. Am J Cardiol 1995;75:308.

40. D'Cruz IA, Holman M, Battu P. Echocardiographic manifestations of esophageal carcinoma. Am Heart J 1992;123:1073.

41. Percy RF, Connetta DA, Miller AB. Esophageal compression of the heart presenting as a extracardiac mass on echocardiography. Chest 1984;85:826.

4

Systemic Great Veins

The superior vena cava (SVC), inferior vena cava (IVC), coronary sinus, and an uncommon variant, the left SVC, all have in common that they drain into the right atrium. They also all develop from the embryonic sinus venosus and ducts of Cuvier. The sinus venosus forms the most caudal part of the primitive cardiac tube and eventually gets absorbed into the right atrium (of the fully developed heart), of which it forms the posterior half. In this process of assimilation, the sinus venosus brings into the right atrium not only the orifices of the SVC, IVC, and coronary sinus but also such vestigal remnants as the eustachian and thebesian valves and the Chiari network.

The anatomy of the systemic great veins entering the heart is therefore intimately related to that of the adult right atrial chamber. Moreover, variants and anomalies of these structures have their origin in aberrant growth of the sinus venosus in early embryonic life.

SUPERIOR VENA CAVA

The superior vena cava (SVC) is a straight tube about 7 cm long formed by the confluence of the right and left innominate (brachiocephalic) veins. It runs vertically downward from the level of the first costal cartilage to the level of the third costal cartilage, behind the right sternal border, to enter the right atrium. There are no valves within the SVC. The upper half of this vessel is extrapericardial; the lower half is intrapericardial. Fortunately, SVC flow is approximately parallel to transducer direction from the supraster-

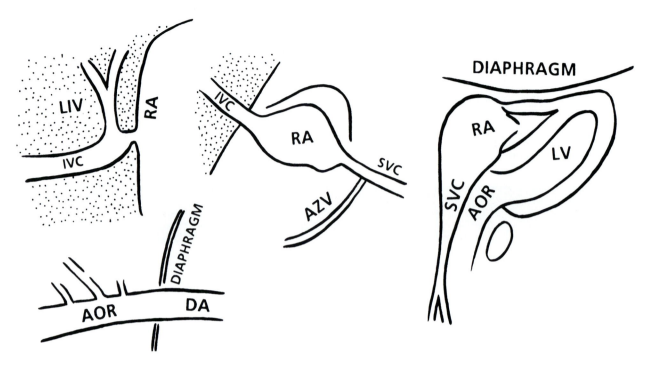

Figure 4–1. Diagram showing venae cavae in various subcostal planes. (Above, left) Sagittal plane showing IVC entering right atrium. (Below, left) Similar though slightly leftward plane showing descending aorta. Note morphologic differences between it and the IVC. (Center) Plane showing IVC, right atrium, and SVC; the azygos vein entering the mid-SVC also may be seen in this plane. (Right) Near-coronal plane showing SVC and right atrium.

nal or right supraclavicular window, facilitating Doppler interrogation of flow patterns in the SVC.

Of the external anatomic relationships of the SVC, two are of importance to the echocardiographer:

1. The *ascending aorta* is closely related to it medially, and both vessels are at this level roughly parallel. Doppler interrogation from suprasternal or right supraclavicular sites therefore detects aortic and SVC flow in close proximity to each other.
2. The *hilum of the right lung* is posterior to the SVC so that hilar neoplastic or lymph node masses can compress or distort the vessel.[1]

Echocardiography of the SVC

The best window for ultrasound visualization of the SVC is the *subcostal*, through the left lobe of the liver. The vessel can be identified by its vertical course and entry into the right atrium (Figures 4-1 to 4-5). Color Doppler imaging or pulse-wave Doppler recording of the typical pattern of caval flow serves to further confirm the identity of the SVC. In some subjects it is possible to image the right atrium with the entry of both the IVC and the SVC.

The SVC is visualized as a narrow tubular sonolucent space, narrowing even further during inspiration. In severe chronic right-sided heart failure, caval dilatation renders SVC caliber obviously wider. A catheter or pacemaker wire within the SVC manifests as a conspicuous intraluminal linear echo. Thrombus in the SVC propagating downstream from an indwelling catheter (perhaps infected) may be detectable,[1-4] especially if it protrudes into the right atrial chamber.

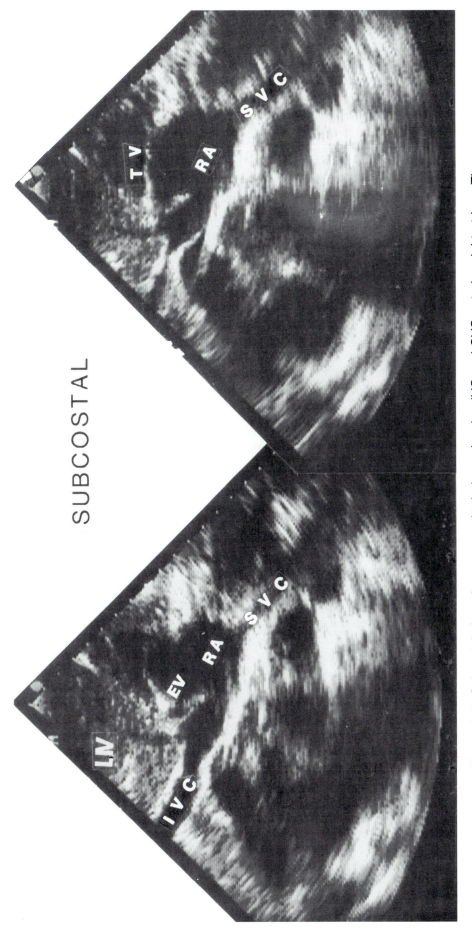

SUBCOSTAL

Figure 4–2. Subcostal views in a parasagittal plane showing IVC and SVC entering right atrium. The eustachian valve (EV) and tricuspid valve (TV) are also seen.

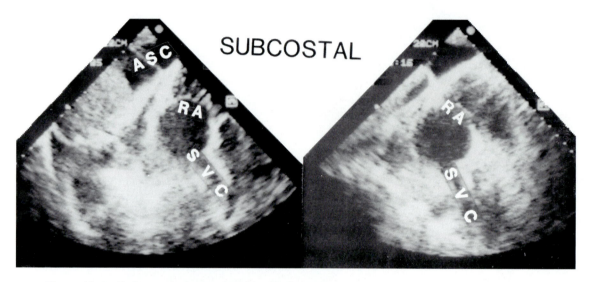

Figure 4–3. Subcostal views showing SVC entering right atrium. A small sonolucent space representing ascites is seen "anterior" to the heart below the diaphragm.

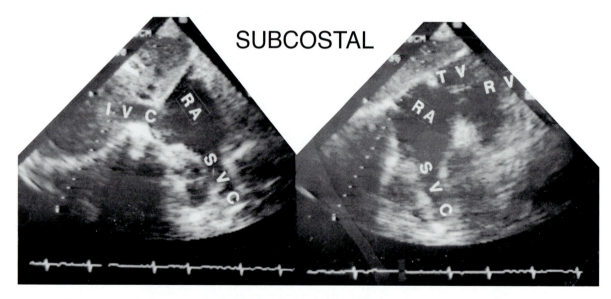

Figure 4–4. Subcostal views showing (left) IVC; at right, IVC is not in view, but the tricuspid valve (TV) is seen, leading into the right ventricle (RV).

SUBCOSTAL

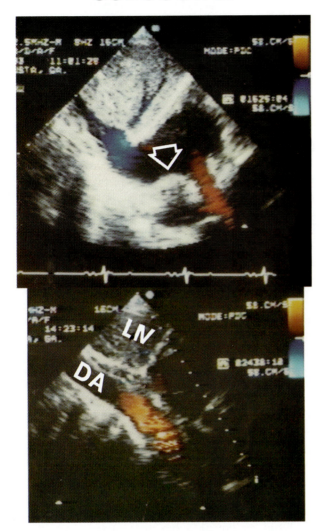

Figure 4–5. (Above) Subcostal view in a plane that includes both the IVC and the SVC with colorflow Doppler demonstrating antegrade flow (blue for IVC, red for SVC). A rounded prominence of the right atrial (RA) posterior wall is a normal variant called the tuber or tubercle of Lower (arrow). (Below) Subcostal view showing descending aorta (DA) passing through diaphragm to become abdominal aorta. Colorflow Doppler shows bright red antegrade aortic flow (LIV, liver).

The *azygos vein* is the only large vein entering the SVC, which it does posteriorly at about the junction of the upper and lower halves of the SVC. This vessel has hitherto been ignored by echocardiographers, but now that it can be identified by transesophageal echocardiographic examination (TEE),[5] its anatomic location becomes relevant because it needs to be differentiated from pulmonary veins and other posterior mediastinal vessels.

It must be admitted that the SVC received little attention from echocardiographers until recently. However, the recognition of diagnostically useful Doppler abnormalities of caval flow in tricuspid regurgitation and in tamponade or pericardial constriction has stimulated the addition of the SVC to the list of cardiac structures interrogated on routine examination. Another reason for gaining expertise in SVC visualization is the uncommon situation where intraluminal pathology or obstruction of this vessel is suspected on clinical grounds.

TEE has made good visualization of the SVC possible. The SVC and ascending aorta are seen as sonolucent spaces, side by side, anterior to the upper left atrium. Several reports have appeared of imaging of thrombus in the SVC by TEE[1,3,4] or of external SVC compression.[1]

It is difficult, if not impossible, to visualize the SVC by two-dimensional (2D) echo from the suprasternal notch or right supraclavicular region in adults. Sometimes dilatation of the SVC due to chronic right-sided heart failure will permit its visualization from this window (Figure 4-6). However, the small Pedoff transducer, with its greater maneuverability, is usually effective in obtaining Doppler signals of SVC from these sites.[6,7] The SVC and ascending aorta are contiguous, parallel, and vertically aligned, the SVC being immediately to the right of the aorta. Obtaining the typical Doppler flow pattern from one of these two vessels, therefore, makes it easy to locate flow in the other vessel by a slight lateral shift in transducer direction.

Anomalous Drainage of the Right SVC into the Left Atrium

This is an extremely rare congenital anomaly, only 11 instances having been reported until 1991. However, some of these have been adults; it is one of the rare causes of central cyanosis with no cardiac murmur. Injection of saline contrast material into either a right or a left arm vein will result in prompt appearance of contrast in left heart chambers; injection into a femoral vein opacifies only the right side of the heart.[8-10]

INFERIOR VENA CAVA

The inferior vena cava (IVC) is formed at the level of the fifth lumbar vertebra by joining of the right and left common iliac veins. It courses vertically upward, anterior to the spine, and in the upper abdomen occupies a deep groove (or sometimes a tunnel) on the posterior aspect of the liver. The IVC then passes through the central tendinous part of the diaphragm to the right of the midline to enter the right atrium about 2 cm above the diaphragm.

The echocardiographer is concerned with that part of the IVC which lies behind the liver and the short intrathoracic segment between diaphragm and right atrium. The latter consists of an extrapericardial part related to the right pleura and lung and an upper intrapericardial part invested with a reflection of visceral pericardium anteriorly but not posteriorly.

The IVC receives many venous tributaries in the abdomen, but the only ones relevant to echocardiography are the hepatic veins. They comprise (1) a superior group, right, middle, and left from the right, caudate, and left hepatic lobes, respectively, and (2) an inferior group, smaller in size than the superior group and variable in number, which drain the right and caudate lobes. Liver tissue has a typical solid, finely stippled ultrasonic texture, against which the hepatic veins and IVC are clearly seen as sonolucent tubular channels.

The IVC in its thoracic part is very short and receives no venous tributaries. Yet it has important anatomic relations, well seen in the subcostal sagittal view: First, as it ascends through the diaphragm, the IVC sometimes shows a local narrowing or "pinching" effect, which increases as the diaphragm contracts during inspiration. The IVC caliber should not be measured at this site. Second, the short intrathoracic IVC is covered anteriorly by pericardium, while to the right and posteriorly it is in contact with the right pleura. These anatomic relationships may be well depicted when a large pericardial effusion and/or right pleural effusion is present; the IVC and the serous effusions manifest as well-defined sonolucent spaces.

Echocardiography of the IVC

The IVC is imaged most clearly from the *subcostal* view, in a sagittal plane; the transducer is placed on the epigastrium, just below the xiphoid process. Thus the IVC is imaged through the liver and appears as a sonolucent tubular space in or just posterior to the solid, homogeneous ultrasound texture of the liver (Figures 4-1, 4-2, 4-4, 4-5, 4-7, and 4-8).

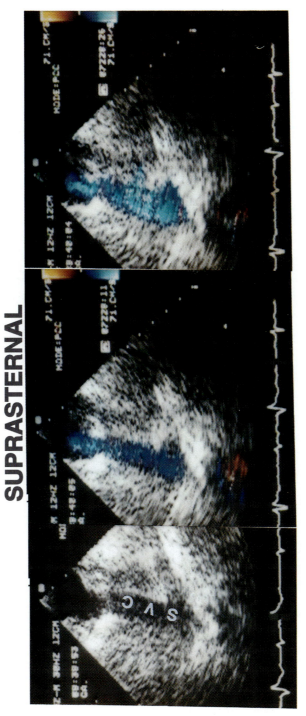

Figure 4–6. Suprasternal view (above medial end of right clavicle) in a patient with severe right-sided heart failure showing a dilated superior vena cava (SVC). Colorflow Doppler (center) demonstrates antegrade SVC flow. In a premature ventricular beat (right), the SVC becomes even more distended.

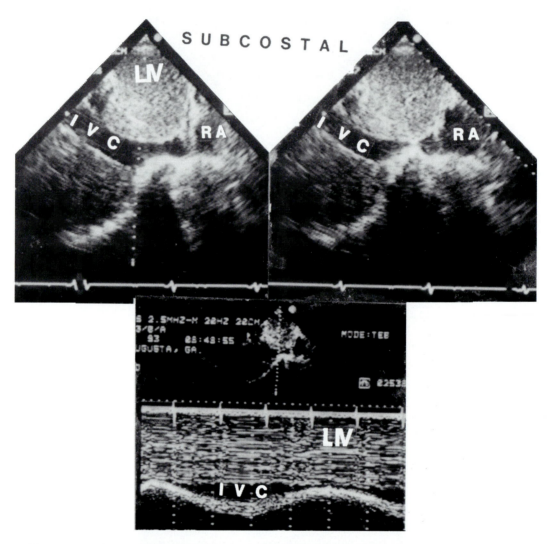

Figure 4–7. Subcostal view showing normal IVC entering the right atrium. During expiration (left), the IVC is wider than during inspiration (right), particularly at the site where it passes through the diaphragm.

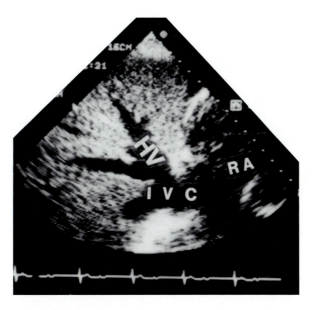

Figure 4–8. Subcostal view showing dilated IVC and hepatic veins in a patient with severe long-standing heart failure.

Another tubular structure in the same general area and nearly parallel to the IVC is the descending abdominal aorta (Figures 4-1 and 4-5). These two large vessels can be differentiated as follows: (1) The IVC ends abruptly by opening into the right atrium, whereas the aorta continues superiorly as the descending thoracic aorta behind the heart, (2) the IVC receives the hepatic veins that course in typical pattern through the liver, whereas the abdominal aorta gives off various anterior branches (celiac, superior, and inferior mesenteric arteries) that are well outside the liver, and (3) the aorta exhibits one strong systolic pulsation with every cardiac cycle, whereas the IVC, by contrast, normally shows two pulsations per heartbeat (corresponding to *a* and *v* waves, which are smaller and "softer" than the aortic systolic expansion).

The IVC also can be visualized in other 2D echo views: the *parasternal short-axis* and the *right heart inflow* views. In both, the IVC is seen to enter the inferior aspect of the right atrium, its recognition facilitated by color Doppler depicting an upward red or orange stream representing IVC flow (Figure 4-9). The eustachian valve, in the anterior rim of the IVC orifice, is a helpful anatomic marker.

The hepatic veins are imaged in about the same plane and from the same epigastric site as the IVC. The right superior hepatic vein is of special interest because its direction is nearly parallel to the ultrasound beam so that flow toward the IVC or away from it (i.e., antegrade or retrograde, respectively) in this vein is easily recorded by pulsed Doppler or colorflow Doppler (Figure 4-10).

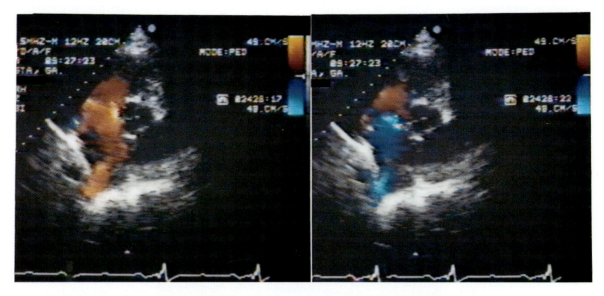

Figure 4–9. Colorflow Doppler in parasternal short-axis view showing antegrade flow through IVC into right atrium (left) and retrograde flow into IVC (right).

SUBCOSTAL

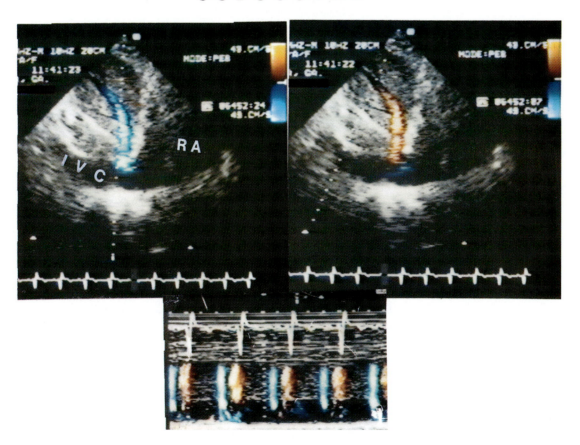

Figure 4–10. Subcostal view showing right superior hepatic vein (HV) opening into IVC. Retrograde flow (blue) in the hepatic vein occurs in early diastole, but retrograde flow (red-orange) occurs in presystole, as seen on colorflow Doppler 2D (above) and M-mode (below).

Reynolds et al.[11] have pointed out that if suitable imaging of the hepatic veins from the epigastrium cannot be obtained, it may be achieved by (1) sliding the transducer rightward along the costal margin as far as the right midclavicular line or, alternatively, (2) with the patient on his or her left side and the transducer in the midaxillary line at the xiphoid level. In both approaches, the liver itself is used as a "window" for ultrasound.

The IVC diameter near its entry into the right atrium ranges from 1.2 to 2.3 cm (mean 1.7 ± 0.3 cm); the hepatic vein caliber ranges from 0.6 to 1.1 cm (mean 0.8 ± 0.2 cm) according to the normal statistics of Weyman.[12]

Normally, the caliber of the IVC undergoes striking phasic fluctuations with respiration, being much narrower (or even completely collapsed) in inspiration than during expiration (Figure 4-10). Himelman et al.[13] use the term *IVC plethora* to refer to cases where the IVC does not narrow to less than 50% of its maximal expiratory diameter. Simonson and Schiller[14] found that the IVC segment between 5 and 30 mm distal (inferior) to the right atrium–IVC junction was more responsive to increased inspiratory pressure change than other parts of the IVC.

Moreno et al.[15] measured IVC caliber in 80 normal subjects "below the level of the hepatic veins and a few centimeters inferior to its junction with the right atrium." IVC diameter was measured in expiration (maximal diameter) and inspiration (minimal diameter). These authors found that the normal IVC diameter was 18.2 mm/m^2 of body surface area (mean) in expiration (range 9 to 28 mm) and 9.2 mm (mean) in inspiration (range 5 to 18 mm). Moreno et al. calculated a *collapsibility index* (inspiratory decrease in IVC diameter) that equaled maximal IVC diameter on expiration minus minimal IVC diameter on inspiration, divided by maximal IVC diameter on expiration, times 100. In their normal subjects, the collapsibility index was mean 55.8% (range 37% to 100%). A low collapsibility index has a similar significance to what Himelman et al.[13] termed *IVC plethora.*

The presence of IVC plethora and dilatation suggests abnormally high central venous pressure. The two abnormalities are usually present concomitantly in patients with right-sided heart failure, severe pulmonary hypertension, constrictive pericarditis, etc., but sometimes IVC dilatation may be found without plethora, and vice versa. Severe tricuspid regurgitation can cause gross IVC dilatation (often without much plethora), presumably because of the effect of massive reflux into the IVC during every systole (Figures 4-11 to 4-13). Moreno et al.[15] found that elevated right atrial pressure correlated much better with IVC collapsibility index than with IVC diameter.

Why does the IVC narrow so much during inspiration under normal conditions? Intrathoracic pressure falls during inspiration, blood flow toward the heart increases, and pressure falls in the IVC during this respiratory phase; the IVC content of blood therefore sharply decreases, and it appears to "collapse." The reverse changes take place in the IVC during expiration: Flow into the right atrium decreases, IVC pressure rises, and the vessel expands in size. It is supposed that when right atrial pressure elevation and pulmonary hypertension exist, normal increase in venous return with inspiration is attenuated so that IVC collapse in inspiration is slight or absent.

Mintz et al.[16] also found that the IVC normally narrows in quiet inspiration to less than 50% of its maximum caliber. They found that the IVC caliber at end-diastole in their normal subjects was 7 ± 3 mm/m^2. They also noted a phasic dilatation of the IVC, in every cardiac cycle, corresponding to *a* and *v* waves. The former did not exceed 125% and the latter 140% of the end-diastolic caliber.[16] In an attempt to correlate IVC diameter with right atrial pressure, these authors found that IVC end-diastolic caliber per square meter of body surface area correlated with mean right atrial pressure ($r = 0.72$). They came up with the following useful statistics: The *a*-wave IVC caliber did not exceed 125% of IVC end-diastolic caliber in any patient with right ventricular end-diastolic pressure less than 10 mmHg; the *v*-wave IVC caliber exceeded 140% of IVC end-diastolic caliber in 75% of severe tricuspid regurgitation; and no inspiratory narrowing of IVC caliber was seen in patients with a right ventricular ejection fraction of less than 25%, as well as in constrictive pericarditis.

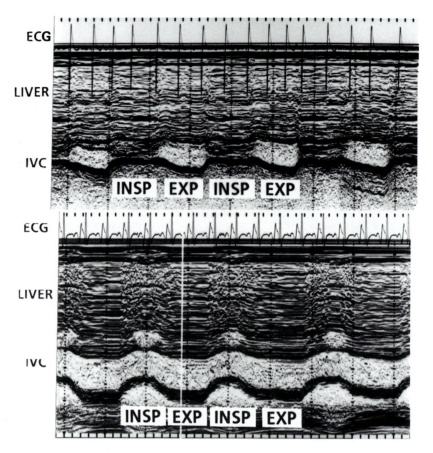

Figure 4–11. M-mode echogram through the liver and IVC in a normal individual (above) and in a patient with high right atrial pressure (below). In normal subjects, the IVC "collapses" in inspiration, but it shows little change in caliber if the central venous pressure is very high.

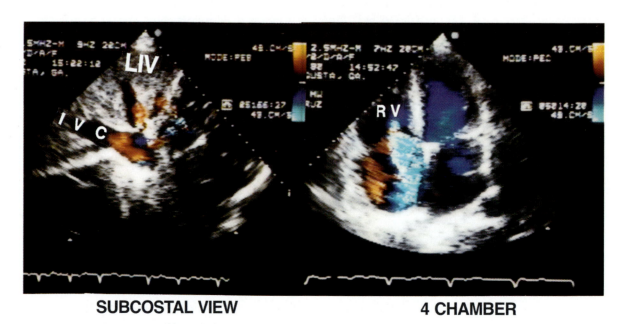

SUBCOSTAL VIEW　　　　　　　**4 CHAMBER**

Figure 4–12. Subcostal view (left) showing retrograde systolic flow in IVC and hepatic veins attributable to 3+ tricuspid regurgitation. The latter is seen as a turquoise jet in the right atrium in the four-chamber apical view (right).

SUBCOSTAL

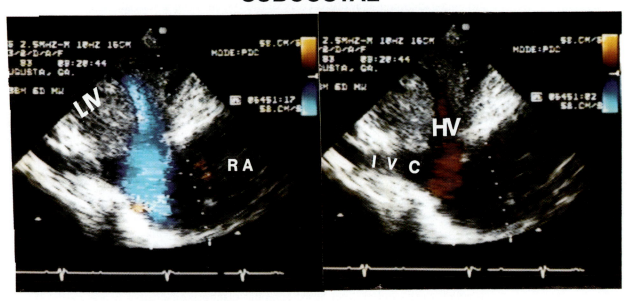

Figure 4–13. Subcostal view showing much dilated IVC and hepatic veins (HV) with antegrade flow in diastole (left) but retrograde flow in systole (right).

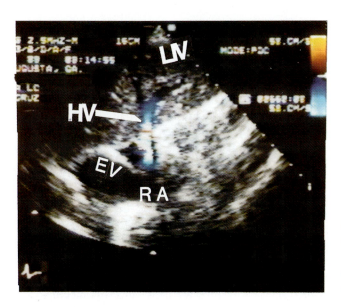

Figure 4–14. Subcostal view showing rare anomaly of drainage of a hepatic vein directly into the right atrium. The eustachian valve (EV) is located between this abnormal orifice and the IVC, which enters the right atrium normally.

Congenital Anomalies

Interruption of the IVC. In this anomaly, the hepatic veins enter the right atrium directly; no connection is seen between the hepatic veins and any vessel in the usual IVC position.[17,18] The IVC is present in the lower abdomen but continues upward as a large posterior venous channel, either the azygos (on the right) or hemiazygos (on the left) vein. The former empties into a right SVC; the latter, into a left SVC. Rarely, a single anomalous hepatic vein can drain into the right atrium directly, with the IVC normal (Figure 4-14).

IVC Draining into the Left Atrium. An extremely rare anomaly causing cyanosis and digital clubbing in adults is entry of the IVC into the left atrial chamber, unassociated with other intracardiac anomalies.[19,20] The atrial septum is intact. It is thought that this "developmental abnormality is confined to the proximal (hepato-cardiac) segment of the IVC, which normally represents the termination of the right vitelline vein."

Tumor Invasion

It is not uncommon for renal cell carcinoma to propagate through the renal vein into the IVC[21-23] (an incidence of 4% to 10%); of these cases, 25% are said to grow upward into the right atrium. Venography has been the method of choice for diagnosing IVC invasion and obstruction. However, the echocardiographer may be required to examine the IVC for tumor invasion in two situations: (1) in patients diagnosed as having renal tumors (carcinoma, Wilm's tumor in children) on clinical/radiologic grounds and (2) in patients with a right atrial mass on echocardiography, to distinguish intrinsic right atrial masses (such as myxoma) from neoplastic masses propagating through the IVC. The latter include not only renal tumors but also pelvic neoplasms such as leiomyomas or leiomyosarcomas. Such neoplasms also can arise from the wall of the IVC itself.

Visualization of normal IVC sonolucency by the subcostal 2D approach excludes gross invasion by tumor, but sometimes the normal IVC is quite narrow or not well visualized, in which case a definite echocardiographic diagnosis of normal versus partial IVC invasion may be difficult. TEE has been used recently to visualize the upper IVC to detect invasion by renal carcinoma.[24] In 3 of 5 patients, the upper level of the intracaval extension was better visualized by TEE than by CT or MRI.

CORONARY SINUS AND LEFT SUPERIOR VENA CAVA

This structure, the main venous channel of the heart, is a short tubular structure 2 to 3 cm long that runs in the coronary sulcus, a groove between the left atrium and ventricle posteriorly. It is a continuation of the great cardiac vein, and it receives several veins draining the ventricles as well as a small (but developmentally important) vein, the oblique vein of the left atrium (of Marshall), which is continuous above with the ligament (of Marshall). This venous remnant persists as a patent vessel in 0.5% of individuals (3% to 10% of those with congenital heart disease) as a left SVC; the latter drains into the right atrium through a dilated coronary sinus.

Echocardiography of the Coronary Sinus

The normal coronary sinus often can be identified as a small sonolucent space at the posterior left atrial-ventricular junction in the parasternal long-axis view (Figures 4-15 and 4-16). When dilated, this sonolucent space is larger and circular or oval in this view, but it is longer and crescentic in short-axis view, posterior to the left atrium (Figure 4-17). Its continuity with the left SVC may be discerned in the same view. As a sonolucent space just behind the left atrium or atrial-ventricular junction, a dilated coronary sinus could be mistaken for a posterior pericardial echo and moves with the neighboring cardiac structures, whereas a descending aorta or pericardial effusion does not participate in cardiac motion.

The coronary sinus can be imaged in a modified four-chamber apical view (Figure 4-18). The transducer is tilted posteriorly from the standard view so as to lose the mitral valve yet keep the right atrium in view. The coronary sinus appears as a transverse sonolucent space 4 to 8 mm in width[25] at the left atrial-ventricular junction opening into the right atrial chamber (see Figure 4-18). The thebesian valve, at the coronary sinus orifice, occasionally may be seen as a small, thin flap. The coronary sinus also may be visualized in a subcostal short-axis view.[26] The contiguous walls of coronary sinus and left atrium appear as a well-defined linear echo between the sonolucencies of these two chambers, and entry of the coronary sinus into the right atrium is also clearly seen.

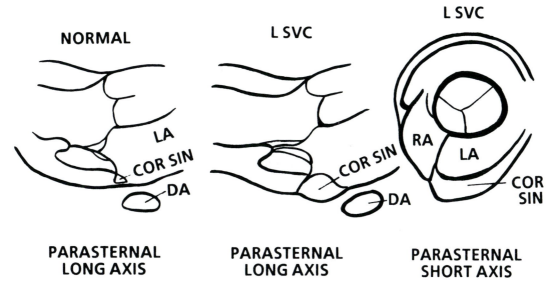

Figure 4–15. (Left) Diagram to show normal appearances of coronary sinus as a small round sonolucency at the junction between the LA and the LV posteriorly. (Center) Same view showing dilated coronary sinus in a patient with persistent left SVC. Note that the descending aorta (DA) is in a more posterior plane. (Right) In short-axis view, the dilated coronary sinus appears as a tubular space posterior to the left atrium and continuous with the left SVC.

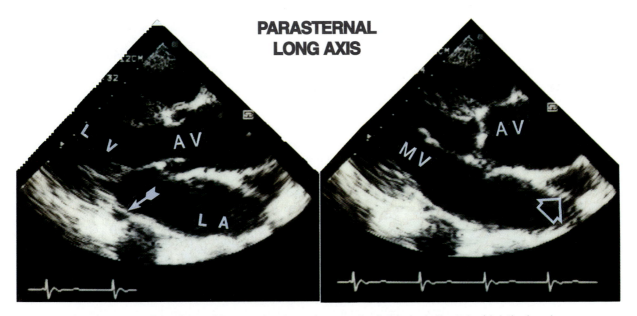

Figure 4–16. Parasternal long-axis views in systole (left) and diastole (right) showing a normal coronary sinus as a small sonolucent space (small thin arrow) and the right pulmonary artery (open arrow) at opposite ends of the left atrium longitudinal section.

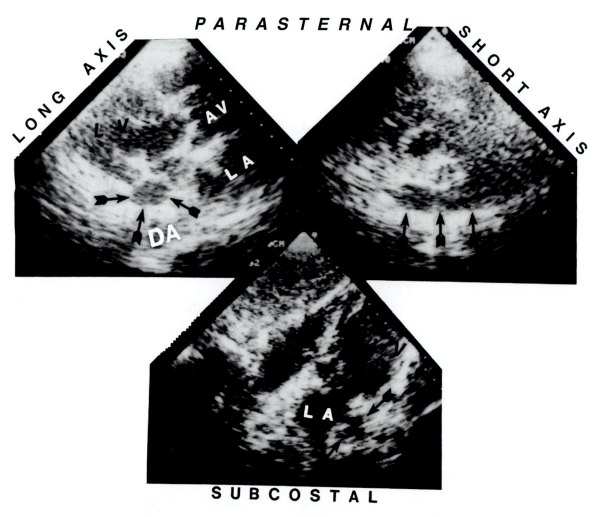

Figure 4–17. Parasternal long- and short-axis views (above) and subcostal view (below) showing dilated coronary sinus (arrows) (AV, aortic valve; LA, left atrium; DA, descending aorta).

The persistent SVC, or bilateral SVC, with or without a bridging transverse vein, may be imaged successfully from the suprasternal notch in children but not usually in adults. Colorflow Doppler reveals an inferior direction of flow in such a left SVC. However, a venous channel in the same general area draining anomalous pulmonary veins into a left SVC or left innominate vein can simulate a left SVC on 2D echo, but flow in it is in a superior direction, i.e., away from the heart, to drain circuitously via the innominate vein and right SVC.

Abnormalities of the coronary sinus are numerous and fascinating. They can be categorized as follows[27]:

1. The most common cause by far of coronary sinus dilatation is persistent left SVC. Several groups have described the echocardiographic findings in children as well as in adults,[28-30] the dilated coronary sinus manifesting as a sonolucent space posterior to the left atrial-ventricular junction in parasternal long- and short-axis views. Cohen et al.[28] showed that injection of saline into a left arm vein selectively opacified the coronary sinus, thus noninvasively identifying not only the anatomic abnormality but also the abnormal flow pattern.

2. Anomalous pulmonary venous drainage into the coronary sinus or left SVC also will manifest with dilated coronary sinus.[27]

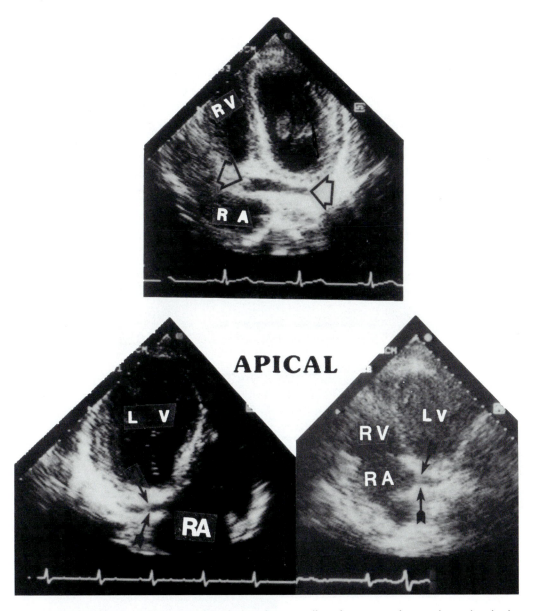

Figure 4–18. (Above) Unconventional view intermediate between short-axis and apical four-chamber view showing coronary sinus (arrows) as a tubular sonolucency. (Below) Apical views in two other patients in a plane such that the coronary sinus (arrows) and its entry into the right atrium are visualized.

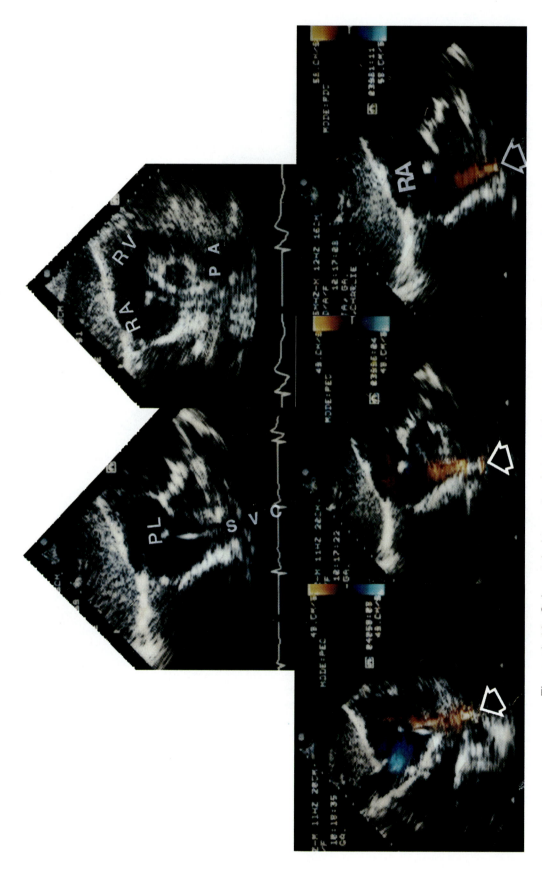

Figure 4–19. Subcostal views showing superior vena cava (SVC) entering the right atrium (RA). A pacemaker lead (PL) is seen in the SVC and RA (above). Colorflow Doppler shows a red-orange stream in the SVC (below).

SUBCOSTAL

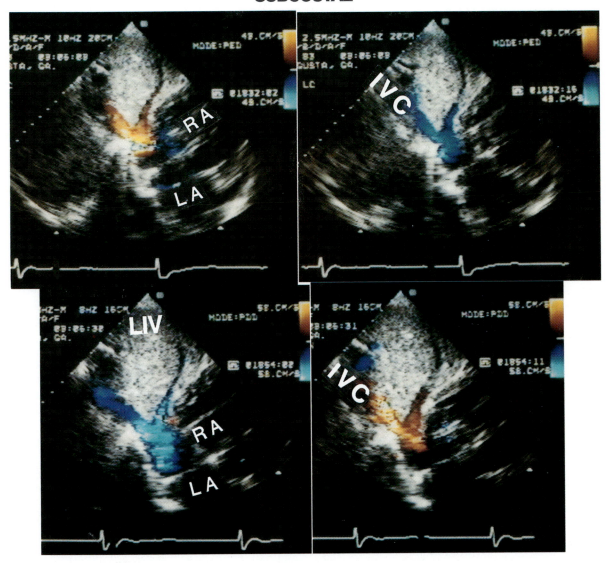

Figure 4–20. Subcostal views in a sagittal plane showing the inferior vena cava (IVC) being joined by the right superior hepatic vein before it enters the right atrium (RA). Colorflow Doppler shows antegrade venous flow in diastole (above, right and below, left) but retrograde flow in systole (above, left and below, right) due to tricuspid regurgitation.

3. Another venous anomaly associated with coronary sinus dilatation is absence of the upper IVC. There is hemiazygos continuation of the IVC that drains into a persistent left SVC and then into the right atrium through the dilated coronary sinus.[34]

4. Other variants with a left SVC include bilateral SVC, with or without a bridging vein; in addition, the right SVC may be atretic, the left SVC and coronary sinus carrying the entire upper body venous flow. In expert hands, all these variations of abnormal venous anatomy can be diagnosed with a very high degree of accuracy, at least in children.[31]

5. Coronary arteriovenous fistulas can result in a large left-to-right shunt. The dilated coronary sinus as well as the dilated artery feeding the fistula may be visualized in suitable imaging planes.

6. Another abnormality is unroofing of the coronary sinus such that it opens directly into the subjacent left atrium through a fenestration of variable size[35-37] (minute to total absence of septation); the anterior wall of the coronary sinus as well as the posterior left atrial wall are defective at this site. A left-to-right shunt at the atrial level results. Unroofing of the coronary sinus can be visualized in apical four-chamber or subcostal short-axis views.[26] In infancy, a coronary sinus–left atrial communication may play a vital compensatory role by providing an alterative route for blood flow in the predicament of mitral or tricuspid atresia with intact atrial septum (sealed foramen ovale).

7. Atresia or severe stenosis of the ostium of the coronary sinus into the right atrium is a rare anomaly. Gerlis et al.[37] described such a case in a 43-year-old woman who died suddenly from myocardial infarction 4 months after angiography had shown normal coronary arteries. These authors reviewed six other previously reported instances.

Raghib et al.[38] in 1965 called attention to a combination of three anomalies: termination of a left SVC into the left atrium, absence of the coronary sinus, and an atrial septal defect in an unusual location—in the posteroinferior corner of the atrial septum, where the coronary sinus orifice normally would be. They postulated that all three abnormalities result from a single embryologic fault—the failure of formation of the left atriovenous fold, a normal fold that develops along the left side of the junction of the sinus venosus with the primitive atrium. The hemodynamic/clinical picture is that of a left-to-right shunt with some oxygen desaturation of arterial blood.

TEE provides excellent imaging of normal as well as dilated coronary sinus; the left SVC also may be well visualized.[40-42] Contrast-enhanced and colorflow Doppler can facilitate identification of these structures. Chaudry and Zabalgoitia[40] have shown that the sequence of opacification on contrast injection is diagnostically helpful. Injection into a right arm vein results in right atrial opacification before coronary sinus opacification, but injection into a left arm vein causes contrast to appear in the coronary sinus before the right atrium, if a left SVC is present.

Colorflow Doppler is very useful in identifying the SVC, IVC, and hepatic veins (Figures 4-19 and 4-20) and in ascertaining direction of flow at different phases of the cardiac cycle; abnormal flow patterns can shed light on pathophysiology (see Figure 4-20).

REFERENCES

(Right) Superior Vena Cava

1. Ayala K, Chandrasekaran K, Karalis DG, et al. Diagnosis of superior vena caval obstruction by transesophageal echocardiography. Chest 1991;101:874.
2. Dick AE, Gross CM, Rubin JW. Echocardiographic detection of an infected superior vena cava thrombus presenting as a right atrial mass. Chest 1989;96:212.
3. Podolsky LA, Manginas A, Jacobs LE, et al. Superior vena caval thrombosis detected by transesophageal echocardiography. J Am Soc Echocardiogr 1991;4:189.

4. Mugge A, Daniel WS, Haver A, et al. Diagnosis of noninfective cardiac mass lesions by two-dimensional echocardiography: Comparison of the transthoracic and transesophageal approaches. Circulation 1991;83:70.

5. Nanda NC, Pinheiro L, Sanyal R, et al. Transesophageal echocardiographic examination of left-sided superior vena cava and azygos and hemiazygos veins. Echocardiography 1991;8:731.

6. Appleton CP, Hatle LK, Popp RL. Superior vena cava and hepatic vein Doppler echocardiography in healthy adults. J Am Coll Cardiol 1987;10:1032.

7. Gindea AJ, Slater J, Kronzon I. Doppler echocardiographic flow velocity measurements in the superior vena cava during the Valsalva maneuver in normal subjects. Am J Cardiol 1990;65:1387.

8. King RE, Plotnick GD. Isolated right superior vena cava into the left atrium detected by contrast echocardiography. Am Heart J 1991;122:583.

9. Park HM, Summerer MH, Preuss K, et al. Anomalous drainage of the right superior vena cava into the left atrium. J Am Coll Cardiol 1983;2:358.

10. Truman JA, Rao PS, Kulangara RJ. Use of contrast echocardiography in anomalous connection of right superior vena cava to left atrium. Br Heart J 1980;44:718.

Inferior Vena Cava

11. Reynolds T, Szymanski K, Langenfeld K, et al. Visualization of the hepatic veins: New approaches for the echocardiographer. J Am Soc Echocardiogr 1991;4:93.

12. Weyman A. Cross-Sectional Echocardiography. Philadelphia: Lea & Febiger, 1982.

13. Himelman RB, Lee E, Schiller NB. Septal bounce, vena cava plethora and pericardial adhesion: Informative two-dimensional echocardiographic signs in the diagnosis of pericardial constriction. J Am Soc Echocardiogr 1988;1:333.

14. Simonson JS, Schiller NB. Sonospirometry: A new method for non-invasive estimation of right atrial pressure based on two-dimensional echographic measurements of the inferior vena cava during measured inspiration. J Am Coll Cardiol 1988;11:557.

15. Moreno FL, Hagan AD, Holmen JR, et al. Evaluation of size and dynamics of the inferior vena cava as a index of right-sided cardiac function. Am J Cardiol 1984;53:579.

16. Mintz GS, Kotler MN, Parry WR, et al. Real-time inferior vena cava ultrasonography: Normal and abnormal findings and its use in assessing right heart function. Circulation 1981;64:1018.

17. Huhta JC, Smallhorn JF, Macartney FJ, et al. Cross-sectional echocardiographic diagnosis of systemic venous return. Br Heart J 1982;48:388.

18. Snider AR, Ports TA, Silverman NH. Venous anomalies of the coronary sinus. Circulation 1979;60:721.

19. Gardner DC, Cole L. Long survival with inferior vena cava draining into left atrium. Br Heart J 1955;17:93.

20. Meadows WR, Bergstrand I, Sharp JT. Isolated anomalous connection of a great vein to left atrium. Circulation 1961;24:669.

21. Ney C. Tumor thrombus of inferior vena cava associated with malignant renal tumors. J Urol 1946;55:583.

22. Svane S. Tumor thrombus of inferior vena cava resulting from renal carcinoma. Scand J Urol Nephrol 1969;3:245.

23. McCullough DL, Talner LB. Inferior vena caval extension of renal carcinoma. AJR 1974;121:819.

24. Treiger BF, Humphrey LS, Peterson CV, et al. Transesophageal echocardiography in renal cell carcinoma: An accurate diagnostic technique for intracaval neoplastic extension. J Urol 1991;145:1138.

Coronary Sinus and Left SVC

25. Andrade J, Somerville J, Corval RO, et al. Echocardiographic routine analysis of the coronary sinus by an apical view: Normal and abnormal features. Texas Heart Inst 1986;13:197.

26. Yeager S, Chin A, Sanders S. Subxyphoid two-dimensional echocardiographic diagnosis of coronary sinus septal defects. Am J Cardiol 1984;54:686.

27. Mantin E, Grondin CW, Lillehei CW, et al. Echocardiographic findings in patients with left superior vena cava and dilated coronary sinus. Am J Cardiol 1979;6:158.

28. Cohen BE, Winer HE, Kronzon I. Echocardiographic findings in patients with left superior vena cava and dilated coronary sinus. Am J Cardiol 1979;66:158.

29. Stewart JA, Franker TD, Scosky DA, et al. Detection of persistent left superior vena cava by two-dimensional contrast echocardiography. J Clin Ultrasound 1979;7:357.

30. Snider AR, Porta JA, Silverman NH. Venous anomalies of the coronary sinus. Circulation 1979;60:721.

31. Hibi N, Fukui Y, Nishimura K, et al. Cross-sectional echocardiographic study of persistent left superior vena cava. Am Heart J 1980;100:69.

32. Paquet M, Gutgssell H. Echocardiographic features of total anomalous venous connection. Circulation 1975;51:599.

33. Aziz KU, Paul MH, Bharati S, et al. Echocardiographic features of total pulmonary venous drainage into the coronary sinus. Am J Cardiol 1978;42:108

34. Campbell M, Deuchar DC. The left sided superior vena cava. Br Heart J 1954;16:423.

35. Freedom RM, Culham JAG, Rowe RD. Left atrial to coronary sinus fenestration (partially unroofed coronary sinus). Br Heart J 1981;46:63.

36. Huhta JE, Smallhorn JF, Macartney FJ, et al. Cross-sectional echocardiographic diagnosis of systemic venous return. Br Heart J 1982;48:388.

37. Rose AG, Beckman CB, Edwards JE. Communication between coronary sinus and left atrium. Br Heart J 1974;36:182.

38. Gerlis LM, Gibbs JC, Williams GJ, et al. Coronary sinus orifice atresia and persistent left superior vena cava. Br Heart J 1984;52:648.

39. Raghib G, Ruttenberg HD, Anderson RC, et al. Termination of left superior vena cava in left atrium, atrial septal defect and absence of coronary sinus: A developmental complex. Circulation 1965;31:906.

40. Chaudry F, Zabalgoitia M. Persistent left superior vena cava diagnosed by contrast transesophageal echocardiography. Am Heart J 1991;122:1175.

41. Nanda NC, Pinheiro L, Sanyal R, et al. Transesophageal echocardiographic examination of left-sided superior vena cava and azygos and hemiazygos veins. Echocardiography 1991;8:731.

42. Hilton T, Castello R, Ohar J, et al. Persistent left superior vena cava in Turner's syndrome: A transesophageal echocardiographic study. Am Heart J 1992;123:234.

5

Right Atrium

The right atrial chamber can be divided neatly (for purposes of description) in two parts, anterior and posterior, which are very different from each other in internal appearance and developmental origin (Figure 5-1). The posterior half, developed from the sinus venosus of the embryo, is a smooth, rounded channel, a half-cylinder into which the superior and inferior venae cavae enter such that all three structures (SVC, right atrium, IVC) are all in the same vertical axis. On the other hand, the anterior right atrium, developed from the primitive atrium, is lined by transverse parallel ridges (pectinate bands) and opens near its upper pole into the right atrial appendage. The latter is a small blind pouch, the inner surface of which is made uneven by irregular, small corrugations. Its chief significance to the clinician is that it is a common site for small thrombi to form if atrial blood flow is rendered sluggish by atrial fibrillation, gross atrial dilatation, or tricuspid valve stenosis.

At the junction of the posterior and anterior halves of the right atrium are certain anatomic landmarks representing persistent remnants of an embryonic structure—the right valve of the sinus venosus—which in the early embryo is a large structure regulating the passage of blood from the sinus venosus to the primitive atrium: (1) The crista terminalis is a ridge that starts above at the junction of the SVC and the right atrium and then runs vertically downward along the lateral (right) atrial wall almost as far as the anterior edge of the IVC opening. The sinus node is located at the upper end of the crista. On the external right atrial surface, a groove (sulcus terminalis) corresponds to the crista terminalis inside. (2) The eustachian valve, a crescentic fold of endocardium, is located at the anterior rim of the IVC orifice. (3) The thebesian valve, a smaller but otherwise similar endo-

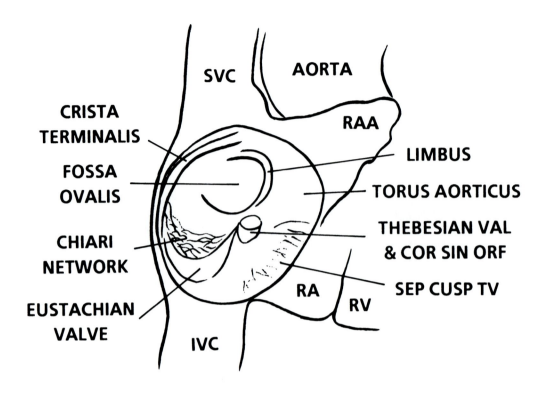

INTERIOR OF RIGHT ATRIUM

Figure 5–1. Diagram showing interior of right atrial chamber after removal of the anterior right atrial wall (RAA, right atrial appendage; RA, right atrium; RV, right ventricle).

cardial fold, guards the opening of the coronary sinus into the right atrium. Whereas these structures are normally present, another structure, (4) the Chiari network, also derived from the right valve of the sinus venosus, is a rare "abnormal" finding.

The eustachian valve, first described 430 years ago, has been studied in detail by several anatomists.[1-6] These observations have revealed an immense variability in size, shape, thickness, and texture of this structure, and even in the extent to which it encroaches on neighboring atrial structures such as the atrial septum. At one end of the spectrum, the embryonic eustachian valve disappears completely or is represented only by a thin ridge; at the other extreme, it persists as a large, mobile flap projecting several centimeters into the right atrial cavity. Most commonly it is a crescentic fold of endocardium arising from the anterior rim of the IVC orifice. The lateral horn of the crescent tends to meet the lower end of the crista terminalis; the other (medial) horn of the crescent joins the thebesian valve, a small semicircular or crescentic fold at the orifice of the coronary sinus. At the eustachian valve–thebesian valve junction or commissure, a small subendocardial cord originates that dips in deeply to attach to the central fibrous body (also called the *right fibrous trigone*) located at the center of the fibrous cardiac skeleton. This cord, called the *tendon of Todaro,* forms one side of Koch's triangle, the other two sides being the coronary sinus opening and the attachment of the septal tricuspid leaflet to the tricuspid annulus. This small triangle is an anatomic landmark of much interest to electrophysiologists and cardiac surgeons because it contains the atrioventricular (A-V) node.

ECHOCARDIOGRAPHIC APPEARANCE AND SIGNIFICANCE OF THE EUSTACHIAN VALVE

The eustachian valve is best identified in the subcostal sagittal view, imaging the IVC entering the right atrium (Figures 5-2 to 5-5). The eustachian valve appears as a linear, partly mobile echo attached to the anterior rim of the IVC orifice.[7,9] Extension of some atrial myocardium into the substance of the eustachian valve probably accounts for its motion and phasic variation in length during the cardiac cycle (see Figure 5-4).

The eustachian valve also may be seen in the parasternal short-axis or parasternal right heart inflow view alongside the entry of the IVC into the right atrium. In the apical four-chamber view, the base of the eustachian valve may be visualized as a transverse fixed linear echo across the right atrial width (see Figure 5-2). Occasionally, the tip of a long valve may "peep" into the imaging plane as a slightly mobile echo, raising the possibility of a right atrial mass; thus a prominent eustachian valve can simulate a right atrial thrombus or myxoma or transcaval spread of a renal or pelvic neoplasm.

Endocarditis producing bacterial vegetations located on the eustachian valve has been reported.[10] An association between unduly large eustachian valves and prolapse of mitral and tricuspid valves has been claimed.[11]

A dense linear echo in the right atrium running transversely across its posterior wall to meet the atrial septum is often encountered in the apical four-chamber or subcostal four-chamber view. This could be the tendon of Todaro or, alternatively, a medial extension of the eustachian valve that encroaches on the atrial septum as far as the limbus of the fossa ovalis.

CHIARI NETWORK

Like the eustachian valve, the Chiari (Figure 5-6) network represents persistence of the right valve of the sinus venosus and is in fact attached to the former inferiorly (Figures 5-7 and 5-8). It is a lace- or filigree-like network of variable size and thickness attached above to the crista terminalis or forming an untethered, free upper edge. The eustachian valve itself is sometimes perforated by multiple fenestrations near its free edge and appears very similar on the echocardiogram, although anatomists make a distinction between eustachian valve fenestrations and a true Chiari network, the latter being more rare. In both cases, multiple small, very mobile linear echoes are detected in the right atrium, flickering in and out of view; close scrutiny may reveal that motion of these small wisps is not random but connected to the eustachian valve region.[12] A right atrial mass can be simulated.[13] Persistence of the entire right sinus venosus valve can form a large, obstructive flap or septum across the right atrium.[14] This extremely rare anomaly, which is visible on two-dimensional (2D) echo, has been called a *right-sided cor triatriatum.*

THE INFEROMEDIAL FOSSA

A fairly deep fossa exists between the eustachian valve and the tricuspid valve ring situated in the inferomedial part of the right atrium. This pouchlike space has in fact been called the *inferomedial fossa* by McAlpine,[15] but it, or part of it, also bears the eponyms of two illustrious anatomists, Sir Arthur Keith and Wilhelm His. When viewed from the outside of the heart, the fossa appears as a bulge or pouch and has even been called the *posterior auricular appendage* (of His). What is commonly termed the *right atrial appendage* or *auricle* is a blind pouch at the anterosuperior part of the right atrium, continuous with the rough corrugated anterior section of the right atrial chamber. This au-

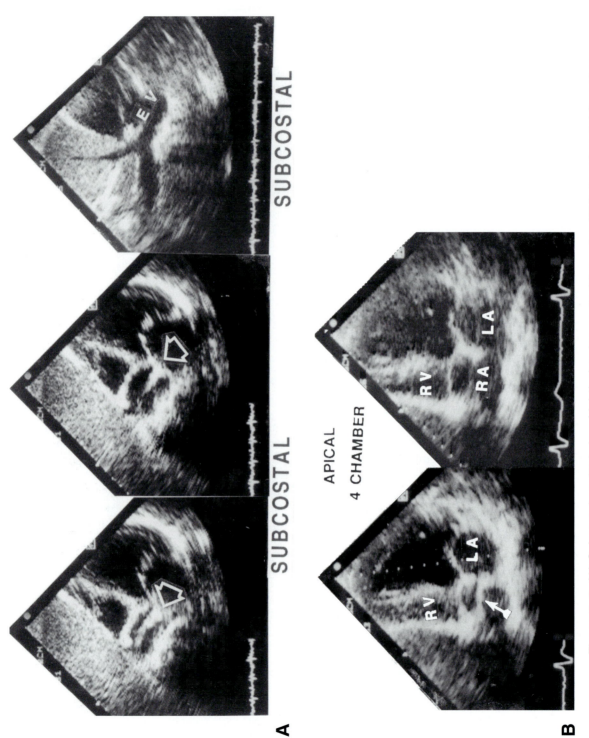

SUBCOSTAL

SUBCOSTAL

A

APICAL
4 CHAMBER

B

Figure 5–2. (A) Subcostal sagittal view (right) showing eustachian valve (EV). In subcostal four-chamber view, the eustachian valve appears as a transverse band (arrows) across the posterior right atrium. (B) Apical four-chamber view (right) shows no intraatrial structure, but in a slightly more posterior plane (left), a transverse band echo (arrow) comes into view, representing the eustachian valve and the anterior rim of the IVC orifice.

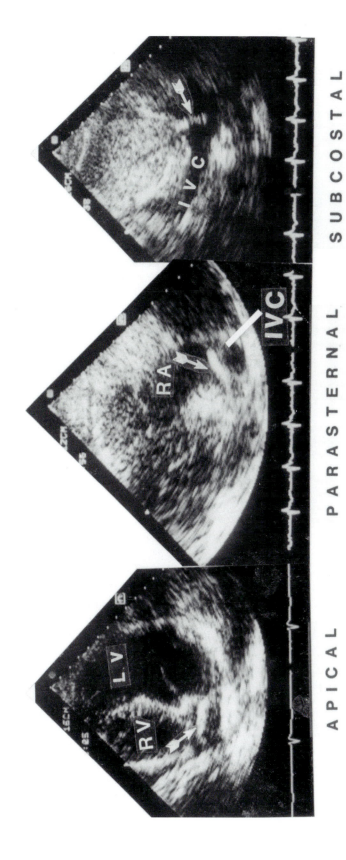

APICAL   PARASTERNAL   SUBCOSTAL

Figure 5–3. Apical view (posterior plane) (left), parasternal right heart inflow view (center), and subcostal sagittal view (right). The band echo (arrows) represents the eustachian valve projecting from the anterior rim of the IVC orifice into the right atrium (RA).

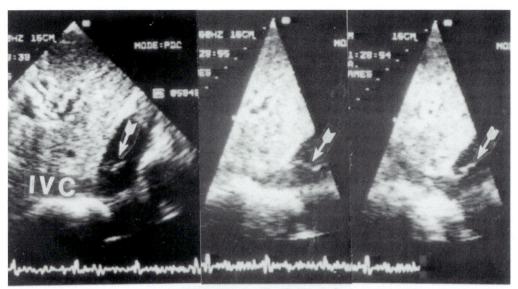

SUBCOSTAL

Figure 5–4. Subcostal view in sagittal plane showing long eustachian valve attached to the anterior edge of the inferior vena cava (IVC) orifice. Note varying contour of the linear eustachian valve echo due to its undulations.

ricular appendage is difficult to visualize on echocardiography. On the other hand, the inferomedial fossa is well seen in the parasternal right heart inflow view as a space in the right atrium between the IVC and the eustachian valve (to the right, posteriorly and inferiorly) and the tricuspid annulus (to the left, superiorly and anteriorly) (Figure 5–9A). The orifice of the coronary sinus, located at the junction of the medial and inferior walls of the right atrium, is also closely related to the inferomedial fossa.

MEDIAL WALL OF THE RIGHT ATRIUM

Unlike the lateral wall of the right atrium, which is related only to the pericardium and right pleura, the medial wall possesses important anatomic landmarks or contiguity with several important cardiac structures.[16] This somewhat complex anatomy can be better understood if it is divided into the following sections: (1) the tricuspid valve, opening into the right ventricle anteroinferiorly, (2) the interatrial septum, facing the left atrium posterosuperiorly (these will be described in detail later), and (3) the anterior part of the right atrium medial wall, which is mainly related to the ascending aorta above and the left ventricular outflow tract below. The normal ascending aorta, slightly dilated just above the aortic valve into the sinus of Valsalva, is closely related to the right atrial wall (Figure 5–9B) and may in fact form a bulge or rounded prominence at this right atrial location called the *torus aorticus*. Of the three sinuses of Valsalva, the right coronary sinus and noncoronary sinus are related to the right atrium. Other adjacent structures at this level include the infundibulum of the right ventricle, the right coronary artery, and the transverse sinus (pericardial recess). Below the level of the aortic valve, the right atrium is related to the left ventricular outflow tract; in fact, the left ventricle and right atrium are separated only by the thin membranous ventricular septum at this site.

These medial-right atrial relationships explain the manifestations of some important cardiac entities. Thus aneurysms of the right coronary or noncoronary sinus of Valsalva may protrude into the right atrium and present as a "right atrial mass" on echocardiography. If such an aneurysm should rupture, the resulting shunt between the aorta and the right atrium is evident on colorflow Doppler.

SUBCOSTAL

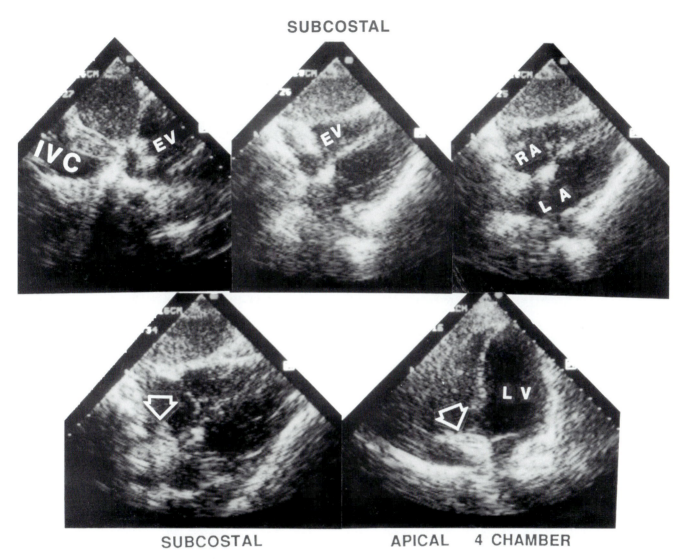

SUBCOSTAL   APICAL   4 CHAMBER

Figure 5–5. Subcostal view (above) showing eustachian valve (EV) in left and central frames. In same patient, subcostal (below, left) shows large lipomatous "hypertrophy" of interatrial septum (arrow). In apical four-chamber view, this unusual variant of lipomatous configuration extends into (or is superimposed on) the eustachian valve, simulating an intraatrial mass.

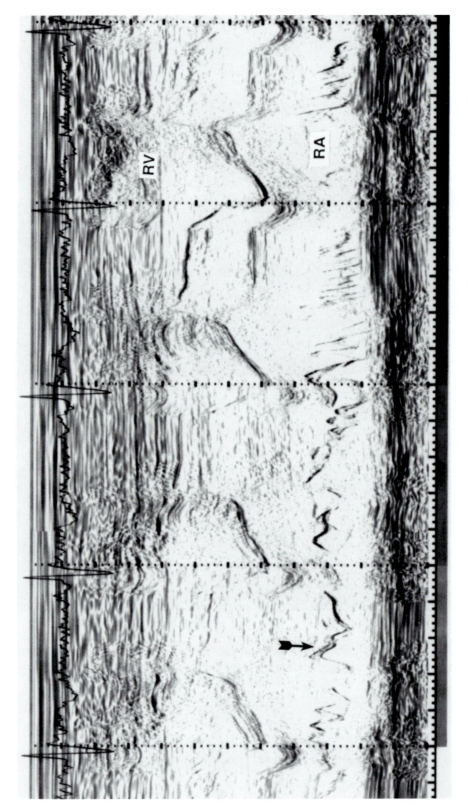

Figure 5–6. M-mode echocardiogram showing rapid irregular motion of a linear echo in the right atrium (RA) representing the Chiari network.

SUBCOSTAL

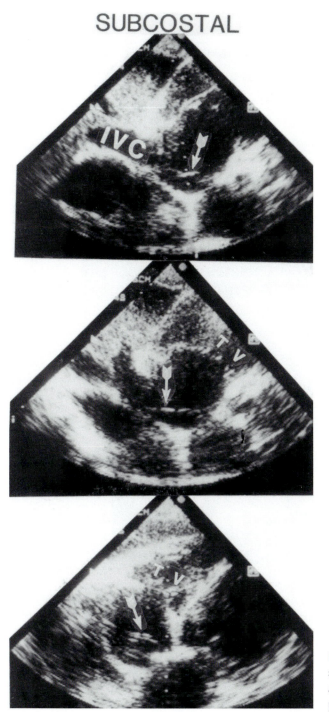

Figure 5–7. Subcostal views in slightly different planes showing a linear filamentous echo (arrows) in the right atrium that showed brisk motion in real-time viewing. It was presumed to represent a variant of the Chiari network.

The left side of the membranous ventricular septum is located just below the aortic valve in the uppermost left ventricle. However, on its right side, the membranous ventricular septum is partly in the right atrium and partly in the right ventricle. This apparently confusing fact is the result of the tricuspid valve's septal attachment being a little closer than the septal mitral valve's attachment to the cardiac apex. If only the right atrial portion of the membranous septum is deficient, a left ventricle–right atrium communication results.

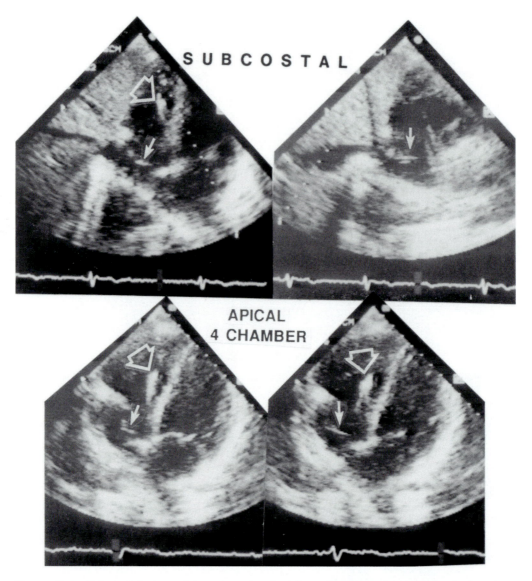

Figure 5–8. Subcostal views (above) and apical four-chamber views (below) showing Chiari filaments in the right atrium (small arrows) as well as a thick dense echo in the right ventricle representing a pacemaker lead (open arrow).

In this rare variety of congenital septal defect, sometimes called the *Gerbode defect,* a left-to-right shunt occurs directly from the left ventricle to the right atrium without involvement of the right ventricle. Similarly located defects of iatrogenic cause have complicated tricuspid or mitral valve surgery.

Systolic flutter of the tricuspid valve (septal leaflet) may be noted on M-mode echo. The defect may be visualized by careful imaging in an appropriate plane; colorflow Doppler demonstrates a high-velocity jet into the right atrium at this site.

RIGHT ATRIUM: NORMAL SIZE AND DILATATION

The right atrium can be visualized in the parasternal short-axis view as well as the parasternal right heart inflow view. Although gross dilatation of this chamber is readily appreciated in these views, the lateral wall of the right atrium is often ill-defined, so accurate measurements of the right atrial dimensions may not be obtainable. Better definition of right atrial borders is possible in the apical four-chamber and subcostal four-chamber views.

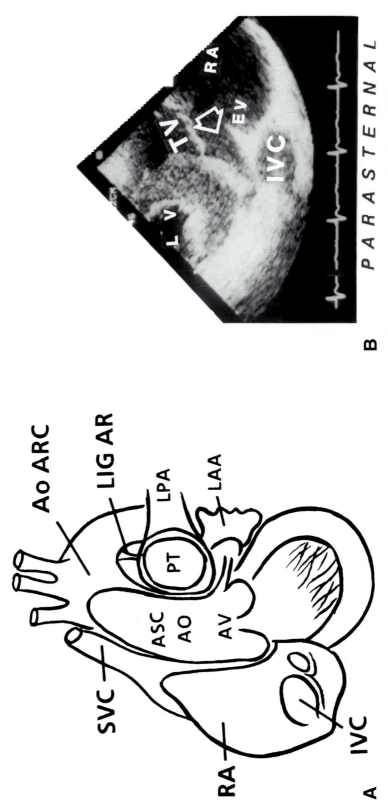

A IVC

B *PARASTERNAL*

Figure 5–9. (A) Parasternal right heart inflow view demonstrating the fossa (arrow) named after His or Keith between the eustachian valve and the tricuspid valve. (B) Diagram of coronal section through heart showing intimate relation of aortic root to medial wall of right atrium.

Published values for right atrial dimensions (measured at end-systole) were measured by Weyman[17] in these views:

	Mean (cm)	Range (cm)
Apical four-chamber view		
Superior-inferior (roof to base) dimension	4.2 ± 0.4	3.4-4.9
Medial-lateral (transverse) dimension		
Largest dimension	3.7 ± 0.4	3.1-0.45
Middle dimension	3.7 ± 0.4	2.9-4.5
Tricuspid annulus	2.2 ± 0.3	1.7-2.8
Right atrial area (by planimetry)	14 ± 1.5 cm^2	11.3-16.7 cm^2
Subcostal view		
Medial-lateral dimension	4.0 ± 0.4	3.3-4.7

The normal (mean) values of Bommer et al.[18] in apical four-chamber view are similar:

Right atrial short axis	3.6 ± 0.1 cm
Right atrial long axis	4.2 ± 0.1 cm
Right atrial area by planimetry	13.9 ± 0.7 cm^2
Short axis × long axis	15 ± 0.7 cm^2

Bommer et al.[18] studied 50 subjects and validated the measurements and estimated volumes of the right atrium in 8 patients who died by making casts of the chamber on autopsy specimens. These authors defined their long axis as the base (tricuspid valve attachment) to roof right atrial dimension in the plane of the atrial septum, and the right atrial short axis as the maximum distance between the inner borders of the atrial septum and the right atrial free wall.

When the left atrial size is normal, moderate to severe right atrial dilatation will be obvious in the apical four-chamber or subcostal four-chamber view because of the disparity between the two chambers as they lie side by side. Right atrial enlargement (without left atrial enlargement) is present in one of the following categories of cardiac conditions: (1) pure right heart volume overload, as in atrial septal defect, (2) pure right ventricular pressure overload, due to pulmonary hypertension of varied causes or pulmonic stenosis, (3) significant tricuspid regurgitation of any etiology, and (4) abnormally weak right ventricular myocardial function, either acquired (RV infarction) or congenital as in Ebstein's anomaly, Uhl's anomaly, arrhythmogenic RV dysplasia, etc.

RIGHT ATRIAL SHAPE

External RA contours are rounded in transverse as well as medial-lateral directions. The right atrium (RA) may be compared with a barrel with a flat surface inferiorly where it opens into the tricuspid valve. The RA wall does not exhibit much motion because a vacuum effect between visceral and parietal pericardium holds it in contact with the latter unless a pericardial effusion exists adjacent to the right atrium, in which case the RA wall is allowed an augmented amplitude of motion during the cardiac cycle. Such exaggeration of RA wall mobility in patients with pericardial effusions should not be mistaken for RA wall indentation (infolding), which is characterized by a conspicuous concavity, often with sharp inward angulation, and is one of the signs of tamponade.

Regional large loculation of pericardial fluid can distort and compress the RA considerably, reducing it to a narrow slit in some imaging planes. Most of the reported cases have occurred as a complication of cardiac surgery.

Some narrowing of the RA chamber also may be seen with an unduly high right diaphragm secondary to hepatomegaly. Uncommonly, a very large right pleural effusion can produce a similar impingement and narrowing of the RA.

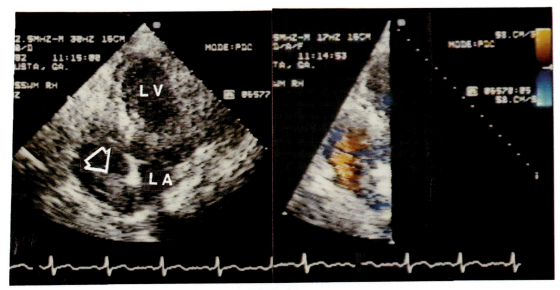

APICAL

4 CHAMBER

Figure 5–10. (Left) Apical four-chamber view of patient with renal cell carcinoma showing transcaval extension of the tumor into the right atrium (arrow). (Right) Colorflow Doppler of same view showing inflow into the right atrium displaced rightward by the tumor mass.

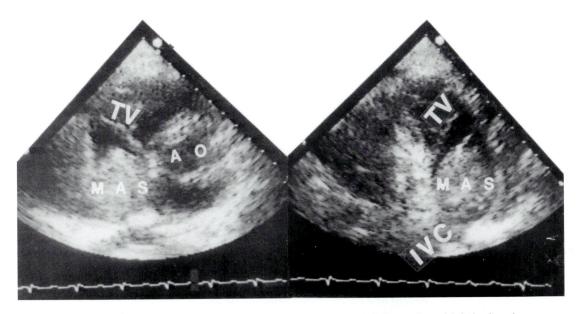

Figure 5–11. Parasternal short-axis view (left) and RV inflow view (right) showing a large mass (MAS) growing into the right atrium through the IVC. The mass was a leiomyosarcoma (TV, tricuspid valve).

Idiopathic RA Dilatation

This rare condition of uncertain etiology was first described 30 years ago by Pastor and Forte[19] in three patients. Subsequently, similar cases were reported by several other groups, among them Sumner et al.,[20] who used the following diagnostic criteria: (1) disproportionate RA enlargement compared with the other cardiac chambers and (2) absence, after systematic exclusion, of all cardiovascular lesions known to produce RA en-

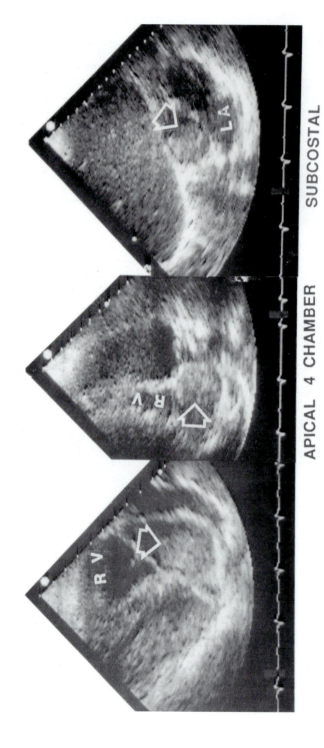

APICAL 4 CHAMBER

SUBCOSTAL

Figure 5-12. RV inflow view (left), apical four-chamber view (center), and subcostal view (right) showing the same right atrial mass (leiomyosarcoma) growing through the IVC.

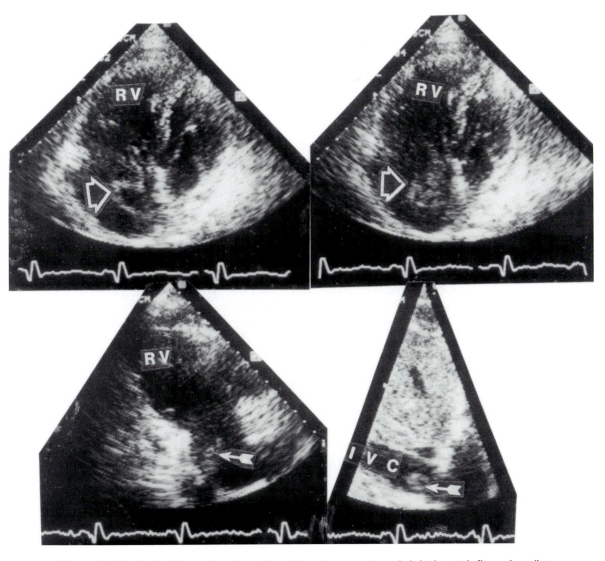

Figure 5–13. Apical four-chamber view (above), parasternal right heart inflow view (below, left), and subcostal view (below, right). An abnormal sinuous mobile echo (arrows) is seen in the right atrium; it was no longer present 2 weeks later and presumably was a thrombus. The right heart chambers are markedly dilated secondary to severe pulmonary hypertension of thromboembolic etiology.

largement. Ayasama et al.[21] used M-mode echocardiography to image the dilated RA; a maximum dimension of 11.6 cm was recorded in their patient.

An even rarer condition, large atrial diverticulum, has been reported in association with supraventricular tachycardia. The very few patients described have been infants; however, the patient of Morrow and Behrendt[22] was a 23-year-old woman who was cured of recurrent supraventricular tachycardia by resection of the diverticulum.

RA MASSES

From the echocardiographer's viewpoint, RA masses can be divided into false and true "masses" (Figures 5-10 to 5-13). False masses include (1) *normal structures* or variants such as the eustachian valve and Chiari network, (2) *artifacts* from strongly reflective objects in neighboring chambers, such as metallic prosthetic aortic valves, and (3) strong echoes from *foreign objects* in the RA, such as pacemaker leads or Swan-Ganz catheters, or reverberations from similar sources. Pacemaker leads often appear thicker than one would expect, perhaps due to fibrous sheathlike formations around the wires in long-standing pacemakers. Echocardiography may in fact be used to verify that a pacemaker lead is in a proper location[23] (tip near the RV apex) or to detect the rare instances of RV wall perforation by the lead.[24,25] Other rare pacemaker lead complications detectable by 2D echo include attached thrombi[26,27] and attached bacterial vegetations.[28]

True masses in the RA are either neoplasms or thrombi. Most common of the primary neoplasms is the *myxoma,* said to comprise 15% of all cardiac masses. They are usually pedunculated, attached to the atrial septum near the foramen ovale, and vary considerably from small to huge.[29-31] Obstruction of tricuspid valve flow, when present, is demonstrated by Doppler.[32]

Neoplasms growing into and up the IVC into the RA are encountered more frequently than primary atrial tumors.[33-35] Hypernephromas and Wilm's tumors of renal origin are notorious in this respect. Uterine leiomyomas are also known for transcaval spread into the RA. These tumor masses growing into this chamber through the IVC are of two types: (1) a large, stiff, unyielding mass which, though it protrudes massively into the RA, remains immobile and fixed, with no participation in normal atrial wall motion, and (2) a flexible, more mobile mass that may grow into the tricuspid orifice and in its motion pattern resemble an atrial myxoma. *Right atrial thrombi*[36-40] are of three main types: (1) mural thrombi, which are flat or at least sessile, with little or no mobility other than that of the atrial wall itself[36] (the patient usually has a much dilated RA and chronic congestive failure), (2) thrombi that have developed on a central venous line (possibly infected) and have propagated downstream into the RA, and (3) mobile, unattached, elongated thrombi,[37-40] sausage or serpentine in shape, that are in transit through the right side of the heart from the leg or pelvic veins to embolize into a pulmonary artery. The appearance of such highly mobile echo masses is often as spectacular as it is unexpected. Their stay in the right heart chamber is very transient because they are soon swept into the pulmonary artery. However, occasionally such an elongated thrombus gets stuck in a patent foramen ovale and thus proceeds into the LA to cause a paradoxical embolism. Yet another possibility is that the sinuous thrombus gets entangled or trapped in the RV chordae tendineae–papillary muscle–trabeculation network.[38]

REFERENCES

1. Yater WM. Variations and anomalies of the venous valves of the right atrium of the human heart. Arch Pathol 1929;7:418.
2. Doucette J, Knoblich R. Persistent right valve of the sinus venosus. Arch Pathol 1963;75:105.
3. Wright RR, Anson BJ, Cleveland HC. The vestigial valves and the interatrial foramen of the adult human heart. Anat Rec 1948;100:331.
4. Hickie JB. The valve of the inferior vena cava. Br Heart J 1956;18:320.
5. Powell EDU, Mullaney JM. The Chiari network and the valve of the inferior vena cava. Br Heart J 1960;22:579.
6. Drury RAB. Persistent venous valves. J Pathol 1978;161.
7. Battle-Diaz J, Stanley P, Kratz C, et al. Echocardiographic manifestations of persistence of the right sinus venosus valve. Am J Cardiol 1979;850.
8. Limacher MC, Gutgesell HP, Vick GW, et al. Echocardiographic anatomy of the eustachian valve. Am J Cardiol 1983;57:363.
9. Bommer WJ, Kwan OL, Mason DT, et al. Identification of prominent eustachian valves by M-mode and two-dimensional echocardiography. Am J Cardiol 1980;45:402.
10. Edwards AD, Vickers MA, Morgan CJ. Infective endocarditis affecting the eustachian valve. Br Heart J 1986;56:561.
11. Schrem SS, Freedberg RS, Gindea AJ, et al. The association between unusually large eustachian valves and atrioventricular valve prolapse. Am Heart J 1990;120:204.

12. Werner JA, Cheitlin MD, Gross BW, et al. Echocardiographic appearance of the Chiari network: Differentiation from right heart pathology. Circulation 1980;63:1104.

13. Katz ES, Freeberg RS, Rutkovsky L, et al. Identification of an unusual right atrial mass as a Chiari network by biplane transesophageal echocardiography. Echocardiography 1992;9:273.

14. Jones RN, Niles NR. Spinnaker formation of sinus venous valve: Case report of a fatal anomaly in a 10-year-old boy. Circulation 1968;38:468.

15. McAlpine WA. Heart and Coronary Arteries. New York: Springer-Verlag, 1975, p 93.

16. Walmsey R, Watson H. The medial wall of the right atrium. Circulation 1966;34:400.

17. Weyman AE. Cross-Sectional Echocardiography. Philadelphia: Lea & Febiger, 1982, p 501.

18. Bommer W, Weinert L, Neumann A, et al. Determination of right atrial and right ventricular size by two-dimensional echocardiography. Circulation 1979;60:91.

19. Pastor BH, Forte AL. Idiopathic enlargement of the right atrium. Am J Cardiol 1961;8:513.

20. Sumner RG, Phillips JG, Jacoby WJ, et al. Idiopathic enlargement of the right atrium. Circulation 1965;32:985.

21. Ayasama J, Matsuura T, Endo N, et al. Idiopathic enlargement of the right atrium. Am J Cardiol 1977;40:620.

22. Shah K, Walsh K. Giant right atrial diverticulum: An unusual cause of Wolff-Parkinson-White syndrome. Br Heart J 1992;68:58.

23. Drinkovic N. Subcostal echocardiography to determine right ventricular pacing catheter position and control advancement of electrode catheters in intracardiac electrophysiologic studies. Am J Cardiol 1981;47:1260.

24. Chazal RA, Feigenbaum H. Two-dimensional echocardiographic identification of epicardial pacemaker wire perforation. Am Heart J 1984;107:165.

25. Gondi B, Nanda NC. Real-time two-dimensional echocardiographic features of pacemaker perforation. Circulation 1981;64:97.

26. Nicolisi GL, Charmet PA, Zannettini D. Large right atrial thrombosis. Br Heart J 1980;43:199.

27. Perry RA, Clarke DB, Shiu MF. Entanglement of embolised thrombus with an endocardial lead causing pacemaker malfunction and subsequent pulmonary embolism. Br Heart J 1987;57:292.

28. Vilacosta I, Zamorano J, Camino A, et al. Infected transvenous permanent pacemakers: Role of transesophageal echocardiography. Am Heart J 1993;125:904.

29. Turlapati RV, Jacobs LE, Kotler MN. Right atrial myxoma causing total destruction of the tricuspid valve leaflets. Am Heart J 1990;120:1227.

30. Panidis IP, Kotler MN, Mintz GS, et al. Clinical and echocardiographic features of right atrial masses. Am Heart J 1984;107:745.

31. Rey M, Tunon J, Compres H, et al. Prolapsing right atrial myxoma evaluated by transesophageal echocardiography. Am Heart J 1991;122:875.

32. Goli VD, Thadani U, Thomas SR, et al. Doppler echocardiographic profiles in obstructive right and left atrial myxomas. J Am Coll Cardiol 1987;7:17.

33. Maurer G, Nanda NC. Two-dimensional echocardiographic identification of intracardiac leiomyomatosis. Am Heart J 1982;103:915.

34. Politzer F, Kronzon I, Wieczorek R, et al. Intracardiac leiomyomatosis. J Am Coll Cardiol 1984;4:629.

35. Gonzalez-Lavin L, Lee RH, Falk L, et al. Tricuspid valve obstruction due to intravenous leiomyomatosis. Am Heart J 1984;108:1544.

36. Lim SP, Hakim SZ, Vander Bel-Kahn JM. Two-dimensional echocardiography for detection of primary right atrial thrombus and pulmonary embolism. Am Heart J 1984;106:1547.

37. Rosenzweig MS, Nanda NC. Two-dimensional echocardiographic detection of circulating right atrial thrombi. Am Heart J 1981;103:435.

38. Starkey IR, DeBono DP. Echocardiographic identification of right sided cardiac intracavitary thromboembolus in massive pulmonary embolism. Circulation 1982;66:1322.

39. Goldberg SM, Pizarello RA, Goldman MA, et al. Echocardiographic diagnosis of right atrial thromboembolism resulting in massive pulmonary embolization. Am Heart J 1984;108:137.

40. Starr SK, Pugh DM, O'Brien-Ladner A, et al. Right atrial mass biopsy guided by transesophageal echocardiography. Chest 1993;104:969.

6

Tricuspid Valve

NORMAL ANATOMY

The *tricuspid valve annulus* is oval rather than circular and faces anteriorly and to the left. Its inferomedial location within the right atrium (RA) and proximity to RA structures such as the eustachian valve, thebesian valve (at orifice of coronary sinus), inferior strip of atrial septum (between the limbus of the fossa ovalis and the tricuspid annulus), atrio-ventricular (A-V) node located deep to Koch's triangle (formed by the tricuspid annulus, coronary sinus, and tendon of Todaro) were described in Chapter 5. The normal circumference of the tricuspid annulus is 11.2 to 11.8 cm in men and 10 to 11.1 cm in women.[1] Its three leaflets, commonly called *anterior, septal,* and *posterior,* also may be properly named *anterosuperior, medial,* and *inferior,* respectively, according to McAlpine[2] (Figure 6-1). There are not always three distinct leaflets; for example, the posterior leaflet may be absent, or there may appear to be an extra (fourth) leaflet. The three leaflets are separated from each other by three commissures, which (unlike the mitral valve) may be almost as long as the posterior or septal leaflet.

The *anterior leaflet* is the longest and is roughly quadrangular or semicircular in shape. Its average length is 22 mm, and its average width (at its base) is 37 mm. The *septal leaflet* is tongue-shaped or half-oval in shape and, on average, is 16 mm long and 36 mm wide. It shows a fold on its atrial surface where the leaflet attachment passes from posterior right ventricular (RV) wall to the membranous septum. The *posterior leaflet* is an average of 20 mm long and 75 mm wide at its base. Its contour is often scalloped, with clefts or indentations of variable depth on its free edge.

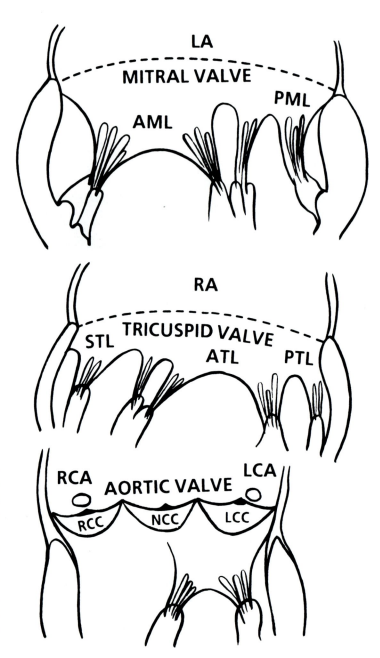

Figure 6–1. Diagram showing the mitral, tricuspid, and aortic valves. The heart has been opened longitudinally and spread apart so that the annuli (dotted lines) of the three valves are seen as flat horizontal bands. Note the differences between the mitral and tricuspid valves in number, location, and size of the leaflets and papillary muscles (AML and PML, anterior and posterior mitral leaflets; STL, ATL, and PTL, septal, anterior, and posterior leaflets; RCC, NCC, and LCC, right, non-, and left coronary cusps; RCA and LCA, right and left coronary artery ostia).

Chordae tendineae, 17 to 36 in number (average 25), are attached to the ventricular surface of the leaflets. Chordae of distinct morphology (fan-shaped or triradiate) tether the commissural areas of the tricuspid valve and therefore help to identify the separation between the three valve leaflets. Tricuspid chordae tendineae vary from 3 to 22 mm in length and 0.5 to 1.5 mm in thickness. These leaflet and chordae measurements are taken from the descriptions by Silver et al.[3]

In a study of 95 normal autopsy specimens by Rosenquist and Sweeney,[4] it was found that in 39 the commissure between the anterior and the septal (medial) leaflets was absent or very incomplete. The authors suggest that if a membranous ventricular septal defect (VSD) should be present in such a patient, the tricuspid anatomy would favor a direct LV-RA left-to-right shunt with no LV-RV shunting.

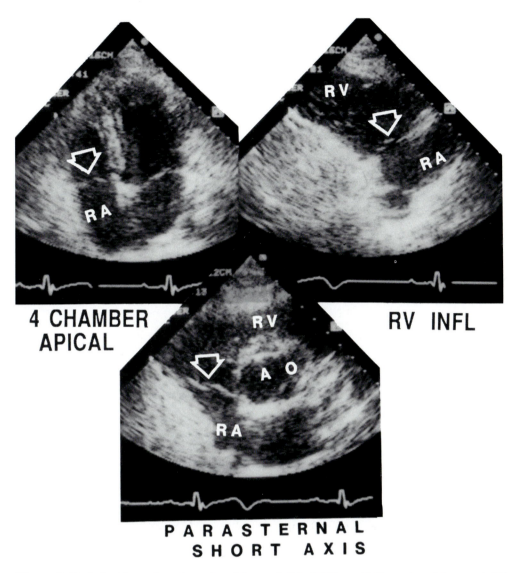

Figure 6–2. Apical four-chamber view (above, left), right heart inflow view (above, right), and parasternal short-axis view (below) showing normal tricuspid valve (arrows).

Unlike the mitral valve, which is supported by only two papillary muscles, the tricuspid leaflets get chordae tendineae from at least three papillary muscles; often a group of mini-papillary muscles replaces a single full-sized one. The anterior papillary muscle is the biggest and is situated beneath the commissure between the anterior and posterior tricuspid leaflets. It arises from the free anterior RV wall and partly from the moderator band, a unique transverse muscular band crossing the RV chamber. The posterior papillary muscle is located below the commissure between the posterior and septal leaflets. The septal or conus papillary muscle, higher in the RV than the others, arises from the septal edge of the infundibulum; it sometimes may be absent or represented only by several chordae.

Chordae from all these papillary muscles insert on the ventricular surface of the tricuspid leaflets. The RV aspect of the ventricular septum below the infundibulum is near to or contiguous with the papillary muscles, chordae tendineae, or trabeculations; on echocardiography, these intracavitary linear or band echoes may be mistaken for the right border of the ventricular septum, in which case septal thickness would appear erroneously increased.

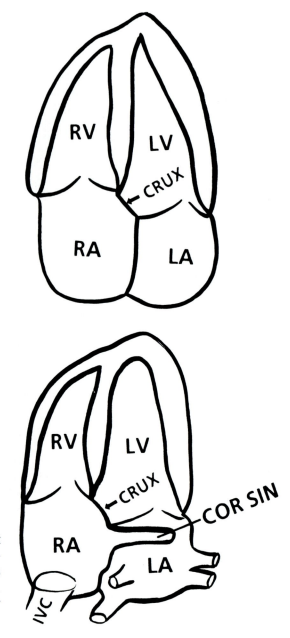

Figure 6–3. Diagram of four-chamber apical view in different planes to depict position of crux of the heart. Note that the attachment of the tricuspid valve (septal leaflet) on the septum is closer to the apex than that of the mitral valve (anterior leaflet). Note locations at which coronary sinus (COR SIN) and inferior vena cava (IVC) enter the right atrium.

ECHOCARDIOGRAPHY OF THE TRICUSPID VALVE

The tricuspid valve is best visualized in three views (Figure 6–2):

1. The parasternal right heart inflow view reveals the anterior and posterior rims of the tricuspid annulus, to which are attached the anterior and posterior tricuspid leaflets, respectively. Leaflet motion is well appreciated, as is forward and regurgitant tricuspid flow. The parasternal short-axis view shows all the tricuspid leaflets at suitable transducer angulation and can demonstrate vegetations on them, but the leaflets are not seen from edge to attachment.

2. The apical four-chamber view reveals the anterior tricuspid leaflet laterally and the septal leaflet medially. The thickness and motion of these leaflets are well seen, as is the position of leaflets with reference to the annulus (to detect or exclude systolic prolapse). The site of attachment of the septal leaflet to the septum, with reference to anterior mi-

tral leaflet septal attachment, is also best appreciated in this view (Figure 6–3), a vital consideration in the diagnosis of Ebstein's anomaly.

3. The subcostal four-chamber view is the third view that permits a good visualization of tricuspid leaflets and also of tricuspid regurgitation (TR), particularly in thin individuals with low diaphragms, where the distance from the transducer to the right ventricle is not too large. In emphysematous patients it may be the only adequate echo window.

In a study of 147 patients with rheumatic valve disease, Guyer et al.[5] found tricuspid leaflets adequately visualized in 95% in the apical four-chamber view, 68% in the parasternal view, and 39% in the subcostal view.

RHEUMATIC TRICUSPID VALVE DISEASE

Autopsy studies in several series of hearts with rheumatic heart disease, published five or six decades ago, mention a prevalence of 30% to 50% of tricuspid valve involvement.[6-8] In a more recent series, studied by 2D echo, of 372 patients with rheumatic heart disease, only 23 (6.2%) had tricuspid valve abnormalities indicative of rheumatic changes.[9] These included increased leaflet thickening, restricted motion, encroachment of leaflets into the RV inlet area, and diastolic doming configuration (rather than normal mobile divergent motion). The lower incidence by 2D echo than in the older autopsy series can be explained by (1) the milder degree of leaflet abnormality not being detected on echo and (2) the rheumatic process not being as severe in recent years as it was in the early decades of this century (and still is in developing countries).

Tricuspid valve stenosis is infrequently encountered at the present time; a rheumatic cause continues to be the rule, and rheumatic mitral stenosis is usually present. Tricuspid stenosis has been reported in 4% to 33% of patients with rheumatic valve disease.[9-13] Cusp thickening and diastolic doming are typical on 2D echo.[14] Other causes of tricuspid valve stenosis include carcinoid and atypical Ebstein's disease.

The tricuspid orifice also may be obstructed by neoplastic right atrial (RA) masses, such as myxomas or sarcomas originating de novo in that chamber, or abdominal neoplasms invading the RA through IVC spread. Extrinsic pressure on the RA-RV junction by intrapericardial hematomas or loculated effusions also has been reported. Pacemaker leads forming loops in the RV with fibrotic adhesions to sub-tricuspid valve structures may prevent valve opening and thus cause stenosis in rare cases, detectable on 2D echo.[15] All these varieties of tricuspid stenosis are well visualized by 2D echo in apical and subcostal views.

TRICUSPID REGURGITATION

Of the numerous causes of tricuspid regurgitation (TR), some common ones and other rarer varieties are described below.

Tricuspid Valve Prolapse

The anatomic basis for tricuspid valve prolapse is redundancy, which in turn is secondary to myxomatous degeneration, as with mitral valve prolapse (MVP). In fact, tricuspid valve prolapse (TVP) usually occurs in patients with MVP.[16-20] Rare instances of isolated TVP with no detectable MVP do occur.

M-mode visualization of TVP was reported by several groups in the mid-1970s[21,22] based on undue posterior sagging of the opposed tricuspid leaflets during systole. Better appreciation of TVP subsequently was possible by 2D echo by imaging the tricuspid valve in multiple views,[18,19,23] such as apical four-chamber, parasternal right heart inflow, and subcostal views. In any given patient, one of these views may demonstrate TVP to better advantage than the others. The diagnostic criterion of TVP is systolic sagging or protrusion of the convexity (belly) of the leaflets below a line joining the attachments of the leaflets to the valve ring (Figures 6–4 and 6–5).

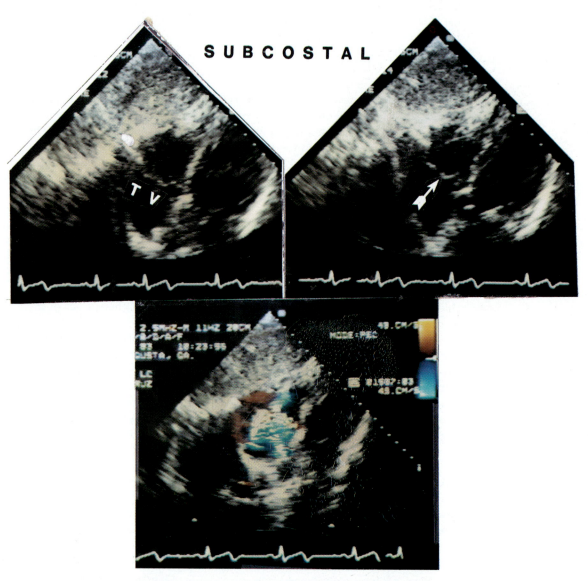

Figure 6–4. Subcostal view showing tricuspid valve (TV) prolapse in the upper frames; the leaflets bulge toward the right atrium, beyond the plane of the tricuspid annulus. The lower frame shows the TR jet.

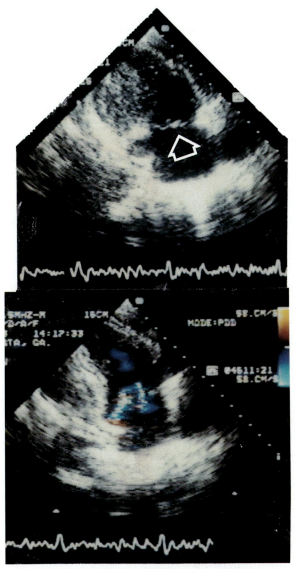

RV INFL

Figure 6–5. (Above) Parasternal right heart inflow view showing mild tricuspid valve prolapse in the upper frame. (Below) Colorflow Doppler reveals the uncommon variant of the two TR jets.

Tricuspid Regurgitation Due to Flail Leaflet

Rupture of tricuspid chordae tendineae results in nonapposition and flail motion of the affected untethered leaflet or part of a leaflet,[24-30] i.e., abnormal motion, especially systolic motion into the right atrium. The most common cause of tricuspid chordal rupture is bacterial endocarditis, with trauma a less frequent etiology and rupture of a RV papillary muscle an even rarer possibility.[29]

On M-mode echo, flail tricuspid leaflet motion manifests as abnormally wide diastolic amplitude of motion with an erratic or coarse diastolic flutter.[23] Systolic flutter also may be seen, as can RV dilatation with paradoxical septal motion if the TR is severe.

On 2D echo, an even more diagnostic appearance is visualized: the flail leaflet fails to coapt with the normal leaflet, and its free edge projects into the RA in systole.[25-28,30]

Carcinoid Tricuspid Valve Disease

In this rare syndrome, fibrotic changes occur in the tricuspid and pulmonic valves in patients with carcinoid tumor metastases in the liver from an intestinal primary.[31-34] A few cases have occurred in association with ovarian carcinoid primaries. In both cases, the carcinoid tissue produces vasoactive substances that are carried to the heart through the IVC and damage right heart endocardium. A peculiar "young collagen" type of fibrous tissue develops on the endocardium of valves and cardiac chambers in diffuse or patchy distribution. Histologically, these fibrous plaques are separated from the cusp structure (which remains essentially intact) by the internal elastic membrane.[32]

The 2D echo appearances of the tricuspid leaflets are highly characteristic,[35-37] in accord with the pathologic descriptions. The leaflets are uniformly thickened, shortened, and stiff. Motion is restricted, and in severe cases the cusps are virtually immobile; lack of coaptation may be evident, with short, stumpy valve leaflets. Papillary muscle involvement renders it unduly echogenic. Doppler manifestations of TR or stenosis or a combination of both (fixed orifice) are the rule.

In a recent series from the Mayo Clinic, the tricuspid valve was abnormal in 97% of 74 patients.[37] TR was present in all and of moderate or severe degree in 90%. Diastolic doming of the valve was not encountered, unlike rheumatic tricuspid stenosis.

"Functional" Tricuspid Regurgitation

In patients with structural disease of the tricuspid leaflets or chordae, lack of proper closure of the leaflets in systole is readily attributable to imperfect apposition of the valve leaflets or, rarely, leaflet perforation. However, when significant TR is present in patients with no intrinsic abnormality of leaflets or chordae, the mechanism or mechanisms responsible for TR remain controversial. These patients usually have pressure and/or volume RV overload.

Pressure overload is not as well tolerated by the RV as by the LV, possibly because the right heart–pulmonary arterial circuit is normally a low-pressure one; the tricuspid annulus is "weaker" than the mitral annulus so that under undue stress it gets easily stretched.[38,39] It has even been suggested that TR may act as a safety valve for a RV chamber striving to cope with pressure overload; the enhanced volume load due to TR then causes greater RV wall stretch and increased systolic performance (Starling's law).

Several groups have used either angiographic or echocardiographic methods to show that patients with significant TR tend to have tricuspid annulus dilatation.[40-43] In an angiocardiographic study, Ubago et al.[40] found that a critical tricuspid annulus diameter of 27 mm/m² of body surface area separated those without TR from those with moderate to severe TR. Mikami et al.[43] found good correlation between the area of the tricuspid annulus (by 2D echo measurement of the annulus in two orthogonal views) and anterior displacement of the tips of the tricuspid leaflets into the RV inlet area.

Some of their patients exhibited lack of coaptation of tricuspid leaflets (separation between the tips of the leaflets throughout systole) or malaligned coaptation (deviation of the tips of the leaflets from each other in systole without distinct separation). It was concluded that "functional" TR results from (1) suboptimal coaptation due to dilatation of the annulus directly and (2) prevention of adequate leaflet coaptation (Figure 6–6) by traction of chordae tendineae secondary to the RV walls drawing apart in a dilated RV chamber.

Tricuspid Valve Endocarditis

Bacterial endocarditis of the tricuspid valve is a major complication of intravenous drug abuse and is seen frequently in large urban medical centers (Figures 6-7 to 6-9). The earliest published echocardiographic reports were based on the M-mode technique (see Figure 6-7), but studies comparing M-mode and 2D echo methods concluded that the latter was diagnostically superior.[44,45] Several studies in the echocardiographic literature attest to the wide spectrum of echo appearances,[44-50] with much variation in size, density, and number of vegetations, as well as in extent of cusp or chordal destruction. The 2D echo manifestations of flail tricuspid leaflets have already been discussed. A vegetation adherent to a flail cusp or ruptured chord renders the abnormal motion of the latter even more conspicuous. In general, tricuspid valve vegetations (Figures 6-9 and 6-10) tend to grow to

RV INFL   APICAL

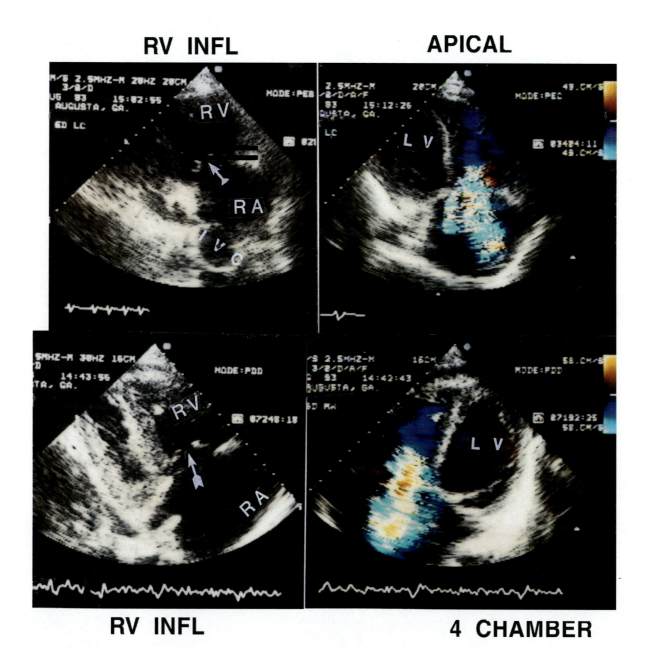

RV INFL   4 CHAMBER

Figure 6–6. Right heart inflow views of two different patients, both of whom had dilated cardiomyopathy and severe TR. The tricuspid leaflets do not appose in systole. The two right frames are apical views demonstrating severe TR on colorflow Doppler.

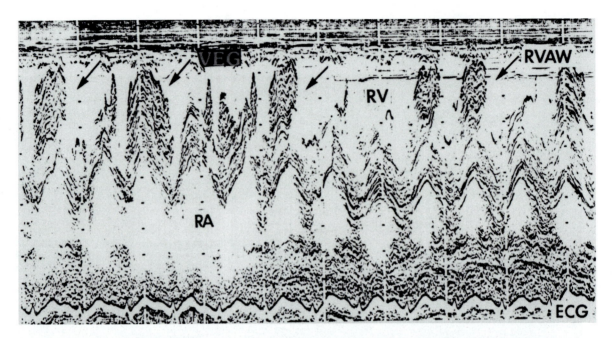

Figure 6–7. M-mode echo of a patient with tricuspid valve endocarditis (*Streptococcus viridans*). The normal tricuspid pattern is replaced by large, mobile masses (arrows).

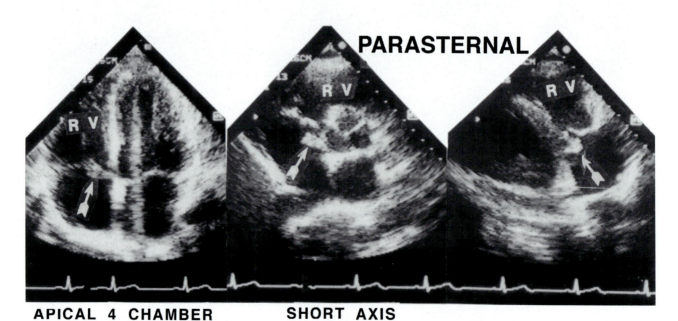

APICAL 4 CHAMBER   SHORT AXIS

Figure 6–8. Apical four-chamber view (left), parasternal short-axis view (center), and RV inflow view (right) showing a vegetation (arrows) on the septal leaflet of the tricuspid valve.

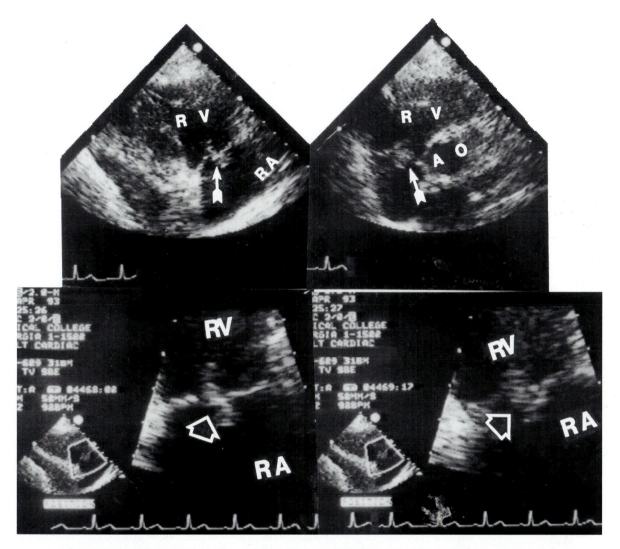

Figure 6–9. (Above) Parasternal RV inflow view (left) and parasternal short-axis view (right) showing a tricuspid vegetation. (Below) Magnified images of the vegetation in slightly different planes.

a larger size than mitral vegetations and may even simulate right atrial masses of neoplastic or thrombotic nature.[48]

The diagnostic sensitivity of 2D echo (transthoracic) for tricuspid vegetations is on the order of 80% to 100%.[51] The size of tricuspid vegetations (greater or less than 1 cm) has been considered by some an important factor in deciding whether or not to excise the infected valve surgically. These authors are inclined toward surgical intervention if 2D echo shows large vegetations because they believe that the prognosis is significantly worse in such patients,[49,52-54] but others[50,51,55] question this opinion.

Miscellaneous Causes of Tricuspid Regurgitation

Pacemaker wires or *Swan-Ganz catheters* passing through the tricuspid valve can mechanically impede proper systolic closure of a normal valve. This situation is obvious on 2D echo and is well known to echocardiographers. *Right atrial myxomas* or *other RA masses* can cause TR by mechanical interference with tricuspid leaflet apposition, as well as by traumatic damage to the delicate tricuspid leaflet structure. *Eosinophilic "endo-*

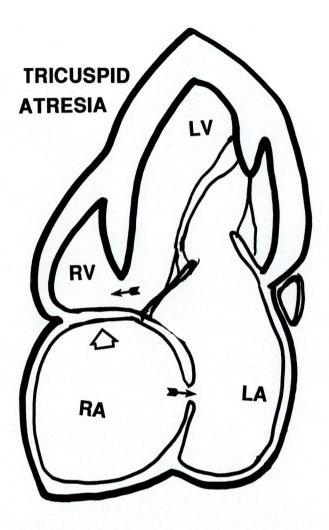

Figure 6–10. Diagram showing apical four-chamber view of tricuspid atresia. The tricuspid orifice is atretic (open arrow). Blood flows from RA to LA through an ASD (thin arrow) and from LV to RV through a VSD (thin arrow).

carditis" of Loeffler and endomyocardial fibrosis are important causes of TR (often severe) in certain African countries. Ebstein's anomaly, an important congenital cause of tricuspid regurgitation, is discussed in Chapter 7. An uncommon cause of tricuspid endocarditis is bacterial infection of a congenital ventricular septal defect getting implanted on a tricuspid leaflet by the jet across the septal defect.

CONGENITAL ABNORMALITIES OF THE TRICUSPID VALVE

Ebstein's anomaly is by far the most important of this group in adults. It is described in detail in Chapter 7 because its main presentation, clinically and echocardiographically, usually is as a cause of gross RV dilatation.

Tricuspid atresia is an important form of cyanotic heart disease in young children, but an exceptional patient survives to adolescence or adulthood. On echocardiography, the tricuspid orifice and leaflets are replaced by an unperforate diaphragm (see Figure 6-9). The RA is dilated and the RV abnormally small; an atrial septal defect is obligatory.

REFERENCES

1. Silver MD. Cardiovascular Pathology. New York: Churchill-Livingstone, 1991, p 23.
2. McAlpine WA. Heart and Coronary Arteries. New York: Springer-Verlag, 1975, p 85.
3. Silver MD, Lam JHC, Ranganathan N, et al. Morphology of the human tricuspid valve. Circulation 1971;43:333.
4. Rosenquist GC, Sweeney LJ. Normal variations in tricuspid valve attachments to the membranous ventricular septum. Am Heart J 1975;89:186.
5. Guyer DE, Gillam LD, Foale RA, et al. Comparison of the echocardiographic and hemodynamic diagnosis of rheumatic tricuspid stenosis. J Am Coll Cardiol 1984;3:1135.
6. Smith JA, Levine SA. The clinical features of tricuspid stenosis. Am Heart J 1942;23:739.
7. Aceves S, Carral R. The diagnosis of tricuspid valve disease. Am Heart J 1947;34:114.
8. Cook WT, White PD. Tricuspid stenosis with particular reference to diagnoses and prognoses. Br Heart J 1941;3:147.
9. Daniels SJ, Mintz GS, Kotler MN. Rheumatic tricuspid valve disease: Two-dimensional echocardiographic, hemodynamic and angiographic correlations. Am J Cardiol 1983;51:492.
10. Kitchin A, Turner R. Diagnosis and treatment of tricuspid stenosis. Br Heart J 1964;26:354.
11. Wanna M, Chandaratna A, Reid C, et al. Value of two-dimensional echocardiography in detecting tricuspid stenosis. Circulation 1983;67:221.
12. Morgan JR, Forker AD, Coates JR, et al. Isolated tricuspid stenosis. Circulation 1971;44:729.
13. El Sherif N. Rheumatic tricuspid stenosis: A hemodynamic correlation. Br Heart J 1971;33:16.
14. Shimada R, Takeshita A, Nakamura M, et al. Diagnosis of tricuspid stenosis by M-mode and two-dimensional echocardiography. Am J Cardiol 1984;53:164.
15. Old WD, Paulsen W, Lewis SA, et al. Pacemaker lead–induced tricuspid stenosis. Am Heart J 1989;117:1165.
16. Gooch AS, Maranhao V, Scampardonis G, et al. Prolapse of both mitral and tricuspid leaflets in systolic murmur-click syndrome. N Engl J Med 1972;287:1218.
17. Werner JA, Schiller NB, Prasquier R. Occurrence and significance of echocardiographically demonstrated tricuspid valve prolapse. Am Heart J 1978;96:180.
18. Morganroth J, Jones RH, Chen CC, et al. Two-dimensional echocardiography in mitral, aortic and tricuspid prolapse. Am J Cardiol 1980;46:1164.
19. Ogawa S, Hayashi J, Sasaki H, et al. Evaluation of combined valvular prolapse syndrome by two-dimensional echocardiography. Circulation 1982;65:174.
20. Rippe JM, Angoff G, Sloss LJ, et al. Multiple floppy valves: An echocardiographic syndrome. Am J Med 1979;66:817.
21. Chandaratna PAN, Lopez JM, Fernandez JJ, et al. Echocardiographic detection of tricuspid valve prolapse. Circulation 1975;51:823.
22. Horgan JH, Beachley MC, Robinson FD. Tricuspid valve prolapse diagnosed by echocardiography. Chest 1975;68:822.
23. Inoue D, Furukawa K, Matsukubo H, et al. Subxiphoid two-dimensional echocardiographic detection of tricuspid valve prolapse. Chest 1979;76:693.
24. Ichikawa T, Okudaira S, Yoshioka J, et al. A case of isolated tricuspid insufficiency. J Cardiogr 1977;7:635.
25. Mintz GS, Kotler MN, Segal BL, et al. Two-dimensional echocardiographic recognition of ruptured chordae tendineae. Circulation 1978;57:244.
26. Brady GH, Talano JV, Meyers FS, et al. Acquired cyanotic heart disease secondary to traumatic tricuspid regurgitation. Am J Cardiol 1979;44:1401.
27. Watanabe T, Katsume H, Matsukubo H, et al. Ruptured chordae tendinae of the tricuspid valve due to nonpenetrating trauma. Chest 1981;80:751.
28. Oliver J, Benito F, Gallego FG, et al. Echocardiographic findings in ruptured chordae tendineae of the tricuspid valve. Am Heart J 1983;105:1033.
29. Gerry JL, Bulkley BH, Hutchins GM. Rupture of the papillary muscle of the tricuspid valve. Am J Cardiol 1977;40:825.
30. Reddy SCB, Rath GA, Ziady GM, et al. Tricuspid flail leaflets after orthoptic heart transplant: A new complication of endomyocardial biopsy. J Am Soc Echocardiogr 1993;6:223.
31. Thorssen A, Biorck G, Bjorkman G, et al. Malignant carcinoid, a clinical and pathological syndrome. Am Heart J 1954;47:795.
32. Roberts WC, Sjoerdsma A. The cardiac disease associated with the carcinoid syndrome. Am J Med 1964;36:5.

33. Teitlebaum SL. The carcinoid: A collective review. Am J Surg 1972;123:564.

34. Ross EM, Roberts WC. The carcinoid syndrome: Comparison of 21 necropsy subjects with carcinoid heart disease to 15 necropsy subjects without carcinoid heart disease. Am J Med 1985;79:339.

35. Baker BJ, McNee VD, Scovil JAS, et al. Tricuspid insufficiency in carcinoid heart disease. Am Heart J 1981;101:107.

36. Callahan JA, Wroblewski EM, Reeder GS, et al. Echocardiographic features of carcinoid heart disease. Am J Cardiol 1982;50:762.

37. Pellikka PA, Tajik AJ, Khandheria BK, et al. Carcinoid heart disease: Clinical and echocardiographic spectrum in 74 patients. Circulation 1993;87:1188.

38. Okene I. Tricuspid valve disease, in JE Dalen, JS Alpert (eds): Valvular Heart Disease, 2d ed. Boston: Little, Brown, 1987, p 354.

39. Carpentier A, DeLoche A, Hanania G, et al. Surgical management of acquired tricuspid valve disease. J Thorac Cardiovasc Surg 1974;67:53.

40. Ubago JL, Figueroa A, Ochoteco A, et al. Analysis of the amount of tricuspid valve anular dilatation required to produce functional tricuspid regurgitation. Am J Cardiol 1983;53:155.

41. Tei C, Pilgrim JP, Shah PM, et al. The tricuspid valve annulus: Study of size and motion in normal subjects and in patients with tricuspid regurgitation. Circulation 1982;66:665.

42. Kuwako K, Tohda E, Ino T, et al. Echocardiographic evaluation of the tricuspid valve and ring. J Cardiogr 1980;10:947.

43. Mikami T, Kudo T, Sakurai N, et al. Mechanisms for development of functional tricuspid regurgitation determined by pulsed Doppler and two-dimensional echocardiography. Am J Cardiol 1984;53:160.

44. Crawford FA, Wechsler AS, Kisslo JA. Tricuspid endocarditis in a drug addict: Detection of tricuspid vegetation by two-dimensional echocardiography. Chest 1978;74:473.

45. Sheikh U, Ali N, Covarrubias EA, et al. Right-sided infective endocarditis: An echocardiographic study. Am J Cardiol 1979;66:283.

46. Come RC, Kurland GS, Vine HS. Two-dimensional echocardiography in differentiating right atrial and tricuspid mass lesions. Am J Cardiol 1979;44:1207.

47. Kisslo J, Von Ramm OT, Haney R, et al. Echocardiographic evaluation of tricuspid valve endocarditis. Am J Cardiol 1976;38:502.

48. Chandaratna PAN, Aronow WS. Spectrum of echocardiographic findings in tricuspid valve endocarditis. Br Heart J 1979;42:528.

49. Ginzton LE, Siegel RJ, Criley JM. Natural history of tricuspid valve endocarditis: A two-dimensional echocardiographic study. Am J Cardiol 1982;49:1853.

50. Berger M, Delfin LA, Jelvch M, et al. Two-dimensional echocardiographic findings in right-sided-infective endocarditis. Circulation 1980;61:855.

51. Chan P, Ogilby JD, Segal B. Tricuspid valve endocarditis. Am Heart J 1989;117:1140.

52. Robbins MJ, Frater RWM, Soeiro R, et al. Influence of vegetation size on clinical outcome of right-sided infective endocarditis. Am J Med 1986;80:165.

53. Wong D, Chandaratna PAN, Wishnow RM, et al. Clinical implications of large vegetations in infectious endocarditis. Arch Intern Med 1983;143:1874.

54. Buda AJ, Zotz RJ, LeMire MS, et al. Prognostic significance of vegetations detected by two-dimensional echocardiography in infective endocarditis. Am Heart J 1986;112:1291.

55. Lutas EM, Roberts RB, Devereux RB, et al. Relation between the presence of echocardiographic vegetations and the complication rate in infective endocarditis. Am Heart J 1986;112:107.

7

Right Ventricle

Unlike the left ventricle (LV), which is almost symmetrical and ellipsoidal in shape, the right ventricle (RV) is so irregular in shape that it does not conform to any simple geometric contour and not even to any combination of geometric shapes. The RV chamber "wraps around" the front of the LV. It consists of an inflow tract into which the tricuspid valve opens and an outflow tract (also called the *infundibular* or *conus portion*) that opens into the pulmonary trunk through the pulmonic valve. Between the inflow and the outflow areas, the central RV chamber is sometimes referred to as the *body* of the RV; others call this the *apical* RV region.

EXTERNAL RV ANATOMY

When looked at from the side, the RV shape is roughly triangular, a large, gently convex anterosuperior surface and a flat inferior surface meeting at a sharp angle (acute or anteroinferior margin of the heart). Both these surfaces are lined by visceral pericardium and are in contact with the parietal pericardium. The left pleura and lung intervene between the anterosuperior RV wall and the chest wall. The flat inferior wall rests on the diaphragm. The ventricular septum forms the left and posterior walls of the RV chamber, and normally, the septum is convex toward the RV cavity.

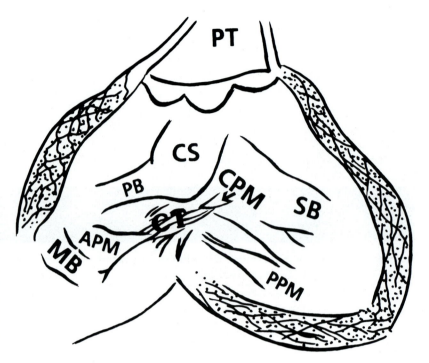

Figure 7–1. Diagram showing the interior of the RV chamber after the RV anterior wall has been cut open and the walls spread out (CS, crista supraventricularis; PB, parietal band; SB, septal band; CPM, conus papillary muscle; APM, anterior papillary muscle; PPM, posterior papillary muscle; MB, moderator band; CT, chordae tendinae; PT, pulmonary trunk; PV, pulmonary valve).

INTERNAL RV ANATOMY

The infundibulum of the RV, developed from the bulbus cordis part of the primitive embryonic heart, has a smooth internal surface. Above, it opens through the pulmonary valve into the pulmonary trunk. At its lower boundary, a massive, thick myocardial arch called the *crista supraventricularis* (supraventricular crest) bridges the space between upper ventricular septum and the RV anterior wall (Figure 7–1). The crista gives off a large parietal band to the RV free wall and a septal band to the ventricular septum; both are important anatomic landmarks. Anomalous development of these components is an essential element of certain common congenital anomalies, notably tetralogy of Fallot.

The pulmonic valve is superiorly (cephalad) located with reference to the aortic valve by about 1.5 cm. Between the attachments of these two valves is interposed a muscular structure called the *conus muscle* within which runs a collagenous band, the conus ligament (or tendon of the infundibulum), which connects the RV infundibulum and pulmonary annulus to the aortic root, specifically the noncoronary sinus of the latter. Inferiorly, the conus ligament blends with the membranous ventricular septum. The conus muscle and ligament cannot be identified individually in echocardiograms but appear in various two-dimensional (2D) echo views as an echogenic area between the aortic and pulmonic valves.

The inflow area and central body of the right ventricle, including the RV apex, are not smooth internally. They are in fact almost entirely covered by trabeculae or papillary muscles (Figure 7–2). The term *trabeculae,* or *trabeculations,* is commonly used to include muscular ridges or columns as well as myocardial bands, variable in thickness, length, and the extent to which they are in contact with the RV wall or ventricular septum. One such rather constant muscular band is the *moderator band,* which can be considered an extension of the parietal band.

The moderator band crosses the RV cavity from the septum and forms an angle of about 60 degrees with it to the base of the anterior papillary muscle. When originally described in the nineteenth century, it was thought that the function of the moderator band was to prevent overdistension of the RV. Later, it was discovered that this band has an-

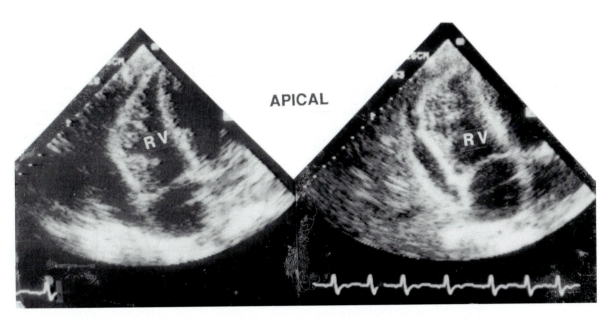

Figure 7–2. Apical four-chamber view in a patient with heavy trabeculation in the RV chamber simulating intraventricular mass lesions.

other important role—it carries the right bundle branch within it. The moderator band is easily and consistently visualized on 2D echo (Figure 7–3); it varies somewhat in thickness and obliquity of direction with respect to the RV long axis, and it is abnormally thick in patients with conspicuous RV hypertrophy. It is attached to the ventricular septum at the junction of its apical and middle thirds, but in this respect too there is a substantial range of variation; rarely, it is double. The moderator band also may give off a trabeculation to the inferior papillary muscle. Branches of the right bundle branch thus convey the cardiac impulse to the papillary muscles slightly in advance of the rest of the RV wall, which is presumably conducive to effective closure of the tricuspid valve in early systole.

The crista supraventricularis can be looked on as being formed by the merging of its septal and parietal bands, thus forming a horseshoe-like "sphincter" (that in reptiles has an important role in controlling pulmonary blood flow). The septal band was mentioned earlier; the parietal band extends across to the tricuspid orifice on the anterior wall, fading out above the level of the anterior papillary muscle. The RV region at and near its apex is sometimes called the *apical recess;* it is even more heavily trabeculated than the rest of the RV chamber.

Permanent pacemaker electrodes are deliberately enmeshed and anchored in these trabeculae, which can be best visualized in apical four-chamber and subcostal four-chamber views. These views are therefore indicated when proper location of pacemaker electrodes is to be ascertained or confirmed. The rare complication of perforation of the electrode wire through the RV wall into the pericardium or through the septum into the LV apical region would be recognized by careful 2D echo scanning of this region.

Extensive trabeculation of the interior of the RV (except for the infundibulum) is an anatomic feature that helps in identifying the "morphologic" RV in certain congenital heart anomalies with ventricular inversion, wherein the morphologic RV is posterior and the morphologic LV is anterior. The LV chamber is much less trabeculated than the RV. Another

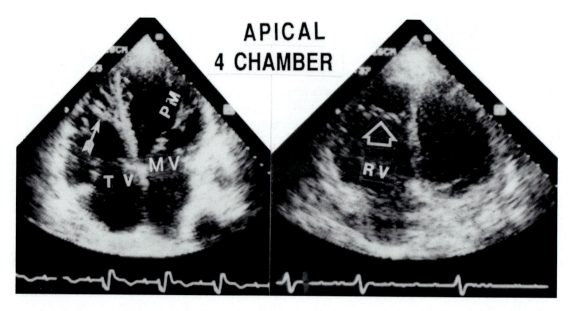

Figure 7–3. Apical four-chamber view of a normal heart (left) and in a dilated RV (right) showing the moderator band (arrows).

echocardiographic aspect of RV trabeculations is that they should not be mistaken for RV mural thrombi. Systolic shortening and thickening of trabeculations serve to distinguish them from thrombi.

RV WALL THICKNESS

The RV wall is only about one-third as thick as the LV wall; 3 to 5 mm is considered the normal range. Pathologists diagnose RV hypertrophy when the RV wall exceeds 5 mm in thickness. Prakash and Matsukubo[2] reported that RV anterior wall thickness of 5 mm or more on M-mode echo, as a criterion of RV hypertrophy, had a sensitivity of 90% and a specificity of 94% (autopsy-echocardiography correlation in 36 patients). They found that RV anterior wall thickness was 3.3 ± 0.6 mm (range 2 to 4 mm) on echocardiography in patients with RV wall thickness of less than 5 mm at autopsy. The latter cutoff point was based on data from several autopsy series. These authors correlated RV wall thickness with RV peak systolic pressure in 75 patients undergoing cardiac catheterization; the end-diastolic RV wall thickness correlated linearly ($r = 0.92$) with the RV systolic pressure; RV wall thickness averaged 3.8 ± 0.9 mm in patients with normal RV pressure.

Normal mean RV wall thickness was 2.4 ± 0.5 mm in the series of Tsuda et al.[3] on parasternal M-mode, and 3.4 ± 0.8 mm in normal subjects studied by M-mode subcostal echocardiography by Matsukubo et al.[4]

In a study correlating RV wall thickness on M-mode echo with RV wall thickness as well as RV mass at autopsy, Baker et al.[5] found that RV wall thickness of greater than 5 mm by echo was 100% specific for anatomic RV hypertrophy. RV mass of greater than 65 g was considered RV hypertrophy; ventricular septum was excluded. However, only 67% of those with anatomic RV hypertrophy had RV wall thickness of greater than 5 mm on echocardiography.

An important practical detail is that the RV wall on M-mode echo is often indistinct or fuzzy so that endocardium and/or epicardium cannot be identified and accurate measurement is not possible. The subcostal approach, using the liver as an ultrasound "window" to the RV, may permit better RV wall definition.

M-MODE RV INTERNAL DIMENSION

During the M-mode echo era (in the 1970s), the only measurable indicator of RV size was the right ventricular internal dimension (RVID), obtained from the left lower parasternal window. It is measured from the RV anterior wall echo to the anterior border of the ventricular septum at the same level that the left ventricular internal dimension (LVID) is measured, i.e., the level of the mitral chordae tendineae. The RVID on M-mode echo has been widely included as a routine measurement in the echocardiogram report since those early years. However, the RVID is not a very reliable parameter of RV size for many reasons:

1. The RV anterior wall echo is often ill-defined.
2. RV trabeculations, tricuspid chordae, or septal papillary muscles produce echoes that can be mistaken for the anterior septal border.
3. Since the RV shape in short axis is crescentic or hemispherical, the ultrasound beam can transect it at its central widest plane or near its narrower periphery, with resulting wide variation in RVID.
4. The RVID is larger when the patient is in the left lateral than in the flat supine position because in the former the beam transverses the RV more obliquely. Since, in actual practice, patients have echocardiography in various decubitus positions in between supine and full left lateral, there is no easy way to correct for this factor.
5. The M-mode ultrasound beam usually transverses the RV outflow rather than the RV inflow region; RVID might not truly reflect RV size if RV dilatation is nonuniform.

2D ECHO OF THE RV

The RV chamber is best visualized in a combination of the following views: parasternal short-axis, parasternal right inflow, apical four-chamber, and subcostal four-chamber and short-axis (Figure 7-4). In the *parasternal short-axis view,* the normal RV chamber appears as a crescentic cavity clasping the anterior and right aspects of the circular left ventricle. In the *parasternal right heart inflow view,* the RV appears as a somewhat triangular chamber (Figure 7-5) with its base inferiorly at tricuspid valve level and its blunted apex pointing upward and to the left; the right atrial (RA) chamber lies below and to the right. In the *apical four-chamber view,* the RV is represented by a triangular space alongside the LV chamber, the apex of the triangle near the LV apex and its base formed by the tricuspid annulus and valve. In the *subcostal four-chamber view,* only the inflow tract is seen as a small triangular space posterior to the liver and anterior to the left ventricle.

In a *high parasternal short-axis view* or in a *subcostal short-axis view* transecting the aortic valve, the entire length of the RV from tricuspid valve to pulmonic valve is depicted, winding round the anterior half of the aortic root. The RV outflow tract is particularly well appreciated in this view, as well as the pulmonic valve and pulmonary trunk (see Chapter 1).

RV contours in various views, with and without RV dilatation, are shown in Figure 7-4. Mild RV dilatation manifests as a modest widening of RV space, with retention of the general shapes of the RV, LV, and ventricular septum. Marked RV dilatation (Figures 7-6 to 7-8) produces much RV widening with alteration of RV contour from roughly triangular to biconvex or even nearly spherical; the LV becomes narrow or even slitlike in extreme cases. The ventricular septum, normally convex toward the RV, becomes flat and in more severe instances convex toward the LV cavity. In apical views it becomes evident that a massively dilated RV displaces the LV from the cardiac apex, pushing the diminu-

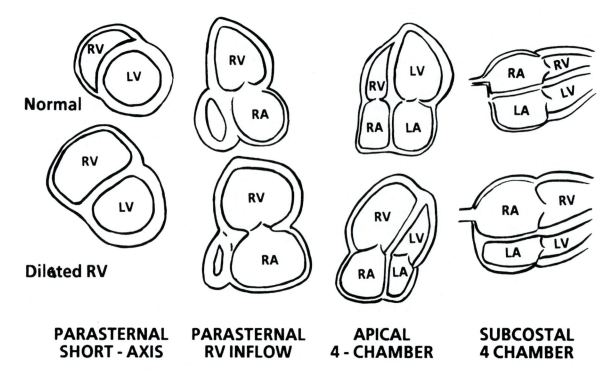

PARASTERNAL SHORT - AXIS **PARASTERNAL RV INFLOW** **APICAL 4 - CHAMBER** **SUBCOSTAL 4 CHAMBER**

Figure 7–4. Diagram showing various 2D echo views in normal subjects (above) and in patients with RV and RA dilatation (below) showing the alteration in configuration of all four chambers.

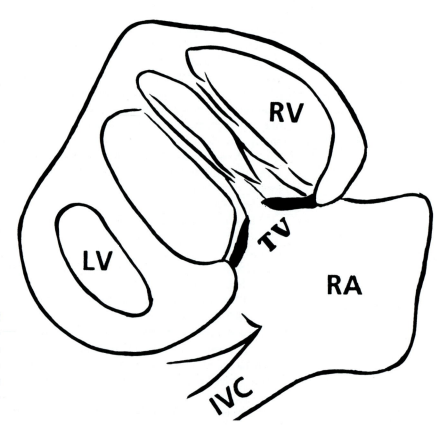

Figure 7–5. Diagram showing right heart inflow view. The IVC is seen entering the right atrium (RA). The tricuspid valve (TV) is well seen opening into the right ventricle (RV). In this view the LV chamber is very attenuated or not seen at all.

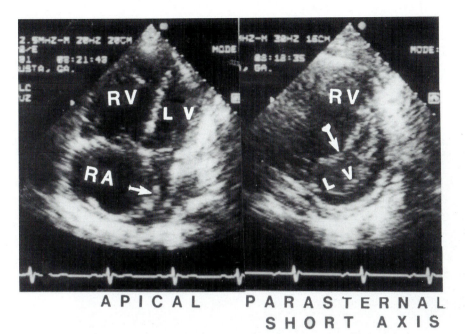

Figure 7–6. Apical four-chamber view (left) and parasternal short-axis view (right) showing marked dilatation of right ventricle (RV) and atrium (RA). Arrows indicate conspicuous bulging of the atrial and ventricular septum toward the left atrium and left ventricle, respectively. The patient had severe chronic pulmonary hypertension (PA pressure 90 mmHg) of thromboembolic etiology.

tive LV chamber to a left posterior position so that the dilated RV forms the entire anterior ventricular surface (see Figures 7-6 and 7-7).

Normal M-Mode RV Internal Dimensions

The first M-mode data on normal RV dimensions (based on 26 adults) were presented by Popp et al.[6]: mean 15 ± 3.9 mm, range 5 to 21 mm. Feigenbaum's normal values, widely used for two decades,[7] for RVID (end-diastolic) were RVID (flat supine): 7 to 23 mm (mean 15 mm), 4 to 14 mm (mean 9 mm) per square meter of body surface area; and RVID (left lateral): 9 to 26 mm (mean 17 mm), 4 to 14 mm (mean 9 mm) per square meter of body surface area.

Normal 2D Echo RV Dimensions

Bommer et al.[8] measured RV dimensions on the 2D echo in 50 normal subjects in the apical four-chamber view. In 8 of them the dimensions were validated from casts of the right heart made from autopsy specimens. Their normal values were RV maximum short-axis: mean 35 ± 2 mm; RV middle short-axis: mean 28 ± 2 mm; and RV area: 18 ± 1.2 cm². Weyman's normal statistics, published in 1982,[9] were as follows:

	Mean (mm)	Range (mm)
Parasternal short-axis view		
RVID (end-diastolic) largest dimension	31 ± 4	25–38
Apical four-chamber view		
RV length, largest dimension	67 ± 6	58–78
RV short axis, largest dimension	29 ± 4	22–36
RV short axis, middle RV level	26 ± 3	20–32
RV area	18.6 cm²	12–22.7 cm²
High short-axis (RV outflow) view		
RV dimension in sagittal plane	27 ± 4	19–22
Pulmonary annulus plane (just below pulmonic valve)	18 ± 2	11–22

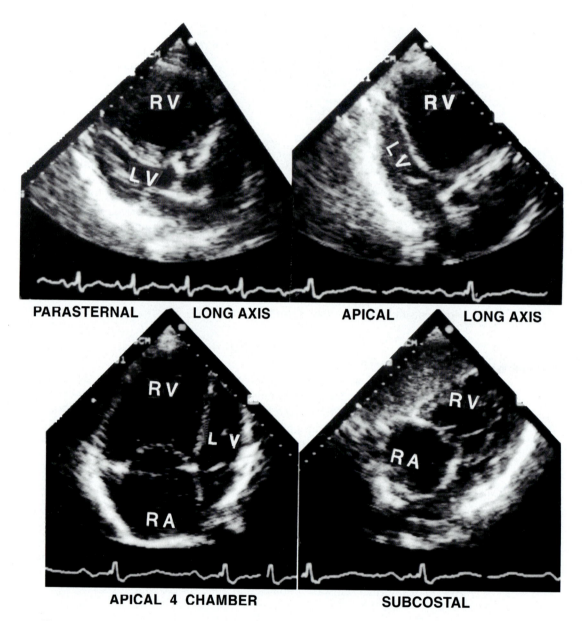

Figure 7–7. Extreme RV and RA dilatation in a patient with severe pulmonary hypertension in parasternal and long-axis views (above, left), apical long-axis view (above, right), apical four-chamber view (below, left) and subcostal four-chamber view (below, right). The LV chamber is reduced in size to a narrow wedge or slit.

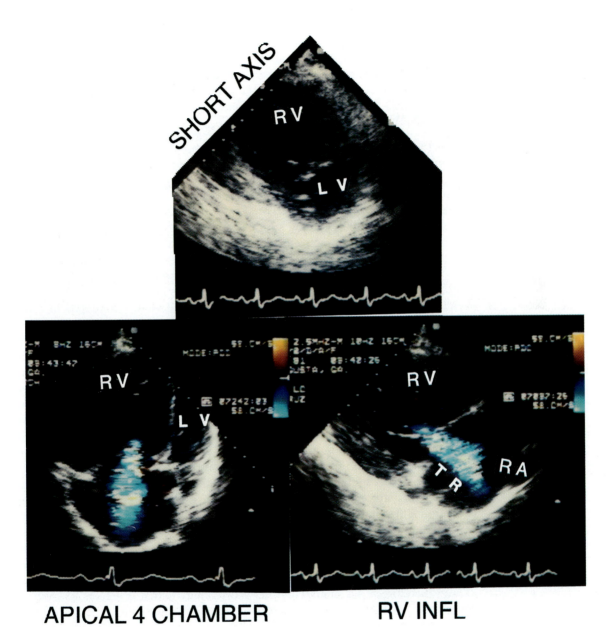

APICAL 4 CHAMBER   **RV INFL**

Figure 7–8. Parasternal short-axis view (above), apical four-chamber view (below, left), and right ventricular inflow view (below, right) showing severe RV dilatation due to cor pulmonale. The tricuspid regurgitant (TR) jet is well seen.

RV VOLUME ESTIMATION

Any attempt to obtain a reliable valid volume estimation of the RV chamber meets with several formidable difficulties:

1. The RV has a complex and asymmetrical shape.
2. Severe RV dilatation is associated with change in shape. Thus geometric formulas for normal RV shape may not be valid for a very dilated RV.
3. RV endocardium is often difficult to identify in a stop frame because of poor acoustic windows or heavy RV trabeculation.
4. It is difficult to standardize the RV planes to be imaged.
5. It is difficult to obtain two orthogonal 2D echo views for valid volume calculations.

Before the 2D echo era, angiographers attempting RV volume estimation struggled with the problem of how best to mathematically represent RV shape.[10] Thus assumptions were made by different groups that the RV was like a pyramid,[11] like stacks of cylinders,[12] like segments of an ellipsoid, etc.

Likewise, several groups endeavored to devise a 2D echo method for estimating RV volume during the 1980s, "fitting" various combinations of geometric shapes to RV chamber shape.[13-18] The merits and shortcomings of these different methods or formulas were well discussed by Levine et al.[14] This latter group imaged the RV in apical four-chamber view and subcostal RV outflow view. Actual volumes of casts of the RV in 12 autopsy hearts were correlated with area-length measurements in these two views. Cast volumes correlated with the formula volume = $\frac{2}{3} \times$ area in one view $\times$ long axis in other view. Further discussion of the topic here would be out of place because of its theoretical complexity, the lack of agreement on method, and the fact that RV volume estimation is seldom, if ever, done in clinical practice (except perhaps in certain research projects).

In view of the technical difficulties in obtaining an accurate, scientifically valid RV volume by 2D echo, it has been suggested that a practically useful idea of RV size might be attained by the simple expedient of planimeterizing the maximal RV area in the apical four-chamber view or even measuring the maximal minor axis dimension in the same view (Figure 7–9). The decrease in RV area (Figure 7–10) from end-diastole to end-systole, divided by end-diastolic area, could be used as a very rough approximation of RV ejection fraction, particularly if the normal range with mean ± 2 SD have been established in that laboratory. Much care must be taken to record the maximal RV area; i.e., the transducer is tilted in an anteroposterior arc until the maximal RV length is obtained and then is rotated around its long axis to image the RV chamber at its widest.

Yet another simple way to assess RV systolic performance was described by Kaul et al.,[17] who measured the systolic excursion of the tricuspid annulus toward the transducer in the apical four-chamber view by placing the M-mode cursor through the tricuspid annulus region (see Figure 7–10). This method reflects long-axis systolic shortening of the RV and therefore of RV contraction. Its shortcoming is that it detects RV systolic shortening in the RV long axis only, whereas RV short-axis shortening is of greater magnitude and contributes more to RV ejection fraction. Foale et al.[18] attempted another simple approach by measuring RV length and various transverse dimensions in apical four-chamber and parasternal right heart inflow views.

RV ENLARGEMENT

The numerous causes of RV dilatation fall into one of the following categories:

1. Pressure RV overload
2. Volume RV overload
3. RV myocardial impairment

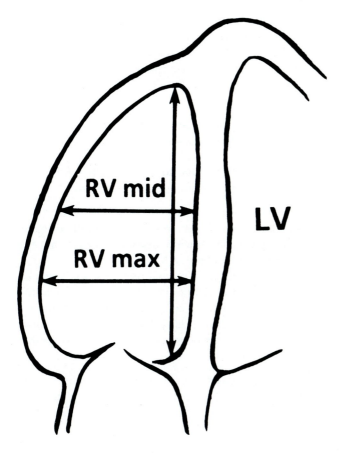

Figure 7–9. Diagram showing RV chamber in apical four-chamber view showing how RV dimensions (length, middle transverse, and maximal transverse) are measured.

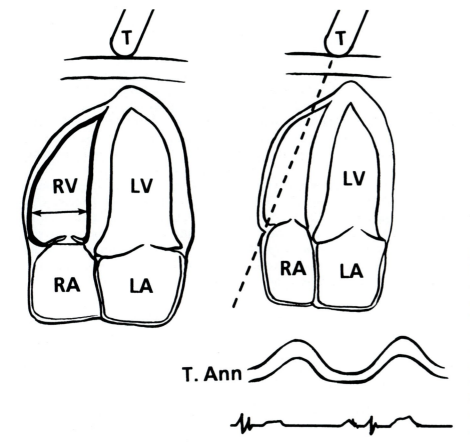

Figure 7–10. Diagram of apical four-chamber view showing how certain RV measurements are made. At left, the RV maximum transverse dimensions (arrows) and RV area (thick line) are shown. At right, the M-mode cursor is directed through the lateral (right) margin of the tricuspid annulus so that the shortening of the LV length (excursions of tricuspid annulus) are recorded on M-mode.

RV pressure overload is due to pulmonary hypertension of any cause or to pulmonary stenosis (RV outflow obstruction below, at, or above the pulmonic valve). Volume overload is due to tricuspid valve regurgitation, pulmonic valve regurgitation, or left-to-right atrial-level shunts. Whereas increased RV chamber size is the rule in moderate to severe pressure as well as volume overload, certain important anatomic and echocardiographic differences are worth noting:

1. RV anterior wall hypertrophy (thickness greater than 5 mm) is the rule in patients with significant RV pressure overload but is absent in pure RV volume overload.
2. In the short-axis view, the ventricular septum is flat, sometimes called the *D sign* because LV shape resembles the letter D rather than the letter O (normal).

In RV pressure overload, this flat septal contour persists in systole as well as diastole. King et al.[19] and Watanabe[20] studied this abnormality quantitatively and found that the change in septal curvature was proportional to the degree of RV hypertension.

In RV volume overload, the systolic septal contour is normal or almost so, but in diastole (especially early diastole), the septum becomes flat or even convex toward the LV. The abrupt change in septal curvature at onset of systole is responsible for the paradoxical systolic septal motion so characteristic of atrial septal defect and severe tricuspid regurgitation.[21] However, this factor may not be the only cause of abnormal septal motion in RV volume overload.[22]

3. RV pressure overload also can be differentiated from volume overload by Doppler estimation of the RV-RA systolic gradient from tricuspid regurgitant jet velocity.

Right Ventricular Dilatation

RV dilatation secondary to impaired RV myocardial function is encountered in several cardiac entities:

RV Infarction.

RV infarction is common, accompanying LV posteroinferior myocardial infarction. Clinical, ECG, and hemodynamic features of RV infarction are frequently (but not always) present.[23-26] The usual 2D echo manifestation is RV dilatation. Paradoxical septal motion and diastolic bulging of the ventricular septum into the LV chamber have been described.[23,24] Regional or selective RV wall motion abnormalities are visualized less commonly, perhaps because they are less diligently sought than LV wall motion abnormalities (Figure 7–11).

As might be expected, severe coronary disease of the right or circumflex coronary artery causing RV infarction also may cause LV wall motion abnormalities. Idiopathic dilated cardiomyopathy typically manifests with diffuse hypokinesis of RV as well as LV chambers. On the other hand, coronary artery disease commonly spares the anterior or lateral RV walls so that it is the rule in so-called ischemic cardiomyopathy for these RV segments to contract well in contrast to generalized LV hypokinesis. This is an important noninvasive means of distinguishing "ischemic" from dilated congestive cardiomyopathy.

Uhl's Anomaly.

This rare and peculiar condition was first described by Uhl in 1952.[27] In the same year, a similar case was reported in the *New England Journal of Medicine.*[28] About 50 instances had been described by 1981, and approximately half the patients survived to adult life.

This anomaly is characterized by total or almost total absence of RV myocardium, especially in the RV inflow area. The RV wall is "parchment-thin," consisting of nothing but endocardium and fibrous tissue. The basic hemodynamic abnormality is ineffective RV

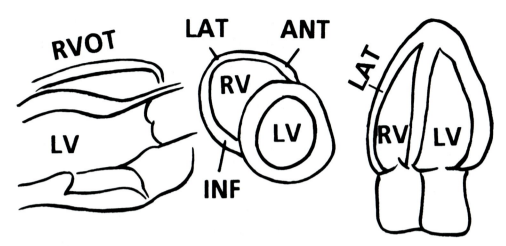

RV REGIONAL WALL SEGMENTS

Figure 7–11. Diagram showing a simple way to designate RV wall segments in parasternal long-axis view (left), parasternal short-axis view (center), and apical four-chamber view (right) (RVOT, right ventricular outflow tract; LAT, lateral; INF, inferior; ANT, anterior).

contraction so that the RV serves as a conduit for blood rather than a pumping chamber. Vigorous septal contraction and a dilated hypertrophic RA attempt to compensate for the inert RV.

On 2D echo,[29-32] the RV and RA are dilated. The RV wall is akinetic and thin, whereas the ventricular septum shows vigorous paradoxical motion. The tricuspid valve appears normal (excluding Ebstein's anomaly) and TR jet velocity is normal (excluding pulmonary hypertension); the LV appears normal.

Arrhythmogenic RV Dysplasia (ARVD). Some believe that this form of heart disease is a partial form of Uhl's anomaly, but whereas the parachment-thin RV wall, devoid of myocardium, in the latter entity is electrically inert, ARVD is characterized by ventricular tachycardia originating from the RV. RV dilatation on 2D echo has been the rule in reported series.[33-35] Regional hyperkinesis or akinesis of part of the RV lateral wall or irregular scalloping (small outpouches) has been demonstrated in the apical four-chamber view in a few cases.[36] The disease is apparently much more common in Europe than in North America.

Ebstein's Anomaly

Wilhelm Ebstein, like Uhl, achieved eponymic immortality by meticulous description of a single autopsied case. It is said to occur in 1 of 20,000 live births and comprises only 0.5% of all congenital heart disease. Nevertheless, it is a major entity for the cardiologist because it is one of the few anomalies that present with sufficient frequency in adult life to be considered in the differential diagnosis of a symptomatic patient with RV dilatation. Although Ebstein's description appeared in 1866, the clinical diagnosis was not achieved until about 1950.

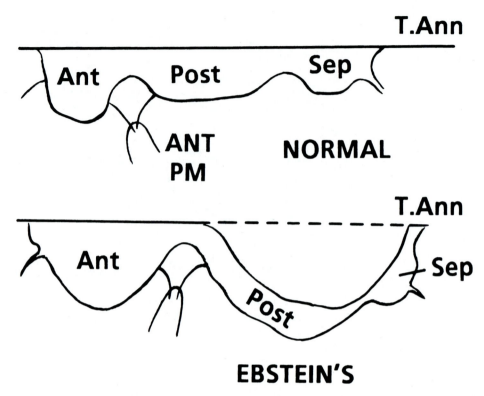

EBSTEIN'S

Figure 7–12. Diagram showing tricuspid annulus and valve stretched horizontally in a normal heart (above) and in Ebstein's anomaly (below) (Ant, anterior leaflet; Post, posterior leaflet; Sep, septal leaflet). The three leaflets are in continuity (through commissures). In Ebstein's anomaly, the anterior leaflet is abnormally large, whereas the posterior and part of posterior leaflet are attached to the RV wall some distance from the tricuspid annulus (T. Ann).

The basic abnormality is displacement of the septal and posterior leaflets of the tricuspid valve downward (Figure 7-12) into the RV chamber.[37-41] The site of maximum displacement is at the commissure between these two leaflets, at the junction of the ventricular septum with the posterior RV wall. A triangular area of RV wall is thus exposed or taken up into the right atrium. In one-third of cases these leaflets are extensively adherent to the RV wall rather than actually displaced. In the other two-thirds the displacement is actual, with no detectable valve tissue on the septum between the true tricuspid annulus and the displaced leaflets (Figure 7-13).

The anterior tricuspid leaflet, though not displaced, is invariably abnormal, often spectacularly so. It is large, perhaps redundant, and sail-like. It is thickened with fibrous strands or even muscular bands in it. It is attached, either by chordae or directly, to a ledge between the inlet and trabecular RV zones and may cover the anterior papillary muscle. Because of the abnormal size and attachments of the anterior leaflet, the latter may in some extreme cases act as a septum in the middle RV, obstructing blood flow (Figure 7-14). Blood entering from the RA can get past the obstruction only at the edges of the leaflet or through perforations in it—an alternative pathway is a right-to-left shunt through an atrial septal defect (ASD) or a patent foramen ovale. A very abnormal anterior leaflet can cause RV outflow obstruction.

The RA is dilated, often enormously. The RV is also often dilated. The "atrialized" upper RV chamber, very variable in extent, is thin-walled. In half the cases, the lower (actual) RV chamber is also abnormally thin. The tricuspid annulus region is abnormally wide.

The genesis of this peculiar anomaly is thought to be failure of the normal delamination process of the inner layers of the inlet zone of the RV, which is responsible for tricuspid valve formation in the embryonic heart.[39] The spectrum of hemodynamic abnor-

EBSTEIN'S ANOMALY

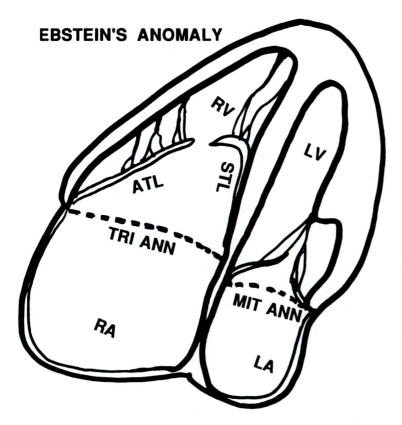

Figure 7–13. Diagram showing apical four-chamber view in a representative patient with Ebstein's anomaly. The septal leaflet of the tricuspid valve is partly fused and partly adherent to the right aspect of the ventricular septum. The anterior leaflet is abnormally large, floppy, and may have abnormal chordal connections to the RV wall. The transverse interrupted lines indicate the tricuspid and mitral annuli (MIT ANN). The RV and RA are dilated.

malities in patients with Ebstein's anomaly is extremely wide so that at one extreme it is fatal in infancy and at the other there have been several reports of patients surviving into the seventh to ninth decades. Tricuspid regurgitation can vary from mild to severe. In a small percentage (10%), the valve is almost imperforate so that tricuspid stenosis is prominent. The right-to-left shunt may be minimal to large so that cyanosis is absent to conspicuous.

The LV chamber is often abnormally small. In patients with corrected transposition, the posterior (morphologic RV) ventricle often has Ebstein's anomaly in this ventricle; this posterior valve is commonly regurgitant with a prominent cleft in the septal leaflet. However, the other valve abnormalities are not as dramatic as with the usual form of the anomaly.

Echocardiography of Ebstein's Anomaly. 2D echo has proved more valuable in the diagnosis of Ebstein's anomaly than in the diagnosis of most other congenital defects.[42-48] This is so because this entity has unique anatomic abnormalities that are easily visualized on 2D echo imaging. In fact, a more reliable and detailed assessment of Ebstein's anomaly can be made by echocardiography than by cardiac catheterization and angiocardiography.

M-mode echo was found useful in diagnosing Ebstein's anomaly in the 1970s.[49-52] Some of the findings, such as RV dilatation and abnormal septal motion, were nonspecific; the most valuable M-mode criteria for Ebstein's were (1) delayed tricuspid valve closure (tricuspid closure following mitral closure by 30 to 70 ms) and (2) the ability to simultaneously record the mitral and tricuspid valve motions easily from the left parasternal area well to the left of the sternal border.

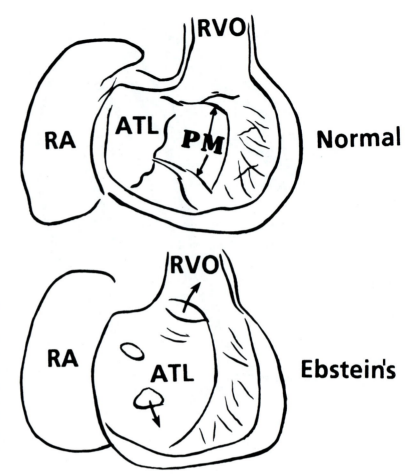

Figure 7–14. Diagram showing anterior tricuspid leaflet (ATL) attached to papillary muscles and interior of RV chamber in normal subjects (above) and in some patients with Ebstein's anomaly (below). In the latter situation, the large anterior leaflet is tethered to the RV wall abnormally, occluding the valve orifice to a large extent and only permitting transvalvar flow at its edges or perforations (RVO, right ventricular outflow tract).

Of the *2D echo* findings, the most important is "displacement of the septal leaflet inferiorly" (toward the RV apex). Normally, the tricuspid septal leaflet is a few millimeters closer to the apex than the anterior mitral leaflet at their septal attachment in the apical four-chamber view, but in Ebstein's anomaly, the septal tricuspid leaflet is displaced 7 to 50 mm (from the tricuspid annulus baseline). The Mayo Clinic group found septal displacements up to 10 mm in normal subjects and up to 15 mm in patients with ASD or severe tricuspid regurgitation. However, the same group found that a septal leaflet inferior displacement exceeding 8 mm/m^2 of body surface area was diagnostic of Ebstein's anomaly. In 5 of 41 patients with Ebstein's anomaly, the septal leaflet was absent on 2D echo.[44]

Leaflet tethering of the anterior or septal leaflet to the adjacent RV wall or septum is another finding detectable on careful 2D echo imaging and correlated with the autopsy finding of anomalous chordae causing such pseudodisplacement; this is distinguishable from true displacement, wherein the septal leaflet is not merely tethered but is very closely adherent to subjacent myocardium. Such aberrant chordal connections are important to the surgeon in deciding between valvoplasty and valve replacement.

The anterior tricuspid leaflet is usually thickened, a nonspecific abnormality, but what is unique to Ebstein's anomaly is impressive elongation and redundancy that results in a whiplike motion.

Certain other 2D echo abnormalities in Ebstein's anomaly are worthy of mention but are also present in other entities presenting with RV dilatation in adult patients, such as ASD and severe tricuspid regurgitation:

1. Dilatation of the tricuspid annulus to 1.5 times or more the size of the mitral annulus (however, a 2 to 2.5 times ratio was almost diagnostic of Ebstein's anomaly)
2. RV dilatation, especially of the RV outflow tract, best seen in parasternal short-axis view at the aortic valve level
3. Augmented tricuspid annulus systolic motion
4. Distortion and diminution of the LV chamber, attributable to RV enlargement
5. Mitral valve prolapse, possibly secondary to LV chamber narrowing

Continuous-wave Doppler of tricuspid regurgitation indicates normal RV systolic pressure. Colorflow Doppler reveals a variable degree of tricuspid regurgitation and origin of the jet within the RV (due to valve displacement) rather than at annulus level.

In conclusion, echocardiography has much to contribute diagnostically in adult patients presenting with symptoms of heart failure and RV dilatation:

1. Unique anatomic and colorflow Doppler findings typical of ASD or of Ebstein's anomaly permit reliable diagnosis of these entities.
2. Severe tricuspid regurgitation is obvious on colorflow Doppler; paradoxical septal motion and conspicuous systolic reflux into the IVC are the rule.
3. Severe pulmonary hypertension is associated with flat septal contour on short axis (D sign); an abnormally thick RV wall and high-velocity TR jet reflect a high RV-RA gradient. It must be added that severe pulmonary hypertension always results in some TR, often moderate to severe TR, so that the hemodynamic situation becomes that of combined RV pressure and volume overload.
4. If none of the preceding echo features are detectable in a patient with definite RV enlargement, RV infarction should be considered if ECG and other clinical findings suggest myocardial infarction, arrhythmogenic RV dysplasia should be considered if ventricular ectopy of a RV origin is present, and Uhl's anomaly should be considered as a remote possibility after all others are excluded.

Ventricular Interaction or Interdependence

This term refers to the mechanisms involved in pathophysiology whereby alteration in pressure or volume or both in one ventricle affects the normal functioning of the other ventricle.[53,54] Bernheim[55] in 1910 postulated that gross LV hypertrophy or enlargement could produce right-sided heart failure because of impaired RV filling secondary to excessive bulging of the ventricular septum into the RV chamber.

Since then, the topic has been studied extensively in animals by various experimental techniques, from those of Henderson and Prince[56] in 1914 to those of Stool et al.[57] in 1975. The advent of echocardiography made it possible to ascertain the position of the ventricular septum and ventricular shape during the various experimental maneuvers.

Dilatation of the RV with leftward displacement of the ventricular septum can be produced acutely by the Müller's maneuver (forced inspiration against a closed glottis).[58] A *reverse Bernheim syndrome* refers to impairment of LV function by extreme RV dilatation; it was suggested by Dexter[59] to explain hemodynamic evidence indicating LV failure in patients with atrial septal defect. Thus, in ASD, LV ejection fraction may be reduced even though LV myocardium contractility is normal. Obviously, the same could apply to other congenital cardiac defects associated with huge RV dilatation[60] and a small LV chamber. In adult cardiology, severe RV dilatation associated with cor pulmonale, Eisenmenger's syndrome, primary pulmonary hypertension, etc. may compress and distort the LV chamber to a narrow or even slitlike configuration. The pericardium, by limiting cardiac expansion, has an important role in determining how RV dilatation can reduce LV size and diastolic filling.[61] Significant changes in RV shape occur; from a somewhat triangular-crescentic chamber, it tends to become spherical.

RV dilatation, especially if accompanied by pulmonary hypertension, can have an impact on LV function in several ways: (1) by compression and distortion of the LV through changes in RV diastolic volume and geometry, (2) by increased RV diastolic pressures, exceeding LV diastolic pressures, causing the ventricular septum to bulge into the LV, and impairing its filling, and (3) by pulmonary hypertension associated with marked prolongation of RV systole so that TR is seen on colorflow Doppler even beyond LV isovolumic relaxation and mitral valve opening, thus interfering with early LV filling.

RV dilatation is a prominent feature of many other congenital cardiac anomalies encountered in adults: (1) pulmonary stenosis (at the infundibular, valvar, or supravalvar level), (2) atrial septal defect and other atrial-level left-to-right shunts, including anomalous pulmonary venous drainage into the right atrium, (3) Eisenmenger's syndrome, severe pulmonary hypertension complicating a congenital septal defect or patent ductus, and (4) tetralogy of Fallot, double-outlet RV transposition of great vessels, and related anomalies. Salient features of Fallot's tetralogy are shown in Figure 7-15.

Acquired RV dilatation is commonly due to chronic cor pulmonale, i.e., pulmonary hypertension resulting from lung disease of various etiologies. Acute or subacute RV dilatation following pulmonary embolism is a valuable sign in assessment of the latter common condition; chronic thromboembolic pulmonary hypertension or primary pulmonary hypertension can result in very impressive RV dilatation (see Figure 7-6).

RV MASSES

The echocardiographic literature contains many case reports of metastatic RV masses originating from a variety of primary neoplastic sites, including carcinoma of the skin, cervix, or rectum; lymphomas; hepatoma; melanoma; etc.[62-68] In some of these, the RV mass has interfered with RV function by (1) causing RV outflow obstruction,[63,66] (2) involving and immobilizing tricuspid leaflets, and (3) filling most of the RV cavity by its very bulk, displacing blood.

The presence of RV outflow obstruction can be diagnosed by Doppler techniques. If the mass is mistaken for myocardium, septal hypertrophy can be simulated. Opacification of the RV chamber by contrast microbubbles may reveal small masses not otherwise seen clearly.[68]

Primary RV neoplasms such as myxomas or rhabdomyomas had been detected even as early as the M-mode era.[69] Hemangiomas of the heart are rare, with only 40 cases recorded in world literature until 1993.[71] Only a very few of these have been detected on 2D echo,[70,71] appearing as a cystic (sonolucent) or partly cystic RV mass. Other such round sonolucent intracardiac masses to be considered in the differential diagnosis include benign cyst, hydatid cyst, cystic myxoma, and lipoma.

Another rare benign mass is that of ectopic thyroid tissue, which for an unknown reason has a predilection for the RV and in particular the right side of the ventricular septum. Only 12 cases have been reported until 1993[72]; an RV mass was visualized in 4 patients.[72-75] Several of the well-documented patients have had RV outflow tract obstruction. Rare instances of spectacular nonneoplastic masses protruding into the RV chamber from the myocardium include that of a dissecting intramyocardial hematoma[76] and of a hydatid cyst.[77]

RV Thrombi

Mobile clots in transit from the IVC to the lungs might get entrapped or snagged among chordae or trabeculations. Mural thrombi (Figure 7-16) are rare, apart from those attached to pacemaker leads (Figure 7-17) or complicating RV infarction. Calcified RV thrombi have been reported.[78]

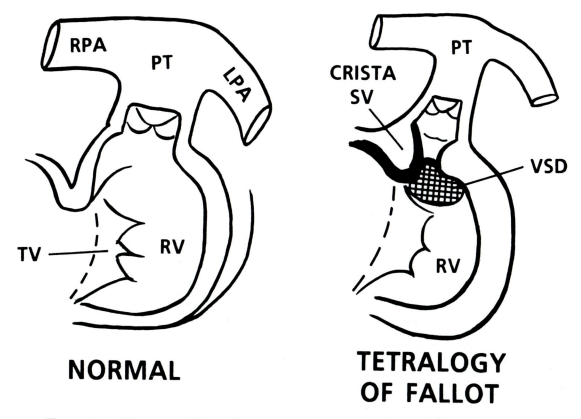

Figure 7–15. Diagram of RV outflow anatomy in normal subjects (left) and in tetralogy of Fallot (right). In the latter, the RV outflow tract is narrower, and infundibular stenosis is caused by a hypertrophied crista supraventricularis (CRISTA SV) and its parietal band. The site of the ventricular septal defect (VSD) is shown (hatched area). The pulmonary trunk and arteries are also small.

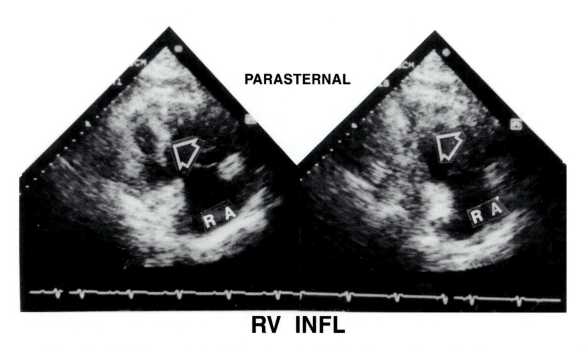

Figure 7–16. Right ventricular inflow views in slightly different planes showing a mass in the RV chamber near its apex, presumably a thrombus. The patient had dilated cardiomyopathy (Ejection fraction 25%) and documented pulmonary embolism.

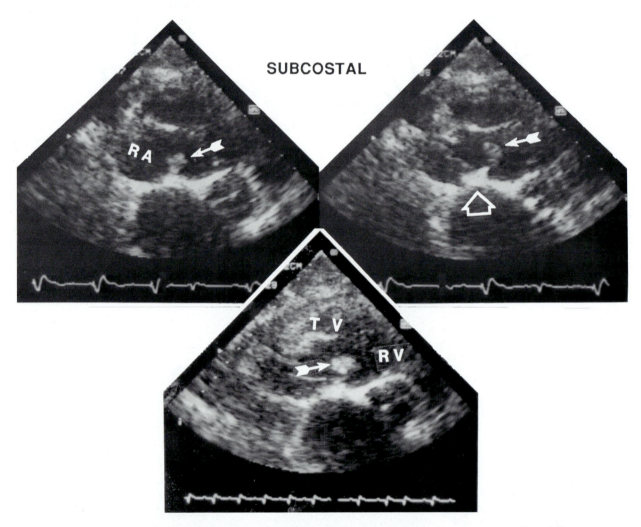

Figure 7–17. Subcostal views of a patient with a pacemaker showing a small mobile thrombus (thin arrow) attached to the pacemaker lead (open arrow). The thrombus was no longer seen on repeat echo a few days later.

REFERENCES

1. St. John Sutton M, Oldershaw PJ. Textbook of Adult and Pediatric Echocardiography and Doppler. Boston: Blackwell, 1989, p 161.
2. Prakash R, Matsukubo H. Usefulness of echocardiographic right ventricular measurements in estimating right ventricular hypertrophy and right ventricular systolic pressure. Am J Cardiol 1983;51:1036.
3. Tsuda T, Sawayama T, Kawai N, et al. Echocardiographic measurement of right ventricular wall thickness in adults by anterior approach. Br Heart J 1980;44:55.
4. Matsukubo H, Matsuura T, Endo N, et al. Echocardiographic measurement of right ventricular wall thickness: A new application of subxiphoid echocardiography. Circulation 1977;56:278.
5. Baker BJ, Scovil JA, Kane JJ, et al. Echocardiographic detection of right ventricular hypertrophy. Am Heart J 1983;105:611.
6. Popp RL, Wolfe SB, Hirata T, et al. Estimation of right and left ventricular size by ultrasound. Circulation 1969;24:523.
7. Feigenbaum H. Echocardiography, 4th ed. Philadelphia: Lea & Febiger, 1986, pp 163, 622.
8. Bommer W, Weinert L, Neumann A, et al. Determination of right atrial and right ventricular size by two-dimensional echocardiography. Circulation 1979;60:91.
9. Weyman AE. Cross-Sectional Echocardiography, 2d ed. Philadelphia: Lea & Febiger, 1994, pp 1291–1294.
10. Goerke RJ, Carlson E. Calculation of right and left ventricular volumes. Invest Radiol 1967;2:360.
11. Ferlinz J, Gorlin R, Cohn PF, et al. Right ventricular performance in patient with coronary artery disease. Circulation 1975;2:608.
12. Gentzler RD, Briselli MF, Gault JH. Angiographic estimation of right ventricular volume in man. Circulation 1974;50:324.
13. Pandidis IP, Ren JF, Kotler MN, et al. Two-dimensional echocardiographic estimation of right ventricular ejection fraction in patients with coronary artery disease. J Am Coll Cardiol 1983;2:911.
14. Levine RA, Gibson TC, Aretz T, et al. Echocardiographic measurement of right ventricular volume. Circulation 1984;69:497.
15. Starling MR, Crawford MH, Sorensen SG, et al. A new two-dimensional echocardiographic technique for evaluating right ventricular performance in patients with obstructive lung disease. Circulation 1982;66:612.
16. Gibson TC, Miller SW, Aretz T, et al. Method for measuring right volume by planes applicable to cross-sectional echocardiography. Am J Cardiol 1985;55:1584.
17. Kaul S, Tei C, Hopkins JM, et al. Assessment of right ventricular function using two-dimensional echocardiography. Am Heart J 1984;107:526.
18. Foale R, Nihoyannopoulos P, McKenna W, et al. Echocardiographic measurement of the normal adult right ventricle. Br Heart J 1986;56:33.
19. King ME, Braun H, Goldblatt A, et al. Interventricular septal configuration as a predictor of right ventricular systolic hypertension in children: A cross-sectional echocardiographic study. Circulation 1983;68:68.
20. Watanabe K. Evaluation of right ventricular pressure by two-dimensional echocardiography. Jpn Heart J 1984;25:523.
21. Weyman AE, Wann S, Feigenbaum H, et al. Mechanism of abnormal septal motion in patients with right ventricular volume overload. Circulation 1976;54:179.
22. Kerber RI, Dippel WF, Abboud FM. Abnormal motion of the interventricular septum in right ventricular volume overload. Circulation 1973;48:86.
23. D'Arcy B, Nanda NC. Two-dimensional echocardiographic features of right ventricular infarction. Circulation 1982;65:167.
24. Jugdutt BI, Sussex BA, Sivaram CA, et al. Right ventricular infarction: Two-dimensional echocardiographic evaluation. Am Heart J 1984;107:505.
25. Lopez-Sendon J, Garcia-Fernandez MA, Coma-Canella I, et al. Segmental right ventricular function after acute myocardial infarction. Am J Cardiol 1983;51:390.
26. Vannucci A, Cecchi F, Zuppiroli A, et al. Right ventricular infarction: Clinical, hemodynamic, mono- and two-dimensional echocardiographic features. Eur Heart J 1983;4:854.
27. Uhl HSM. A previously undescribed congenital malformation of the heart: Almost total absence of the myocardium of the right ventricle. Bull Johns Hopkins Hosp 1952;91:197.

28. Castleman B, Towne VW. Case record of the Massachusetts General Hospital, no 38201. N Engl J Med 1952;246:785.
29. Vecht RJ, Carmichael JS, Gopal R, et al. Uhl's anomaly. Br Heart J 1979;41:676.
30. Hoback J, Adicoff A, From AHL, et al. A report of Uhl's disease in identical adult twins. Chest 1981;79:306.
31. Gaffney FA, Nicod P, Lin JC, et al. Noninvasive recognition of the parchment right ventricle (Uhl's anomaly, arrhythmogenic right ventricular dysplasia) syndrome. Clin Cardiol 1983;6:235.
32. Child JS, Perloff JK, Froncoz R, et al. Uhl's anomaly (parchment right ventricle): Clinical, echocardiographic radionuclear, hemodynamic and angiographic features in 2 patients. Am J Cardiol 1984;53:635.
33. Marcus FI, Fontaine GH, Guirandon G, et al. Right ventricular dysplasia. Circulation 1982;65:384.
34. Rowland E, McKenna WJ, Sugrue D, et al. Ventricular tachycardia of left bundle branch block configuration in patients with isolated right ventricular dilatation. Br Heart J 1984;51:15.
35. Fitchett DH, Sugrue DD, MacArthur CG, et al. Right ventricular dilated cardiomyopathy. Br Heart J 1984;51:25.
36. St. John Sutton M, Oldershaw PJ. Textbook of Adult and Pediatric Echocardiography and Doppler. Boston: Blackwell, 1989, p 166.
37. Yater WM, Shapiro MJ. Congenital displacement of the tricuspid valve (Ebstein's disease). Ann Intern Med 1937;11:1043.
38. Anderson KR, Lie JT. Pathologic anatomy of Ebstein's anomaly of the heart revisited. Am J Cardiol 1978;41:739.
39. Anderson KR, Zuberbuhler JR, Anderson RH, et al. Morphological spectrum of Ebstein's anomaly of the heart: A review. Mayo Clin Proc 1979;54:174.
40. Lev M, Liberthson RR, Joseph RH, et al. The pathologic anatomy of Ebstein's disease. Arch Pathol 1970;90:334.
41. Engle MA, Payne TPB, Bruins C, et al. Ebstein's anomaly of the tricuspid valve: Report of three cases and analysis of clinical syndrome. Circulation 1950;1:1246.
42. Ports TA, Silverman NH, Schiller NB. Two-dimensional echocardiographic assessment of Ebstein's anomaly. Circulation 1978;58:336.
43. Nihoyannopoulos P, McKenna WJ, Smith G, et al. Echocardiographic assessment of the right ventricle in Ebstein's anomaly. J Am Coll Cardiol 1986;8:627.
44. Shiina A, Seward JB, Edwards WD, et al. Two-dimensional echocardiographic spectrum of Ebstein's anomaly: Detailed anatomic assessment. J Am Coll Cardiol 1984;3:356.
45. Matsumoto M, Matsuo H, Nagata S, et al. Visualization of Ebstein's anomaly of the tricuspid valve by two-dimensional and standard echocardiography. Circulation 1976;53:69.
46. Hirschklau MJ, Sahn DJ, Hagan AD, et al. Cross-sectional echocardiographic features of Ebstein's anomaly of the tricuspid valve. Am J Cardiol 1977;40:400.
47. Gussenhoven WJ, Spitaels SEC, Bom N, et al. Echocardiographic criteria for Ebstein's anomaly of tricuspid valve. Br Heart J 1980;43:31.
48. Kambe T, Ischimiya S, Toguchi M, et al. Apex and subxiphoid approaches to Ebstein's anomaly using cross-sectional echocardiography. Am Heart J 1980;100:53.
49. Lundstrom NR. Echocardiography in the diagnosis of Ebstein's anomaly of the tricuspid valve. Circulation 1973;47:597.
50. Farooki ZQ, Henry JG, Green EW. Echocardiographic spectrum of Ebstein's anomaly of the tricuspid valve. Circulation 1976;53:63.
51. Yuste P, Minguez I, Aza V, et al. Echocardiography in the diagnosis of Ebstein's anomaly. Chest 1974;66:273.
52. Daniel W, Rathsack P, Walpurger G, et al. Value of M-mode echocardiography for non-invasive diagnosis of Ebstein's anomaly. Br Heart J 1980;43:38.
53. Bove AA, Santamore WP. Ventricular interdependence. Progr Cardiovasc Dis 1981;23:286.
54. Santamore WP, Lynch PR, Meier GM, et al. Myocardial interaction between the ventricles. J Physiol 1976;41:362.
55. Bernheim PI. De l'asystolie venous dans l'hypertrophie du coeur gauche par stenose concomitante due ventricle droit. Rev Med 1910;39:785.
56. Henderson Y, Prince AL. The relative systolic discharges of the right and left ventricles and their bearing on pulmonary congestion and depletion. Heart 1914;5:217.
57. Stool EW, Mullins CB, Leshin SJ, et al. Dimensional changes of the left ventricle during acute pulmonary arterial hypertension in dogs. Am J Cardiol 1974;33:868.

58. Brinker JA. Leftward septal displacement during right ventricular loading in man. Circulation 1980;61:626.
59. Dexter L. Atrial septal defect. Br Heart J 1956;18:209.
60. Popio KA, Gorlin R, Teichholtz LE, et al. Abnormalities of left ventricular function and geometry in adults with an atrial septal defect. Am J Cardiol 1975;36:302.
61. Shabetai R, Mangiardi L, Bargava V, et al. The pericardium and cardiac function. Progr Cardiovasc Dis 1979;22:107.
62. Steffens TG, Mayer HS, DAS SR. Echocardiographic diagnosis of a right ventricular metastatic tumor. Arch Intern Med 1980;140:122.
63. Norell MS, Sarvasvaran R, Sutton GC. Solitary tumor metastasis: A rare cause of right ventricular outflow tract obstruction and sudden death. Eur Heart J 1984;5:684.
64. Itoh K, Matsubara T, Yanagisawa K, et al. Right ventricular metastasis of cervical squamous cell carcinoma. Am Heart J 1984;108:1369.
65. Moosa YA, Lewis JE. Rare metastatic tumors of the right ventricular cavity. Echocardiography 1989;6:289.
66. Schaefer S, Shohet RV, Nixon JV, et al. Right ventricular obstruction from cervical carcinoma. Am Heart J 1987;113:397.
67. Rey M, Alfonso F, Torrecilla E, et al. Right heart metastatic endocardial implants. Am Heart J 1990;119:1217.
68. Schmidt DR, Johns JP, Linville KW. Detection of intracavitary right ventricular polypoid masses due to metastatic lymphoma using contrast echocardiography. Am Heart J 1990;120:446.
69. Ports TA, Schiller NB, Strunk BL. Echocardiography of right ventricular tumors. Circulation 1977;56:439.
70. Ryan TJ, Aretz TH. A fifteen-year-old girl with a right ventricular mass. N Engl J Med 1983;308:206.
71. Cunningham T, Lawrie GM, Stavinoha J, et al. Cavernous hemangioma of the right ventricle: Echocardiographic-pathologic correlates. J Am Soc Echocardiogr 1993;6:335.
72. Shemin RJ, Marsh JD, Schoen FJ. Benign intracardiac thyroid mass causing right ventricular outflow tract obstruction. Am J Cardiol 1985;56:828.
73. Greco-Lucchina P, Ottino GM, Avonto L, et al. Ectopic thyroid remnants within the myocardium. Am Heart J 1988;115:195.
74. Doria E, Agostoni P, Fiorentini C. Accessory thyroid tissue in the right ventricle. Chest 1989;96:424.
75. Ansani L, Percoco G, Zanardi F, et al. Intracardiac thyroid heterotopia. Am Heart J 1993;125:1797.
76. Mohan JC, Agarwala R, Khanna SK. Dissecting intramyocardial hematoma presenting as a massive pseudotumor of the right ventricle. Am Heart J 1992;124:1641.
77. Limacher MC. Cardiac echinococcal cyst: Diagnosis by two-dimensional echocardiography. J Am Coll Cardiol 1983;2:574.
78. Patel AK, Kronke GM, Heltne CE, et al. Multiple calcified thrombi (rocks) in the right ventricle. J Am Coll Cardiol 1983;2:1224.

8

Pulmonary Valve and Artery

NORMAL ANATOMY

Pulmonary Valve

The pulmonary valve consists of three cusps, two anterior (left and right) and one posterior (Figure 8-1). The valve plane faces superiorly, slightly to the left, and posteriorly. The pulmonary valve lies in a plane above and anterior to that of the aortic valve and is in fact separated by about 1.5 cm from the "fibrous skeleton of the heart" by right ventricular (RV) conus myocardium.

Each cusp is essentially a thin fold of endocardium strengthened by a lamina fibrosa. The latter is thicker near the free edge and at the cusp attachment than in the rest of the cusp. In the center of the free edge of each cusp is a fibrocartilaginous nodule (nodule of Arantius), from which collagen fibers radiate to the cusp periphery (Figure 8-2). On either side of the nodule of Arantius is a narrow strip near the free edge of the cusp, thinner than the rest of the cusp, called the *lunule*. Rarely, a fourth rudimentary cusp is present; bicuspid pulmonary valves are also quite rare.

Clinicians commonly regard the pulmonary valve as being attached to a pulmonary annulus. The word *annulus* implies a circular ringlike structure, and strictly speaking, the pulmonary valve attachment is not ringlike; each cusp is attached to a U-shaped margin. Thus the cusps are attached not to a ring but to three half-ellipses, an arrangement that may be described as coronet-like or tricrenate (see Figure 8-2). From the lowest point of attachment to the free edge, each cusp is about 1.5 cm high.

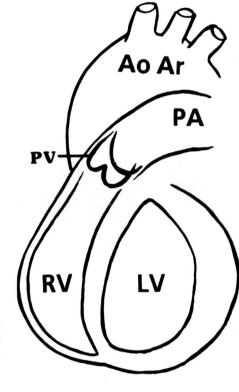

Figure 8–1. Diagram of the heart in sagittal plane to show position of pulmonary valve (PV) with respect to right ventricle (RV) and pulmonary trunk [main pulmonary artery (PA)] (Ao AR, aortic arch).

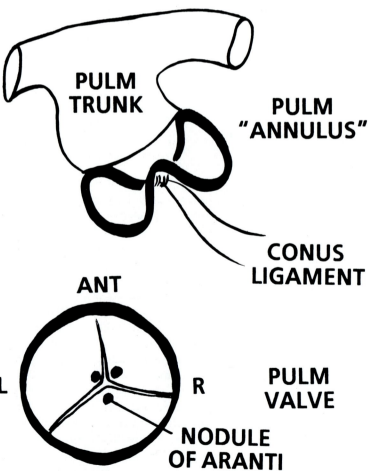

Figure 8–2. (Above) Diagram to show the coronet-like configuration of the pulmonary valve "annulus" interposed between pulmonary trunk and RV outflow tract. The conus ligament connects the pulmonary valve annulus to the aortic valve annulus. (Below) Diagram to show the orientation of the three pulmonary valve cusps, each of which has a small nodular thickening in the center of its free edge.

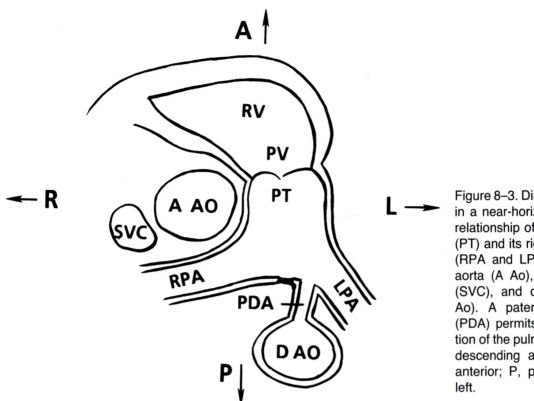

Figure 8–3. Diagrammatic depiction in a near-horizontal plane to show relationship of the pulmonary trunk (PT) and its right and left branches (RPA and LPA) to the ascending aorta (A Ao), superior vena cava (SVC), and descending aorta (D Ao). A patent ductus arteriosus (PDA) permits flow to the bifurcation of the pulmonary trunk from the descending aorta. Orientation: A, anterior; P, posterior; R, right; L, left.

The *pulmonary trunk* (main pulmonary artery) is a short, wide vessel about 5 cm long and 2.5 to 3 cm in caliber. It arises from the RV infundibulum anterior to the ascending aorta and runs backward, upward, and slightly to the left, forming an angle of only 30 degrees with the horizontal. The pulmonary trunk is entirely intrapercardial. Anteriorly, it is related to a thin wedge of left lung and pleura behind the second left intercostal space. The pulmonary trunk is anterior to the ascending aorta at its origin and then to its left; the bifurcation of the pulmonary trunk lies under the concavity of the aortic arch. Posterior to the pulmonary trunk is the left main coronary artery and left atrium. The right and left atrial appendages lie on either side of the pulmonary trunk. Just above the pulmonary trunk is the tracheal bifurcation and tracheobronchial lymph nodes.

The short pulmonary trunk divides into the right and left pulmonary arteries, the former being longer and slightly larger than the latter (Figure 8-3). These two vessels do not run symmetrically; the right pulmonary artery comes off the pulmonary trunk at an angle of about 90 degrees and courses horizontally rightward across the midline to reach the hilum of the right lung. The left pulmonary artery runs in almost the same direction as the pulmonary trunk and then curves upward and posteriorly over the left main bronchus before turning inferiorly to lie in proximity to the left lower lobe bronchus.

The *right pulmonary artery* (Figure 8-4) is related, near its origin, to the ascending aorta, superior vena cava (SVC), and right upper pulmonary vein, all of which are anterior to it. Superior to it is the tracheal bifurcation, and inferior to the right pulmonary artery is the left atrium (Figure 8-5). Posteriorly, it is related to the esophagus and right main bronchus. At the right hilum, the right pulmonary artery bifurcates into a larger lower and smaller upper branch.

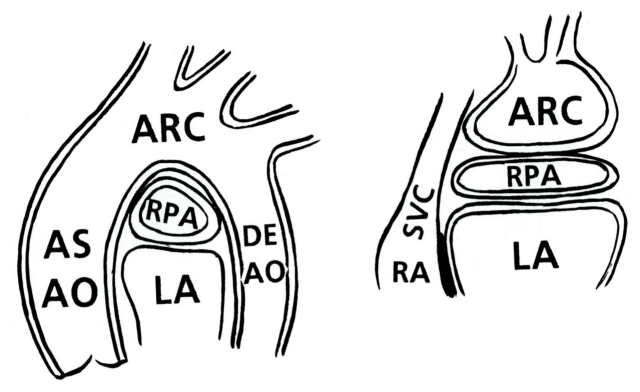

Figure 8–4. Diagram showing relationship of right pulmonary artery (RPA) to aortic arch (ARC) in long-axis of latter (left) and short-axis (right) in suprasternal views (DE Ao, descending aorta; As Ao, ascending aorta; SVC, superior vena cava; LA, left atrium; RA, right atrium).

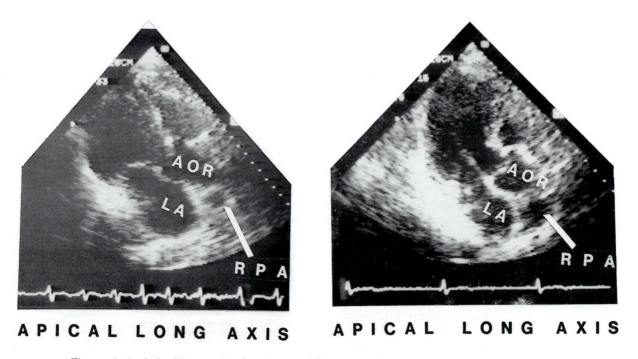

Figure 8–5. Apical long-axis view in two different patients showing the location of the right pulmonary artery (RPA): anterior and above the superior pole (roof) of the left atrium and posterior to the ascending aorta. The lumen of the right pulmonary artery is larger in the patient shown on the right than in the patient shown on the left.

The *left pulmonary artery* descends anterior to the left main bronchus and descending thoracic aorta to reach the hilum of the left lung where it bifurcates. The ligamentum arteriosum (or ductus arteriosus in intrauterine life) is attached at one end to the concavity of the aortic arch and at its other to the left pulmonary artery near the bifurcation of the pulmonary trunk. Immediately to the left of this ligamentum arteriosum, the left recurrent laryngeal nerve loops around the aortic arch, lying between it and the pulmonary artery at this site.

Echocardiography of the Pulmonary Valve and Pulmonary Trunk

In the M-mode echo era, the pulmonary valve echogram was obtained in a "blind" manner, with the transducer directed posteriorly, upward, and to the left from the second or third left intercostal space. Only the posterior leaflet could be visualized as a linear echo that moved posteriorly as the valve opened in systole.

This opening motion is preceded by a small transient posterior dip named the *a* wave; this is the result of the impact of the "atrial kick" on the ventricular surface of the pulmonary valve, causing the latter to bulge briefly into the pulmonary trunk. In the presence of pulmonary hypertension, the atrial kick cannot achieve this effect, so the pulmonary valve *a* wave is absent. On the other hand, in pulmonary valve stenosis, the combination of low pulmonary artery pressure and a powerful atrial kick (due to right atrial hypertrophy) causes an unusually large *a* wave or even premature opening of the pulmonary valve.[1] Other cardiac entities associated with considerably elevated diastolic pressure in the right heart chambers (but normal pulmonary artery pressure) such as severe tricuspid regurgitation, Ebstein's anomaly, and constrictive pericarditis also may manifest exaggerated pulmonary valve *a* waves.

Two-dimensional (2D) echo visualization of the pulmonary valve can be done in one of two ways:

1. In a high parasternal short-axis view containing the aortic valve, the pulmonary valve leaflets are seen as small, mobile echoes slightly above and to the right of the aortic root and interposed between the RV outflow tract and pulmonary trunk.
2. In a subxiphoid near-sagittal short-axis view (Figure 8-6), the configuration of cardiac structures resembling somewhat the parasternal short-axis view, the RV outflow tract–pulmonary trunk appears as a vertical tubular sonolucent space. The pulmonary valve can be detected as a small, mobile echo within this space.

Doppler recordings of flow across the pulmonary valve can be made from each of these windows because, fortunately, the axis of the ultrasound beam is almost the same as the direction of blood flow. The commencement of the pulmonary regurgitant jet helps mark the location of the pulmonary valve (Figure 8-7).

Pulmonary Valve Stenosis

Isolated pulmonary valve stenosis (PVS), unassociated with any other cardiac defects, is of two anatomic types: (1) The common type in adolescents and adults is caused by fusion of the three cusps to form a dome with an orifice of varying diameter at the summit of the dome. The pulmonary annulus and subpulmonic RV outflow tract are of normal size. The pulmonary trunk is usually dilated (poststenotic dilatation), but the dilatation is not proportional to the severity of stenosis. If PVS is severe, the RV may be hypertrophied with increased RV chamber width and flattened ventricular septum. (2) The PVS is similar to that described above, is usually of severe degree, and there is in addition stenosis of the RV outflow (conus region) below the valve because of undue hypertrophy of the myocardium in this region.

In infancy, an additional "hypoplastic" variety of pulmonary stenosis with unduly small pulmonary valve, annulus, and conus RV is common, with unfavorable prognosis. PVS can

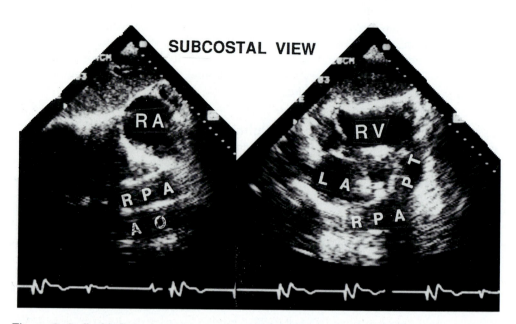

Figure 8–6. (Left) Subcostal views showing relationship of right atrium (RA), right pulmonary artery (RPA), and aortic arch (Ao). (Right) Another plane showing right atrium, right ventricle (RV), pulmonary trunk (PT), and right pulmonary artery (RPA) in continuity.

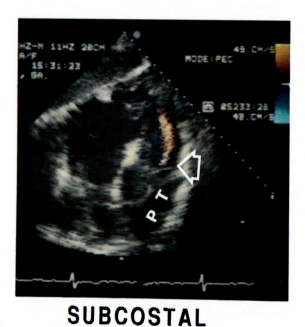

Figure 8–7. Subcostal view with colorflow Doppler showing pulmonary regurgitant jet that starts at the pulmonary valve (arrow) and enters the RV.

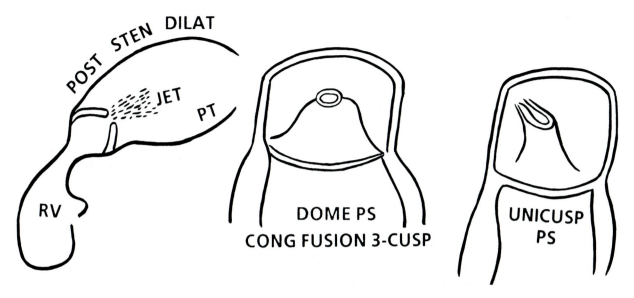

Figure 8–8. Diagram showing features of pulmonary valve stenosis. (Left) Sagittal plane, as projected on angio (lateral) view showing dome-shaped pulmonary valve stenosis between right ventricle (RV) and pulmonary trunk (PT). The latter shows poststenotic dilatation. (Center) Dome-shaped pulmonary valve with small orifice at summit of dome. The stenotic dome results from congenital fusion of a basically three-cusp valve. (Right) Unicuspid pulmonary stenosis, common in infancy.

occur as part of tetralogy of Fallot, transposition of the great vessels, and other complex cyanotic anomalies, in which case the PVS may not be of the domed three-fused-leaflets configuration but bicuspid or unicuspid.

On 2D echo, the normal pulmonary valve cusps move apart at onset of RV ejection, and the valve remains in the fully open position, i.e., the cusps lie parallel and closely applied to the walls of the pulmonary trunk.

In PVS (Figure 8–8), the normal pattern is replaced by an inward curving of the cusps to form a dome.[2] The base of the dome shows more motion than its apex; i.e., the tips of the cusps remain close together, and at this site the stenotic orifice is identified by the high-velocity jet emerging from it (by colorflow Doppler). Continuous-wave Doppler recording of the velocity of the systolic jet thruogh the PVS provides a reliable indicator of the severity of stenosis.[3-5]

Stenosis of the Pulmonary Trunk (Figure 8–9)

Discrete stenosis of the pulmonary trunk can be due to a sclerotic ring or a diaphragm (Figure 8–9); a few instances of this rare anomaly have been documented in children.[6,7] It can be visualized as an abnormal shelf or annular structure within the pulmonary trunk, distal and separate from the pulmonary valve, in the parasternal short-axis or subcostal view.[8] Stenosis of the pulmonary trunk also can take the form of a tubular narrowing of most or all of this vessel; this is usually part of the congenital rubella syndrome and so is often accompanied by valvar aortic or pulmonary stenosis.

Stenosis of the pulmonary artery branches (see Figure 8–9) had long been known as a pathologic curiosity and was demonstrated by cardiac catheterization and angiogra-

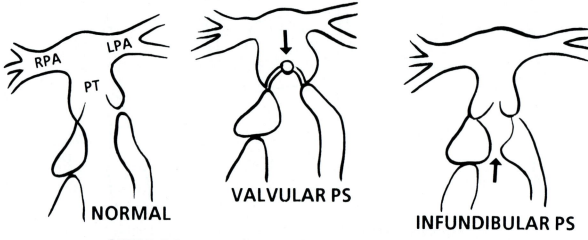

SITES OF PULM (RV OUTFLOW) STENOSIS

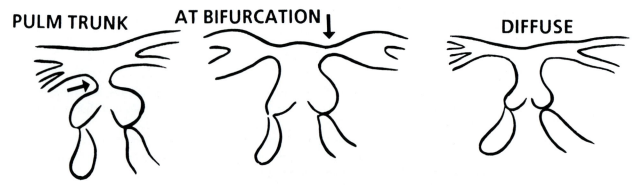

VARIETIES OF PULMONARY ARTERY STENOSIS

Figure 8–9. (Above) Diagram showing normal RV outflow (left), pulmonary valve stenosis (center), and infundibular stenosis (right) (PT, pulmonary trunk; RPA, right pulmonary artery; LPA, left pulmonary artery). (Below) Diagram showing various types of supravalvar pulmonary artery stenosis: at pulmonary trunk level (left), at pulmonary trunk bifurcation (center), the most common type, and diffusely narrow pulmonary artery tree (right).

phy in the 1960s.[9-11] The patient is commonly a child (but occasionally an adult) with a systolic murmur of wide radiation. Severe obstruction to outflow from the right heart is rare.

1. One variety is characterized by local stenosis at or near the bifurcation of the pulmonary trunk with poststenotic dilatation affecting one or both of the main branches. This characteristic angiographic configuration also can be identified on 2D echo[8,12] in the short-axis parasternal view, with the transducer so tilted as to display the pulmonary trunk and its branches to best advantage.

2. In other cases of pulmonary artery branch stenosis, the narrowing is diffuse so that the whole arterial tree appears "spidery" on angiography. In such cases, a quantitative estimation of arterial caliber may be attempted and compared with normal standards.[13] Since the normal range of pulmonary artery caliber in adults of all ages is not established, Tinker et al.[12] used the following 2D echo criteria for diagnosing stenosis of the right or left pulmonary artery:

1. Narrowing by 50% or more of adjacent vessel
2. Right pulmonary artery 25% or less of transverse aortic arch diameter

Poststenotic arterial dilatation, when present, is a useful pointer to the stenosis.

Surgical banding of the pulmonary trunk often was done as palliative therapy in certain infants with defects too complicated to correct directly to reduce torrential pulmonary blood flow. The band is usually placed around the pulmonary trunk at its midlevel, but it can slip or migrate over time, either proximally to near the pulmonary valve or distally to the bifurcation of the artery. On 2D echo, the band is visualized as a dense local constriction[14] of the pulmonary trunk. Although commonly seen in the pediatric domain, survival into adolescence or adult life can occur.

Pulmonary Valve Endocarditis

Bacterial endocarditis of the pulmonary valve accounted for only 1% of autopsy-diagnosed valvar endocarditis until the mid-twentieth century. However, during the last two decades, the following important changes in the clinicopathologic profile of right-sided endocarditis have occurred: (1) Intravenous drug abuse, especially in large urban centers, has sharply increased the incidence of tricuspid and pulmonary valve endocarditis. (2) Formerly in the United States (and even now in countries relatively free of drug addicts), right-sided endocarditis usually occurred in patients with congenital heart disease such as Fallot's tetralogy, pulmonary stenosis, patent ductus arteriosus, etc. Vegetations in such hearts are located on the low-pressure side of the anomalous communication, presumably at the site of endocardial roughening secondary to jet trauma. During the last quarter century, endocarditis on such previously abnormal hearts has been overshadowed by virulent infections afflicting previously normal valves. Concomitantly, *Staphylococcus aureus* has increased in frequency at the expense of *Streptococcus viridans* as the most frequently grown organism from blood cultures in patients with pulmonary valve endocarditis. Despite its rarity, numerous reports of one or two cases (and one series of eight cases from Japan[15]) have established the echocardiographic appearances of pulmonary valve endocarditis.

The M-mode diagnosis was suspected when the normal fine linear pulmonary valve echo was replaced by a thick, "shaggy" echo or a "double" cusp echo.[16] In M-mode echocardiography, only one of the three pulmonary cusps is visualized (the posterior one).

On 2D echo, pulmonary valve vegetations appear as fluffy or irregularly nodular echoes on the pulmonary valve cusps and move along with them.[17-20] Sometimes the vegetations are large and fungating, obscuring cusp structure. Occasionally, the affected cusp becomes flail so that the vegetation on it demonstrates an exaggerated range of motion, prolapsing into the RV outflow tract in diastole. Unlike the other three valves, pulmonary valve endocarditis is very rarely accompanied by a ring (paravalvar) abscess.

Vegetations on the tricuspid and pulmonary valves are often large and friable so that fragments of infected material break off and produce multiple pulmonary emboli. In the patient of Mehlman et al.,[17] a 3-cm pulmonary valve vegetation was found at surgery. The pulmonary manifestations and septicemia may dominate the clinical picture and may or may not respond to antibiotic therapy. In the latter case, surgical resection of the infected valve is the treatment of choice and is well tolerated (at least in short term), even if the valve is not replaced with a prosthetic valve.

The echocardiographic differential diagnosis of pulmonary valve vegetations includes other causes of gross cusp thickening such as congenital valve stenosis or carcinoid disease and benign neoplasms of the valve such as fibroma. Pedunculated RV and even right atrial (RA) myxomas can encroach into the RV outflow area in systole.

PULMONARY ARTERY CALIBER

Quantitative assessment of the width of the pulmonary trunk and of the right main pulmonary artery has been studied by several pediatric cardiology groups.[21-23] The normal range with reference to body surface area was obtained in children and teenagers; the upper end of subject size approached that of adults (2 m^2).[21,22] The pulmonary trunk–aorta diameter ratio was assessed and found to be 0.99 ± 0.06 in normal subjects.

These authors endeavored to correlate pulmonary artery dilatation quantitatively with enhanced pulmonary blood flow in left-to-right shunts. Thus Denef et al.[23] reported an excellent correlation ($r = 0.89$) between the pulmonary trunk–aorta diameter ratio and the QP/QS (pulmonary-to-systemic flow by cardiac catheterization). The pulmonary trunk–aorta diameter ratio was 1.35 ± 0.23 in 42 atrial septal defect (ASD) patients.[23]

Lappen et al.[21] found an excellent correlation ($r = 0.93$) between right pulmonary artery diameter by echocardiography and by angiography. The diameter of this artery was less than the third percentile of normal in 16 of 37 patients with tetralogy of Fallot but greater than the ninety-seventh percentile of normal in 17 of 30 patients with ASD.

Pulmonary Artery Aneurysms

Aneurysms of the pulmonary trunk or its main branches can grow to very large sizes. About half the patients with this rare abnormality have associated congenital defects, either ASD, ventricular septal defect (VSD), patent ductus arteriosus (PDA), or pulmonary stenosis. The other etiologic factors include syphilis (common many decades ago but now rare), trauma, mycotic aneurysm following septic pulmonary embolus, and Marfan's syndrome. An extensive account of the earlier literature on this topic was published by Deterling and Clagett,[24] and a more recent comprehensive review by Bartter et al.[25] has updated it. The diagnosis was formerly dependent on angiography. On 2D echo, a distinction has been made between a fusiform or generalized pulmonary trunk dilatation and a saccular aneurysm characterized by an asymmetrical local bulge. The latter type may contain a thrombus. The aneurysm can be so large that the entire outline of it may not be encompassed within the 2D echo sector image, also so large that some adjacent structures are displaced from their usual location, perplexing the echocardiographer.

Severe pulmonary hypertension due to mitral stenosis, Eisenmenger's syndrome, or primary pulmonary hypertension is often associated with massive dilatation of the pulmonary trunk, extending to some degree into the main branches (Figures 8-10 and 8-11). Rosenson and St. John Sutton[26] described the 2D echo findings in a 59-year-old woman with mitral stenosis who had an 8-cm dissecting aneurysm of the pulmonary trunk. A huge aneurysm containing intimal flaps was demonstrated. It is known that about one-third of patients with severe pulmonary hypertension die suddenly, and it was suggested by these authors that pulmonary trunk dissection might account for this catastrophe. Rupture ensues either into the mediastinum or into the pericardium causing tamponade.

Idiopathic Dilatation of the Pulmonary Artery

This entity has been known to clinicians and radiologists for 70 years. Several small series have documented the existence of this condition,[27-30] but its etiology remains a mystery.

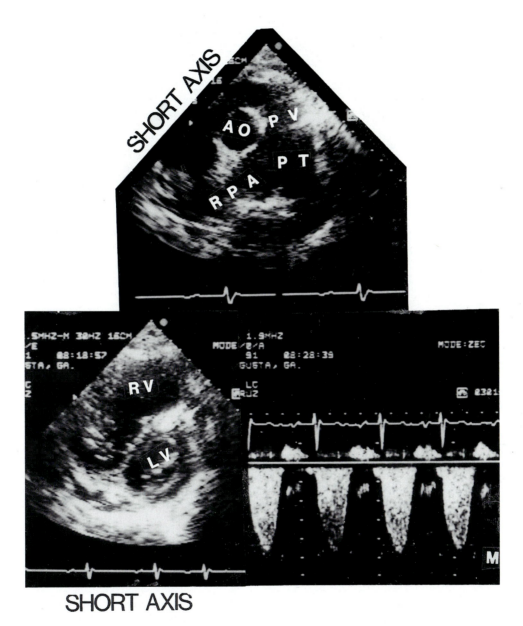

SHORT AXIS

Figure 8–10. (Above) High parasternal short-axis view showing a dilated pulmonary trunk (PT) and right pulmonary artery in a patient with severe chronic pulmonary hypertension of thromboembolic etiology. (Below, left) Low parasternal short-axis view shows RV dilatation. (Below, right) Continuous-wave Doppler of tricuspid regurgitation (4.7 m/s) indicating a pulmonary artery peak systolic pressure of about 100 mmHg.

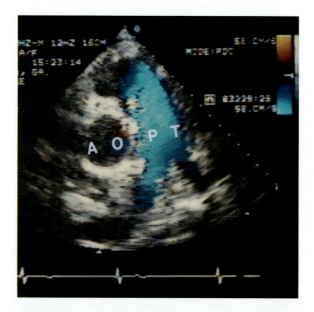

Figure 8–11. Colorflow Doppler in high parasternal short-axis view showing dilated pulmonary trunk (blue) (Ao, aortic root).

The criteria of Greene et al.[30] are essentially (1) simple dilatation of the pulmonary trunk with or without involvement of its branches and (2) absence of shunts, chronic cardiac or pulmonary disease, and syphilis, atherosclerosis, or other arterial disease. The diagnosis is therefore made by a process of exclusion of other causes for pulmonary trunk dilatation. In former decades, this meant cardiac catheterization and angiocardiography, but since the availability of 2D echo and Doppler, these techniques can achieve the same purpose noninvasively. It has been suggested that pulmonary trunk dilatation in this entity is caused by unequal septation of the primitive truncus arteriosus in the embryo; some instances of concomitant "hypoplastic" aorta have been cited in favor of this theory.

Dilatation of the pulmonary trunk in idiopathic dilatation of the pulmonary artery is not as extreme as in pulmonary artery aneurysm. However, it is of sufficient degree to produce a conspicuous bulge on the left border of the cardiac silhouette in the postero-anterior chest radiograph.

EXTRINSIC AND INTRINSIC PULMONARY TRUNK OR ARTERY MASSES

The various anatomic relationships of the pulmonary trunk and its branches have clinical as well as echocardiographic relevance. Marshall and Trump[31] reported three patients with lymphomatous mediastinal masses compressing the pulmonary artery and reviewed 35 cases in the literature previous to 1982. Teratomatous tumors or cysts and Hodgkin's lymphomas were the most common, with about 10 cases each. Large saccular aneurysms of the ascending aorta can compress the pulmonary trunk, whereas aortic arch aneurysms expanding inferiorly can distort and narrow the main pulmonary artery branches.

Fox et al.[32] described compression of the pulmonary trunk by a large mediastinal mass, presumably metastatic from a popliteal sarcoma, in a 25-year-old man. Doppler echo revealed a mild gradient (16 mmHg) across the site. D'Cruz and Chiemmongkoltip[33] reported a mass at a similar location in a 5-year-old child, visualized on echocardiography; at surgery, a mass having the size, shape, and rigidity of a Ping-Pong ball was found to be a cystic chondroma arising from the fourth left costal cartilage.

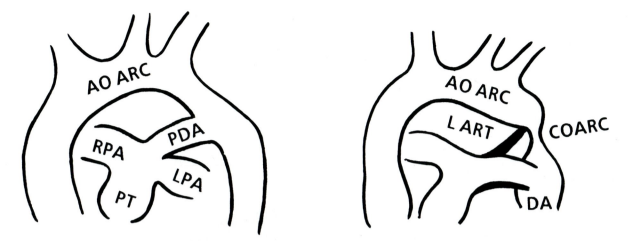

Figure 8–12. (Left) Diagram showing relation of patent ductus arteriosus (PDA) to the aortic arch (Ao ARC) and the pulmonary arteries (RPA and LPA) (PT, pulmonary trunk). (Right) Diagram showing attachments of the ligamentum arteriosum (L ART) to the aorta and to the bifurcation of the pulmonary trunk (DA, descending aorta).

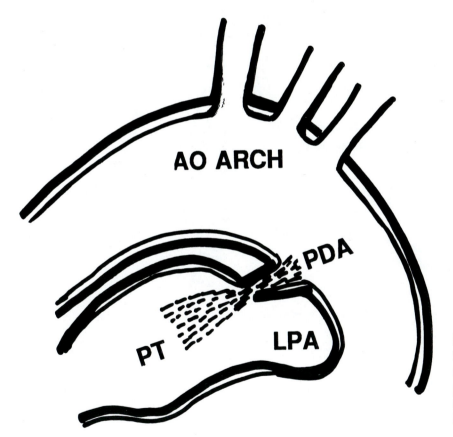

Figure 8–13. Diagram showing relationship of patent ductus arteriosus (PDA) to pulmonary trunk (PT), left pulmonary artery (LPA), and aortic arch (Ao ARCH). The jet through the PDA is shown.

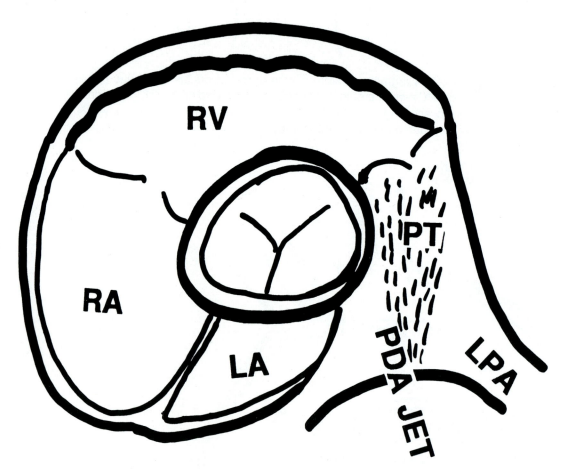

Figure 8–14. Diagram of high parasternal short-axis view showing location of PDA jet into the pulmonary trunk (PT).

Primary or secondary neoplastic masses in the pulmonary trunk or its main branches have manifested as filling defects on angiocardiography encroaching on the normal smooth tubular contour of these vessels.[34-36] The main diagnostic significance of such masses within these large arteries is that they may mimic acute or subacute pulmonary embolism. Transesophageal 2D echo visualization of primary pulmonary artery sarcoma was described in these locations in even finer detail.[40-43]

Pulmonary Artery Embolus

Pulmonary embolism constitutes a major medical emergency. Blood clots originating in leg or pelvic veins float through the inferior vena cava (IVC) into the right heart chambers and then into the pulmonary arteries, where they get impacted. Right ventricular failure results, manifesting as right ventricular dilatation on 2D echo. Until recently, thrombus had not actually been visualized by echocardiography in the pulmonary trunk or its main branches. Kasper et al.[37] performed echocardiography in 105 patients with acute and recurrent pulmonary embolism and visualized thrombi in 13 patients in the right pulmonary artery in the suprasternal view. Others have used a high parasternal short-axis view to image thrombus in the pulmonary trunk or its main branches.[38,39] Transesophageal echocardiography (TEE) has been used to identify such emboli.

PATENT DUCTUS ARTERIOSUS

This very common congenital abnormality (Figure 8–12) is of great importance to pediatric cardiologists, who have documented the 2D echo appearances in detail.[44-46] It is one of the major causes of left-to-right shunt in adults; a series from Edinburgh comprised 32 such individuals who had reached the age of 50.[47] Sahn and Allen[44] described the 2D echo appearances in parasternal short-axis view. Smallhorn et al.[46] considered the suprasternal view (Figure 8–13) superior to the parasternal (Figure 8–14) and emphasized the need to visualize the pulmonary artery end of the ductus as well as the aortic end; the latter is often expanded into a funnel-like shape.

The 2D echo imaging of a PDA is difficult in adults because of impaired resolution due to the large distance from the transducer, which particularly hinders identification of small ducti. However, pulsed-wave Doppler compensates for imperfect 2D echo pictures by the recording of typical "continuous" left-to-right shunt into the pulmonary trunk, corresponding to the well-known continuous "machinery" murmur[45,47] so characteristic of this anomaly. In fact, Stevenson et al.[45] found that attenuation of the diastolic component of such shunt flow into the pulmonary artery correlated with the presence of pulmonary hypertension.

REFERENCES

1. Weyman AE, Dillon JC, Feigenbaum H, et al. Echocardiographic pattern of pulmonary valve motion in valvular pulmonary stenosis. Am J Cardiol 1974;34:644.
2. Weyman AE, Hurwitz RA, Girod DA, et al. Cross-sectional echocardiographic visualization of the stenotic pulmonary valve. Circulation 1977;56:769.
3. Johnson GL, Kwan OL, Handshoe S, et al. Accuracy of combined two-dimensional echocardiography and continuous wave Doppler recordings in the estimation of pressure gradient in right ventricular outlet obstruction. J Am Coll Cardiol 1984;3:1013.
4. Hatle L, Angelsen B. Doppler Ultrasound in Cardiology, 2d ed. Philadelphia: Lea & Febiger, 1985.
5. Lima CO, Sahn DJ, Valdes-Cruz LM, et al. Noninvasive prediction of transvalvular pressure gradient in patients with pulmonary stenosis by quantitative two-dimensional echocardiographic Doppler studies. Circulation 1983;67:866.
6. Hastreiter AR, Joorabchi B, Pujatti G, et al. Cardiovascular lesions associated with congenital rubella. J Pediatr 1967;71:59.

7. Roberts N, Moes CAF. Supravalvar pulmonary stenosis. J Pediatr 1973;82:838.
8. Snider AR, Serwer GA. Echocardiography in Pediatric Heart Disease. Chicago: Year Book Medical Publishers, 1989, p 238.
9. D'Cruz IA, Agustsson MH, Bicoff JP, et al. Stenotic lesions of the pulmonary arteries. Am J Cardiol 1964;13:441.
10. Oram S, Pattison N, Davies P. Postvalvular stenosis of the pulmonary valve and its branches. Br Heart J 1964;26:832.
11. Rios JC, Walsh BJ, Massumi RA, et al. Congenital pulmonary artery branch stenosis. Am J Cardiol 1969;24:318.
12. Tinker DD, Nanda NC, Harris P, et al. Two-dimensional echocardiographic identification of pulmonary artery branch stenosis. Am J Cardiol 1982;50:814.
13. Snider AR, Enderlein ME, Teitel DF, et al. Two-dimensional echocardiographic determination of aortic and pulmonary artery sizes from infancy to adulthood in normal subjects. Am J Cardiol 1984;53:218.
14. Foale R, King ME, Gordon D, et al. Pseudoaneurysm of the pulmonary artery after the banding procedure: Two-dimensional echocardiographic description. J Am Coll Cardiol 1984;3:371.
15. Nakamura K, Satomi G, Sakai T, et al. Clinical and echocardiographic features of pulmonary valve endocarditis. Circulation 1983;67:198.
16. Kramer NE, Gill SS, Patel R, et al. Pulmonary valve vegetations detected with echocardiography. Am J Cardiol 1977;39:1064.
17. Mehlman DJ, Furey W, Phair J, et al. Two-dimensional echocardiographic features diagnostic of isolated pulmonary valve endocarditis. Am Heart J 1982;103:137.
18. Naidoo DP, Seedat MA, Vythilingam S. Isolated endocarditis of the pulmonary valve with fragmentation hemolysis. Br Heart J 1988;60:527.
19. Cremieux AC, Witchitz S, Malergue MC. Clinical and echocardiographic observations in pulmonary valve endocarditis. Am J Cardiol 1985;56:610.
20. Cassling RS, McManus BM. Isolated pulmonic valve infective endocarditis: A diagnostically elusive entity. Am Heart J 1985;109:558.
21. Lappen RS, Riggs TW, Lapin GD, et al. Two-dimensional echocardiographic measurement of right pulmonary artery diameter in infants and children. J Am Coll Cardiol 1983;2:121.
22. Snider AR, Enderlein MA, Teitel DF, et al. Two-dimensional echocardiographic determination of aortic and pulmonary artery sizes from infancy to adulthood in normal subjects. Am J Cardiol 1984;53:218.
23. Denef B, Dumoulin M, VanderHauwert LG. Usefulness of echocardiographic assessment of right ventricular and pulmonary trunk size for estimating magnitude of left-to-right shunt in children with atrial septal defect. Am J Cardiol 1985;55:1571.
24. Deterling RA, Clagett OT. Aneurysm of the pulmonary artery. Am Heart J 1947;34:471.
25. Bartter T, Irwin RS, Nash G. Aneurysms of the pulmonary arteries. Chest 1988;94:1065.
26. Rosenson RS, St. John Sutton M. Dissecting aneurysm of the pulmonary trunk in mitral stenosis. Am J Cardiol 1986;58:1140.
27. Oppenheimer BS. Idiopathic dilatation of the pulmonary artery. Trans Assoc Am Physicians 1933;48:290.
28. VanBuchem FSR, Nieveen J, Marring W, et al. Idiopathic dilatation of the pulmonary artery. Dis Chest 1955;28:326.
29. Deshmukh M, Guvenc S, Bentivoglio H, et al. Idiopathic dilatation of pulmonary artery. Circulation 1960;21:710.
30. Greene DG, Baldwin EF, Baldwin JS, et al. Pure congenital pulmonary stenosis and idiopathic dilatation of the pulmonary artery. Am J Med 1949;6:24.
31. Marshall ME, Trump DL. Acquired extrinsic pulmonic stenosis caused by mediastinal tumors. Cancer 1982;49:1496.
32. Fox R, Panidis IP, Kotler MN, et al. Detection of Doppler echocardiography of acquired pulmonic stenosis due to extrinsic tumor compression. Am J Cardiol 1984;53:1475.
33. D'Cruz IA, Chiemmongkoltip Pinot C. Echocardiographic diagnosis of an unusual anterior mediastinal mass. Clin Cardiol 1982;5:464.
34. Moffat RE, Chang CH, Slave JE. Roentgen considerations in primary pulmonary artery sarcoma. Radiology 1972;104:283.
35. Wright EC, Wellons HA, Martin RP. Primary pulmonary artery sarcoma diagnosed noninvasively by two-dimensional echocardiography. Circulation 1983;67:459.

36. Weyman AE. Principles and Practice of Echocardiography, 2d ed. Philadelphia: Lea & Febiger, 1994, p 893.
37. Kasper W, Meinertz T, Henkel B, et al. Echocardiographic findings in patients with proved pulmonary embolism. Am Heart J 1986;112:1284.
38. Evans BH, Maurer G. Echocardiographic diagnosis of pulmonary embolus. Am Heart J 1990;120:1236.
39. Zaid SJ. Two-dimensional echocardiographic detection of asymptomatic pulmonary thromboembolism. Echocardiography 1992;9:17.
40. Nixdorff U, Erbel R, Drexler M, et al. Detection of thromboembolus of the right pulmonary artery by transesophageal two-dimensional echocardiography. Am J Cardiol 1988;61:488.
41. Klein AL, Stewart WC, Cosgrove DM, et al. Visualization of acute pulmonary emboli by transesophageal echocardiography. J Am Soc Echocardiogr 1990;3:412.
42. Hunter JJ, Johnson KR, Karagianes TG, et al. Detection of massive pulmonary embolus-in-transit by transesophageal echocardiography. Chest 1991;100:1210.
43. Gelernt MD, Mogdater A, Hahn RT. Transesophageal echocardiography to diagnose and demonstrate resolution of an acute massive pulmonary embolus. Chest 1992;102:297.
44. Sahn DJ, Allen HD. Real-time cross-sectional echocardiographic imaging and measurement of the patent ductus arteriosus in infants and children. Circulation 1978;58:343.
45. Stevenson JG, Kawabori, Gunteroth WG. Noninvasive detection of pulmonary hypertension in patent ductus arteriosus by pulsed Doppler echocardiography. Circulation 1979;60:355.
46. Smallhorn JF, Huhta JC, Anderson RH, et al. Suprasternal cross-sectional echocardiography in assessment of patent ductus arteriosus. Br Heart J 1982;48:321.
47. Marquis RM, Miller HC, McCormack RJM, et al. Persistence of the ductus arteriosus with left to right shunt in the older patient. Br Heart J 1982;48:469.

9

The Interatrial Septum

NORMAL ANATOMY

The interatrial (or atrial) septum occupies an area on the right atrial medial wall[1] that in contour can be compared with the blade of a short, broad blunt knife (Figure 9-1). In its center lies the fossa ovalis, bordered by a curved ridge of atrial myocardium called the *limbus.* The shape of the fossa ovalis varies (from circular to oval), as does its size. The prominence and circumferential extent of the limbus are also variable. In shape it may be circular, oval, or shaped like the letter C or an inverted U. The average area of the atrial septum was 8.9 cm², that of the fossa ovalis 2.4 cm², as measured in adult autopsies by Sweeney and Rosenquist.[2] They found the fossa ovalis area to be a mean of 28% of atrial septal area.

Schwinger et al.[3] used transesophageal echocardiography (TEE) to study the thickness of the atrial septum. They found that the latter was thickest peripherally (i.e., near its attachment to the atrial free wall) and most thin at the fossa ovalis. In 82% of their 119 patients, the atrial septum on either side of the fossa ovalis was of approximately uniform thickness, though the actual thickness varied enormously, from 2 to 20 mm (average 6 ± 2 mm). In 18% of their patients, atrial septal thickness tapered gradually from its periphery to the fossa ovalis region.

Atrial septal thickness at the fossa ovalis was only 1.8 ± 0.7 mm (mean). This relative thinness of the fossa ovalis is the reason why it often apparently "drops out," especially when parallel to the ultrasound beam (apical or parasternal view), leading to an erroneous impression that an atrial septal defect (ASD) exists. The fossa ovalis, and in fact, the atrial

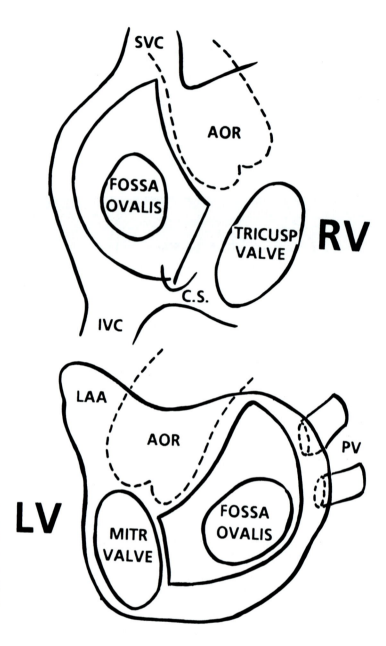

Figure 9–1. Diagram showing anatomic relationships of the atrial septum (AS) to fossa ovalis within it and to neighboring structures viewed from the right atrium (above) and left atrium (below) (SVC, superior vena cava; IVC, inferior vena cava; AOR, aorta; CS, coronary sinus; LAA, left atrial appendage; PV, pulmonary veins). RV and LV signify location of the respective ventricles.

septum as a whole, is best imaged in the subcostal four-chamber view; the ultrasound beam is perpendicular to it so that even the thin fossa ovalis reflects ultrasound adequately, avoiding the pitfall of dropout.

The *superior (or posterosuperior) part of the atrial septum,* sometimes called the *sinus venosus region,* lies above the limbus of the fossa ovalis, anterior to the posterior atrial wall, and posterior to the right atrial appendage. The superior vena cava (SVC) enters the right atrium at this region. The right pulmonary veins are closely related to this region posteriorly and enter the left atrium just to the left of this part of the atrial septum.

The *inferior (or anteroinferior) part of the atrial septum,* also called the *primum part,* is developed partly from the endocardial cushion, and defects of this region are included in the spectrum of endocardial cushion or atrioventricular septal defects. This region of the atrial septum (and defects thereof) must be distinguished from the posteroinferior atrial septum at the coronary sinus area.

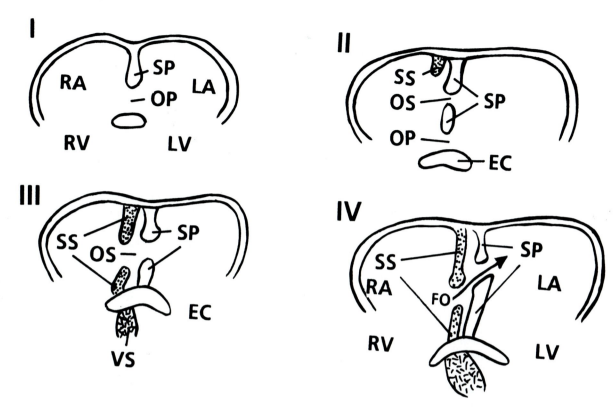

Figure 9–2. Diagram showing successive stages in atrial septal development and explaining the terms primum and secundum with respect to the words septum and ostium (RA, right atrium; RV, right ventricle; LV, left ventricle; VS, ventricular septum; EC, endocardial cushion; SP, septum primum; SS, septum secundum; OP, ostium primum; OS, ostium secundum; FO, foramen ovale).

PATENT FORAMEN OVALE

In the fetus, the interatrial septum consists mainly of the septum secundum, which is a nonmobile, flat structure deficient in its center (Figure 9–2). Immediately to the left of this is the septum primum, a mobile flap that allows blood to flow from right to left if right atrial pressure exceeds left atrial pressure but does not allow flow from the left to the right atrium when left atrial pressure exceeds right atrial pressure. All through intrauterine life blood flows through this valvelike foramen ovale from the right to the left atrium, but at birth the left atrial pressure rises above that of the right atrium, and the flaplike septum primum closes the foramen ovale and forms the floor of the fossa ovalis.

Fusion of the septum primum with the septum secundum occurs at a variable time after birth in the majority of individuals, thus sealing off the two atria from each other permanently. In a minority of otherwise normal persons, such fusion does not occur, though the foramen ovale remains functionally closed. In other words, an oblique, slitlike potential communication persists between the right and the left atrium. In a series of 965 autopsies from the Mayo Clinic,[4] 27% of hearts had a valve-patent foramen ovale, the prevalence being higher (34%) in children and young adults than in the elderly (20%). The size of the foramen ovale slit varied from 1 to 19 mm (mean 4.9 mm). Some clinicians make a distinction between a probe-patent (2 to 5 mm) and a pencil-patent (6 to 10 mm) foramen ovale.

The difference between a true atrial septal defect (ASD), which is in plain terms a hole in the atrial septum, and a patent foramen ovale is that the former permits shunts in either or both directions, whereas a patent foramen ovale allows only right-to-left shunts.

Right-to-left blood flow through a patent foramen ovale may be demonstrable on colorflow Doppler, usually best seen in the four-chamber subcostal view on routine 2D echo or in a two-chamber atrial view transecting the foramen ovale region on TEE. Mosvowitz et al.[5] and Chenzbraun et al.[5a] found the best TEE plane for this purpose to be a vertical plane passing through the fossa ovalis as well as both venae cavae. Ten milliliters of agitated saline solution is injected into an arm vein, resulting in dense right atrial opacification by microbubbles. A right-to-left shunt is judged to be present if microbubbles are found in the left atrium within three cardiac cycles after complete right atrial opacification.[6] Five or more microbubbles must be visualized. Right-to-left shunting through a patent foramen ovale can be enhanced or provoked by the Valsalva maneuver[7] or coughing,[8] both of which cause abrupt transient elevation of right-sided heart pressures.

Between 10% and 18% of apparently healthy normal persons have a patent foramen ovale by contrast TEE echocardiography.[7] In the platypnea-orthodeoxia syndrome, dyspnea is provoked by the upright position and relieved by recumbency (platypnea); arterial oxygen saturation falls when the patient stands and rises in the supine position. It has been demonstrated by contrast echocardiography that a right-to-left shunt across a patent foramen ovale is present in these patients, which is accentuated when the patient is tilted from horizontal to upright position. This unusual syndrome has been encountered in patients with diverse chronic lung diseases such as recurrent pulmonary embolization and pneumonectomy. Intriguingly, pulmonary artery pressures are normal. The mechanism whereby body position affects right-to-left shunting through a patent foramen ovale is uncertain; possible causes include changes in pulmonary vascular resistance, distortion of fossa ovalis anatomy, and altered right ventricular compliance-flow relationships.

Right-to-left shunting can occur in conditions associated with elevated right-sided heart pressures such as chronic obstructive lung disease, pulmonary embolism, positive-pressure ventilation,[9] right ventricular infarction,[10] high-altitude pulmonary hypertension,[11] pneumonectomy,[12] etc.

Using saline-contrast TEE, Langholz et al.[13] have shown that right-to-left shunting across a patent foramen ovale (PFO) can occur even if there is no pulmonary hypertension. They demonstrated three different mechanisms and correlated them with motion of the PFO flap valve (septum primum). These mechanisms included (1) transient phasic reversal of the left atrial–right atrial pressure gradient during part of every cardiac cycle, (2) sustained elevation of right atrial pressure above left atrial pressure by positive-pressure breathing, and (3) a mass in the right atrium that causes preferential intraatrial flow such that a stream is directed toward and through the PFO, even though the mean left atrial pressure exceeds right atrial pressure.

In paradoxical embolization, venous thrombi pass through the foramen ovale into the left heart chambers and then into a systemic artery rather than floating through the pulmonary artery into the lungs. In addition to a communication between the right and left sides of the heart, there also must be a pressure gradient from the right to the left atrium that permits flow in this direction, at least transiently or phasically during some part of the cardiac cycle. Once a septal defect or patent foramen ovale has been demonstrated, the diagnosis of a paradoxical embolus is usually presumptive, except for rare occasions when a thrombus has actually been seen on echocardiography or at autopsy straddling the patent foramen ovale.[10]

An association between transient or permanent cerebrovascular deficits and a patent foramen ovale has been the subject of much interest[14-18] over the last 5 years. The published results are not entirely in accord. Most suggest a definite association, and many are tempted to claim that a stroke (arterial occlusion) in a patient with a patent foramen ovale but no other demonstrable cardiac source of emboli may be presumed to be due to paradoxical embolization. Others cautiously consider the chain of cause and effect implicating the foramen to be tenuous at best.

ANEURYSM OF THE ATRIAL SEPTUM

Abnormal pouchlike protrusions of the fossa ovalis part of the atrial septum were first described as a curiosity at autopsy,[19,20] but a landmark paper by Silver and Dorsey[21] in 1978 established the pathologic anatomy of the entity and the fact that it was not rare. Several echocardiographic descriptions of interatrial septal (IAS) aneurysms appeared during the 1980s,[22-26] including a series of 80 cases from the Mayo Clinic.[26] Awareness of its wide prevalence and of its association with transient ischemic attacks (TIAs) or strokes has recently aroused much interest among clinicians and echocardiographers. Cardiac ultrasound is undoubtedly the method of choice not only to diagnose IAS aneurysms but also to assess their dynamics or associated shunts.

Since the floor of the fossa ovalis is developed from the septum primum of the embryo, aneurysms of this region are sometimes referred to as *septum primum aneurysms.*[21] The floor of the fossa ovalis is commonly taut and flush with the limbus of the fossa and the adjacent atrial septum, or the floor of the fossa may be mildly depressed with the limbus a conspicuous ridge or shoulder. In yet other cases, the thin fossa floor is somewhat lax or floppy on pressure but cannot be pushed far into either atrium; such mild redundancy is considered within the range of normal variance and should not be called an IAS aneurysm. The latter term should be reserved for cases with severe redundancy such that the aneurysmal bulge protrudes far into the atrial cavity.[26]

Quantitative measurements of IAS aneurysms were reported by Silver and Dorsey[21] in their 16 autopsy cases. The diameter of the base of the aneurysm varied from 1.5 to 2.5 cm, and the aneurysm projected 1.1 to 2.4 cm into the atrium (usually the right). The Mayo Clinic's echocardiographic criteria[26] for diagnosis of IAS aneurysm were a 1.5-cm protrusion beyond the plane of the atrial septum and a base diameter of at least 1.5 cm. As seen on routine 2D echo in the apical or subcostal view or on TEE, IAS aneurysms are easily recognized as thin protrusions of the fossa ovalis either into the right or the left atrium (Figures 9–3 to 9–6). In some patients, such aneurysmal bulges are "fixed"; in others, the aneurysm is mobile and moves rapidly to and fro between the two atria with every cardiac cycle, presumably reflecting transient phasic pressure differences between the two chambers (see Figures 9–3 and 9–6). In certain situations, including tamponade, phasic motion of the IAS aneurysm into the left atrium may be respiratory (during inspiration).

Certain aspects of the pathology of IAS aneurysm may have clinical implications[21]: (1) fine fibrin-like tags have been noted on the aneurysm's convexity, causing a rough or ragged appearance of the latter, (2) rarely, small annular thrombi have been seen in the groove formed between the aneurysm and the limbic ridge, (3) multiple small perforations on the order of 1 or 2 mm often occur at the apex of the IAS aneurysm, presumably the result of progressive thinning and eventual fenestration[27] (such tiny holes are not recognizable by conventional echocardiography but have been detected by TEE), and (4) valve-patent patent foramen ovale and (5) mitral valve prolapse are more common in patients with IAS aneurysms than in the general population.

Whereas IAS aneurysms in adults are virtually always restricted to the fossa ovalis, larger aneurysms involving the whole atrial septum have been described in infants or young children with severe congenital anomalies of the hypoplastic right ventricle category.[26] These huge aneurysms protrude into the left atrium and exceptionally into the mitral orifice or even the left ventricular chamber.

Association with Mitral Valve Prolapse

Several authors have drawn attention to an association between IAS aneurysms and mitral valve prolapse.[28-31]

Simulation of Right Atrial Mass

Thompson et al.[32] reported a case of IAS aneurysm under the title of "pseudotumor of the right atrium." On 2D echo, the "pseudotumor" is round or domelike in contour; imaging through the plane of the fossa ovalis reveals the typical IAS aneurysm contour and location.[33,34]

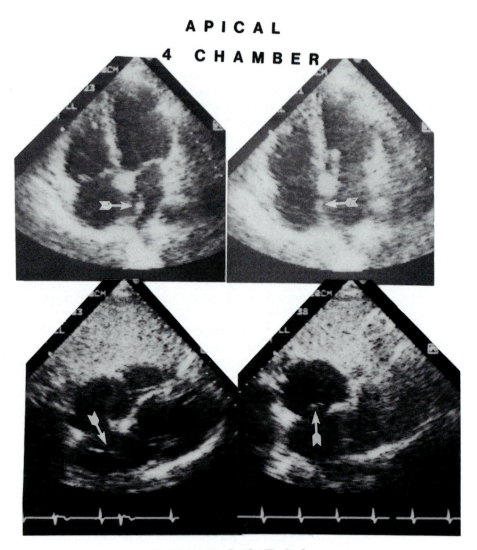

Figure 9–3. Apical four-chamber view (above) and subcostal view (below) showing considerable lateral motion of the atrial septal aneurysm.

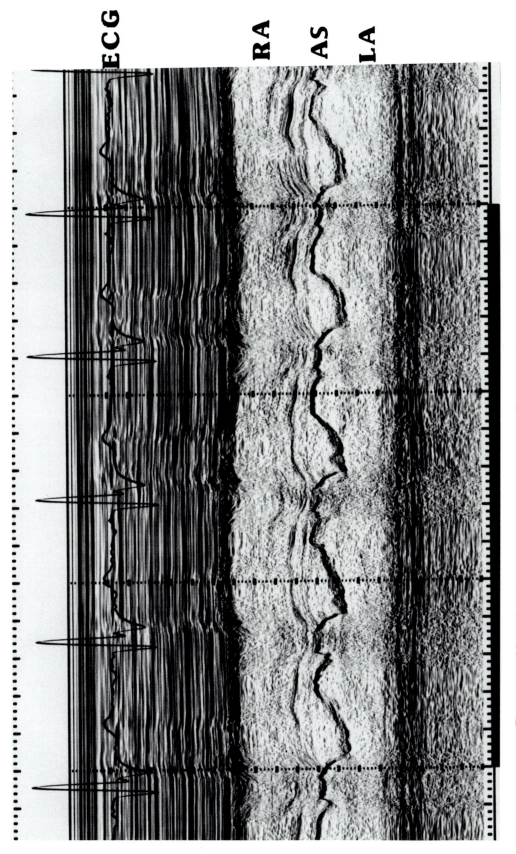

Figure 9–4. M-mode echo view of same patient (see Figure 9–3) showing posterior motion of the atrial septum (toward LA) in systole and anterior position of the septum in diastole.

193

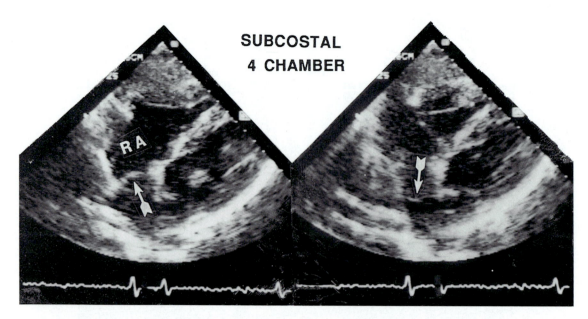

Figure 9–5. Subcostal view of a patient with atrial septal aneurysm. The frame at left shows normal atrial septal contour, but during inspiration (right), an atrial septal aneurysm is seen to protrude far into the left atrium.

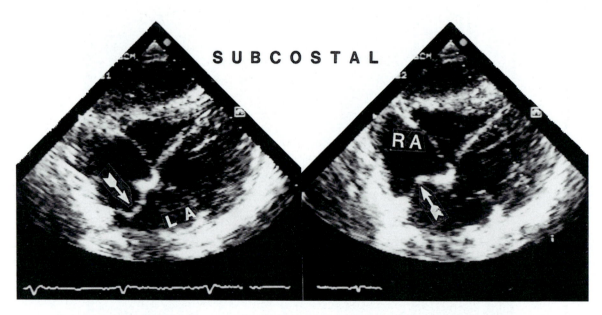

Figure 9–6. Subcostal view of an atrial septal aneurysm (arrows) bulging toward the left atrium during inspiration (left) but toward the right atrium during expiration (right).

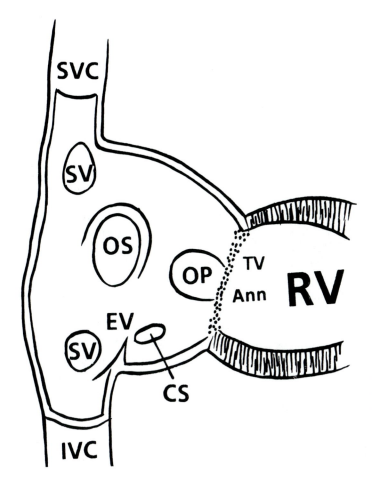

Figure 9–7. Diagram of the right side of the atrial septum showing different ASD locations (SV, sinus venosus type; OS, ostium secundum type; OP, ostium primum type; CS, unroofed coronary sinus). Note the two possible sites of sinus venosus defects, the upper one usual and the lower one very rare. The stippled band indicates the tricuspid annulus.

Association with Strokes

There has been a recent surge of interest in the potential role of IAS aneurysms in the causation of cerebrovascular or other systemic embolism. The issue has been assessed using either conventional 2D echo or TEE.[35-39] These studies have yielded the following findings: (1) TEE is more sensitive than transthoracic 2D echo in detecting IAS aneurysms, (2) these aneurysms are more prevalent in patients with strokes than in those without strokes, and (3) a surprisingly high proportion of IAS aneurysms (about three-quarters) show right-to-left shunting on contrast echocardiography.

How do IAS aneurysms cause strokes? One theory is that small thrombi form in the aneurysm or the groove at the base of the aneurysm and are then swept into the left atrium to embolize. The other theory postulates that venous thrombi pass through the IVC and then through the fenestrations of the IAS aneurysm into the left side of the heart. Although microbubbles from saline contrast injections into an arm vein are seen to pass into the left atrium in many or most of such patients, the fenestrations that permit such small right-to-left shunts are probably too tiny to allow any but the smallest thrombi through.

ATRIAL SEPTAL DEFECT

Abnormal communications between the two atria constitute the most common major congenital heart defect encountered in the adult population. There are several types of atrial septal defects (ASDs), each of which has a particular location, embryologic origin, and certain associated anatomic abnormalities.[40,41] Figure 9-7 is a simplified diagram depicting the various possible ASD locations.

Ostium Secundum ASD

This is by far the most common variety, accounting for about two-thirds of all ASDs. They are restricted to the fossa ovalis region, though variable in size within the area enclosed by the ridge or limbus of the fossa ovalis. An ASD (literally a hole in the atrial septum) can permit flow from the left to the right atrium or in a reversed direction and is a different hemodynamic situation from a valve-patent patent foramen ovale, which allows only right-to-left shunting if right atrial pressure exceeds left atrial pressure.

A secundum ASD can result either from excessive resorption of the septum primum or from deficient growth of the septum secundum. Some believe that gross right atrial dilatation, due to right-sided heart failure in a patient with a patent foramen ovale, can stretch the latter so as to convert it into a true ASD in the sense that a hiatus is formed in part of the fossa ovalis floor.

The size of an ASD has an important bearing on its pathophysiology. On the basis of his hemodynamic studies, Dexter[42] concluded that an "unrestricted" ASD of more than 2 cm^2 in area was associated with marked attenuation or absence of the normal pressure gradient between the atria. A "physiologically common atrium" results; the magnitude of the left-to-right shunt depends entirely on the relative compliances of the two ventricles; i.e., the large left-to-right shunt usually present in a patient with a large ASD is due to the RV being more compliant to diastolic filling than the LV.

A "physiologically common atrium" should not be confused with an "anatomically common atrium," characterized by total or almost complete absence of the atrial septum, an anomaly seldom seen in adults but often noted in infants or young children with endocardial cushion defects and/or visceral heterotaxis.

Secundum ASDs are usually single, but rarely, fenestration of the fossa ovalis with two or more defects can occur.[43] Spontaneous closure of ASDs has been demonstrated, by serial hemodynamic studies, to be not uncommon in infancy but very rare after 1 year of age.[44-46]

It is not widely known that the fossa ovalis is not always in an identical position within the atrial septum and in anatomic relation to various right atrial structures. In a study of 100 cases with ASD located within the fossa ovalis, Ferreira et al.[47] found that in 43 patients the ASD was in the center of the atrial septum and in 51 it was slightly displaced toward the IVC orifice. In 4 patients the fossa ovalis was substantially displaced toward the IVC orifice, and in 2 others it was displaced toward the SVC orifice. Another related anatomic variant with ASD is that of a eustachian valve that is unusually large and extensive so that it forms a "false" inferior margin of the fossa ovalis.[41,47]

The significance of undue proximity of an ASD to the entry of the IVC (less commonly, the SVC) into the right atrium is that streamlining of caval flow into the left atrium through the ASD can sometimes occur,[48] even though the predominant shunt is still left-to-right and there is little or no pulmonary hypertension. A large eustachian valve may facilitate such streaming of IVC blood into the left atrium, which is in fact its normal role in fetal life. This uncommon but important ASD variant, characterized by arterial desaturation and possibly cyanosis and digital clubbing due to streaming of caval blood, needs to be differentiated from the more common situation of ASD with severe pulmonary hypertension and reversed (right-to-left) shunting. The latter predicament (Eisenmenger ASD) is not suitable for surgical closure and carries a serious prognosis; the former (ASD with left-to-right shunt but some right-to-left shunt due to streaming of caval blood into left atrium) can be repaired surgically and has a prognosis on a level with usual secundum ASDs.

Sinus Venosus ASD

The posterior part of the right atrium, into which both venae cavae open, is developed from the sinus venosus. Sinus venosus defects, resulting from maldevelopment of this structure, can be of the SVC or IVC type. The SVC type accounts for 2% to 3% of all ASDs[49]

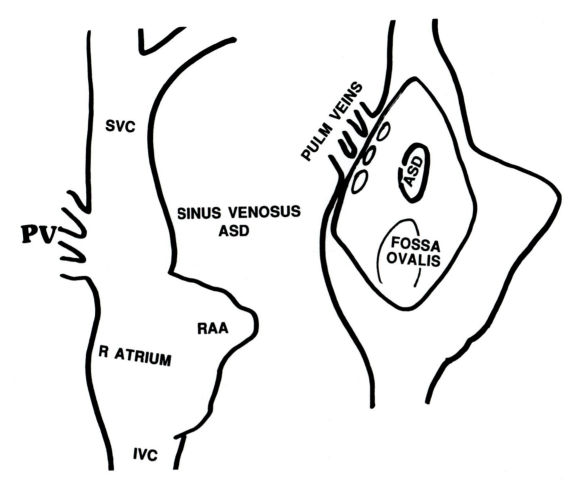

Figure 9–8. Diagram of sinus venosus type of ASD. (Left) Externally, the superior vena cava shows local dilatation of its lower end, which receives anomalous drainage of right pulmonary veins. (Right) Interior of right atrium showing high location of ASD, above intact fossa ovalis; anomalous pulmonary veins open into SVC-RA near the ASD.

and is associated with anomalous connection between the right upper pulmonary vein and the SVC just above the latter's entry into the right atrium in 80% to 90%.[49] The SVC is often dilated at this site to form an ampulla or pouch (Figure 9-8), which is useful as a diagnostic clue when seen on echocardiography or chest radiograph. The site of this type of ASD is above the fossa ovalis (see Figure 9-8), and in fact, the interatrial communication may even be partly above the level of the normal extent of the atrial septum. Only 10% of patients with secundum ASDs have partial anomalous venous connection.[50]

The IVC type of sinus venosus ASD is much rarer than the SVC type; it occurs inferior to the fossa ovalis and merges with the floor of the IVC.

Ostium Primum ASD

These defects constitute one variety of incomplete endocardial cushion defect and occur in the most inferior part of the atrial septum just above the attachment of the mitral and tricuspid valves. They account for 15% to 20% of all ASDs. Almost always the anterior mitral leaflet is cleft; less commonly, the septal leaflet of the tricuspid valve is also cleft. The fossa ovalis is not involved. An extreme form of endocardial cushion defect is the common atrioventricular (A-V) canal (Figure 9-9).

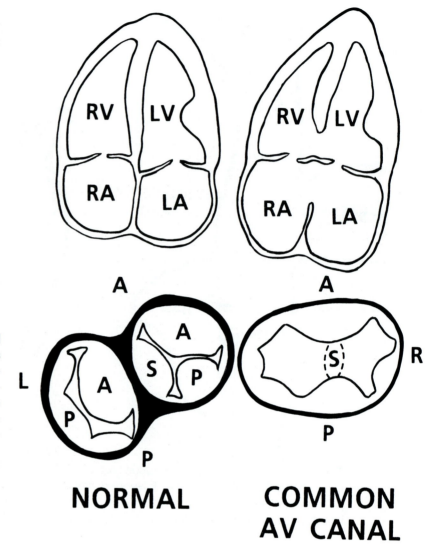

Figure 9–9. Diagram showing apical four-chamber views in normal subjects (above, left) and common atrioventricular (A-V) canal (above, right). The ventricular septum and the atrial septum are deficient in the region of the crux of the heart. Valve tissue spans this septal defect. The lower section shows the anatomy of the mitral and tricuspid valve leaflets and annuli in normal subjects (left) and common A-V canal (right) (A, anterior; P, posterior; L, left; R, right; S, ventricular septum).

Echocardiography of ASD[51-53]

Defects in the atrial septum are visualized in the 2D echo views that depict the atrial septum (Figure 9-10): parasternal short-axis or four-chamber, apical four-chamber, and subcostal four-chamber views. "Dropout" of the normal fossa ovalis region in the parasternal short-axis and apical views is common, thus simulating a secundum ASD. In these views, the ultrasound beam is parallel to the plane of the atrial septum, and the very thin floor of the fossa ovalis does not reflect enough ultrasound to register on the 2D echo image. When present, the T sign is useful in distinguishing an ASD from dropout in the apical four-chamber view: The inferior edge of the ASD has an inverted T contour instead of a tapered appearance typical of dropout.

Caveat: This T sign is not always reliable. Patients with lipomatous hypertrophy of the atrial septum (which always spares the fossa ovalis) may exhibit a T sign because of the abrupt limitation of lipomatous thickening at the edge of the fossa ovalis. The subcostal four-chamber view is the best for imaging the atrial septum[51] and identifying the three varieties of ASD: The common secundum or fossa ovalis defect is seen as a gap in

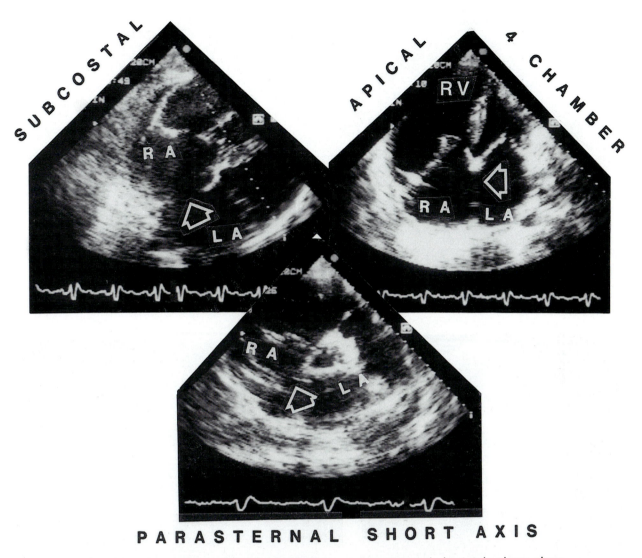

Figure 9–10. Subcostal, apical four-chamber, and parasternal short-axis views show-ing a large defect (arrows) in the atrial septum of secundum type in patient C.R.

the center of the septum; in primum ASDs, the gap is at the lower end of the septum, just above mitral and tricuspid valves; and in sinus venosus (SVC) type of ASDs, septal dis-continuity is located at the most superior part of the atrial septum. Colorflow Doppler confirms the presence and site of ASDs, demonstrating a strong left-to-right stream toward the transducer at the site of septal discontinuity (Figures 9–11 to 9–14).

The subcostal view is useful in patients with ASD for the following additional pur-poses: (1) the entry of the pulmonary veins into the left atrium can be scrutinized, an im-portant consideration because of the frequent association of ASDs with anomalous pul-monary venous drainage, (2) the rare coronary sinus type of left-to-right atrial-level shunt can be visualized in short-axis subcostal views, (3) aneurysms of the atrial septum, which are sometimes associated with ASDs, are best seen in this view, and (4) the subcostal sagit-tal view permits visualization and measurement of an ASD in a plane at right angles to the subcostal four-chamber plane, thus providing more complete information on the actual area of the ASD and the extent of atrial septum bordering the defect, information which is valuable to the surgeon.

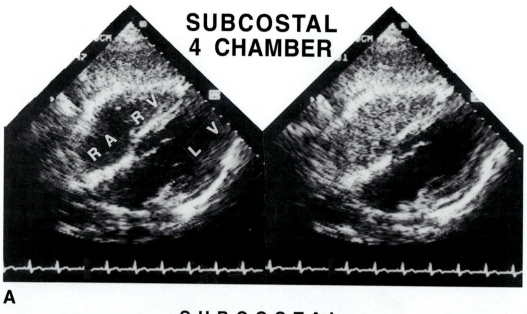

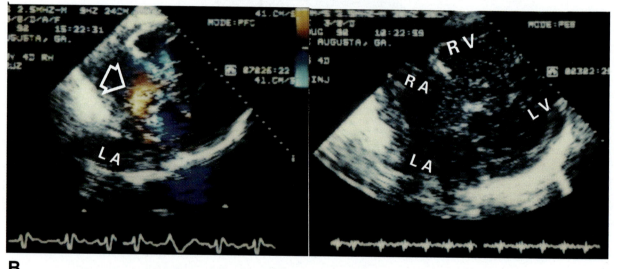

Figure 9–11. (A) Subcostal view showing dense opacification of right atrium and ventricle after agitated saline injection. No shunt is present. (B) Subcostal view in patient C.R. The left-to-right atrial shunt is well seen on colorflow Doppler (left). On injection of saline into an arm vein (right), microbubbles are seen filling RA and RV; a few microbubbles are also seen in left heart chambers.

Contrast echocardiography has been much used in detecting or excluding ASDs. Agitated saline is injected into an arm vein, and the microbubbles it contains opacify the right heart chambers (see Figure 9–11A). A left-to-right shunt across an atrial septal defect shows up as a stream of nonopacified blood in the right atrium.[52,54] Moreover, a few microbubbles transverse the ASD from the right to the left atrium in a high percentage of cases, even in apparently uncomplicated left-to-right ASD cases (see Figure 9–11B).

TEE provides excellent visualization of ASDs[53,53a] and is particularly useful for detecting small shunts when used in conjunction with continuous-wave Doppler or contrast echocardiography. Enhanced resolution by this mode also may permit more accurate mea-

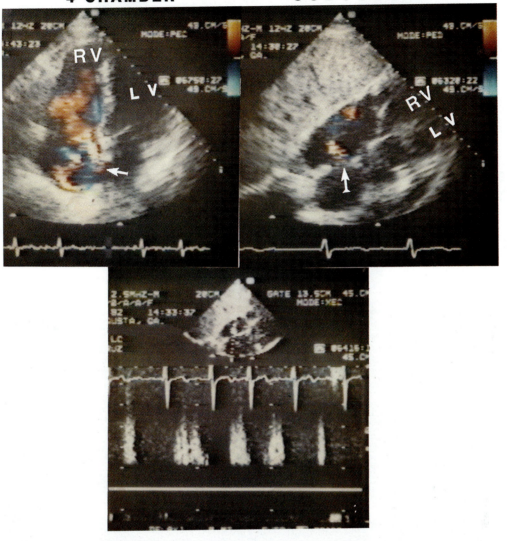

Figure 9–12. Apical four-chamber view (above, left) and subcostal view (above, right) in a patient with a small ASD. Arrows indicate a narrow jet into the right atrium emerging through the fossa ovalis region of the atrial septum. Pulsed-wave Doppler (below) shows phasic left-to-right atrial flow.

surement of the size of the ASD, as well as visualization of associated fossa ovalis pathology such as an aneurysm or fenestration at this site.

Echocardiography in various views also demonstrates right ventricular and right atrial dilatation and abnormal systolic ventricular septal motion resulting from volume overload. These features are so consistently present in secundum ASDs with significant shunts that absence of these features would render the diagnosis of a hemodynamically significant ASD unlikely.

A cleft anterior mitral leaflet, easily identified on the parasternal short-axis view, is consistently present in the primum type of ASD. Thickening of the anterior mitral leaflet, especially its medial half, is common in secundum ASDs; fibrous surface thickening of the cusp makes it white and opaque, in contrast to the normal delicate translucent texture.[55] While such leaflet thickening is of little consequence at an early age, perhaps significant mitral regurgitation may result in later life.[56] Echocardiographic abnormalities of the mi-

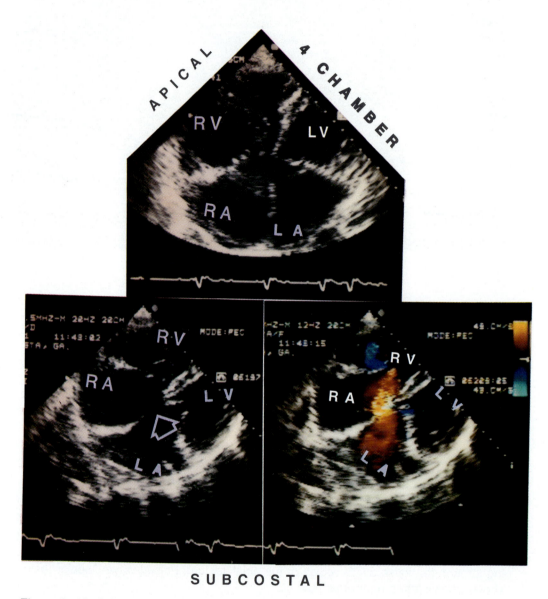

Figure 9–13. Apical four-chamber view (above) and subcostal view (below) in a patient with ostium primum ASD. The lower atrial septum (just above A-V valves) is deficient. Colorflow Doppler shows a large shunt crossing the ASD from the left to the right atrium.

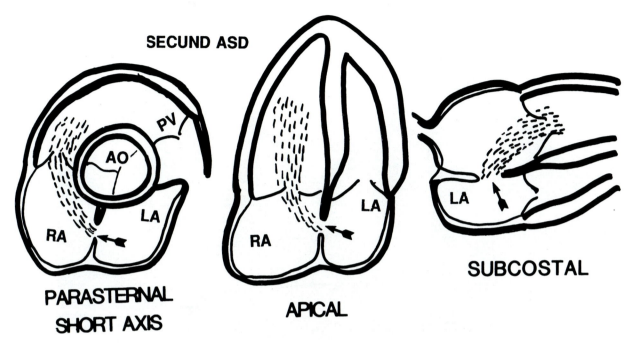

Figure 9–14. Diagram showing streams of flow (red color on colorflow Doppler) in various 2D views in patients with secundum ASD.

tral valve are therefore not unexpected in patients with ASD; rheumatic or other causes need not necessarily be invoked.

It is well known that mitral valve prolapse, especially of the anterior leaflet, is unduly prevalent among ASD patients. It is thought that such prolapse is secondary to geometric changes in left ventricular shape and size caused by marked right ventricular dilatation; thus its pathogenesis would be different from that in usual idiopathic mitral prolapse, wherein prolapse is attributable to inherent weakness of the collagen framework of mitral cusps and chordae with consequent stretching and redundancy.

LIPOMATOUS HYPERTROPHY OF THE ATRIAL SEPTUM

This unusual entity was first described by Prior[57] in 1964, although a few such instances had been reported earlier under the inaccurate label of "atrial lipoma," including one as far back as 1887.[58] Although extensive subepicardial deposits of fat are common, adipose tissue is not found within the myocardium except for the atrial septum, particularly in the elderly of both sexes. The extent of fat within the atrial septum correlates directly with the quantity of subepicardial fat[59] and probably with excess of body fat. In fact, it has been shown that fat in the atrial septum is directly continuous anteriorly with epicardial fat in the transverse pericardial sinus facing the posterior aspect of aortic root and pulmonary trunk and posteriorly with epicardial fat in the posterior groove between the two atria.[59]

An important feature of lipomatous hypertrophy of the interatrial septum (LHIAS) is that it always spares the fossa ovalis. This results in a very characteristic bilobed or dumbbell distribution of the lipomatous atrial thickening: bulbous thickening of the posterosuperior and anteroinferior atrial septum, separated by a small, narrow waist (fossa ovalis) in between. This configuration is evident in an anatomic section at this cardiac level, as well as in corresponding tomographic images on 2D echo (Figures 9–15 and 9–16), CT, or MRI.[60-62]

In younger adults, atrial septal fat is less extensive, often presenting as a wedge-shaped deposit in the posterior atrial septum that extends progressively deeper into the septum with advancing age, insinuating itself between the left atrial and right atrial components

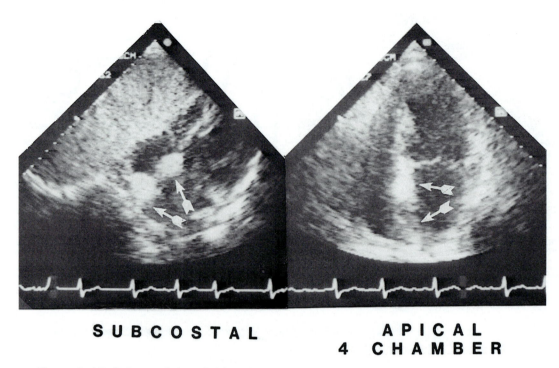

SUBCOSTAL

**APICAL
4 CHAMBER**

Figure 9–15. Subcostal view (left) and apical four-chamber view (right) in a patient with lipomatous hypertrophy of the atrial septum. Note dumbbell-like hypertrophy (arrows) with sparing of the fossa ovalis septal region.

of atrial septal myocardium. A few thin bands of atrial myocardium may be found embedded in the mass of fat; such myocardial fibers may on histology be normal, hypertrophied, or atrophied and may include the specialized pathways of interatrial conduction. Some clinicians think that this may be relevant to atrial arrhythmias or abnormal P waves, sometimes noted in patients with LHIAS.

Parts of the atrial septum affected by LHIAS appear bright and echogenic on echocardiography, more so than ventricular myocardium or epicardial fat. Perhaps this is related to the fact that atrial septal fat is, macroscopically and microscopically, different from epicardial fat; it is brownish rather than yellow and also more firm and compact.

Autopsy studies in normal hearts have shown that the thickest part of the atrial septum is the part posterior to the fossa ovalis.[63] In this region, septal thickness varied from 1.5 to 6 mm (mean 3.4 mm).

In another series, Page[59] found that the atrial septum was substantially thicker in 32 unselected elderly individuals (61 to 90 years), the range being from 2 to 25 mm (mean 12.5 mm). These measurements are relevant to the 2D echo diagnosis of atrial septal hypertrophy. The Mayo Clinic group suggested that the echocardiographic diagnosis of LHIAS should be based on the following criteria in the subcostal view: (1) atrial septal thickness of 15 mm or more, (2) bilobed appearance, the hypertrophy sparing the fossa ovalis, and (3) absence of other causes for atrial wall thickening, such as amyloid or other infiltrative myocardial disease or neoplastic invasion (rare).[60]

The actual distribution of atrial septal fat in LHIAS and of the resulting configuration on 2D echo (or other tomographic imaging) varies to some degree from patient to patient. The dumbbell contour is typical and diagnostically useful. In some, the thick atrial septum appears as a flat slab of uniform thickness. Often the posterosuperior atrial septum (above fossa ovalis) forms a very thick wedge (Figure 9–17), with the anteroinferior atrial septum less conspicuously thickened. Uncommonly, asymmetrical local bulges of LHIAS may mimic an atrial neoplasm or even partly obstruct the SVC. In such cases, as well as in the rare examples of massive LHIAS (maximal septal thickness of 4 to 5 cm or

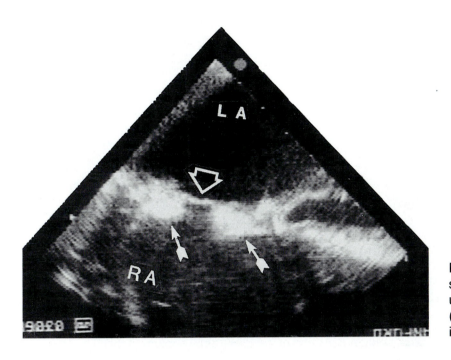

Figure 9–16. TEE view of atrial septum showing lipomatous hypertrophy. The upper and lower atrial septa are thick (small thin arrows), but the fossa ovalis is spared (open arrow).

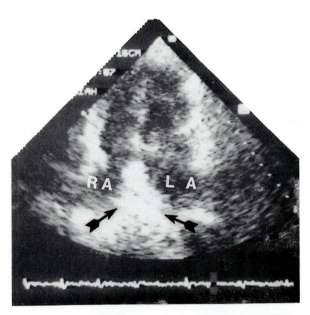

Figure 9–17. Apical four-chamber view of a patient with severe lipomatous hypertrophy of the atrial septum. In this view, the morphology is that of a triangular mass broadest at its upper part (atrial roof).

more), distortion of normal atrial contours may be so extreme and bizarre as to be even more suggestive of a neoplastic atrial mass.[61,64]

In common with other atrial septal abnormalities, LHIAS is best visualized in the subcostal four-chamber view (Figures 9–15 and 9–18) because the ultrasound beam is more perpendicular to the atrial septum in this view than in any other. TEE in a suitable plane also can achieve such optimal alignment of the atrial septum and therefore excellent imaging of LHIAS.[62,65] In two patients with LHIAS, lipomatous tissue was shown by TEE to extend from the atrial septum into the adjacent right wall epicardium.[65]

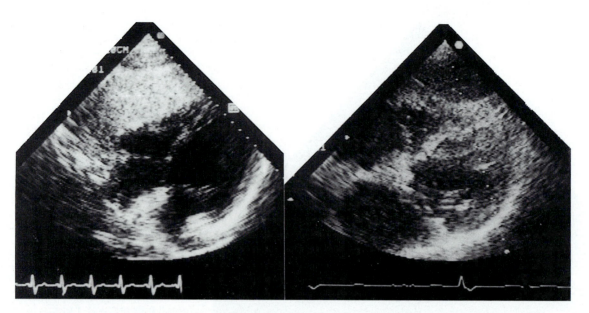

Figure 9–18. Subcostal view in two different patients showing wedge-shaped lipomatous hypertrophy of the upper atrial septum (left) and of the lower atrial septum (right).

REFERENCES

1. Walmsley R, Watson H. The medial wall of the right atrium. Circulation 1966;34:400.
2. Sweeney LJ, Rosenquist GC. The normal anatomy of the atrial septum in the human heart. Am Heart J 1979;98:194.
3. Schwinger ME, Gindea AJ, Freedberg RS, et al. The anatomy of the interatrial septum: A transesophageal echocardiographic study. Am Heart J 1990;119:1401.
4. Hagen PT, Scholtz DG, Edwards WD. Incidence and size of patent foramen ovale during the first 10 decades of life: An autopsy study of 965 normal hearts. Mayo Clin Proc 1984;59:17.
5. Mosvowitz C, Podolsky LA, Meyerowitz CB, et al. Patent foramen ovale: A nonfunctional embryological remnant or a potential cause of significant pathology. J Am Soc Echocardiogr 1992;5:259.
5a. Chenzbraun A, Pinto FJ, Schnittger I. Biplane transesophageal echocardiography in the diagnosis of patent foramen ovale. J Am Soc Echocardiogr 1993;6:417.
6. Siostrzonek P, Zangeneh M, Gossinger H, et al. Comparison of transesophageal and transthoracic contrast echocardiography for detection of a patent foramen ovale. Am J Cardiol 1991;68:1247.
7. Lynch JJ, Schuchard GH, Gross CM, et al. Prevalence of right-to-left shunting in the healthy population: Detection by Valsalva maneuver contrast echocardiography. Am J Cardiol 1984;53:1478.
8. Dubourg O, Bourdarias JP, Farcot JC, et al. Contrast echocardiographic visualization of cough-induced right-to-left shunt through a patent foramen ovale. J Am Coll Cardiol 1984;4:587.
9. Moorthy SS, Lasasso AM. Patency of the foramen ovale in the critically ill patient. Anesthesiology 1974;41:405.
10. Bansal RC, Marsa RJ, Holland D, et al. Severe hypoxemia due to shunting through a patent foramen ovale: A correctable complication of right ventricular infarction. J Am Coll Cardiol 1985;5:188.
11. Levine BD, Grayburn PA, Voyles WF, et al. Intracardiac shunting across a patent foramen ovale may exacerbate hypoxemia in high altitude pulmonary edema. Ann Intern Med 1991;114:569.
12. Holtzman H, Lippman M, Nakhajavan F, et al. Postpneumonectomy interatrial right-to-left shunt. Thorax 1980;35:307.
13. Langholz D, Louie EK, Konstadt SN, et al. Transesophageal echocardiographic demonstration of distinct mechanisms for right to left shunting across a patent foramen ovale in the absence of pulmonary hypertension. J Am Coll Cardiol 1991;18:1112.

14. Loscalzo J. Paradoxical embolism: Clinical presentation, diagnostic strategies and therapeutic options. Am Heart J 1986;112:141.
15. Lechat PH, Mas JL, Lascault G, et al. Prevalence of patent foramen ovale in patients with stroke. N Engl J Med 1988;318:1148.
16. Cujec B, Polasek P, Voll C. Transesophageal echocardiography in the detection of potential cardiac source of embolism in stroke patients. Stroke 1991;22:727.
17. Webster MWI, Chancellor AM, Smith HJ, et al. Patent foramen ovale in young stroke patients. Lancet 1988;2:11.
18. Lee RJ, Bartzokis T, Yeoh T, et al. Enhanced detection of intracardiac sources of cerebral emboli by transesophageal echocardiography. Stroke 1991;22:734.
19. Canavan MM. Two hearts with anomalies in the interauricular septum. J Tech Methods 1940;20:68.
20. Freedom RM, Rowe RD. Aneurysm of the atrial septum in tricuspid atresia. Am J Cardiol 1976;83:265.
21. Silver MD, Dorsey JS. Aneurysms of the septum primum in adults. Arch Pathol Lab Med 1978;102:62.
22. Gondi B, Nanda NC. Two-dimensional echocardiographic features of atrial septal aneurysm. Circulation 1981;63:452.
23. Alexander MD, Bloom KR, Hart P, et al. Atrial septal aneurysm: A cause for mid systolic click. Circulation 1981;63:1186.
24. Vandenbossche JC, Englert M. Effects of respiration on an atrial septal aneurysm of the fossa ovale shown by echocardiographic study. Am Heart J 1982;103:922.
25. Hauser AM, Timmis GC, Stewart JR, et al. Aneurysm of the atrial septum as diagnosed by echocardiography: Analysis of 11 patients. Am J Cardiol 1984;53:1401.
26. Hanley PC, Tajik AJ, Hynes JK, et al. Diagnosis and classification of atrial septal aneurysm by two-dimensional echocardiography: Report of 80 consecutive cases. J Am Coll Cardiol 1985;6:1370.
27. Burston DJ, McEniery PT, Stafford EG. Fenestrated atrial septal aneurysm: Diagnosis by transesophageal echocardiography. J Am Soc Echocardiogr 1990;3:499.
28. Iliceto S, Papa A, Sorino M, et al. Combined atrial septal aneurysm and mitral valve prolapse: Detection by two-dimensional echocardiography. Am J Cardiol 1984;54:1151.
29. Roberts WC. Aneurysm (redundancy) of the atrial septum (fossa ovale membrane) and prolapse (redundancy) of the mitral valve. Am J Cardiol 1984;54:1153.
30. Rahko PS, Xu QB. Increased prevalence of atrial septal aneurysm in mitral valve prolapse. Am J Cardiol 1990;66:235.
31. Abinader EG, Rokey R, Goldhammer E, et al. Prevalence of atrial septal aneurysm in patients with mitral valve prolapse. Am J Cardiol 1988;62:1139.
32. Thompson JI, Phillips LA, Melmon KL. Pseudotumor of right atrium: Report of a case and review of its etiology. Ann Intern Med 1966;64:665.
33. Smith AJ, Panidis IP, Berger S, et al. Large atrial septal aneurysm mimicking a right atrial mass. Am Heart J 1990;120:714.
34. Yeoh JK, Applebe AF, Martin RP. Atrial septal aneurysm mimicking a right atrial mass on tranesophageal echocardiography. Am J Cardiol 1991;68:827.
35. Shenoy MM, Vijaykumar PM, Friedman SA, et al. Atrial septal aneurysm associated with systemic embolism and interatrial right-to-left shunt. Arch Intern Med 1987;147:605.
36. Belkin RN, Hurwitz BJ, Kisslo J. Atrial septal aneurysm: Association with cerebrovascular and peripheral embolic events. Stroke 1987;18:856.
37. Zabalgoitia-Reyes M, Herrera C, Gandhi DK, et al. A possible mechanism for neurological ischemic events in patients with atrial septal aneurysm. Am J Cardiol 1990;66:761.
38. Schneider B, Hanrath P, Vogel P, et al. Improved morphological characterization of atrial septal aneurysm by transesophageal echocardiography: Relation to cerebrovascular events. J Am Coll Cardiol 1990;16:1000.
39. Pearson AC, Nagelhout D, Castello R, et al. Atrial septal aneurysm and stroke: A transesophageal echocardiographic study. J Am Coll Cardiol 1991;18:1223.
40. Edwards JE. Malformations of the atrial septal complex, in SE Gould (ed): Pathology of the Heart and Blood Vessels, 3d ed. Springfield, Ill: Charles C Thomas, 1968, p 262.
41. Bedford DE. The anatomical types of atrial septal defect: Their incidence and clinical diagnosis. Am J Cardiol 1960;6:568.
42. Dexter L. Atrial septal defect. Br Heart J 1956;18:208.
43. Forfar JC, Godman MJ. Functional and anatomic correlates in atrial septal defect: An echocardiographic analysis. Br Heart J 1985;54:193.
44. Cumming GR. Functional closure of atrial septal defects. Am J Cardiol 1968;22:888.

45. Mody MR. Serial hemodynamic observations in secundum atrial septal defect with special reference to spontaneous closure. Am J Cardiol 1973;32:978.

46. Cockerham JT, Martin TG, Gutterez FR, et al. Spontaneous closure of secundum atrial septal defect in infants and young children. Am J Cardiol 1983;52:1267.

47. Ferreira SMAG, Ho SY, Anderson RH. Morphological study of defects of the atrial septum within the oval fossa. Br Heart J 1992;67:316.

48. Gallagher ME, Sperling DR, Swinn JC, et al. Functional drainage of the inferior vena cava into the left atrium. Am J Cardiol 1963;12:561.

49. Davia JE, Cheitlin MD, Bedynek JL. Sinus venosus atrial septal defect. Am Heart J 1973;85:177.

50. Gotsman MS, Astley R, Parsons CG. Partial anomalous pulmonary venosus drainage in association with atrial septal defect. Br Heart J 1965;27:566.

51. Shub C, Dimopoulos IN, Seward JB, et al. Sensitivity of two-dimensional echocardiography in the direct visualization of atrial septal defects utilizing a subcostal approach. J Am Coll Cardiol 1983;4:127.

52. Fraker TD, Harris PJ, Behar VS, et al. Detection and exclusion of interatrial shunts by two-dimensional echocardiography and peripheral venous injections. Circulation 1979;59:379.

53. Hanrath P, Schluter M, Langenstein BA, et al. Detection of ostium secundum atrial septal defects by transesophageal cross-sectional echocardiography. Br Heart J 1983;49:350.

53a. Ishii M, Kato H, Inoue O, et al. Biplane transesophageal echo-Doppler studies of atrial septal defects. Am Heart J 1993;125:1363.

54. Weyman AE, Wann LS, Caldwell RL, et al. Negative contrast echocardiography: A new method for detecting left to right shunts. Circulation 1979;59:498.

55. Davies MJ. Mitral valve in secundum atrial septal defect. Br Heart J 1981;29:317.

56. Hynes KM, Frye RL, Brandenburg RO. Atrial septal defect (secundum) associated with mitral regurgitation. Am J Cardiol 1974;34:333.

57. Prior JT. Lipomatous hypertrophy of the cardiac interatrial septum. Arch Pathol 1964;78:11.

58. Handford H. Fatty tumor (lipoma) of the heart. Trans Pathol Soc Lond 1887;38:108.

59. Page D. Lipomatous hypertrophy of the cardiac interatrial septum: Its development and probable clinical significance. Hum Pathol 1970;1:151.

60. Fyke FE, Tajik AJ, Edwards WD, et al. Diagnosis of lipomatous hypertrophy of the atrial septum by two-dimensional echocardiography. J Am Coll Cardiol 1983;1:1352.

61. Applegate PM, Tajik AJ, Ehman RL, et al. Two-dimensional echocardiographic and magnetic resonance imaging observations in massive lipomatous hypertrophy of the atrial septum. Am J Cardiol 1987;59:489.

62. Kindman LA, Wright A, Tye T, et al. Lipomatous hypertrophy of the interatrial septum: Characterization by transesophageal and transthoracic echocardiography, magnetic resonance imaging and computed tomography. J Am Soc Echocardiogr 1988;1:450.

63. Sweeney LJ, Rosenquist GC. The normal anatomy of the atrial septum in the human heart. Am Heart J 1979;98:194.

64. Menegus MA, Greenberg MA, Spindola-Franco H, et al. Magnetic resonance imaging of suspected atrial tumors. Am Heart J 1992;123:1260.

65. Cohen IS, Raiker K. Atrial lipomatous hypertrophy: Lipomatous atrial hypertrophy with significant involvement of the right atrial wall. J Am Soc Echocardiogr 1993;6:30.

10

Left Atrium

NORMAL ANATOMY

The words *auricle* and *atrium* have been used interchangeably in the past. *Auricle* was the old term used for centuries (attributed to the resemblance of the protruding pointed part of each upper chamber to a dog's ear) to refer to the whole chamber. Earlier this century, the main chamber was commonly called the *atrium,* with *auricle* reserved for the small projecting portion. More recently, the word *auricle* has been dropped completely, *atrium* being used for the entire chamber, and the small *auricular* pouch is known as an *atrial appendage.*

The right and the left atrial appendages differ in shape; the right has a broader base and is very roughly conical in shape, whereas the left is narrower and somewhat tubular. Both end as a blind pouch in a blunt ridge or point. The left atrial appendage (LAA) is often most narrow at its attachment to the main atrial chamber. This becomes important when the surgeon introduces his or her finger into the LAA through a purse-string suture and tries to push it into the main left atrial chamber. The left atrial wall (3 mm) is slightly thicker than the right (2 mm).

The left atrial chamber (excluding the LAA) has been considered as ellipsoidal in shape for purposes of calculating its volume based on long-axis (base to roof) and short-axis (lateral and/or anteroposterior) dimensions. Its shape also may be compared with that of a biconvex lens with anterior and posterior surfaces. Gross left atrial dilatation is associated with change in shape toward the spherical.

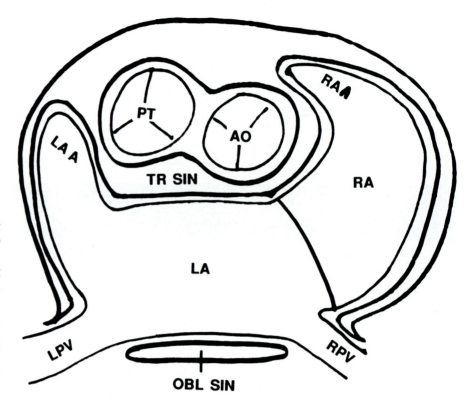

Figure 10–1. Diagram of transverse section through the heart to depict left atrial (LA) relationships, the view is from above (LAA, left atrial appendage; LVP, left pulmonary vein; RPV, right pulmonary vein; RA, right atrium; RAA, right atrial appendage; PT, pulmonary trunk; Ao, aorta; TR SIN, transverse sinus; OBL SIN, oblique sinus).

For the purpose of understanding its anatomic relationships (Figures 10-1 and 10-2), the left atrium may be divided into five walls, although, because of its smooth, rounded contour, these walls are not sharply demarcated from each other: superior, anterior, posterior, left lateral, and right lateral walls. Inferiorly, the chamber opens into the left ventricle through the mitral orifice.

Superiorly, the left atrium is closely related to the right pulmonary artery, which crosses the midline horizontally from left to right to reach the hilum of the right lung. The left pulmonary artery is not in contact with the left atrium or any other part of the heart.

Above the left atrium but not touching it are the tracheal bifurcation and the left bronchus. Elevation of the left bronchus by gross left atrial dilatation is a well-known sign on the chest radiograph.

Anteriorly, the upper left atrium is related to (1) the pulmonary trunk, from which it is separated by the transverse sinus, a pericardial recess lined by visceral pericardium, and (2) the ascending aorta, the transverse sinus intervening between it and the left atrium above, while below that level they are separated by connective adipose tissue. The noncoronary and left coronary sinuses of Valsalva face the left atrium; part of the former faces the right atrium.

Posteriorly, the left atrium is closely related to the esophagus so that left atrial and mitral valve structures are exquisitely visualized by transesophageal echocardiography (TEE). The descending thoracic aorta is adjacent to the esophagus in most of its extent and is therefore also amenable to detailed scrutiny by TEE.

Esophageal carcinoma, commonly located in the retrocardiac segment of the esophagus, can be visualized as a mass behind the left atrium that may impinge on the posterior left atrial wall and should not be mistaken for an intraatrial mass.[1] The same remarks and caveat apply to esophageal dilatation[2,3] and diaphragmatic hiatus hernia.[4-7]

The descending thoracic aorta and its abnormalities, such as dilatation and dissection, can be visualized by transthoracic (parasternal) echocardiography (TTE), but its great distance from the transducer results in poor resolution. TEE allows superb visualization of

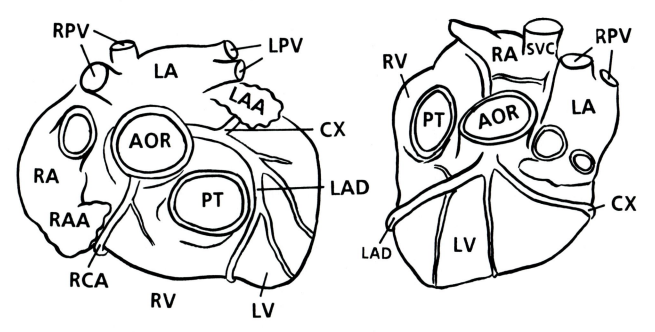

Figure 10–2. (Left) Diagram of superior aspect of the heart, with the large vessels removed near their cardiac attachment. (Right) Left-superior aspect of the heart; the left atrial appendage has been retracted from its normal location over the left coronary artery. Abbreviations as in Figure 10–1 (SVC, superior vena cava; LAD, left anterior descending artery; Cx, circumflex artery).

the descending thoracic aorta all through its length; it has therefore become very important in assessing patients with dissecting aneurysm of this vessel.

Dilatation of the retrocardiac part of the descending aorta may encroach on the left atrium (LA) posteriorly, resulting in an abnormally small anteroposterior LA dimension.[8] A dilated aortic root encroaches on the LA anteriorly and may likewise reduce the anteroposterior (AP) diameter of the LA chamber on the M-mode echocardiogram. In both situations, M-mode assessment of LA size would be grossly fallacious. The coronary sinus is another important structure closely related to the LA posteriorly, about 1 cm above the LA-LV junction.

The left lateral LA wall has no important relationships other than the left pleura and lung. The left atrial appendage (LAA) is a blind pouch that arises from the upper left corner of the chamber near the orifice of the left upper pulmonary vein. The LAA provides a roof or hood for the coronary fossa, a shallow depression in which the left main coronary artery runs as it emerges from the aortic root, embedded in loose adipose tissue. Above the LAA and coronary artery lies the pulmonary trunk. When viewed in parasternal short-axis view, this region, containing the left main coronary artery, is interposed between the large sonolucencies of the pulmonary trunk and the left atrium; it was called the "atriopulmonary sulcus" by Shah and Gramiak during the early years of M-mode echocardiography, but this term did not achieve an enduring usage.

The LAA is quite variable in size and shape. It may be curved or curled into a C or J configuration. Normally, the point of the LAA is directed anteriorly and superiorly, perhaps a little to the left or right. Unusually, the LAA is inverted toward the right so that its tip extends toward or as far as the right coronary artery. Another aberrant position of the LAA is to be inverted into the transverse pericardial sinus. Juxtaposition of the right and left atrial appendages is a rare anomalous situation (not rare, however, in children with severe cardiac defects such as common ventricle, transposition of the great vessels, common truncus arteriosus, etc.) wherein the two atrial appendages lie side by side within the transverse pericardial sinus.

The right wall of the LA is the interatrial septum. It has no special features except for the fossa ovalis and foramen ovale (when patent). Anteriorly, as well as posteriorly, a groove marks the location of the atrial septum; this groove tends to be deeper posteriorly than anteriorly. Epicardial fat is usually seen at these sites and in older patients tends to spread or penetrate into the atrial septum, forming the atrial septal thickening called *lipomatous hypertrophy.*

LEFT ATRIAL SIZE

The estimation of LA size is not merely an academic exercise. It is important to clinicians because it is an important consideration (1) in deciding whether or not to attempt conversion of atrial fibrillation to sinus rhythm, (2) in deciding whether or not to administer long-term anticoagulant therapy, (3) in assessing the severity of mitral stenosis or regurgitation, and (4) in assessing the severity of a left-to-right shunt at the ventricular or aortic level.

LA size estimation by M-mode echo was in wide use in the 1970s.[9-12] The anteroposterior LA dimension by the parasternal approach was measured. The American Society of Echocardiography (ASE) recommended that this dimension should be measured from the leading edge of the posterior aortic root echo to the leading edge of the posterior LA wall echo. In some M-mode echocardiograms, the latter can be closely and sharply defined; in others, there are ill-defined, fuzzy echoes in this vicinity, in which case it is recommended that they should be ignored and only a sharp, dense echo border (the "dominant line") be taken as the LA wall.

Several groups attempted the correlation of electrocardiographic LA enlargement (based on P-wave morphology) with LA dilatation on M-mode echography.[12-14] It was found by these authors that the ECG diagnosis of LA enlargement is reasonably specific but relatively insensitive.[12,13] The incidence of atrial fibrillation in patients with normal and enlarged LA chambers was studied by Henry et al.[15] and Watson et al.[16] In patients with rheumatic valve disease or hypertrophic cardiomyopathy, atrial fibrillation was exceptional if the M-mode LA dimension was less than 40 mm but the rule if it was over 55 mm in Henry's series; paroxysmal atrial fibrillation was frequent if the LA dimension was between 40 and 55 mm.

Whereas the initial studies correlating the M-mode LA dimension with angiographically determined LA volumes showed a good concordance,[9,10] later studies did not.[17,18] It has been demonstrated that LA volume estimations based on measurements of multiple orthogonal dimensions, or dimensions and LA areas, by two-dimensional (2D) echo correlate better with angiographic or with cine-CT imaging than with the M-mode LA dimension.[17-20] The anteroposterior LA dimension, whether obtained by the "blind" M-mode transducer (now seldom used) or by a cursor on the 2D echo long- or short-axis image, has certain shortcomings if used as the sole indicator of LA size: First, the posterior wall of the aortic root and the LA posterior wall are by no means always parallel, nor are all points on the LA posterior wall equidistant from the transducer placed on the chest wall—thus the LA dimension on M-mode can vary substantially in some cases depending on whether it is obtained at the attachment of the aortic valve, at the tips of the open cusps, or at a higher aortic level. Second, dilatation of the aortic root encroaches on the LA space, and the LA dimension in the AP axis becomes unduly small; this is more marked in thin persons with small AP thoracic diameter, perhaps with the straight-back syndrome. Less commonly, the descending thoracic aorta is so dilated that it encroaches on the LA posteriorly so as to reduce the AP dimension of the chamber to abnormally low levels. Third, severe LA enlargement is associated with change in LA shape (normally somewhat ellipsoidal) toward the spherical; i.e., very dilated LA chambers tend to be globular with little difference in orthogonal diameters. Therefore, extrapolation of any one dimension (such as the M-mode AP dimension) to actual LA volume size is prone to error in patients with severe LA dilatation. Figures 10–3 to 10–6 are examples of gross LA dilatation.

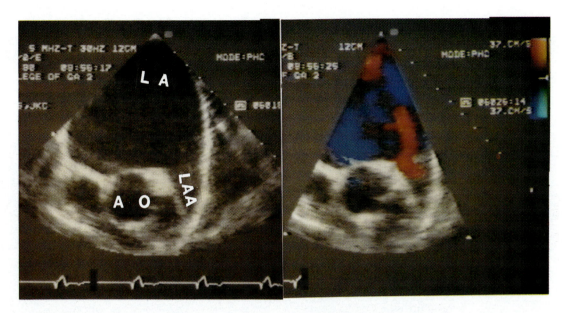

Figure 10–3. TEE showing a dilated left atrium (including atrial appendage LAA) in a patient with mitral stenosis.

NORMAL LEFT ATRIAL MEASUREMENTS

As measured on the original "blind" M-mode tracings, the normal range of LA dimension, based on 133 adults, was stated by Feigenbaum[21] to be 19 to 40 mm (mean 29 mm); corrected for body surface area, 12 to 22 mm/m² (mean 16 mm).[21] As obtained from 2D echo in parasternal long- and short-axis views in 50 normal subjects, the same LA dimension (anteroposterior dimension) was 21 to 37 mm in range (12 to 20 mm/m² of body surface area).

A more complicated but informative graphic depiction of the range of normal values for the LA M-mode dimension, taking into consideration the variables of age and body surface area, was published by Gardin et al.[22] It was based on measurements by standard ASE method in 136 adults of all ages with no clinically detectable heart disease or obesity. The statistics[22] reveal that older persons in the 40- to 80-year range tend to have larger LA dimensions than younger adults. Moreover, the upper limit of normal range in adults above age 40 and especially age 60 is well into the 40- to 50-mm range, which is the age and LA size category containing many of the patients with heart disease referred for LA size assessment.

Left Atrial Dimensions

In addition to the anteroposterior (AP) dimension measured on M-mode echo, the LA chamber has two other important dimensions that can be measured easily on 2D echo: the transverse or mediolateral dimension, on the parasternal short-axis or apical four-chamber view, and the superoinferior roof-to-base dimension (also called the *long* or *major LA axis*), on the apical four- or two-chamber view (Figure 10–7).

Normal values for all three dimensions, which are approximately orthogonal to each other, have been published by various authors[22-24]:

	Anteroposterior		Mediolateral		Superoinferior	
	Range	Mean	Range	Mean	Range	Mean
Weyman[14]	29–43 mm	35 mm	25–45mm	37mm	42–61 mm	51 mm
Schnittger et al.[15]	16–24 mm/m² BSA				23–35 mm/m² BSA	

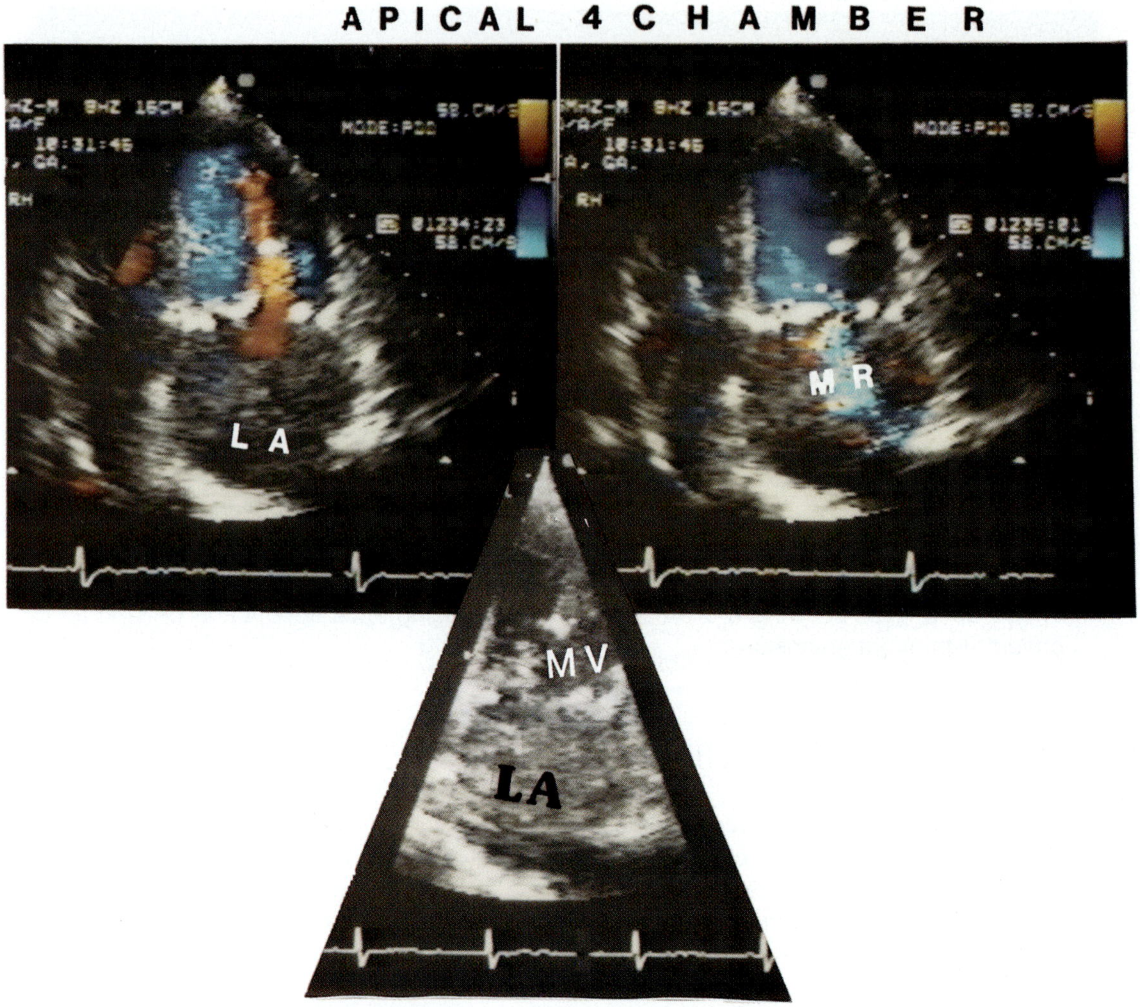

APICAL 4 CHAMBER

Figure 10–4. Apical four-chamber view: Dilated spherical left atrium in a patient with mitral stenosis. (Top Left) Colorflow Doppler shows a narrow inflow stream into the left ventricle; in systole (top right) a mitral regurgitant (MR) jet emerges at the same site. The left atrium is full of spontaneous echo contrast resulting from stagnant flow (below).

Pearlman et al.[16] measured LA dimensions in a population of 196 children and 72 adults without detectable heart disease. The three LA dimensions were plotted against body surface area. They demonstrated that LA dimensions increase as a function of body size, and the extent of variance also increases with body size. Whereas the transverse (mediolateral) and superoinferior (roof-to-base) LA dimensions are not usually measured in routine clinical echocardiography, it seems more scientific and thorough to measure all three LA dimensions when LA size is an important factor in a clinical study[25] or when an important clinical decision regarding anticoagulation or cardioversion will be made on the basis of LA size.

Recently, Stoddard et al.[25] have measured anteroposterior LA dimension by TEE and compared it with the conventional transthoracic echocardiography (TTE)–derived LA dimension. The LA plane imaged for this purpose was one that passes also through the aortic root and valve. These authors found that in normal subjects this TEE LA dimension was 33 ± 7 mm (range 20 to 45 mm) and 17 ± 3 mm/m^2 of body surface area (range 11 to 22 mm/m^2). The LA dimension by TEE was consistently and proportionately less than that by TTE: LA dimension (TTE) = LA dimension (TEE) $\times 0.6 \pm 15$ mm.

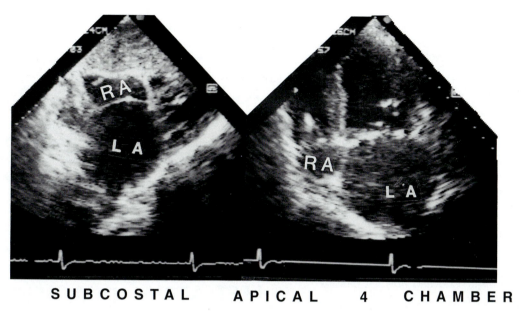

SUBCOSTAL   APICAL   4   CHAMBER

Figure 10–5. Subcostal view (left) and apical four-chamber view with a giant left atrium. Note spherical left atrial shape with bulging of the atrial septum toward the right atrium.

PARASTERNAL

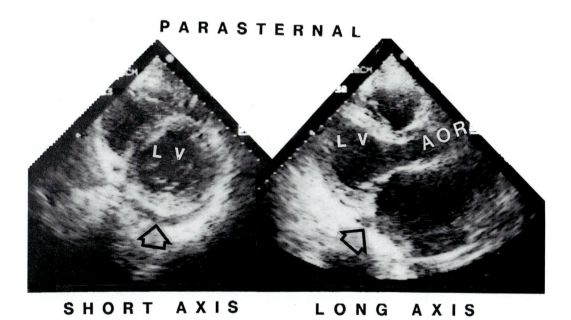

SHORT   AXIS   LONG   AXIS

Figure 10–6. Parasternal long-axis view (right) in a patient with severe left atrial dilatation. The left atrial chamber shows a small protrusion (arrow) behind the posterobasal left ventricular wall. In the parasternal short-axis view (left) this small sonolucent space mimics a small pericardial effusion.

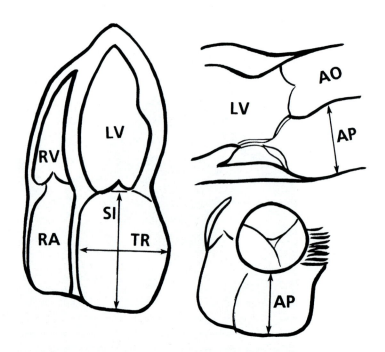

Figure 10–7. Diagram showing how LA dimensions are measured on 2D echo.

LEFT ATRIAL DIMENSIONS

Left Atrial Area

Using computerized electronic callipers and light pens, LA areas in the apical and subcostal views can be measured easily and quickly. Hofstetter et al.[26] measured LA areas at end-systole by inner-edge convention in the apical and subcostal views in infants and children (30 subjects aged 4 days to 7.5 years, mean 2.5 years) and found that these areas correlated very closely with the angiocardiographic LA area in the frontal plane ($r = 0.91$ for the apical view and $r = 0.98$ for the subcostal view).

Left Atrial Volume

It is not surprising that LA volume estimations in normal and diseased hearts have been attempted by several groups[10,18-20] because of the importance of ascertaining the presence and degree of LA dilatation in clinical cardiology. Schiller and associates[27] have pioneered the 2D echo assessment of left atrial and ventricular volume. In a series of 52 normal volunteers, LA volumes (end-diastolic as well as end-systolic) were measured by a modified Simpson's rule formula in apical four- and two-chamber views.[27] Gutman et al.[27] found a normal LA end-systolic volume of 37 ± 11.7 ml (mean ± SD) or 21 ± 6.6 ml/m^2 of body surface area; in the same study, the LA end-diastolic volume was 13 ± 5.7 ml, or 7.3 ± 3.2 ml/m^2 of body surface area. Kircher et al.[28] found excellent echo-angiocardiographic correlation for LA volumes under 300-ml size.

The mean value of Gutman et al.[27] for normal end-systolic LA volume was almost the same as that obtained by Gehl et al.[29] in 9 normal subjects—36 ± 11 ml. These estimates of normal LA volume are substantially less than those obtained in previous angiocardiographic studies published in the 1960s,[30,31] which were on the order of about 60 ml.

Some practical details in the 2D echo procedure for estimating LA volume[27] are worth mentioning: (1) patients were in the extreme left lateral position, (2) video recordings were made with the breath held in end-expiration, (3) the transducer was angled or tilted such that the maximal LA area was imaged, and (4) the inferior LA border was taken as a straight line joining the attachments of the anterior and posterior mitral leaflets and not the leaflets themselves.

Other Formulas for Left Atrial Volume Calculation

Schiller's group[17] and Wade et al.[18] used the Simpson rule or a modified Simpson rule method for calculating LA volume; Hofstetter[26] used the modification of Arcilla et al.[32] of the area-length formula of Sauter et al.[33] By the formula of Arcilla et al.,[32]

$$\text{Volume} = \frac{8}{3}\pi \times A_{fr} \times \frac{A_{lt}}{D_s}$$

where A_{fr} is the area in the frontal plane, A_{lt} is the area in the lateral plane, and D_s is the shorter of the long diameters in both planes. Yet others have used the ellipsoid formula:

$$\text{Volume} = \frac{4}{3} \times \pi \times \frac{L}{2} \times \frac{D_1}{2} \times \frac{D_2}{2}$$
$$= 0.523 \times L \times D_1 \times D_2$$

where L is the long axis, and D_1 and D_2 are the two minor axes.

GIANT LEFT ATRIUM

Extreme LA dilatation was described 90 years ago at autopsy,[34] and subsequently, several other excellent postmortem or radiographic descriptions of massively enlarged LA chambers were published.[35-40] Extreme LA dilatation is not only a spectacular finding in itself but also is sometimes associated with symptoms caused by compression or encroachment of the huge LA on adjacent anatomic structures.

Although quite rare, such pressure effects of a giant LA reflect the central position of this chamber in the posterior thorax such that it abuts against several important mediastinal structures. Thus dysphagia due to esophageal compression has been recorded, as well as hoarseness of the voice resulting from pressure on the left recurrent laryngeal nerve[38,39] and partial or complete bronchial obstruction.[38-40] Even back pain caused by vertebral erosion has been described.[41]

Recently, Minagoe et al.[42] made detailed Doppler observations of flow in the venae cavae and right atrium in patients with mitral stenosis. They found that mild obstruction to flow coming in through the inferior vena cava (IVC) was present in 18 patients with "giant LA." Severe rightward bulging of the atrial septum resulted in conspicuous narrowing of the right atrium so that Doppler (pulsed-wave and colorflow) demonstrated increased velocity at this site: between the atrial septal convexity and the anterior atrial wall just above the entry of the IVC. However, in this paper and in others, Japanese authors seem to apply the term *giant LA* to all LA chambers exceeding 65 mm of M-mode dimension. Most Western echocardiographers would restrict the adjective *giant* to larger LA chambers, perhaps over 80 mm, but this is admittedly an arbitrary cutoff point. The first M-mode echocardiogram of a patient with a giant LA was published by Kronzon and Mehta[43] in 1974. In subsequent papers by several groups on LA dimensions by M-mode echo in their respective series of patients with mitral valve disease, the upper end of the range varied from 72 to 87 mm. We reported the radiographic, CT, and 2D echo appearances of a patient with a prosthetic mitral valve and an LA chamber of enormous proportions[44] (M-mode AP dimension, 11 cm; superoinferior dimension, 11 cm; subcostal view, 13 cm). We estimated the LA volume to be approximately 1 liter. In this patient, the LA extended up to the right chest wall so that it was possible to visualize the atria from the right midaxillary line.

ANEURYSM OF THE LEFT ATRIUM OR ATRIAL APPENDAGE

Thirty-four cases of this rare anomaly, the diagnosis confirmed at surgery or autopsy, were reported by 1990.[45] In most instances, the left atrial appendage was dilated into a large to huge aneurysmal sac; in the remaining cases, some other part of the left atrial wall was the site of aneurysmal change. Williams[46] divided left atrial appendage aneurysms (LAAA) into extra- and intrapericardial categories. In the former, the primary defect is thought to be a local or partial absence of the left side of the pericardial sac through which the LAAA protrudes and progressively enlarges. In the latter, the pericardium is intact, but the left atrium or auricle wall is congenitally weak at one spot that dilates continuously over years under the distending force of intraatrial pressure.

LAAA is one of the few cardiac anomalies that mainly present in adult life. The mean age of the 34 reported cases collected by Frambach et al.[45] was 24 years (range 2 to 68 years). The condition remains asymptomatic until the patient presents with a supraventricular tachyarrhythmia, an episode of systemic embolism, or occasionally heart failure.

The left border of the cardiac silhouette has been distorted by a bulge in all cases. LAAA was first visualized by echocardiography in 1975, and more recent instances have used 2D echo to reveal typical morphology.[47,49] LAAAs can grow to enormous proportions (maximum diameter up to 20 cm). At surgery, 9 of the 22 LAAAs explored contained a thrombus. In about three-fourths of cases the atrial appendage is the site of aneurysmal dilatation; in the rest the aneurysm originates in the body of the left atrium.

On 2D echo, LAAA appears as a large sonolucent space adjacent to the left ventricle,[47-49] within the pericardium, extending toward the apex. The LAA indents the LV wall anterolaterally (or posteriorly if the aneurysm arises from the posterior left atrium). Thrombus may be suspected within the LAAA. The differential diagnosis includes other large left paracardiac spaces, including loculated pericardial effusion, pleural effusion, left ventricular pseudoaneurysms, pericardial or other mediastinal cysts, dilated coronary sinus, and massive coronary A-V fistula. TEE is particularly suited to excellent imaging of an LAAA, its communication with the main left atrial chamber, and the presence of intra-aneurysmal thrombus.[50,51]

COR TRIATRIATUM

Cor triatriatum is a rare congenital anomaly characterized by a fibromuscular septum within the left atrium dividing it into a posterior compartment that receives the pulmonary veins and an anterior compartment that includes the left atrial appendage and opens through the mitral valve into the left ventricle (Figure 10-8). The two chambers communicate through one or more orifices, usually small so that there is partial obstruction to flow into the left ventricle; the hemodynamic situation and symptoms are therefore similar to mitral stenosis.

The anomaly was first described in 1868[52] but remained a pathologic curiosity until angiographic diagnosis and surgical correction became possible in the 1950s and 1960s. The patient is usually an infant or young child, but sometimes the diagnosis is not made until adult life or even old age.[53,54] Despite its rarity (0.1% of all congenital heart disease),[55] cor triatriatum is worth bringing to the attention of echocardiographers because it has to be considered whenever abnormal linear left atrial echoes are seen on echocardiography.

The posterior part of the normal left atrium is developed from the common pulmonary vein, which is an embryonic vessel that normally gets incorporated fully into the true atrial chamber. Cor triatriatum is the result of failure of this process to take place. Strictly speaking, cor triatriatum is not due to development of a septum in the left atrium but to persistence of an embryologic structure; Van Praagh and Corsini[56] called the abnormal proximal chamber the "common pulmonary vein chamber of cor triatriatum," and Belcher[57] termed the anomaly "stenosis of the common pulmonary vein." Some therefore feel that using the synonym *subdivided left atrium*[58] is not entirely appropriate.

In typical or "classic" cor triatriatum, the proximal chamber is larger and thicker-walled than the anterior distal chamber. The abnormal septum separating the two chambers is usually thick and fibromuscular with one or more openings. The fossa ovalis is

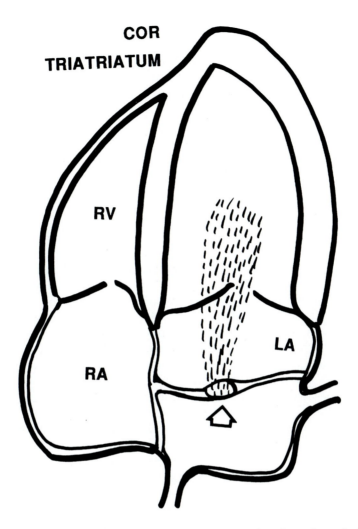

Figure 10–8. Diagram of cor triatriatum in apical four-chamber view. A diaphragm or septum separates the LA chamber into two parts, which communicate through a narrow opening (arrow).

more often between the proximal chamber and the right atrium than between the distal chamber and the right atrium. An atrial septal defect (ASD) is present in 70% of cases, though perhaps only a stretched foramen ovale.

Partial anomalous pulmonary venous drainage may be present. Part or all of the left lung may drain into the left innominate vein. Thilenius et al.[58] described a subvariety in which left pulmonary veins drained into the distal chamber but right pulmonary veins entered the proximal chamber.

Thus there are two modes of presentation of cor triatriatum: (1) with no interatrial shunt and narrow communicating orifice between the proximal and distal chamber, presenting like mitral stenosis, and (2) with a left-to-right shunt "decompressing" the obstructed proximal chamber, which resembles an ASD hemodynamically and clinically. This form is more conducive to longevity.

Echocardiography of Cor Triatriatum

M-mode echocardiography showed a linear echo in the left atrium and diastolic flutter on the mitral leaflets, but these findings are nonspecific. On the 2D echo, the abnormal septum is seen in multiple views.[53-55,59,60] In the parasternal short-axis view, it forms a linear echo more or less parallel to and near the posterior border of the aortic root; in the parasternal long-axis view, the linear echo tends to curve inferiorly toward the posterior mitral orifice but stopping short of it; and in the apical views, it manifests as two or even three linear arcs. In diastole, the abnormal septum moves toward the mitral valve. Doppler demonstrates a high velocity across it, indicating severity of stenosis. Colorflow Doppler shows an abnormal pattern of flow, perhaps a helpful clue when the abnormal septum itself is inconspicuous. TEE provides enhanced definition of the septation in the left atrium and also facilitates identification of entry of pulmonary veins into the posterior chamber, anomalous drainage of pulmonary veins (if present), and interatrial shunt (if present).

LEFT ATRIAL MASSES

Tumors

Primary benign tumors are by far more common than metastatic neoplasms; of these, myxomas are by far the most frequent.[61-64] Left atrial myxomas constitute 70% or more of all cardiac myxomas. The typical myxoma is a friable, soft, almost jelly-like tumor attached by a pedicle to the atrial septum. Its surface is smooth and glistening. Its size varies considerably, as does its shape, from spherical to oval to elongated (egg-, cigar-, or finger-like). Usually very mobile, they prolapse into the mitral orifice in diastole but get pushed back into the left atrium in systole. Thus they tend to obstruct mitral flow so that the symptoms, murmurs, and hemodynamics resemble those of rheumatic mitral stenosis. Occasionally, the impact on the mitral leaflets is traumatic enough to seriously damage the valve, making mitral valve replacement necessary at the time of tumor resection.

A minority (10%) of left atrial myxomas are sessile and nonmobile or almost so. Some myxomas are so large that they are too bulky to pass into the mitral orifice. On the other hand, very small myxomas are found at autopsy (or, recently, by TEE) as an incidental finding, having caused no symptoms or mitral obstruction.

The most important secondary change in an LA myxoma is breaking off of a fragment of it that embolizes. Surgical removal of such a tumor-embolus from the occluded artery and histologic identification of myxoma serve to establish or confirm the diagnosis. Other changes in the tumor that can sometimes be suspected on 2D echo include bacterial infection, intratumor hemorrhage or cystic change, and calcification. Although myxomas are usually nonmalignant, about 5% recur after surgical removal. Bilateral myxomas, growing from the atrial septum into both the LA and the RA, have a similar incidence. The echocardiographic diagnosis of LA myxomas was well established even in the M-mode era.[65-67] The tumor mass appears abruptly between the mitral leaflets in early diastole just after anterior motion of the anterior mitral leaflet and disappears abruptly as the mitral valve closes (Figures 10-9 to 10-11). This same to-and-fro motion into and out of the mitral orifice is even better appreciated on 2D echo.[68-71] Frequently, the tumor mass is pervaded by a speckled texture; however, myxomas vary much in echo density, and occasionally, the tumor mass is so fluffy or nebulous that it may be overlooked and suspected by an alert echocardiographer by mitral leaflet flutter (due to turbulence), by a filling defect in the mitral inflow colorflow Doppler stream, or by Doppler patterns of mitral stenosis without a mitral leaflet configuration of stenosis.

The pedicle with site of attachment (usually to the atrial septum) is commonly difficult to visualize well on TTE, but TEE is more successful in this respect; the contour and motion of the tumor are, expectedly, better appreciated by TEE.[72-74]

Sessile LA myxomas have been encountered on 2D echo.[75] Differentiation of these from malignant neoplasms or LA thrombi is difficult. Unusual echographic features of the tumor itself, suggesting cystic change,[71] intramass hemorrhage,[77] or infection,[78,79] have been reported. Doppler features of mitral obstruction are present in most cases. Colorflow Doppler findings indicating local turburlence are common adjacent to tumor masses during mitral inflow.

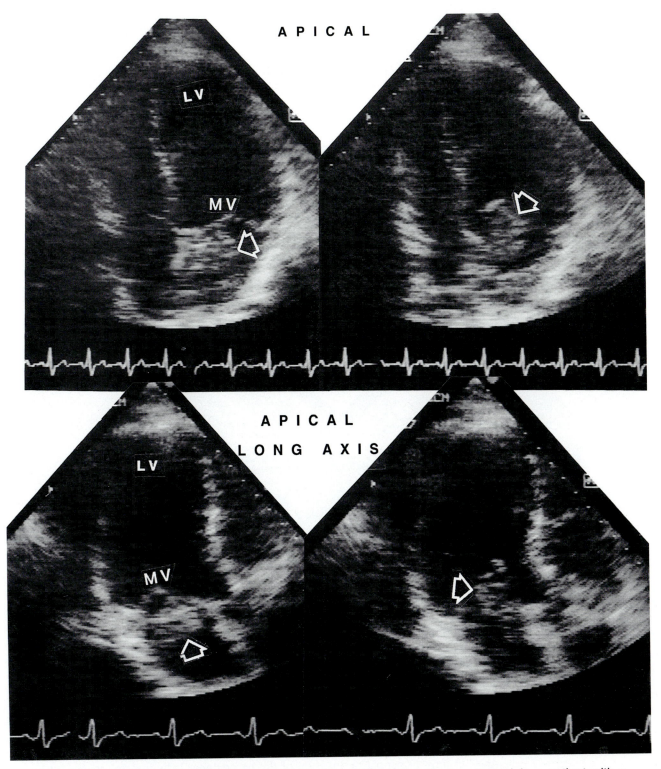

Figure 10–9. Apical four-chamber view (above) and apical long-axis view (below) in a patient with a left atrial myxoma. In systole (left frames) the mass (arrows) is seen in the left atrium, against the closed mitral valve (MV). In diastole (right frames) the mass protrudes into the left ventricle through the open mitral valve.

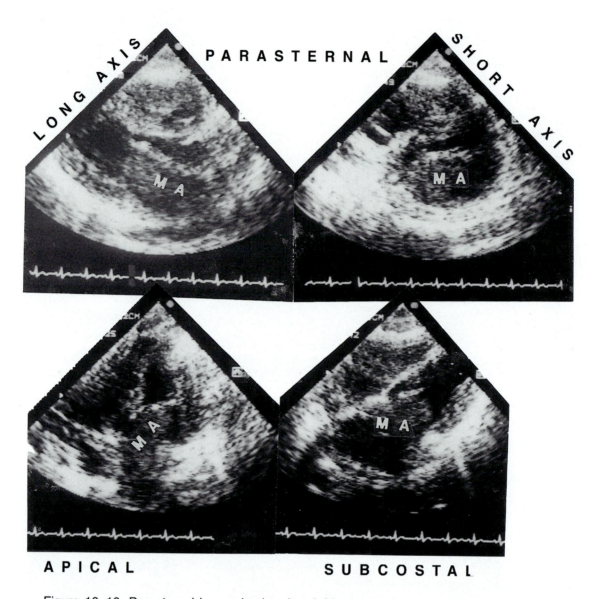

Figure 10–10. Parasternal long-axis view (top left), short-axis view (top right), apical four-chamber view (bottom left) and subcostal four-chamber view (bottom right) in a patient with a left atrial myxoma. In all views the mass protrudes through the open mitral valve in diastole.

Neoplasms other than myxomas have been reported as single case reports[80-84]; though rare, they may be suspected if a large, solid, rigid tumor mass projects into the LA from a fixed base in the LA wall. Sarcomas have a strong tendency to recur after excision. Another form of neoplastic invasion of the LA chamber is by invasive malignant lung tumors (primary or metastatic) that grow into the LA through a pulmonary vein; these tend to have some mobility and may be easily mistaken for LA myxomas.[80,83]

Left Atrial Thrombi

Mural thrombi in the main LA chamber are typically broad based with little mobility. In most cases, mitral valve stenosis or a prosthetic mitral valve is present.[85-88] Frequently, the thrombus is dense and perhaps calcified. On the LV posterior wall it may need to be

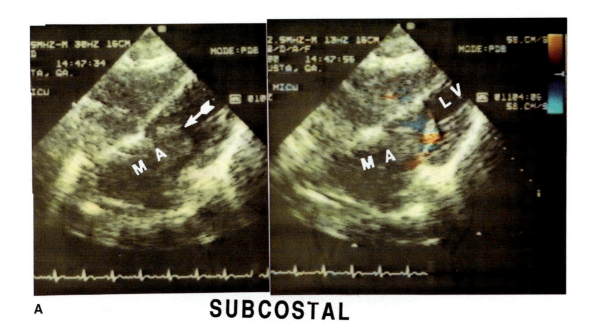

SUBCOSTAL

PARASTERNAL LONG AXIS

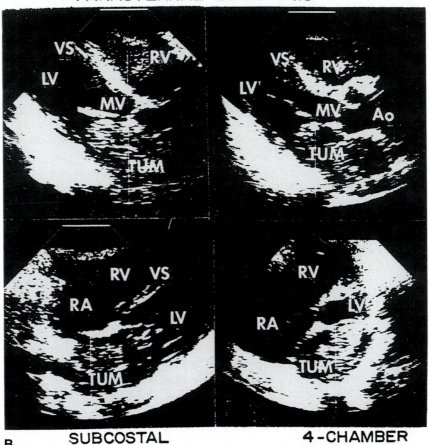

SUBCOSTAL　　　　　　**4-CHAMBER**

Figure 10–11. (A) Subcostal view of patient with left atrial myxoma (arrow) protruding into the mitral orifice and obstructing flow. Colorflow Doppler (right) shows narrow mitral inflow stream at the tumor's edge. (B) Parasternal, subcostal, and modified apical four-chamber view showing mobile LA mass, apparently typical of myxoma. It was in fact spread of lung malignancy through a bronchial vein.

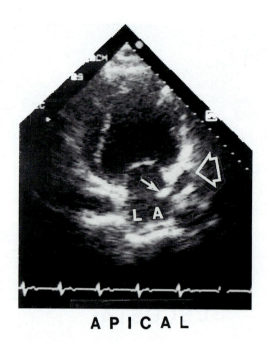

A P I C A L

Figure 10–12. Small projection or ridge (small arrows) at site of entry of left lower pulm onary vein (open arrow) into the left atrium (LA) is a normal variant. It should not be mistaken for a LA thrombus.

differentiated from a plaque associated with rheumatic mitral regurgitation (MR) (McCallum's patch). Autopsy studies indicate that, in mitral stenosis, thrombi in the left atrial appendage outnumber those in the main LA chamber.[85] Thrombi in the left atrium are occasionally encountered in patients with dilated and poorly functioning left ventricles, accompanied by mild to moderate LA dilatation. LA thrombi do not occur in individuals with normal LA, LV, and mitral valves.

On 2D echo, LV thrombi are variable in shape, size, and density. Ultrasound artifacts, normal variants such as the ridge between the orifice of the left lower pulmonary vein and the LA appendage (Figure 10-12), atypical mitral annulus calcification, and normal corrugations of the LA appendage can all mimic LA thrombi. Extrinsic masses (commonly hiatus hernia) can simulate LA masses (Figure 10-13). An unusual distortion of cardiac anatomy at the LV-LA junction by an LV pseudoaneurysm can simulate an LA mass (see Figure 10-14).

Although the visualization of thrombi in the LA appendage by conventional TTE has been reported,[92] it is very seldom that such a diagnosis can be made confidently in actual practice. However, TEE has revolutionized this aspect of echocardiography and has demonstrated that thrombi in the body or appendage of the LV chamber are not rare (see Figure 10-13), so TEE is now being routinely used for this purpose.[93]

Ball thrombi are rare but dramatic in appearance. They are found in the LA in patients with mitral valve stenosis or prosthetic valves. A large, smooth, free-floating thrombus cannot exit the chamber because of mitral stenosis. The theoretical danger of the mobile thrombus getting impacted in the mitral orifice causing syncope or "sudden death" is a notorious by extremely infrequent complication.

Spontaneous slow-moving contrast echoes swirling within the LA chamber were observed by TTE[102] several years ago but have been noted with much greater frequency on TEE in various conditions associated with stasis of blood within this chamber. There is little doubt that such findings predispose to and herald the formation of LA clots. This fact is important in deciding whether to start long-term anticoagulant therapy.

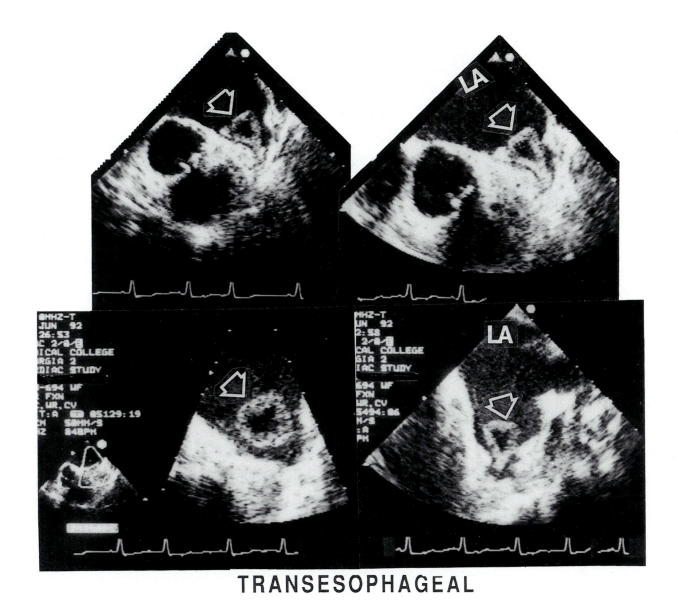

TRANSESOPHAGEAL

Figure 10–13. TEE view showing LA thrombus in a patient with mitral stenosis.

PULMONARY VEINS

Normal Anatomy

Each pulmonary lobe is drained by one vein; the right upper and middle lobe veins usually join to form one vein. Thus there are four pulmonary veins, two on each side, which pierce the pericardium separately to enter the left atrium. Of the many variants of this basic pattern, one is the joining of the two left pulmonary veins to form a common left vein; another variant is that of the three right pulmonary veins entering the LA separately.

APICAL

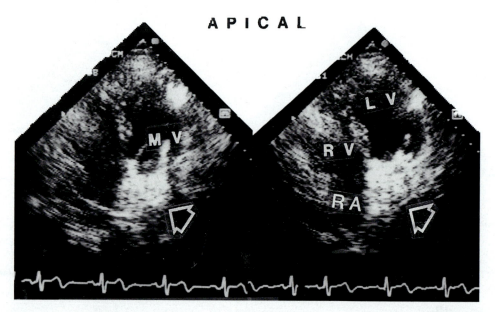

Figure 10–14. Apical four-chamber views in a patient with a diaphragmatic hiatus hernia. The latter encroaches on the left atrium, simulating a mass filling that chamber.

The pulmonary veins enter the LA chamber on its posterior aspect, nearer to its upper than to its lower border. The left upper pulmonary vein ostium is very close to the mouth of the LA appendage so that the junction between the two orifices may form a ridge projecting into the LA (Figures 10-12, 10-17, and 10-19). In the hilum of each lung, the upper pulmonary vein is anteroinferior to the respective pulmonary artery; the lower pulmonary vein is still more inferior. On the right side, the upper pulmonary vein runs posterior to the SVC, and the lower pulmonary vein runs posterior to the right atrium. On the left side, both pulmonary veins run anterior to the descending aorta.

Abnormalities of Pulmonary Veins

These are of major importance to pediatric cardiologists, but this is seldom true in adult practice. Abnormalities include (1) *anomalous drainage* into the right rather than left atrium, either directly or indirectly via one of the large systemic veins, and (2) *stenosis* of one or more pulmonary veins.[103] Anomalous pulmonary venous drainage may be *total,* all the veins joining to form a common vessel that empties into the SVC, IVC, coronary sinus, or a tributary of the former. Partial anomalous pulmonary venous drainage can involve one or more of the pulmonary veins. Volume overload of the right ventricle results, so the RV findings on echo resemble ASD. The systemic vein into which the pulmonary vein or veins drain is dilated and so may possibly be imaged in suprasternal or TEE views. Stenosis may accompany anomalous drainage or may be an isolated abnormality. Another cause is that resulting from certain operations performed to partly correct transposition of the great vessels (Mustard's or Senning's operation).

Echocardiography of Pulmonary Veins (Figures 10–16 to 10–19)

In the apical four-chamber view, the two left pulmonary veins can be imaged in suitable planes entering the LA chamber on its lateral (left) aspect. The right upper pulmonary vein enters the LA at its roof near the atrial septum. In infancy and childhood, the identification of normal entry of these veins into the LA chamber is important to exclude anom-

PARASTERNAL

LONG AXIS

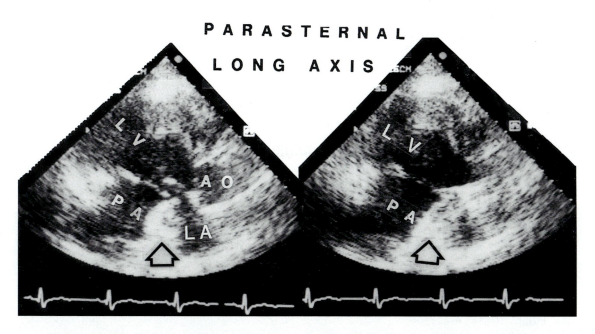

Figure 10–15. Parasternal long-axis views of patient with LV pseudoaneurysm follow-ing post-myocardial rupture of the LV posteroinferior wall. (Left) The posterobasal LV wall is displaced forward and upward by the pseudoaneurysm (PA), mimicking a large mass in the LA. In an unconventional off-center view (right) this "mass" seems to fill almost the whole LA chamber.

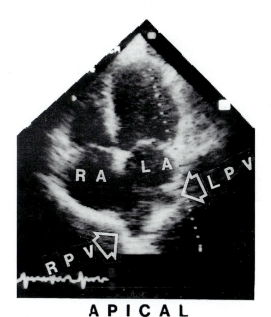

APICAL

4 CHAMBER

Figure 10–16. Apical four-chamber view showing entry of left upper pulmonary vein (arrow) and of right upper pulmonary vein (arrow) into the left atrium.

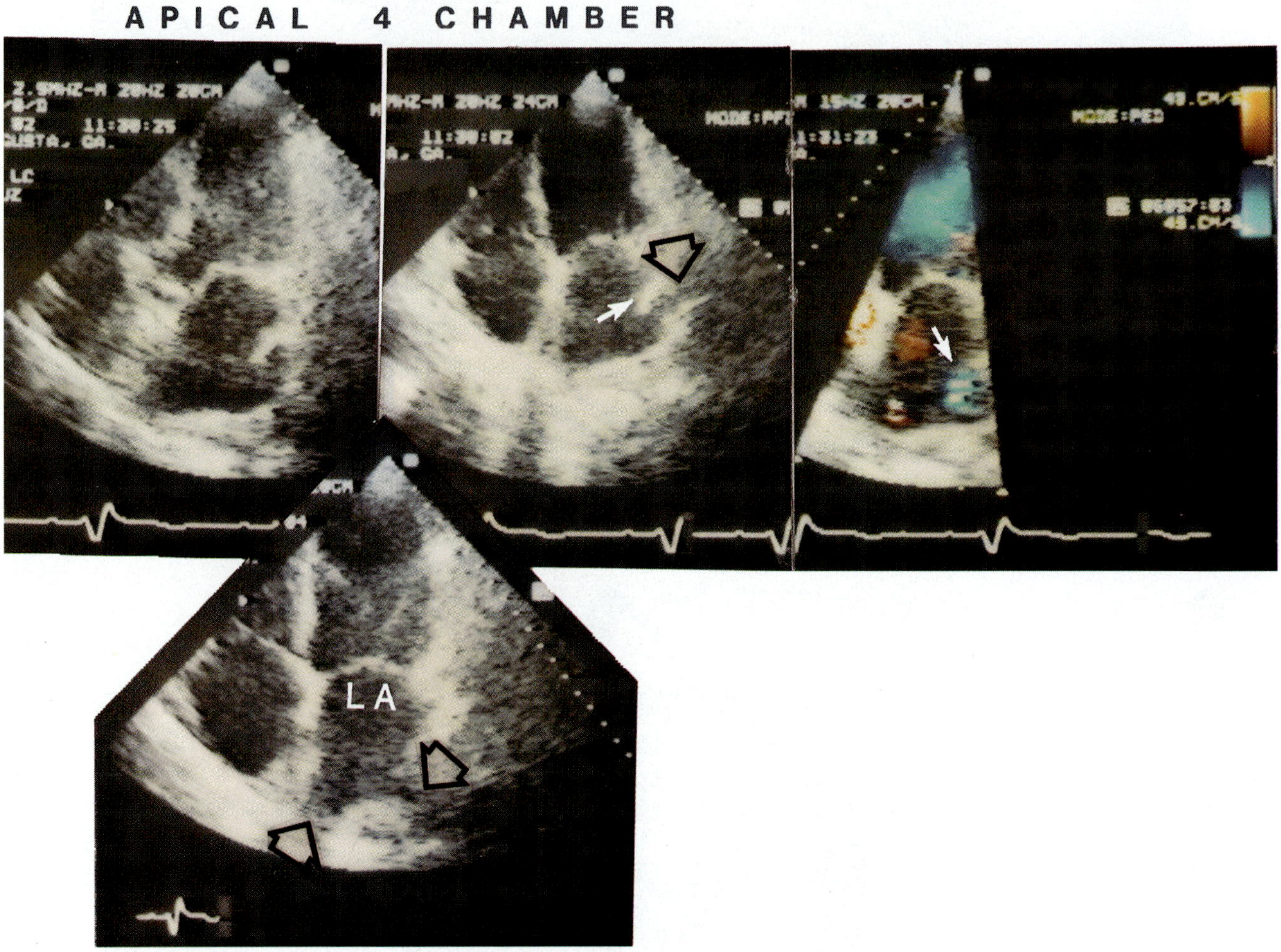

APICAL 4 CHAMBER

Figure 10–17. (Left) Apical "five-chamber" view showing apparently abnormal object attached to left atrial wall. (Center) In a more posterior plane, it is evident that this structure (arrow) is at the margin of the pulmonary vein ostium. (Right) Colorflow Doppler shows flow into the LA (arrow) through this vein. (Below) A more posterior plane showing the left upper and right upper pulmonary veins entering the LV chamber.

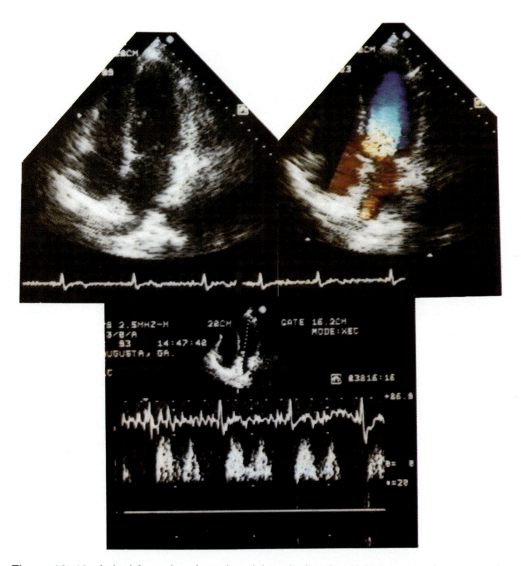

Figure 10–18. Apical four-chamber view (above) showing right upper pulmonary vein (arrow) near its entry into the left atrium. Colorflow Doppler confirms site of drainage of this vein into left atrium. Pulse-wave Doppler sampling at the mouth of the vein shows typical pattern of pulmonary venous flow.

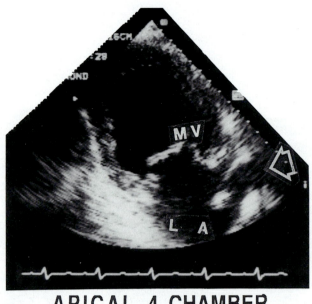

APICAL 4 CHAMBER

Figure 10–19. Apical four-chamber view in a patient with dilated cardiomyopathy and severe congestive heart failure. Arrow indicates dilated left lower pulmonary vein. Apparent small mass adjacent to it is the fold separating this vein from the left atrial appendage.

alous drainage. In adults, the right upper pulmonary vein is worth locating because pulsed-wave Doppler recording of its flow is valuable in assessing mitral regurgitation severity.[104] Suprasternal imaging of all four pulmonary veins entering the LA may sometimes be possible in children, the so-called "crab view" imaging the posterior mediastinum.

The pulmonary veins are prominent features in the TEE scene. Doppler recordings of pulmonary vein flow are easily recorded. Stenosis of pulmonary veins may be visualized on 2D TEE; increased velocity of flow and turbulence where the veins enter the LA are evidence of pulmonary vein stenosis.[105] The intrapericardial course of pulmonary veins is short, but in the presence of large pericardial effusions (especially large posterior high-pressure loculated effusions), the pulmonary veins appear stretched and conspicuous against the sonolucent background of the effusion.[106]

REFERENCES

Left Atrium

1. D'Cruz IA, Holman M, Battu P. Echocardiographic manifestations of esophageal carcinoma. Am Heart J 1992;123:1703.
2. Percy RF, Conetta DA, Miller AB. Esophageal compression of the heart presenting as an extracardiac mass on echocardiography. Chest 1984;85:826.
3. Hoit BD, Eppert D. Presbyesophagus masquerading as a extracardiac mass on echocardiography. Am Heart J 1989;118:419.
4. Nishimura RA, Tajik AJ, Schattenberg TT, et al. Diaphragmatic hernia mimicking an atrial mass: A two-dimensional echocardiographic pitfall. J Am Coll Cardiol 1985;5:992.
5. Baerman JM, Hogan L, Swiryn S. Diaphragmatic hernia producing symptoms and signs of a left atrial mass. Am Heart J 1988;116:198.
6. D'Cruz IA, Hoffman PK, Ewald FW. Echocardiography of posterior mediastinal masses encroaching on the left atrium. Echocardiography 1989;6:485.

7. D'Cruz IA, Holman M, Battu P, et al. Noninvasive imaging of a retrocardiac spleen. Chest 1992;101:1159.

8. D'Cruz IA, Callaghan WE. Imaging of the aorta: II. Doppler and two-dimensional echocardiography of descending thoracic aortic abnormalities. Am J Cardiac Imaging 1987;1:331.

9. Hirata T, Wolfe SB, Popp RL, et al. Estimation of left atrial size using ultrasound. Am Heart J 1969;78:43.

10. Ten Cate FJ, Kloster FE, Van Dorp WG, et al. Dimensions and volumes of left atrium and ventricle determined by single beam echocardiography. Br Heart J 1974;36:737.

11. Brown OR, Harrison DC, Popp RL. An improved method for echocardiographic detection of left atrial enlargement. Circulation 1974;50:58.

12. Waggoner AD, Adyanthaya AV, Quinones MA, et al. Left atrial enlargement: Echocardiographic assessment of electrocardiographic criteria. Circulation 1976;54:553.

13. Rubler S, Shah NN, Moallem A. Comparison of left atrial size and pulmonary capillary pressure with P wave of electrocardiogram. Am Heart J 1976;92:93.

14. Josephson ME, Kastor JA, Morganroth J. Electrocardiographic left atrial enlargement: Electrophysiologic, echocardiographic and hemodynamic correlates. Am J Cardiol 1977;39:967.

15. Henry WL, Morganroth J, Pearlman AS, et al. Relation between echocardiographically determined left atrial size and atrial fibrillation. Circulation 1976;53:273.

16. Watson DC, Henry WL, Epstein SE. Effects of operation on left atrial size and the occurrence of atrial fibrillation in patients with hypertrophic subaortic stenosis. Circulation 1977;55:178.

17. Schabelman S, Schiller NB, Silverman NH, et al. Left atrial volume estimation by two-dimensional echocardiography. Cathet Cardiovasc Diagn 1981;7:165.

18. Wade MR, Chandaratna PAN, Reid CL, et al. Accuracy of nondirected and directed M-mode echocardiography as an estimate of left atrial size. Am J Cardiol 1987;60:1208.

19. Hiraishi S, Disessa TG, Jarmakani JM, et al. Two-dimensional echocardiographic assessment of left atrial size in children. Am J Cardiol 1983;52:1249.

20. Kircher B, Abbott JA, Pau S, et al. Left atrial volume determination by biplane two-dimensional echocardiography: Validation by cine computed tomography. Am Heart J 1991;121:864.

21. Feigenbaum H. Echocardiography, 4th ed. Philadelphia: Lea & Febiger, 1986, pp 622, 636.

22. Weyman AE. Cross-Sectional Echocardiography. Philadelphia: Lea & Febiger, 1982.

23. Schnittger I, Gordon EP, Fitzgerald PJ, et al. Standardized intracardiac measurements of two-dimensional echocardiography. J Am Coll Cardiol 1983;2:934.

24. Pearlman JD, Triulzi MO, King ME, et al. Left atrial dimensions in growth and development: Normal limits for two-dimensional echocardiography. J Am Coll Cardiol 1990;16:1168.

25. Stoddard MF, Liddell NE, Vogel RL, et al. Comparison of cardiac dimensions by transesophageal and transthoracic echocardiography. Am Heart J 1992;124:675.

26. Hoffsteter R, Bartz-Bazzanella P, Kentrup H, et al. Determination of left atrial area and volume by cross-sectional echocardiography in healthy infants and children. Am J Cardiol 1991;68:1073.

27. Gutman J, Wang YS, Wahr D, et al. Normal left atrial function determined by two-dimensional echocardiography. Am J Cardiol 1983;51:336.

28. Kircher B, Abbott JA, Pau S, et al. Left atrial volume determination by biplane two-dimensional echocardiography: Validation by cine computed tomography. Am Heart J 1991;121:864.

29. Gehl LS, Mintz GS, Kotler MN, et al. Left atrial volume overload in mitral regurgitation: A two-dimensional echocardiographic study. Am J Cardiol 1982;49:33.

30. Hawley RR, Dodge HT, Graham TP. Left atrial volume and its changes in heart disease. Circulation 1966;34:989.

31. Murray JA, Kennedy JW, Figley MM. Quantitative angiocardiography: II. The normal left atrial volume in man. Circulation 1968;37:826.

32. Arcilla RA, Thilenius O, Chiemmongtip P, et al. Left atrial volume calculation by angiocardiography in children. Chest 1973;63:189.

33. Sauter HJ, Dodge HT, Johnson RR, et al. The relationship of left atrial pressure and volume in patients with heart disease. Am Heart J 1964;67:635.

34. Owen I, Fenton WJ. A case of extreme dilatation of the left auricle of the heart. Trans Clin Soc Lond 1901;34:183.

35. Shaw HB. A case of extreme dilatation of the left auricle. Lancet 1924;2:493.

36. Parkinson J. Enlargement of the heart. Lancet 1936;1:1391.
37. Parsonnet AE, Bernstein A, Maitland HS. Massive left auricle with special reference to its etiology and mechanism. Am Heart J 1946;31:438.
38. Daley R, Franks R. Massive dilatation of the left auricle. Q J Med 1949;18:81.
39. DeSanctis RW, Dean DC, Bland EF. Extreme left atrial enlargement. Circulation 1964;29:14.
40. Bach F, Keith TS. Enlargement of the left auricle of the heart. Lancet 1929;2:766.
41. Ashworth H, Jones AM. Aneurysmal dilatation of the left auricle with erosion of the spine. Br Heart J 1946;9:207.
42. Minagoe S, Yoshikawa J, Yoshida K, et al. Obstruction of inferior vena caval orifice by giant left atrium in patients with mitral stenosis. Circulation 1992;86:214.
43. Kronzon I, Mehta A. Giant left atrium. Chest 1974;65:677.
44. D'Cruz IA, Haverty HO, Pallas CW. Noninvasive imaging of a giant left atrium. Am J Cardiac Imaging 1989;3:149.
45. Frambach PJGM, Geskes GG, Cheriex EC, et al. Giant intrapericardial aneurysm of the left atrial appendage. Eur Heart J 1990;11:848.
46. Williams WG. Dilatation of the left atrial appendage. Br Heart J 1963;25:643.
47. Foale RA, Gibson TC, Guyer DE, et al. Congenital aneurysms of the left atrium: Recognition by cross-sectional echocardiography. Circulation 1982;66:1065.
48. Labarre TR, Stamato NJ, Hwang MH, et al. Left atrial appendage aneurysm with associated anomalous pulmonary venous drainage. Am Heart J 1987;114:1243.
49. Pinamonti B, Alberti E, Buttignol G, et al. Echocardiographic diagnosis of congenital left atrial aneurysm. Am Heart J 1986;111:406.
50. Comess KA, LaBate DF, Winter JA, et al. Congenital left atrial appendage aneurysm with intact pericardium: Diagnosis by transesophageal echocardiography. Am Heart J 1990;120:992.
51. Burke RP, Mark JB, Collins JJ, et al. Improved surgical approach to left atrial appendage aneurysm. J Cardiac Surg 1992;52:104.
52. Church WS. Congenital malformation of the heart: Abnormal septum in left auricle. Trans Pathol Soc Lond 1867/8;19:188.
53. Fagan LF, Penick DR, Williams GA. Two-dimensional, spectral Doppler and color flow imaging in adults with acquired and congenital cor triatriatum. J Am Soc Echocardiogr 1991;4:177.
54. Patel AK, Ninneman RW, Rahko PS. Surgical resection of cor triatriatum in a 74-year-old man: Review of echocardiographic findings with emphasis on Doppler and transesophageal echocardiography. J Am Soc Echocardiogr 1990;3:402.
55. Ostman-Smith I, Silverman NH, Oldershaw P, et al. Cor triatriatum sinistrum: Diagnostic features on cross-sectional echocardiography. Br Heart J 1984;51:211.
56. Van Praagh R, Corsini I. Cor triatriatum. Am Heart J 1969;78:379.
57. Belcher JR, Somerville W. Cor triatriatum (stenosis of the common pulmonary vein). Br Med J 1951;1:1280.
58. Thilenius DG, Bharati S, Lev M. Subdivided left atrium: An expanded concept of triatriatum sinistrum. Am J Cardiol 1976;37:743.
59. De Belder MA, Argano V, Burrell CJ. Cor triatriatum sinister, not mitral stenosis, in an adult with previous Sydenham's chorea. Br Heart J 1992;68:9.
60. Lengyel M, Arvay A, Biro V. Two-dimensional echocardiographic diagnosis of cor triatriatum. Am J Cardiol 1987;59:484.
61. Nasser WK, Davis RH, Dillon JC, et al. Atrial myxoma: I. Clinical and pathologic features in nine cases. Am Heart J 1972;83:694.
62. Greenwood WF. Profile of atrial myxoma. Am J Cardiol 1968;21:367.
63. Newman HA, Cordell AR, Pritchard RW. Intracardiac myxomas. Am Surg 1966;32:219.
64. Bulkley BH, Hutchins GM. Atrial myxomas: A fifty-year review. Am Heart J 1979;97:639.
65. Finegan RE, Harrison DC. Diagnosis of left atrial myxoma by echocardiography. N Engl J Med 1970;282:1022.
66. Bass NM, Sharratt GP. Left atrial myxoma diagnosed by echocardiography with observations on tumor movement. Br Heart J 1973;35:1332.
67. Kostis JB, Moghadam AN. Echocardiographic diagnosis of left atrial myxoma. Chest 1970;58:550.
68. Moses HW, Nanda NC. Real-time two-dimensional echocardiography in the diagnosis of left atrial myoma. Chest 1980;78:788.
69. Lappe DC, Bulkley BH, Weiss JL. Two-dimensional echocardiographic diagnosis of left atrial myxoma. Chest 1978;74:55.

70. Perry LS, King JF, Zeft HO, et al. Two-dimensional echocardiography in the diagnosis of left atrial myxoma. Br Heart J 1981;45:667.

71. Nomeir AM, Watts LE, Seagle R, et al. Intracardiac myxomas. J Am Soc Echocardiogr 1989;2:139.

72. Obeid AI, Marvasti M, Parker F, et al. Comparison of transthoracic and transesophageal echocardiography in diagnosis of left atrial myxoma. Am J Cardiol 1989;63:1006.

73. Reeves WC, Chitwood WR. Assessment of left atrial myxoma using transesophageal two-dimensional echocardiography and color-flow Doppler. Echocardiography 1989;6:547.

74. Thier W, Schluter M, Krebber J, et al. Cysts in left atrial myxomas identified by trans-esophageal cross-sectional echocardiography. Am J Cardiol 1983;51:1793.

75. Lee YC, Magram NY. Nonprolapsing left atrial tumor. Chest 1980;78:332.

76. Mugge A, Daniel WG, Haverich A, et al. Diagnosis of noninfective cardiac mass lesions by two-dimensional echocardiography. Circulation 1991;83:70.

77. Rahilly GT, Nanda NC. Two-dimensional echocardiographic identification of tumor hemor-rhages in atrial myxomas. Am Heart J 1981;101:237.

78. Tunick PA, Fox AC, Culliford A, et al. The echocardiographic of an atrial myxoma vegeta-tion. Am Heart J 1990;119:679.

79. Quinn TJ, Codini MA, Harris AA. Infected cardiac myxoma. Am J Cardiol 1984;53:361.

80. Mich RJ, Gillam LD, Weyman AE. Osteogenic sarcoma mimicking left atrial myxomas. J Am Coll Cardiol 1985;6:1422.

81. Shecter M, Glikson M, Agranat O, et al. Echocardiographic demonstration of mitral block caused by left atrial spindle cell sarcoma. Am Heart J 1992;123:232.

82. Hui G, McAllister HA, Angelini P. Left atrial paraganglionoma. Am Heart J 1987;113:1230.

83. D'Cruz IA, Roth P. Left atrial extension of pulmonary adenocarcinoma mimicking left atrial myxoma. Echocardiography 1987;4:89.

84. Pasquale M, Katz NM, Caruso AC, et al. Myxoid variant of malignant fibrous histiocytoma of the heart. Am Heart J 1991;122:248.

85. Jordan RA, Scheifley CH, Edwards JE. Mural thrombosis and arterial embolism in mitral stenosis. Circulation 1951;3:363.

86. Boyrne G. Embolism in mitral stenosis. Br Heart J 1950;12:263.

87. Wallach JB, Lukash L, Angrist AA. An interpretation of the incidence of mural thrombi in the left auricle and appendage with particular reference to mitral commisurotomy. Am Heart J 1953;45:252.

88. Bansal RC, Heywood IT, Applegate PM, et al. Detection of left atrial thrombi by two-dimen-sional echocardiography and surgical correlation in 148 patients with mitral valve disease. Am J Cardiol 1989;64:243.

89. Okun M, Plotnick GD, Salmon D, et al. Two-dimensional echocardiographic detection of bia-trial thrombi. Am Heart J 1987;114:184.

90. DePace NL, Soulen RL, Kotler MN, et al. Two-dimensional echocardiographic detection of intraatrial masses. Am J Cardiol 1981;48:954.

91. Mikel FL, Asinger RW, Rourke T, et al. Two-dimensional echocardiographic demonstration of left atrial thrombi in patients with prosthetic mitral valves. Circulation 1979;60: 1183.

92. Herzog CA, Bass D, Kane M, et al. Two-dimensional echocardiographic imaging of left atrial appendage thrombi. J Am Coll Cardiol 1984;3:1340.

93. Schweitzer P, Bardos P, Erbel R, et al. Detection of left atrial thrombi by echocardiography. Br Heart J 1981;45:148.

94. Olson JD, Goldenberg IF, Pedersen N, et al. Exclusion of atrial thrombus by transesophageal echocardiography. J Am Soc Echocardiogr 1992;5:52.

95. Manning WJ, Reis GJ, Douglas PS. Use of transesophageal echocardiography to detect left atrial thrombus before percutaneous balloon dilatation of the mitral valve. Br Heart J 1992;67:170.

96. Aschenberg W, Schluter M, Kremer P, et al. Transesophageal two-dimensional echocardiog-raphy for the detection of left atrial appendage thrombus. J Am Coll Cardiol 1986;7:163.

97. Hwang JJ, Kuan P, Lin SC, et al. Reappraisal by transesophageal echocardiography of the sig-nificance of left atrial thrombi in the prediction of systemic arterial embolization in rheumatic mitral valve disease. Am J Cardiol 1992;70:767.

98. Furukawa K, Katsume H, Matsukubo H, et al. Echocardiographic findings of floating throm-bus in the left atrium. Br Heart J 1980;44:599.

99. Gottdiener JS, Temeck BK, Patterson RH, et al. Transient occlusion of the mitral valve ori-fice by a free-floating left atrial ball thrombus. Am J Cardiol 1984;53:1730.

100. Wrisley D, Giambartolomei A, Lee T, et al. Left atrial ball thrombus. Am Heart J 1991;121:1784.
101. Rey M, Tunon J, Vinolas X, et al. Free-floating left atrial thrombus and its mechanical interaction with mitral regurgitant jet assessed by color Doppler echocardiography. Am Heart J 1992;123:1067.
102. Garcia-Fernandez MA, Moreno M, Banuelos F. Two-dimensional echocardiographic identification of blood stasis in the left atrium. Am Heart J 1985;109:600.
103. Sade RM, Freed MD, Mathews EC, et al. Stenosis of individual pulmonary veins. J Thorac Cardiovasc Surg 1974;67:953.
104. Smallhorn JF, Pauperio H, Benson L, et al. Pulsed Doppler assessment of pulmonary vein obstruction. Am Heart J 1985;110:483.
105. Samdarshi TE, Morrow WR, Helmcke FR, et al. Assessment of pulmonary vein stenosis by transesophageal echocardiography. Am Heart J 1991;122:1495.
106. D'Cruz IA, Macander PJ, Gross CM, et al. Distension of the oblique pericardial sinus in tamponade due to loculated posterior pericardial effusion. Am J Cardiol 1990;65:1520.

11

Mitral Valve

NORMAL ANATOMY

In common parlance, the words *mitral valve* usually refer to the mitral leaflets. However, when considering the functional integrity of this vital cardiac structure, it is important to think in terms of the mitral valve apparatus, which includes not only the mitral leaflets but also the mitral annulus, the chordae tendineae, and the papillary muscles.[1-6] Thus mitral stenosis is usually due to rheumatic leaflet scarring, but chordal sclerosis also may contribute to orifice narrowing. Mitral regurgitation can be due to abnormalities of leaflets, chordae, papillary muscles, or mitral annulus.

The cardiac chambers on either side of the mitral valve—the left atrium and ventricle—especially the latter, also have a role to play in mitral function. The papillary muscles are not only seated on the LV wall but also are continuous and integrated with the ventricular myocardium so that hypocontractility or infarction of the LV wall underlying the papillary muscles or LV dilatation altering papillary muscle alignment can cause or aggravate mitral regurgitation.

This chapter will first describe each component of the mitral valve apparatus and then discuss how all these components are thought to act together in accomplishing efficient valve closing and opening; finally, the common lesions altering mitral anatomy and function (causing stenosis or regurgitation) will be reviewed.

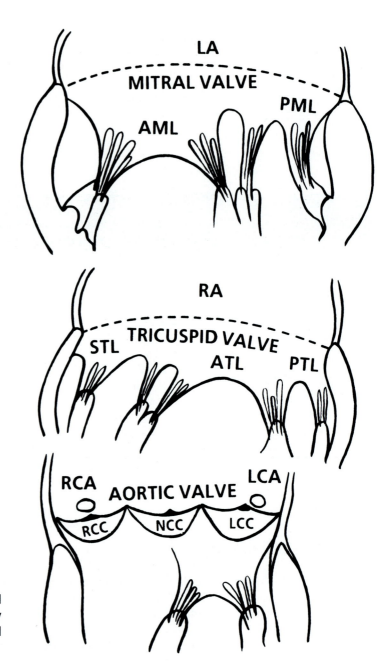

Figure 11–1. Diagram showing anatomy of mitral leaflets; the LV has been cut open longitudinally and spread apart (AML and PML, anterior and posterior mitral leaflets, respectively).

Mitral Valve Leaflets

The mitral leaflets (Figure 11-1) must be thought of not merely as two flaps coming together in systole and moving apart in diastole but rather as a continuous veil or curtain of valve tissue suspended from the entire 360-degree circumference of the mitral valve "ring." In addition to the two leaflets, there are two commissures that connect the leaflets at each end. The anterior and posterior mitral leaflets are, of course, the principal components of the mitral valve. The anterior leaflet, sometimes in the past called the *antero-medial* or *aortic leaflet* (because of its proximity to the aortic valve), is narrower at its base but longer from attachment to free edge than the posterior leaflet. The latter, also called the *posterolateral, mural,* or *ventricular leaflet* in the past (because of its close relation to the left ventricular posterior wall), is short from base to free edge but extends over twice as much of the mitral ring circumference as the anterior leaflet.

The free edges of the anterior and posterior mitral leaflets do not extend all the way to the annulus. In other words, the two leaflets are connected to each other by segments of valve tissue known as *commissures:* posteromedial and anterolateral.

The anterior mitral leaflet is roughly triangular or semicircular in shape; its free edge is not significantly indented, unlike the posterior leaflet. Its average length (attachment to free edge) and width are both about 3 cm. The leaflet divides the basal left ventricle (LV) into inflow and outflow tracts, thus becoming part of both.

On its atrial surface can be discerned a ridge 8 to 10 mm from its free edge—the line of leaflet closure. Between this line and the free edge is the *rough zone* of the leaflet; it is thicker than the rest of the leaflet and widest at its center (at the tip or apex of the leaflet) and is the area receiving insertion of the chordae tendineae. It is also the part of the leaflet that opposes the posterior leaflet during systole. The rest of the anterior leaflet, between the rough zone and leaflet attachment, is the *clear zone,* translucent on transillumination and devoid of chordal attachment. At its broadest (center of leaflet), the clear zone of the anterior mitral leaflet is twice as broad as the rough zone.

The posterior mitral leaflet is only 1.2 mm long but 4.8 cm wide on average, thus occupying much more of the annulus circumference than the anterior leaflet though being "low profile" compared with the latter. The free edge of the posterior leaflet exhibits two prominent indentations. The leaflet is thus divided, in 90% of hearts, into three scallops, a large central scallop with a smaller scallop on either side. In the past, semantic confusion has been caused by some authors calling the lesser scallops "accessory" or "commissural mitral cusps" or even "junctional tissue."

Proceeding from free edge to attachment of the posterior leaflet, three zones can be distinguished: (1) as with the anterior leaflet, the *rough zone* between free edge and line of closure, receiving the insertions of the main chordae tendineae, and wider at the center than at the end of each scallop, (2) the *clear zone,* devoid of chordae and much narrower than the corresponding zone of the anterior leaflet, and (3) the *basal zone,* a narrow 2-mm area between the clear zone and leaflet attachment, restricted mainly to the large middle scallop. The basal zone has no counterpart in the anterior mitral leaflet.

Barlow's measurements of the mitral leaflets in his South African autopsy subjects are anterior leaflet, 2.5 to 4.5 cm, and posterior leaflet: central scallop, 2.0 to 4.0 cm, lateral scallop, 1.0 to 1.8 cm, medial scallop, 0.8 to 1.6 cm.[6]

Structure of Leaflets.

Under the surface lining of endocardium, the leaflet consists of three layers: (1) a thin fibrous layer facing the left atrium—the *atrialis,* (2) a tough collagenous layer facing the left ventricle—the *ventricularis* (this provides the real tensile strength of the leaflet), and (3) a thin loose spongy layer—the *spongiosa,* which lies between the atrialis and ventricularis. In valves with myxomatous degeneration, the spongiosa increases much in thickness, invading and replacing the fibrous or collagenous framework and weakening the latter. Leaflet redundancy and systolic prolapse result.

Atrial myocardial fibers have been described as often extending into the substance of the anterior mitral leaflet (very rarely the posterior one). It has been speculated that this myocardial valvar component may have a role in normal mitral closure; another suggestion is that undue strain or traction on this myocardium is a possible cause of arrhythmias or chest pain in patients with mitral valve prolapse.

Chordae Tendineae of the Mitral Valve

True chordae tendineae arise from a papillary muscle and insert on a valve leaflet. Tendinous bands or filaments other than these are commonly encountered in the left ventricle at echocardiography or autopsy and are referred to as *false tendons* (they will be discussed in Chapter 12).

The traditional classification of LV chordae tendineae, as described by the anatomists Tandler and later Quain,[7] was into three orders: The first order of chordae inserted into the free edge of a mitral leaflet, the second order inserted 6 to 8 mm from the free edge on the LV surface of the leaflet, and third (on posterior leaflet only) inserted into the basal portion of the leaflet. Rusted et al.[2] drew attention to commissural chordae that run from papillary muscles to the two (posteromedial and anterolateral) mitral commissures and showed that the tips of the two papillary muscles can be used as landmarks to identify such commissural chordae.

The introduction of mitral valve surgery stimulated interest in mitral anatomy, and an eminent cardiac surgeon, Russell Brock,[8] reassessed the topic. He emphasized the functional importance of certain mitral chordae that were thicker than the rest, later called *strut chordae*.

More recently, the classification of Silver[5] of Toronto has been much used. Silver divided chordae into four main types: (1) rough zone chordae, comprising the main bulk of chordae inserted on and near the free edges of both mitral leaflets, including the mechanically essential strut chordae, (2) basal chordae, attached to the basal strip of the posterior mitral leaflet only (they arise not from papillary muscles but from small ridges on surface of the posterior LV wall itself, and they vary from 0 to 5 in number), (3) commissural chordae, and (4) cleft chordae. The latter two subvarieties can be better understood after the commissures themselves are described. The anterior and posterior mitral leaflets are continuous with and connected by leaflet-like tissue called the *posteromedial* (or *medial* or *superior*) and *anterolateral* (or *lateral* or *inferior*) *commissures.* They are integral parts of the mitral valve apparatus, participating in valve opening and closure along with the leaflets themselves. Chordae tendineae of a distinctive fanlike morphology insert into each of the two mitral commissures. These (commissural chordae) are similar to cleft chordae, which insert into the two clefts that divide the posterior mitral leaflets into three scallops.

On average, 25 chordae insert into the mitral valve. An average of 9 pass to the anterior mitral leaflet (7 rough zone and 2 strut chordae), 14 to the posterior mitral leaflet (10 rough zone, 2 cleft chordae, and 2 basal chordae), and 2 commissural chordae.

Variation in chordal branching is great; some chordae remain unbranched—branching into three chords before insertion into the leaflet is most common. Collagen fibers in chordae fan out into the collagenous framework of the leaflet; however, some chordae seem to traverse the substance of the leaflets as cords that terminate at or near the leaflet attachment.

Chordae muscularis (see Figure 12-6) constitute another uncommon variant of chordal configuration. Instead of being a tendinous structure, a chord may be muscular and fleshy, either in its whole length or "sausage-shaped" with a muscular central segment and tendinous origin and insertion. This variant is also known as *muscularization of the chorda,* and it may appear (on autopsy, at surgery, or during echocardiography) that the papillary muscle inserts directly on a leaflet with no intervening chorda tendinea. The substitution of myocardium for tendon in the chorda is not surprising if the embryologic development of papillary muscles, chordae tendineae, and valve leaflets is considered. All these structures arise by "delamination" of the primitive ventricular myocardium, followed by subsequent differentiation into the various components of the mitral apparatus.

Strut chordae are two of the thickest and largest mitral chordae tendineae, inserted on the anterior leaflet. They are present in 90% of hearts, arise from the tips of each of the two papillary muscles, and remain unbranched or bifurcate only at or inside the leaflet edge. They are obviously of great mechanical importance in supporting the leaflet, so rupture by endocarditis would have much greater consequences than other chordal rupture.

Basal chordae that insert into the posterior mitral leaflet near its attachment are responsible for small linear echoes (often multiple) on the M-mode tracing. These lines are near and somewhat parallel to the endocardial echo of the LV posterior wall. The practical importance of this to the echocardiographer is that these basal chordae echoes could be mistaken for the endocardial echo, thus overestimating LV posterior wall thickness (and therefore LV mass). The basal chordae of the posterior cusp tend to expand into a triangular attachment to the ventricular surface of the leaflet. On echocardiography, they can add to the confusing multiple echoes often visualized on M-mode or 2D echo at the base of the posterior mitral leaflet.

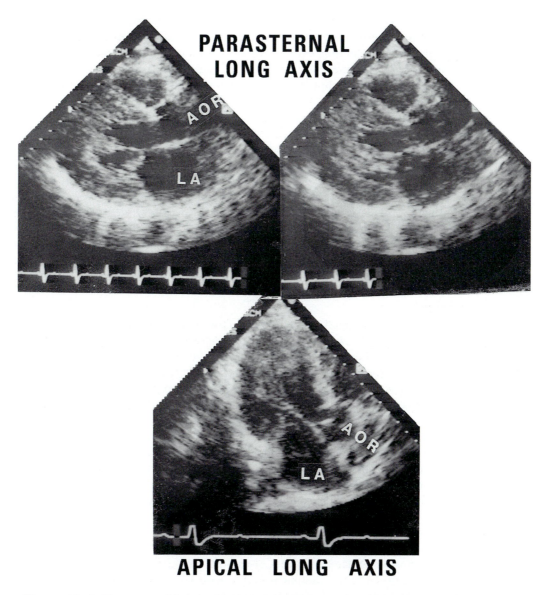

Figure 11–2. Parasternal long-axis view (above) and apical long-axis view (below) in a hypertensive patient showing LV hypertrophy and hypertrophied papillary muscle and mitral chordae with leaflets.

LV Papillary Muscles

The LV usually has two papillary muscles (PMs), the posteromedial and the anterolateral. Both arise from the LV free wall; unlike the right ventricle (RV), no LV papillary muscles arise from the septum. The anterolateral PM originates from the midconcavity of the LV free wall, and the posteromedial PM originates near the junction of the LV posteroinferior wall with the ventricular septum. Both PMs are attached by broad bases to the middle third of the LV wall (Figure 11–2), although occasionally accessory PMs may arise in the apical third. The two PMs are of approximately equal size, conical in shape, and at their apex or tip divide into two or more heads or columns; the posteromedial PM does so more frequently than the anterolateral one. Rusted et al.[2] found that the posteromedial PM was split into two or more heads in over 60% of hearts, whereas the anterolateral PM was usually undivided. These authors pointed out that the two PMs have a consistent anatomic relationship to the two mitral valve commissures, the former being located directly below the latter: the posteromedial PM just below the posteromedial commissure and the anterolateral PM in line with the anterolateral commissure.

The two LV papillary muscles are cone-shaped with their apices or tips projecting into the basal third of the LV, the anterolateral PM extending slightly closer to the mitral annulus level than the posteromedial PM. Both PMs give chordae to both leaflets. Chordae tendineae to the posterior mitral leaflet tend to run vertically upward, parallel to the LV long axis, whereas chordae to the anterior leaflet run obliquely across the LV long axis.

The PMs are rooted in the subjacent LV wall by myocardial continuity and the confluence of multiple adjacent trabeculations. It is not uncommon for the PMs to be connected to each other or the LV wall (elsewhere in the LV chamber) or septum by muscular bands or by tendinous "strings" of varying thickness. The latter are known as *false tendons* or *chordae* and are noted frequently on routine 2D echo.

The anterolateral PM is supplied by the second septal branch of the left anterior descending artery and usually also a circumflex artery branch. The posteromedial PM is supplied by the posterior branch of the right coronary artery (RCA) and often also a circumflex artery branch. Occlusion of these arteries causing infarction also can involve the PM in its territory. The arterial supply of each PM is so structured that its apex (tip) is very vulnerable to ischemia. This may be the reason why echocardiographers often see undue brightness (presumably sclerocalcific changes) at the tips of either or both PMs.

Mitral Valve Ring (Annulus)

This is a thin, curved fibroelastic structure that forms part of the cardiac skeleton. It is not a true ring because it is incomplete anteriorly. It is connected to the atrial myocardium superiorly and the ventricular myocardium inferiorly and can be identified in the embryo as early as the eighth week of intrauterine life. The mitral valve leaflets, particularly the posterior one, are attached to the circumference of the mitral annulus. Externally, the annulus is closely related to the circumflex coronary artery; 1 cm above it lies the coronary sinus.

The mitral annulus faces anteriorly, inferiorly, and to the left. Its circumference is 8.5 to 11.5 cm (mean 10 cm) in men and 8 to 10.5 cm (mean 9 cm) in women. The mitral valve ring proper is deficient anteriorly, where the anterior mitral leaflet is continuous directly with the aortic valve by means of the intervalvar fibrosa (trigone or ligament).

Although the mitral ring itself is nonmuscular, the subjacent ventricular muscle is believed to exert a sphincter-like action in systole, effectively narrowing the mitral orifice and thus playing a part in closure of the normal mitral valve in systole. The mitral annulus corresponds externally to the deepest trough of the atrioventricular groove between posterior-posterolateral aspects of the left atrium and ventricle. The sphincter-like contraction of the mitral annulus is said to reduce the mitral orifice area by 20% to 50%.[10,11]

Although a true annulus in the form of a distinct ring does not suspend or anchor the anterior mitral leaflet, there are certain definite collagenous areas (trigones) in this vicinity which are elements of the cardiac skeleton binding together important structures such as the aortic valve and root, anterior mitral leaflet, and membranous ventricular septum (Figure 11-3). The right fibrous trigone is closely related to the membranous ventricular septum, aortic root, and tricuspid valve; the left trigone is related to the intervalvar fibrous ligament (membrane) linking the anterior mitral leaflet to the aortic cusps.

Closure of the Normal Mitral Valve

To understand the mechanics of systolic mitral closure, it is necessary to know that the combined surface area of the two mitral leaflets (and commissures) is about 2 to $2\frac{1}{2}$ times that of the mitral valve ring in diastole.[12] In systole, the mitral leaflet area is even more in excess of the mitral orifice area because the latter decreases as a result of sphincter-like contraction of the underlying ventricular muscle.

The mitral leaflets coapt in systole not only by their free edges but come into extensive apposition (i.e., the atrial surfaces of the leaflets are in contact over several millimeters of their length), thus sealing the orifice "watertight" and supporting each other. The appositional parts of the leaflets are at right angles to the nonappositional parts.

The process of mitral closure can be conveniently divided into three phases: (1) The mitral leaflets approach each other and come into loose contact following the atrial fill-

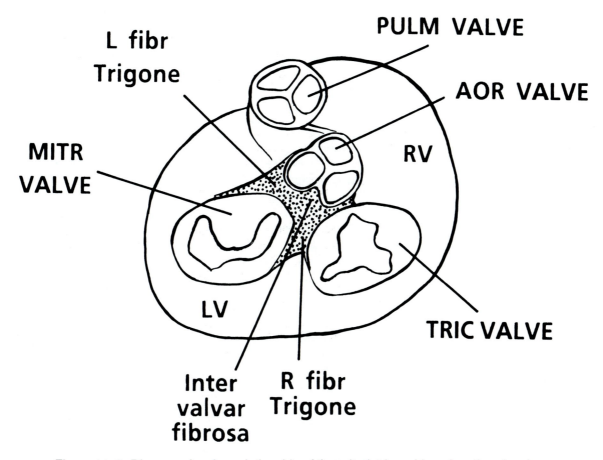

Figure 11–3. Diagram showing relationship of the mitral, tricuspid, and aortic valve rings to each other and to components of the cardiac skeleton (view from above, after removal of atria).

ing phase. This may be considered the atriogenic phase caused by a large circular vortex and produced by reflection of the atrial kick from the apical LV chamber driving the mitral leaflets toward each other. However, loss of atrial contraction as in atrial fibrillation or other arrhythmias does not by itself cause mitral regurgitation. (2) The second phase begins with the onset of ventricular systole (isovolumic contraction). The mitral leaflets bulge toward the atria like parachutes and oppose each other firmly in response to the steep rise in intraventricular pressure. Simultaneously, the LV papillary muscles contract, assisting in holding the leaflet edges in leakproof contact; the integrity of the PMs and chordae tendineae is essential in preventing eversion of the free edges of the leaflets into the left atrium under the considerable LV pressure. (3) In the systolic ejection phase, LV chamber size decreases, and the mitral leaflets increase their area of apposition so that the apposed areas of both leaflets are vertical and parallel to each other and to the LV long axis. Next, systole ends, and the mitral leaflets open abruptly.

ECHOCARDIOGRAPHY OF THE NORMAL MITRAL VALVE

The mitral valve was the first cardiac structure to arouse the interest of pioneers of cardiac ultrasound 30 years ago and continues to be of great importance to present-day echocardiographers (Figures 11–4 and 11–5). Because of its central location in the heart and distinctive motion pattern, it is the easiest cardiac valve to visualize and can be well imaged in numerous 2D planes: parasternal long-axis and short-axis, apical four-chamber, two-chamber, and long-axis, subcostal views.

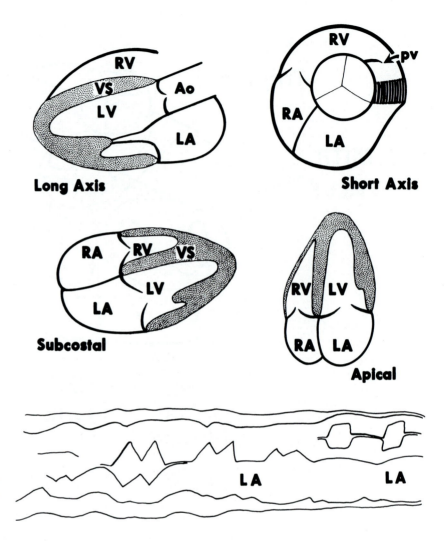

Figure 11–4. Diagram showing various 2D echo views (above) and M-mode sweep (below).

In the *parasternal long-axis 2D view,* the anterior mitral leaflet appears as a mobile linear echo attached to the anterior wall of the aortic root at one end, while the other end moves freely in the LV chamber during diastole and apposes the posterior leaflet in systole. The posterior mitral leaflet is much shorter and less conspicuous than the anterior one; it is attached to the mitral annulus posteriorly, and the other end moves freely in a manner qualitatively similar to the anterior leaflet, though of lesser amplitude. The linear echoes representing the mitral leaflets are continuous with the linear chordal echoes, and it is not always easy to be sure where leaflet ends and chorda tendineae begins.

The *M-mode mitral valve echo* shows the well-known typical pattern: anterior leaflet M-shaped, posterior leaflet W-shaped in diastole; in systole, the apposed leaflets merge into a linear straight or slightly convex echo.

In *parasternal short-axis view,* the open mitral leaflets form a continuous "fish mouth" ellipse, its long axis horizontal. Scanning gradually toward the LV apex, the chordae tendineae and then the two papillary muscles come into view; the latter mark the locations of the two commissures (posteromedial and anterolateral). In systole, the apposed leaflets close, and their respective echoes merge into a single thick horizontal echo closer to the posterior than the anterior wall of the LV chamber.

In the *apical views (four-chamber, two-chamber, and long-axis),* the mitral leaflets appear as linear mobile echoes, the anterior longer than the posterior. As the valve opens, the normal mitral leaflets abruptly fly apart so that their tips (free edges) point toward the body or apex of the LV chamber and show brisk undulatory motion corresponding to the

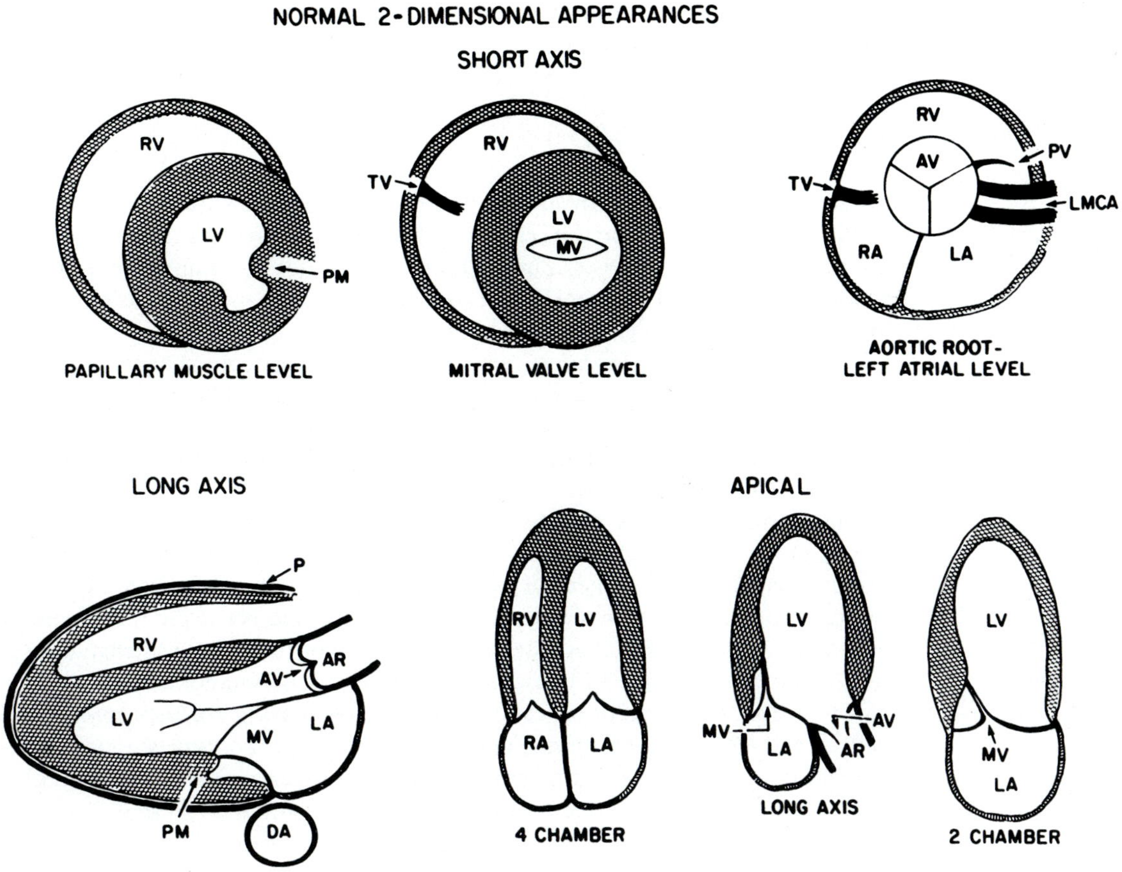
NORMAL 2-DIMENSIONAL APPEARANCES
SHORT AXIS
RV
LV
PM
PAPILLARY MUSCLE LEVEL
TV
RV
LV
MV
MITRAL VALVE LEVEL
RV
AV
TV
PV
LMCA
RA
LA
AORTIC ROOT-
LEFT ATRIAL LEVEL
LONG AXIS
P
RV
AR
AV
LV
MV
LA
PM
DA
APICAL
RV
LV
RA
LA
4 CHAMBER
LV
MV
AV
LA
AR
LONG AXIS
LV
MV
LA
2 CHAMBER

Figure 11–5. Diagram showing further 2D echo views.

early rapid and atrial filling phases of diastole. In mitral prolapse, redundant mitral leaflets may exhibit an exaggerated or floppy quality to this diastolic motion. In mitral stenosis, the mitral leaflets move toward the LV chamber in diastole but do not fly apart; they remain attached to each other, forming an inverted-U contour or dome.

In the apical views, the two mitral leaflets are seen to appose near their free edges, forming an obtuse angle. It is important to note that the point of leaflet apposition, as well as the leaflets themselves, remain on the ventricular side of the mitral annulus plane in systole. The annulus plane is represented by a straight line joining the attachments of the anterior and posterior mitral leaflets. In mitral prolapse, the body or belly of one or both leaflets bulges toward the left atrium across this plane; with a flail mitral leaflet it is the free edge of the affected leaflet that projects abnormally into the left atrium.

Regarding the *subcostal views,* mitral leaflet morphology in the four-chamber subcostal view is similar to what is seen in the apical four-chamber view; the subcostal short-axis view is very much like the parasternal short-axis view.

Doppler recordings of mitral valve flow are best made from the apical window, because in apical views the axis of the Doppler beam is very close to the direction of antegrade mitral flow and usually of regurgitant mitral flow. In a small minority of patients with mitral regurgitation (especially mitral prolapse), the regurgitant jet runs in an oblique or even almost horizontal direction in the apical view; fortunately, colorflow Doppler reveals the presence of such unusual jets. Another echocardiographic problem is caused by prosthetic mitral valves, which produce large reverberatory artifacts obscuring left atrial flow patterns on pulsed-wave Doppler and colorflow Doppler, rendering the diagnosis of mitral regurgitation virtually impossible. If such patients are subjected to transesophageal echocardiography (TEE), the regurgitant mitral jet is clear of artifactual interference because it is now between transducer and prosthetic valve rather than on the far side of the valve where reverberations are.

MITRAL STENOSIS (Figures 11–6 to 11–14)

Mitral valve stenosis is nearly always due to previous rheumatic valve damage. Although mitral stenosis (MS) can be the result of other disease processes (mentioned at the end of this section), they are all very rare and together do not account for more than 1% or 2% of adult MS. Supravalvar stenosis, due to congenital anomalies such as cor triatriatum and stenotic supravalvar ring, is discussed in Chapter 10.

Rheumatic MS[13-17] manifests several decades after acute rheumatic carditis, except in developing countries, where the intervening interval can be a few years.[18] In early or mild MS, the anterior and posterior mitral leaflets fuse at their two commissures, and concomitantly, there is obliteration of the clefts in the posterior mitral leaflet so that this leaflet is short and puckered.

In normal adults, the mitral valve orifice area is about 4 to 5 cm^2. In mild MS, it is 2 cm^2 or more; in moderate MS, around 1.5 cm^2; and in critical MS (hemodynamically important, needing valve surgery or balloon valvoplasty), it is less than 1 cm^2. In mild MS, the mitral orifice is oval in shape, and leaflet thickening is usually not severe. Increasing severity of MS takes place because of one or more of the following changes: (1) contraction of the mitral orifice to a *slitlike "buttonhole"* configuration due to progression in leaflet scarring or in extent of leaflet fusion, (2) *increasing stiffness and sclerosis* of the leaflets, and (3) in some patients, *rheumatic scarring involving the chordae tendineae* in addition to the leaflets. Stiffness and sclerotic changes are described by the pathologist or surgeon as thickening, sclerosis or dense fibrosis, and heavy calcification, in order of increasing severity. In men, calcification occurs more extensively and at an earlier age than in women. A funnel-shaped mitral valve configuration is common (Figure 11–6), the severity of MS being dependent on the cross-sectional area of the narrow (lower) end of the funnel. In patients with MS, the severity of sclerocalcific changes in the leaflets correlates with the severity of MS in a general way, but by no means in every case.[19] Thus in younger women one often encounters severe MS with little calcification and with pliable leaflets; conversely, in elderly patients large calcific plaques or nodules in one or both mitral leaflets may coexist with mild to moderate MS. Verrucae or multiple nodular thickening is common in younger patients with MS but are replaced by large sclerotic or calcific plaques in the elderly. In patients with rheumatic scarring of the chordae tendineae, subvalvar sclerocalcific changes then aggravate the MS by adding an element of *subvalvar stenosis* to the valvar MS. Since calcification is easily appreciated on 2D echo, the location and extent of mitral calcific deposits are important to ascertain.

Thrombi in the left atrium are not rare in patients with MS. Thrombi in the LA appendage (a common site) are virtually never visualized on conventional transthoracic echocardiography (TTE) but are well seen by TEE. Forty years ago, 20% of MS patients suffered systemic embolism at least once during their lives.[20] Mural thrombi in the main LA chamber, especially on the posterior LA wall (on MacCallum's patch[21]), are not uncommon in MS and are also detectable on TEE with much greater sensitivity than TTE. A rare but spectacular type of LA thrombus, peculiar to MS and prosthetic mitral valves, is a free-floating large ball thrombus[22]; such a clot cannot exit the LA chamber because it cannot pass through a narrow slitlike stenotic mitral orifice.

However, the ball thrombus can produce syncope or even "sudden death" by transiently occluding the stenotic mitral orifice. Change of patient position is presumed to dislodge the ball thrombus from its occlusive site over the stenotic orifice and thus restore mitral blood flow.

Nonrheumatic mitral stenosis has been described in a variety of rare lesions:

1. Congenital MS is not rare in infancy, usually along with other anomalies.
   Distinctive anatomic findings such as parachute mitral valve with a single

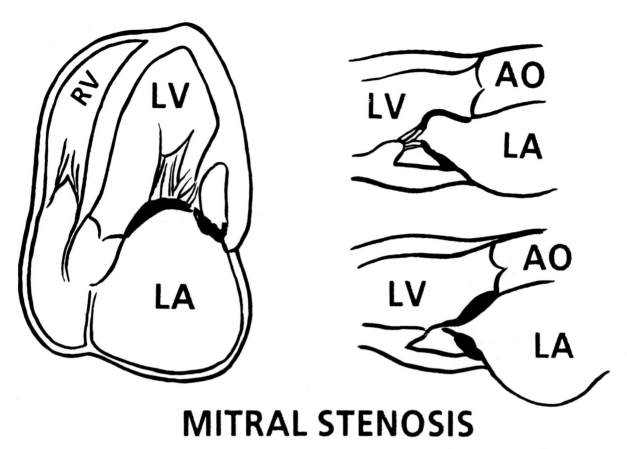

MITRAL STENOSIS

Figure 11–6. Diagram showing typical 2D echo configurations in apical four-chamber view (left) and in parasternal long-axis view (right). At right, the upper diagram depicts the diastolic mitral contour of a noncalcific pliable mitral valve; the lower diagram, that of a more calcified mitral valve with more limitation of mobility.

papillary muscle and mitral arcade are well known to pediatric cardiologists. Congenital MS is rarely diagnosed in older children or teenagers but virtually never in adults.

2. Mitral annulus calcification is extremely common in the elderly, but it is extremely rare for it to produce significant MS. Patients with end-stage renal disease on long-term dialysis can exceptionally develop a progressive calcific MS.

3. Large LA masses, such as myxomas and sarcomas, and even large mitral vegetations can mechanically obstruct the mitral orifice.

4. A miscellany of uncommon syndromes reported to have caused MS include Fabry's disease,[23] Hurler's syndrome (gargoylism),[24] Whipple's disease,[25] and methysergide therapy.[26] Carcinoid metastases in the liver are well known to cause tricuspid and pulmonary valve stenosis; mitral stenosis has been documented in such cases if an atrial septal defect is present or as a complication of carcinoid tumor of the lung.

Echocardiography of Mitral Stenosis

M-Mode.[27–30]   The ultrasound appearances of anterior mitral echoes were the first application of reflected ultrasound to cardiology. The initial abnormalities described—low

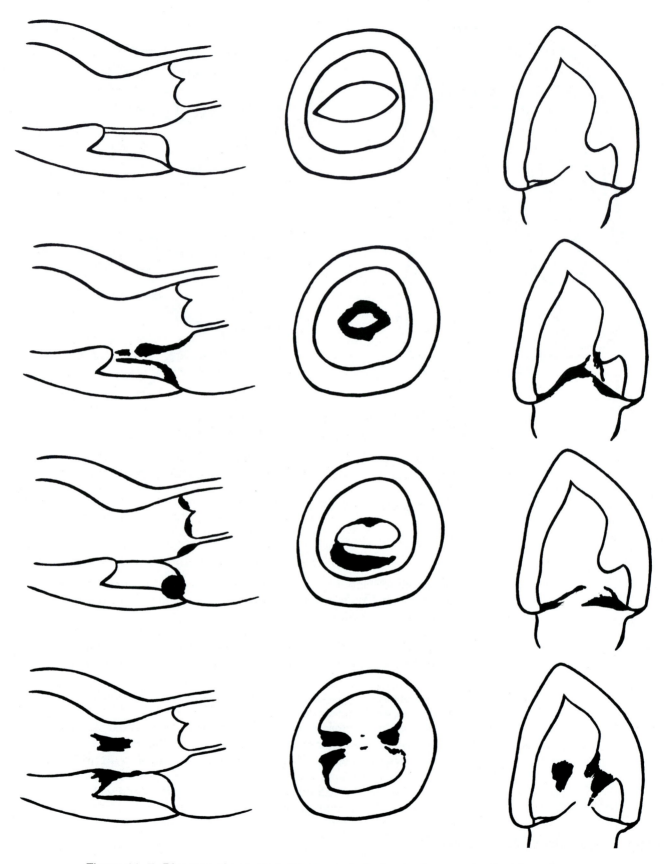

Figure 11–7. Diagram of parasternal long- and short-axis views and apical four-chamber views (transversely) in normal individuals, mitral stenosis, mitral annulus calcification, and papillary muscle calcification.

EF slope and small anterior diastolic excursion—were later found not to be quite specific for MS; abnormally small but constant separation between the two mitral leaflets in diastole is a more reliable sign of MS. In other words, the normal diastolic contour, M-shaped and W-shaped for the anterior and posterior leaflets, respectively, alters to a rectangular "box" shape. Usually the posterior leaflet moves anteriorly, except in very mild MS. Diastolic movement of both leaflets in tandem is due to their adherence at the commissures. The larger and longer anterior leaflet is believed to carry the shorter posterior leaflet anteriorly along with it, explainable as the result of the displacing forces (torques) of blood on the two leaflets.[26a]

Sclerotic change in leaflet structure is the rule, varying from slightly thickened, pliable leaflets to almost immobile, heavily calcified masses. Raj et al.,[31] correlating echocardiographic appearances with assessment of leaflet calcification by radiography and calcium extraction of surgically excised valves, found that a single thin mitral diastolic echo excludes calcification. All valves containing more than 80 mg of calcium exhibited multiple linear leaflet echoes. The work of Zanolla et al.[32] and Wong et al.[33] showed that echocardiography was very sensitive in detecting mitral valve calcification but not very specific.

Two-Dimensional Echocardiography[34] *(Figures 11–6 to 11–11).* The mitral leaflets exhibit typical configuration and motion in all standard views. The most common abnormality is that the free edges of the mitral leaflets cannot open freely; being tethered to each other, the tip of the anterior leaflet is relatively fixed, while its belly is allowed to bulge anteriorly in diastole and then move back to appose the posterior leaflet in systole.

In the long-axis view, the anterior mitral leaflet billows or bulges toward the LV chamber during all of diastole and then abruptly slams closed as systole begins. Posterior leaflet abnormalities are less spectacular because of its short length; in fact, this leaflet is often sclerotic and immobile. In diastole, the mitral valve has a funnel contour in long-axis view, its wider rim being the mitral annulus, while the narrow lower end is the effective or hemodynamic mitral orifice. When the mitral leaflets are heavily calcified, the pliable funnel configuration may be replaced by dense, thick masses with little mobility (see Figures 11–7 and 11–8). Such valves are invariably stenotic to a critical degree.

In the short-axis view, the thickened mitral valve appears circular or oval; the size of the opening depends on whether the imaging plane intersects the valve funnel nearer its base or at its lower narrow orifice. It is important to obtain good images at the latter level by sweeping upward from papillary muscle level until the complete mitral circumference first appears. If the mitral valve is imaged closer to the wide end of the funnel, the severity of MS will be underestimated.

The area of the mitral orifice (area enclosed by inner border of the thick valve echo) correlates very well with the mitral valve orifice area measured at surgery or estimated hemodynamically by the Gorlin formula.[35-37] Mitral valve orifice area is the most important index of MS severity, superior to the mitral pressure gradient obtained by cardiac catheterization because the latter is determined also by the variables of cardiac output and presence of associated mitral regurgitation (MR).

In the apical views, the stenotic mitral valve presents a highly typical inverted-U or "basket" configuration during diastole, also called *diastolic doming* (Figures 11–6 and 11–7). This is very different from the normal springing apart of the tips of the leaflets followed by brisk undulations corresponding to the phases of early rapid and later (atrial) LV filling.

Doppler interrogation of forward mitral flow is performed from the apical window, since the ultrasound beam axis in this view is very close to the direction of flow. In moderate to severe MS, a significant pressure gradient between LA and LV persists through all of diastole. This is what maintains diastolic doming of the leaflets throughout diastole and what causes a slow decrease (decay) of velocity of forward mitral flow during diastole. The latter can be quantified by the pressure half-time estimation, from which the mitral

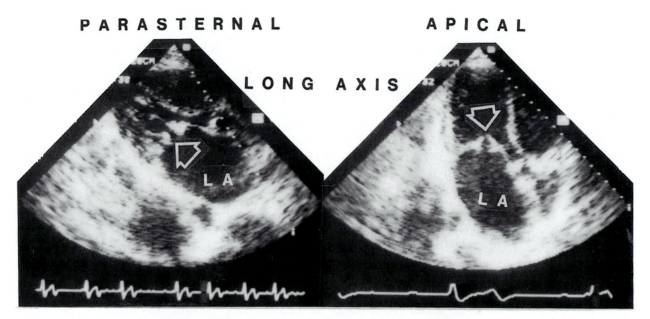

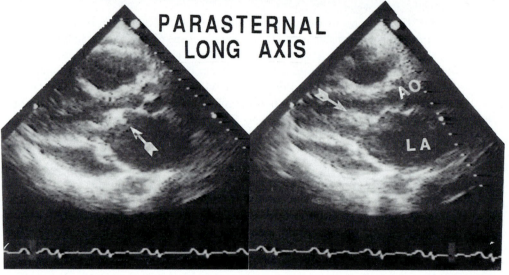

A

Figure 11–8. (A) (Above) Parasternal long-axis view (left) and apical long-axis view (right) in a patient with mitral stenosis. The mitral leaflets are calcified at their tips, i.e., at the valve orifice (arrows). The left atrium is dilated. (Below) In a different patient, parasternal long-axis view with mitral stenosis showing calcification of mitral leaflets (left) and sclerocalcific changes in subvalvar mitral apparatus (right).

APICAL 4 CHAMBER

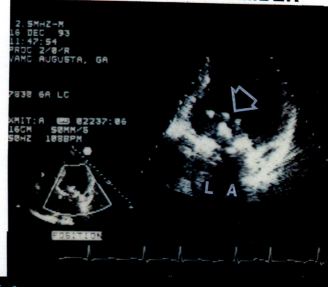

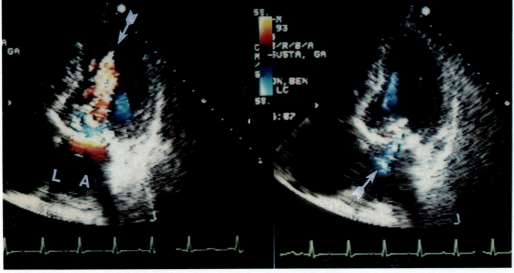

B

(B) Apical four-chamber view showing prominent subvalvar mitral sclerocalcification (open arrow). A turbulent though wide jet (arrow) of mild mitral stenosis is seen at bottom left, and a small jet of MR is seen at bottom right.

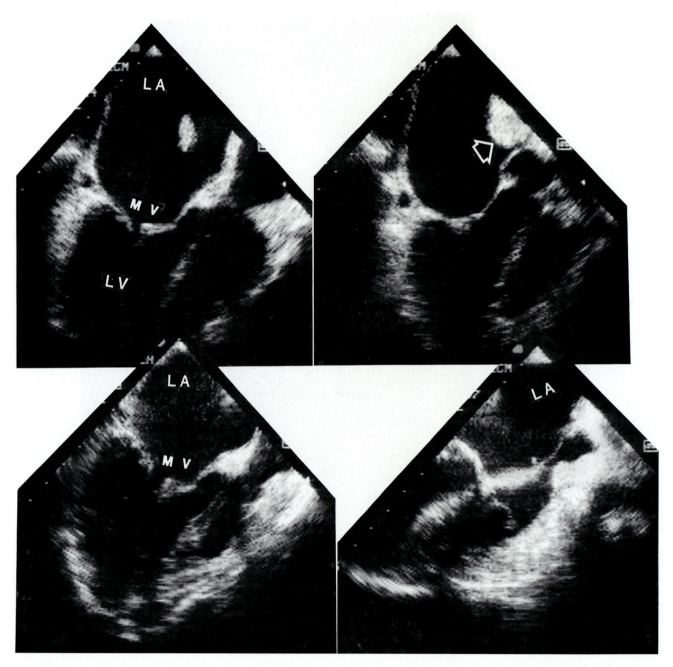

Figure 11–9. TEE in a patient with noncalcific mitral stenosis. The left atrial chamber is dilated and contains a thrombus (arrow).

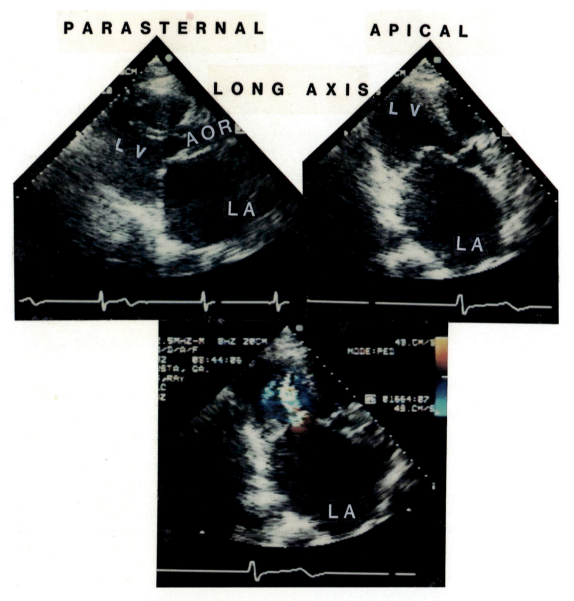

Figure 11–10. Parasternal long-axis view (above, left) and apical long-axis view (above, right) showing a tight mitral stenosis. The left atrium is severely dilated. Colorflow Doppler shows a narrow diastolic jet entering the left ventricle.

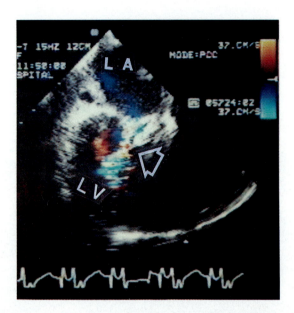

Figure 11–11. TEE of a patient with mitral stenosis showing the jet (arrow) through the stenotic mitral orifice into the left ventricle.

valve area can be reliably estimated by the formula 220/pressure half-time (ms). Colorflow Doppler reveals typical features of the high velocity turbulent diastolic jet (Figures 11–10 to 11–14).

MITRAL REGURGITATION

The causes of mitral regurgitation (MR) are many and comprise abnormalities not only of the leaflets, chordae, and papillary muscles but also of the mitral annulus and LV chamber. In any particular patient, more than one component of the mitral apparatus may be at fault, and more than one mechanism of MR may operate.

Rheumatic mitral valve damage was the leading cause of MR due to leaflet and/or chordae tendineae disease in this country until a quarter of a century ago but since then has been increasingly overtaken by mitral valve prolapse (MVP).[38] The most common cause of severe MR at present is not lesions of valve leaflets or chords but myocardial disease: dilated cardiomyopathy or ischemic heart disease. Extensive calcification in the posterior mitral annulus region and/or papillary muscles is seldom the sole cause of severe MR but probably contributes to MR associated with ischemic, hypertensive, or cardiomyopathic myocardial disease.

From the echocardiographer's viewpoint, it is important to know not only the long list of cardiac disease known to be associated with MR but also the various pathologic mechanisms that permit regurgitation to occur. The following categorization of MR according to whether the mitral leaflet is excessive, restricted, or normal was used by Stewart et al.[39] and was itself adapted from that of Carpentier et al.[40] It forms an excellent basis for an echocardiographic approach to any patient presenting with significant MR.

MR with Excessive Leaflet Motion

Exaggerated leaflet motion is due to either (1) redundancy of the leaflet or chordae (i.e., too much length for that LV chamber), attributable to myxomatous degeneration and weakening of these structures, or (2) rupture of one or more chords or (rarely) papillary mus-

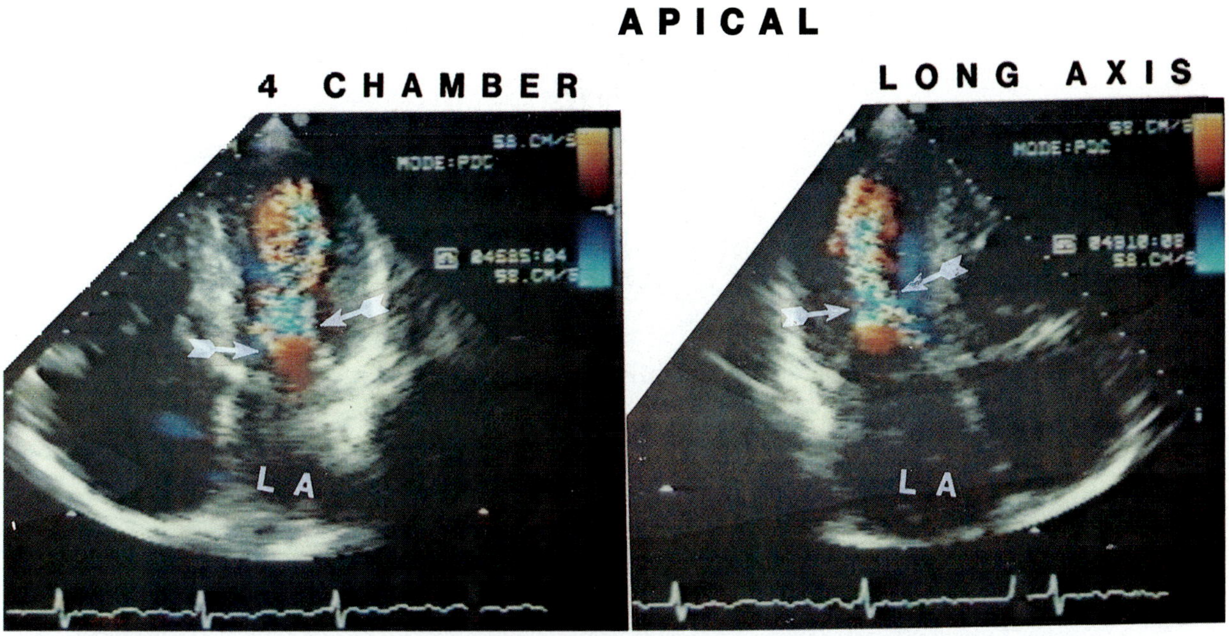

APICAL

4 CHAMBER

LONG AXIS

Figure 11–12. Apical four-chamber view (left) and apical long-axis view (right) in a patient with mild mitral stenosis. Colorflow Doppler shows the mitral diastolic jet (arrows) entering the left ventricle; however, this jet is not very narrow, consistent with mild mitral stenosis.

cles. Some consider that focal infarction involving a papillary muscle can sometimes belong in this category. Mitral prolapse involves systolic bulging of any portion of a mitral leaflet past the level of the mitral annulus, i.e., on the atrial side of the annulus plane. In the majority of patients with MVP, one of the leaflets prolapses to a greater degree than the other, and in 93% of such instances (in the series of Stewart et al.), the MR jet is directed toward the contralateral side of the left atrial chamber, i.e., in a direction away from the abnormal leaflet.[38,41-43] When both mitral leaflets prolapse to the same extent, the MR jet is usually central.

MR with Restricted Leaflet Motion

This is typical of rheumatic scarring of mitral leaflets and chordae. Commonly, the posterior leaflet is shrunken or curled up so that the anterior leaflet overrides it. The MR jet is directed posteriorly, in the same direction as the abnormal leaflet.

Massive mitral annulus calcification can immobilize the posterior mitral leaflet but also pushes it upward and anteriorly. Such abnormal anatomy might contribute to MR in these patients; however, the mechanics are somewhat different from the rheumatic regurgitant valve. In patients with combined rheumatic MS and MR, Veyrat et al.[44] showed that the MR jet was central in 80%.

MR with Normal Leaflet Motion[45]

Uncommon though surgically correctable causes include cleft anterior mitral leaflet (usually but not always associated with ostium primum atrial septal defect), leaflet perforation (complicating bacterial endocarditis), and trauma (complicating penetrating wounds).

However, by far the most common basis for severe MR with normal mitral leaflet motion is what Stewart et al.[39] call "ventricular annulus dilatation." This is a broad category that includes mitral annulus dilatation and LV chamber dilatation associated with dilated cardiomyopathy or coronary heart disease. Although dilatation of both the annulus and the LV chamber is often present, one can exist without the other.

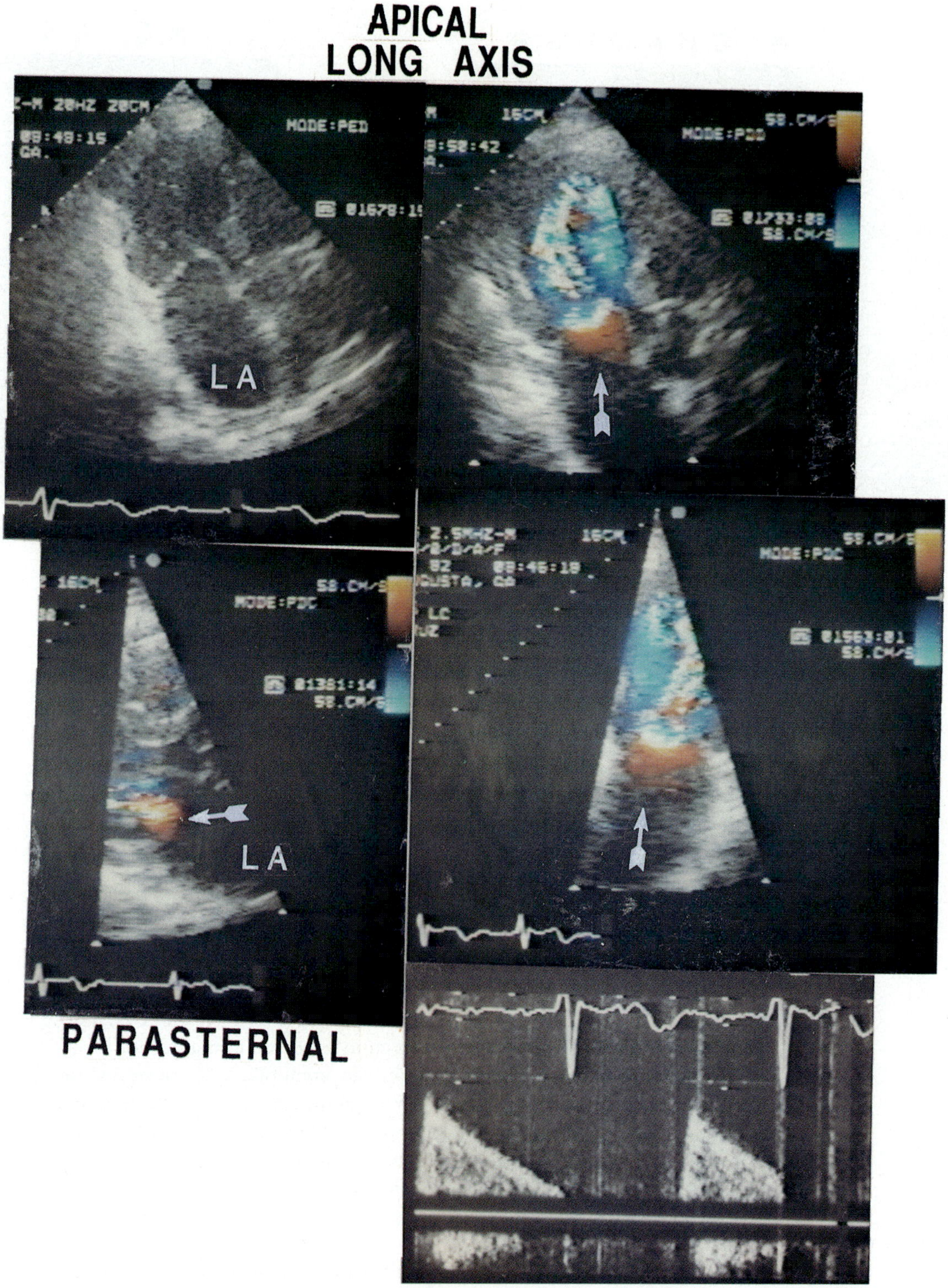

APICAL
LONG AXIS

PARASTERNAL

Figure 11–13. Apical long-axis view (above) showing a narrow high-velocity diastolic jet entering the LV chamber. Note that the jet starts on the ventricular side of the stenotic mitral valve (arrow). This phenomenon is also evident on the parasternal long-axis view (below, left) and the apical four-chamber views (below, right). Below this the continuous-wave Doppler shows a contour of mitral stenosis.

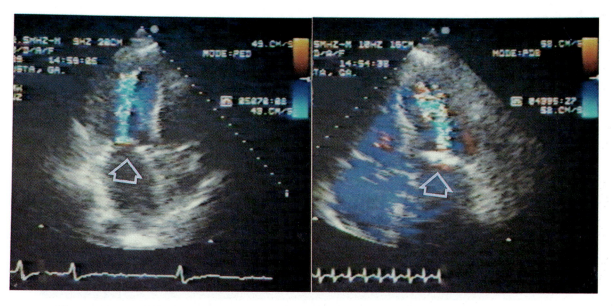

Figure 11–14. Colorflow Doppler of apical long-axis view (left) and apical four-chamber view in patient with mitral stenosis showing a high-velocity turbulent diastolic jet emerge into the left ventricle through a calcified mitral valve.

In an autopsy study, Bulkley and Roberts[46] found that in 24 patients with normal hearts, the average mitral annulus circumference was 9 cm (range 7 to 11 cm); in 15 with severe rheumatic MR, the average circumference was 11 cm; in 10 with floppy mitral valve and severe MR, the average circumference was 15.5 cm. In many patients with MVP the LV chamber is not dilated; i.e., there is selective dilatation of the mitral annulus region.

In dilated dysfunctioning left ventricles, it has been suggested that altered geometry within the chamber, i.e., change in position of the papillary muscles with respect to leaflet position, may be a major factor in causing MR. Such LV chambers are abnormally wide, with a shape change from the ellipsoidal to the spherical. It is supposed that outward displacement of the papillary muscles tends to draw the mitral leaflets further apart, impeding complete systolic apposition.[47,48] Poor LV contraction might worsen the situation by decreasing the normal motion of the papillary muscles toward the center of the LV chamber and the valve leaflets. The MR jet is usually centrally located in the left atrium. Sixty years ago, Paul D. White[49] commented, "displacement downward of the papillary muscles as a result of the ventricular dilatation is a more important factor in causing mitral regurgitation than is dilatation of the valve ring."

MR associated with dilated, poorly contracting left ventricles, as discussed in the preceding paragraph, is sometimes loosely referred to as due to "papillary muscle dysfunction." The same name has been used to refer to MR accompanying infarction or ischemia of the LV posteroinferior wall, a syndrome first described about 25 years ago.[50] It is open to question as to whether one or the other papillary muscle should be blamed whenever a patient with myocardial infarction is found to have MR. However, there are undoubtedly a few patients with posteroinferior infarction, severe MR, and normal contraction of the rest of the LV who present with cardiac failure and benefit from mitral valve replacement.

The PMs contract just before the LV wall, so they exert traction on the mitral chordae and leaflets during all of systole, preventing overshoot or eversion of the leaflets and thus avoiding MR. If PM contraction is absent or very impaired, this tensing effect is lost, the chordae remain lax, and MR results.

In describing and commenting on papillary muscle dysfunction, Burch et al.[50] and later Shelbourne et al.[51] hypothesized that LV infarction including the PM site either failed

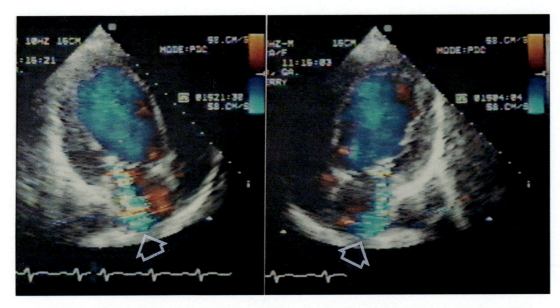

Figure 11–15. Colorflow Doppler of apical long-axis view (left) and apical four-chamber view (right) showing a posterior-posterolateral MR jet (arrows).

to anchor the PM properly or, by causing regional dyskinesis or aneurysm, altered papillary muscle alignment with the chordae and leaflets.

However, it has been shown experimentally that damage strictly limited to a PM may not cause MR, unless the subjacent LV wall is also damaged. Functionally, the PM should not be thought of in isolation but as part of a larger myocardial unit including the complex LV spiral muscle bundle system, which extends into the PM and physiologically as well as anatomically forms a continuous integral whole.

Recently, 2D echo has been used to assess PM function directly by measuring the fractional shortening of the LV papillary muscle: 27% ± 8% for the anterolateral and 30% ± 8% for the posteromedial papillary muscle; in patients with prior infarction, fractional shortening was 19% ± 17% and 15% ± 14%, respectively.[51a]

Colorflow Doppler Jet Area in MR

Colorflow Doppler was introduced for the estimation of severity of MR in the mid-1980s and quickly became the most widely used noninvasive method for this purpose, supported by several studies that indicated a good correlation between severity of MR and MR jet length, jet area, or jet area/LA area.[52-54] However, hemodynamic factors such as LV-LA pressure gradient, jet velocity, and jet momentum also influence jet area.[55-57] Later work showed that these determinants of MR jet area apply to central MR jets, but eccentric jets along the LA wall are much less affected by MR regurgitant volume.[58-60] The latter tend to remain thin, and if they expand, they do so in flat manner along the LA wall so that in any one 2D echo plane the jet does not appear impressively broad. This type of MR jet is common in patients with prolapse or flail motion of the mitral valve, whereas central MR jets are the rule in patients with "functional" MR or MR secondary to ischemic heart disease.

Figure 11-15 shows a posterior (posterolateral) MR jet, Figure 11-16 shows an anterior (anteromedial) MR jet, and Figure 11-17 shows a massive MR jet filling the LA due to severe 4+ MR.

MITRAL VALVE PROLAPSE (MVP)

This very common clinical-echocardiographic entity has been recognized by cardiologists for only about three decades. Long before that, the auscultatory manifestations—midsys-

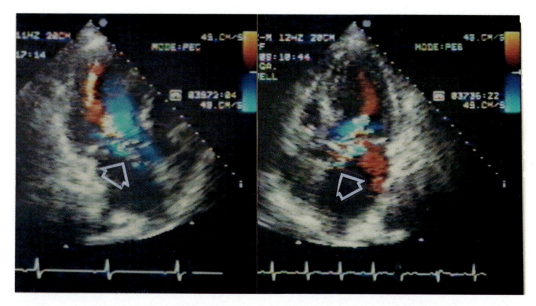

Figure 11–16. Colorflow Doppler of apical long-axis view (left) and apical four-chamber view (right) showing an anterior-anteromedial MR jet (arrows).

tolic click and/or late systolic murmur—had been described, but their anatomic basis had not been understood; in fact, many thought them extracardiac in origin. Barlow, whose name deservedly has been associated with mitral prolapse, played a major role in correlating the anatomic, auscultatory, and angiocardiographic findings, although many others in the 1960s and 1970s also did important work in elucidating the nature of the abnormal mitral valve structure and function.

In addition to the term *Barlow's disease* or *syndrome,* the terms *mitral valve prolapse* (MVP) and *ballooning, billowing, floppy,* or *redundant mitral valve* have been used synonymously until the present day. Barlow uses the qualifying words *billowing, prolapse, floppy,* and *flail* to denote increasing levels of abnormal mitral motion and function, generally associated with increasing severity of echocardiographic appearances and of mitral regurgitation.[61] However, such nuances of meaning, though scientifically commendable, have not yet received widespread acceptance.

Another point needing clarification is use of the word *syndrome* in conjunction with MVP.[61] Barlow uses it to signify the presence of symptoms (chest pain, palpitations, dizziness, fatigue, syncope), ECG changes including ectopic beats or rhythms, anxiety or panic attacks, or transient ischemic neurologic or retinal episodes, in any combination, in patients who have auscultatory and/or echocardiographic findings indicating MVP.

The morphologic changes in the mitral valve at surgery or autopsy in MVP, often designated *myxomatous,* are characterized by an excess of myxomatous tissue in the spongiosa layer, which encroaches on or invades the strong collagenous layer (fibrosa) so that the leaflet weakens, then stretches, and becomes "redundant," i.e., too long for that LV chamber.[61,62] The posterior mitral leaflet is more often affected than the anterior; the former consists of three scallops, any or all of which may be affected while the rest of the valve is relatively unaffected. Fibrous or fibroelastic thickening of the superficial atrial or ventricular surface of the valve cusps may be superimposed on the myxomatous changes mentioned above; even calcification is noted on occasion, usually restricted to the basal attachment of the posterior mitral leaflet (so-called mitral annulus calcification). However, commissural fusion of the mitral leaflets and valve orifice stenosis does not occur.

The replacement or invasion of the fibrosa layer may be diffuse, being spread apart by finger-like prolongations of spongiosa, or may be focal. Thus the redundant mitral leaflet might balloon into the atrium in a smooth "umbrella-like" curve or form smaller local bulges or protrusions depending on whether the leaflet is diffusely or locally weakened.

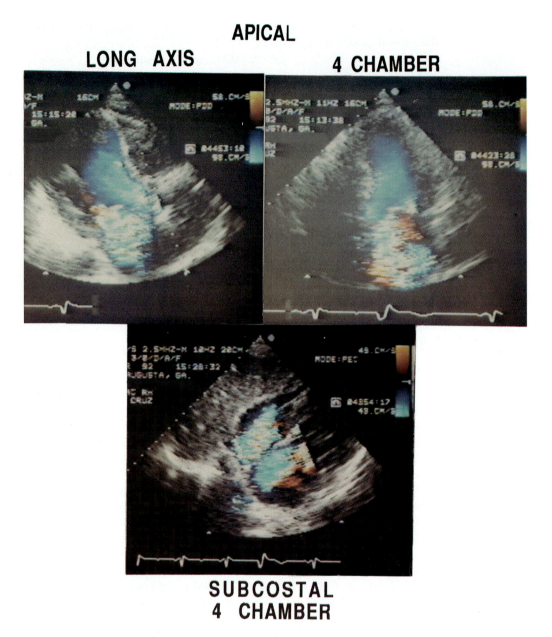

Figure 11–17. Apical long-axis and four-chamber views (above) and subcostal view (below) showing severe mitral regurgitation with large regurgitant jet (MR) filling almost the entire left atrium.

Dilatation of the mitral annulus in MVP has been described and is of interest as a possible cause for mitral regurgitation.[63]

The mitral chordae in MVP may appear normal or may be elongated, the weakening of the central fibrous chordal core with subsequent stretching occurring for the same reason that the leaflets elongate, i.e., myxomatous change. Even more important than chordal redundancy is spontaneous chordal rupture,[64,65] which results in the affected segment of mitral leaflet becoming abruptly flail, thus initiating or seriously aggravating MR. Although this complication is uncommon (less than 5% of MVP), the high prevalence of MVP renders severe MR due to MVP (with or without chordal rupture) the most common indication for mitral valve replacement in this country.

Mitral regurgitation (MR) is common on colorflow Doppler in MVP; apical systolic murmurs may be prominent, soft, or absent. The mechanism of MR is complex and probably varies from patient to patient. Mitral annulus dilatation, chordal rupture, and abnormal leaflet apposition are possible factors. Malapposition of leaflets is often due to the more redundant leaflet prolapsing to a greater extent toward the left atrium so that the regurgitant jet is directed away from the more prolapsed leaflet toward the contralateral left atrial wall.

Yet another anatomic lesion in MVP that could contribute to MR is fusion of the LV mural endocardium (just below attachment of the posterior mitral leaflet) to the chordae tendineae inserting into the base of this leaflet.[66] This process starts with linear fibrous thickening of the endocardium due to friction against the adjacent chordae; the endocardial thickening increases, coalesces, and may proceed to fuse with the chordae, perhaps shortening them and restricting posterior mitral leaflet motion.

MVP is one of the major cardiac entities predisposing to bacterial endocarditis.[67,68] This complication is said to befall about 5% to 8% of patients with MVP followed prospectively, but its incidence in the general population is probably less. The necessity for administering antibiotic prophylaxis at the time of dental or other bacteremia-causing procedures in otherwise healthy young adults with a murmur or click is one of the most common indications for echocardiography in office practice.

Transient ischemic neurologic or retinal episodes, often recurrent, constitute another common reason for referral to the echocardiography laboratory.[69-71] Such patients frequently do have MVP on 2D echo, but seldom is a thrombus or even a fibrinous wisp or strand ever demonstrated by conventional echocardiography.[72] TEE may yield more tangible evidence that solid material (possibly platelet thrombi or fibrinous strands) can form on myxomatous mitral valves. Rare reports of such material being detected at autopsy in the angle between the posterior leaflet and the LA wall have appeared.[71]

Pomerance[73] noted "fibrinous endocarditis" in 10 of her 35 autopsy cases of MVP. She suggested that undue stretch of the weakened mitral leaflets led to rupture of subendocardial connective tissue and loss of overlying endothelial continuity, with secondary deposition of fibrin in the traumatized endocardium. It is possible that fragments of this fibrin embolize into small cerebral or retinal arteries causing transient ischemic attacks (TIAs) that soon regress as the fibrin is lysed or dispersed.

Echocardiography of Mitral Valve Prolapse (Figures 11–18 to 11–27)

On M-mode echo,[74-78] MVP was diagnosed when the apposed mitral leaflets were displaced 3 mm or more posterior to the *CD* line, the *C* and *D* points being, respectively, where the mitral leaflets abruptly come into contact soon after onset of systole and where they abruptly move away at the moment of valve opening. The abnormal systolic posterior mitral valve motion can vary from late to middle to early systole. Generally, the more severe cases of MVP exhibit "hammocking" or sagging during almost all of systole (Figure 11–19), and in extreme instances the posterior leaflet displacement is 1 cm or more so that it may abut the posterior atrial wall or atrioventricular junction.

On 2D echo,[78-83] the appearances indicating MVP are observed in the parasternal long-axis and apical views (Figure 11–20). The main findings (visualized from both these windows) are posterior (superior and cephalad) displacement of one or both mitral leaflets to the atrial side of the plane of the mitral annulus. The latter can be identified easily by a line joining the attachments of the anterior leaflet (to the aortic wall posterior root) and the posterior leaflet (to the posterior LV wall–LA wall junction). In MVP, the belly of the prolapsing leaflet bulges toward the atrial chamber, but its free edge points toward the ventricle, and the two mitral leaflets appear apposed. Although both mitral leaflets may sometimes prolapse to the same degree, more often one leaflet prolapses to a greater extent than the other. Borderline MVP or not quite typical MVP (Figure 11–21) is common.

It has been pointed out by Weyman et al. that the mitral annulus is not a flat uniplanar circle but is somewhat saddle-shaped when imaged as a three-dimensional (3D) object.[83a] These authors claimed that this rendered the apical four-chamber view less reli-

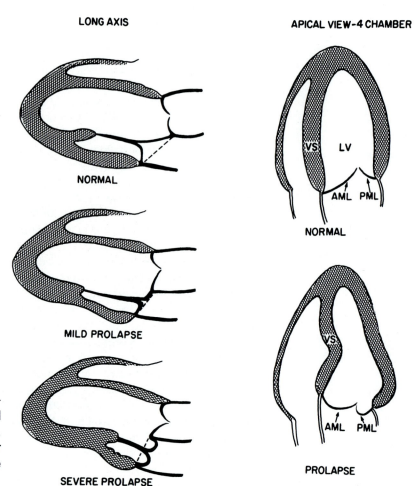

MITRAL PROLAPSE: 2D ECHO

LONG AXIS

APICAL VIEW-4 CHAMBER

NORMAL

NORMAL

MILD PROLAPSE

SEVERE PROLAPSE

PROLAPSE

Figure 11–18. Diagram showing parasternal long-axis view (left) of normal mild MVP and severe MVP configuration. (Right) The normal apical four-chamber view (above) and the contour of prolapse (below).

able than the parasternal long-axis view for diagnosis of MVP. However, this view has not been accepted by all echocardiographers. Any intervention that transiently reduces LV size, such as a change in position from supine to standing or inhalation of amyl nitrite, permits the redundant mitral valve to prolapse further into the left atrium. This fact can be used to advantage by the echocardiographer to enhance the M-mode or 2D echo manifestation of MVP.[84-86]

Morganroth et al.[80] called attention to the location of the point of coaptation of the mitral leaflets with respect to the plane of the mitral annulus in the apical four-chamber view. In normal persons, the leaflets themselves as well as the coaptation point are on the ventricular side of the annulus plane. In mild MVP, the point of coaptation is in the annulus plane, though the leaflets themselves bulge or bow slightly on the atrial side of this plane. In severe MVP, the prolapsing leaflets as well as their coaptation point are all on the atrial side of the annulus plane in systole. Redundancy of mitral leaflets or chords may be prominent (Figures 11-22 and 11-23) and even simulate vegetations on cursory viewing. There is a wide spectrum of echo Doppler appearances of this very common and important mitral abnormality (Figures 11-24 to 11-28). The diagnosis is best made on the combined basis of systolic leaflet contour, leaflet thickness, leaflet redundancy, and colorflow Doppler MR jet.

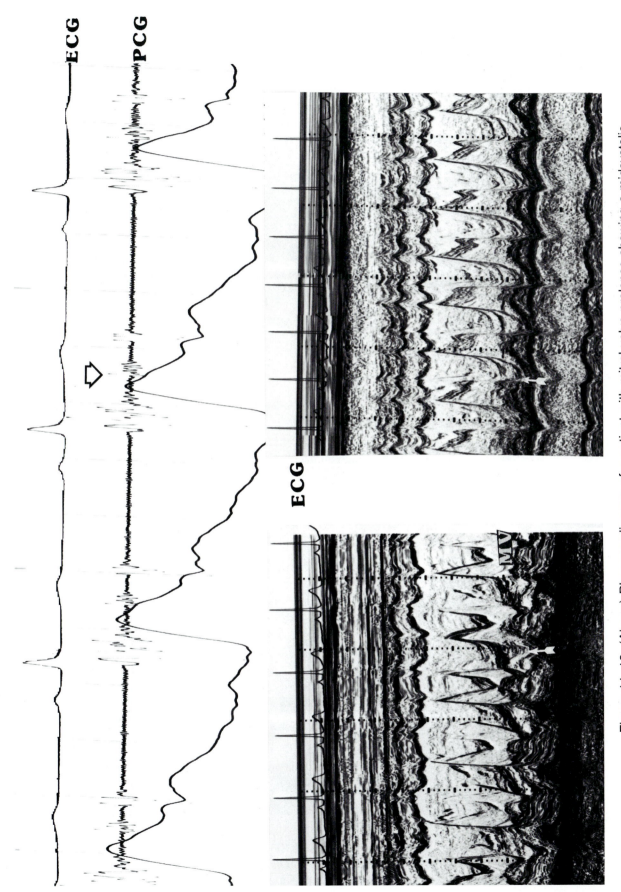

Figure 11–19. (Above) Phonocardiogram of a patient with mitral valve prolapse showing a midsystolic click. (Below) M-mode echo showing late-systolic mitral prolapse in supine position (left). Standing position (right) shows that prolapse begins earlier in systole.

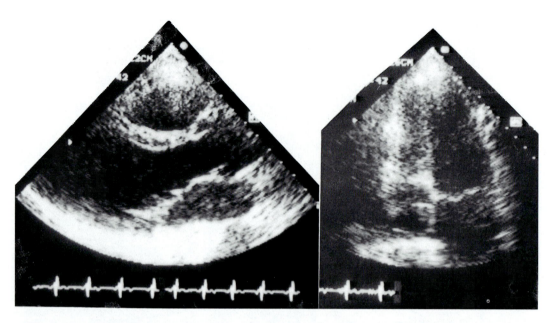

Figure 11–20. Parasternal long-axis view (left) and apical four-chamber view (right) of a patient with typical mild mitral prolapse.

CALCIFICATION IN THE MITRAL ANNULUS REGION

Echocardiographers are all familiar with the fact that mitral annulus calcification (MAC) is common in elderly patients. Conflicting reports of its predilection for the female sex have been resolved by the Framingham data,[87] which demonstrated that MAC is twice as common in women as in men. Age is undoubtedly the major predisposing factor. In the

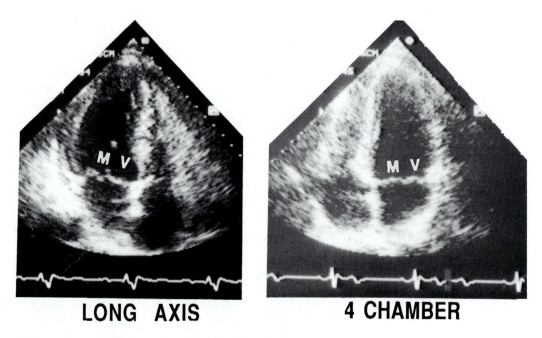

Figure 11–21. Apical long-axis and four-chamber views showing a small local protrusion of the posterior mitral leaflet but no typical prolapse.

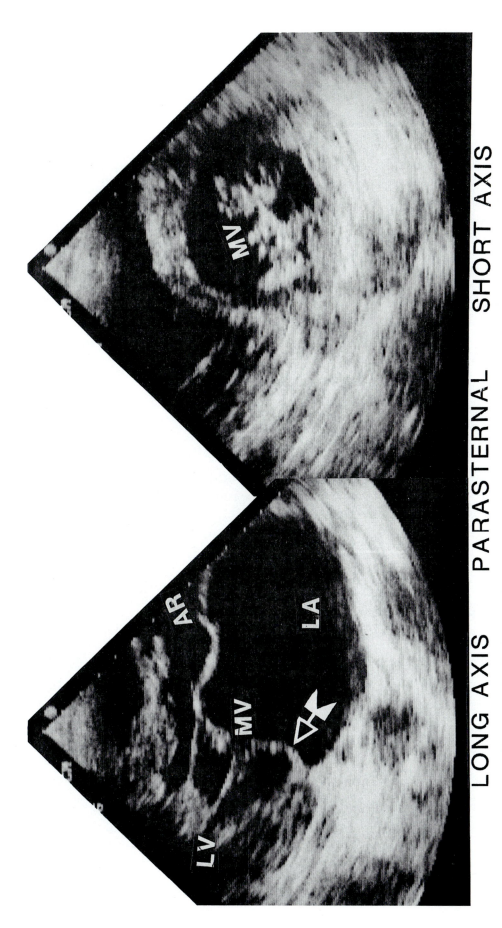

LONG AXIS   PARASTERNAL   SHORT AXIS

Figure 11–22. Parasternal long-axis view (left) and short-axis view (right) showing conspicuous redundancy of the mitral leaflets resulting in a bizarre configuration (right).

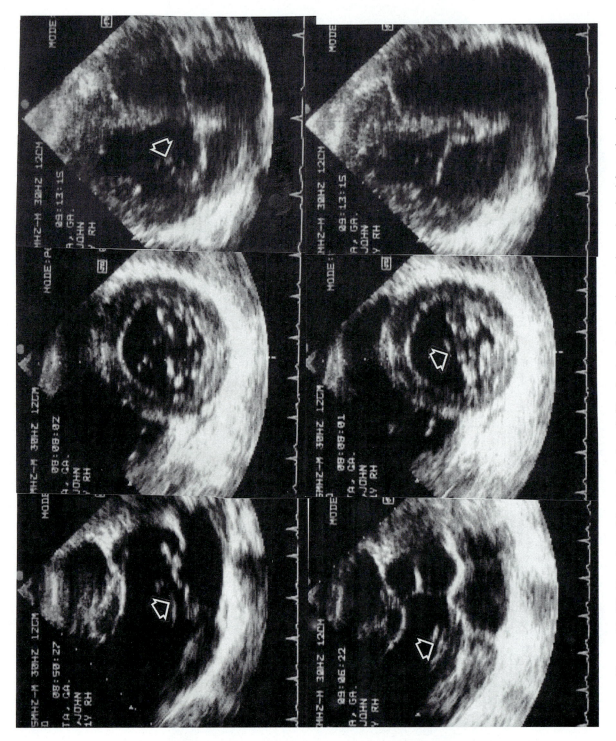

Figure 11–23. Parasternal long-axis view (left), short-axis view (center), and apical four-chamber view (right) in a patient with mitral prolapse showing redundancy with anterior buckling of mitral chordae tendineae (arrows).

APICAL LONG AXIS   APICAL 4 CHAMBER

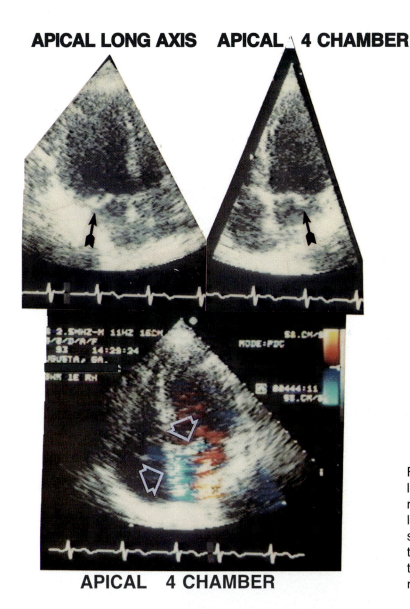

APICAL   4 CHAMBER

Figure 11–24. Apical long-axis view (above, left) and apical four-chamber view (above, right) showing prolapse of the posterior mitral leaflet (arrows). Colorflow Doppler (below) shows MR jet that runs first parallel to the anterior mitral leaflet and then along the atrial septum (arrows). Thus the MR jet is opposite in direction to the prolapsed posterior leaflet.

Framingham study, a prevalence of 11.9% was found in women and 6.2% in men in the 70 to 79 age group and 22.4% in women and 6.0% in men in the over-80 population. Under age 60, it was encountered in well below 1%.

Although well studied in autopsied hearts by numerous authors since 1910, clinicians remained virtually ignorant about MAC, except for its occasional appearance on chest radiographs or fluoroscopy as a C- or J-shaped opacity within the posteroinferior part of the cardiac shadow.

The location of MAC is important, especially to echocardiographers. MAC is restricted to the vicinity of the posterior mitral annulus, i.e., that part of the circumference of the mitral valve to which the posterior mitral leaflet is attached. Kirk and Russell[88] were the first to point out that MAC occurred in one or both of two possible locations: (1) in the true fibrous mitral annulus at the junction of the atrial and ventricular myocardium on the posterior and posterolateral LV aspects and (2) at the base of the posterior mitral leaflet, which is the more common site. Echocardiography can easily distinguish between these two locations; in fact, cardiac ultrasound is far more sensitive than radiography in detecting the presence of calcification.[89]

MAC begins as one or more small hard nodules at the base of the posterior mitral leaflet, commonly the middle of this leaflet. As it increases in size, the small calcific nod-

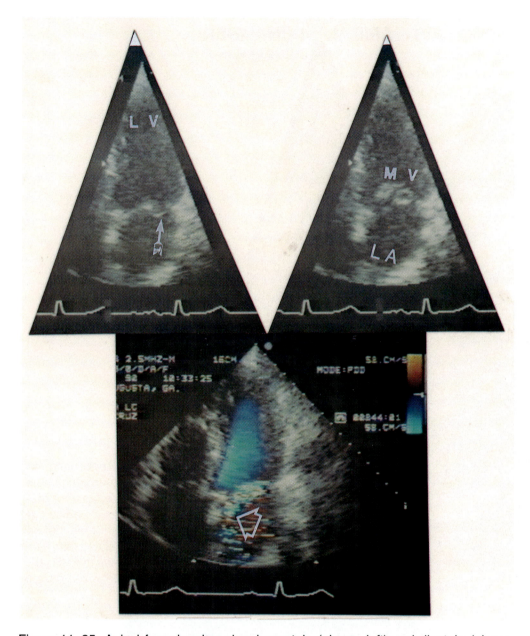

Figure 11–25. Apical four-chamber view in systole (above, left) and diastole (above, right). Systolic prolapse of the posterior mitral leaflet is seen (arrow); in diastole this redundant leaflet appears "curled up." Colorflow Doppler (below) shows an anterior (medial) MR jet directed away from the prolapsed posterior leaflet.

ules coalesce to form a continuous bar or ridge projecting into the angle between the posterior mitral leaflet and LV posterior wall. On palpation, it usually becomes evident that the rigid MAC is partly embedded in the myocardium of this region. When severe, MAC is not only extensive in circumferential extent (under the entire posterior leaflet attachment and also posteromedial commissure) but also thicker and bulkier. The posterior leaflet may be displaced and even immobilized by massive MAC. Calcific spurs may ulcerate the endocardium on the atrial side; rare instances of thrombi[90] or vegetations forming on such sites have been reported, and even of calcified material from MAC embolizing to multiple systemic arteries, with fatal outcome.[91]

A fibrotic reaction may surround the actual calcific area and add to its bulk. Microscopically, MAC appears as solid, amorphous masses arising in the fibrosa of the

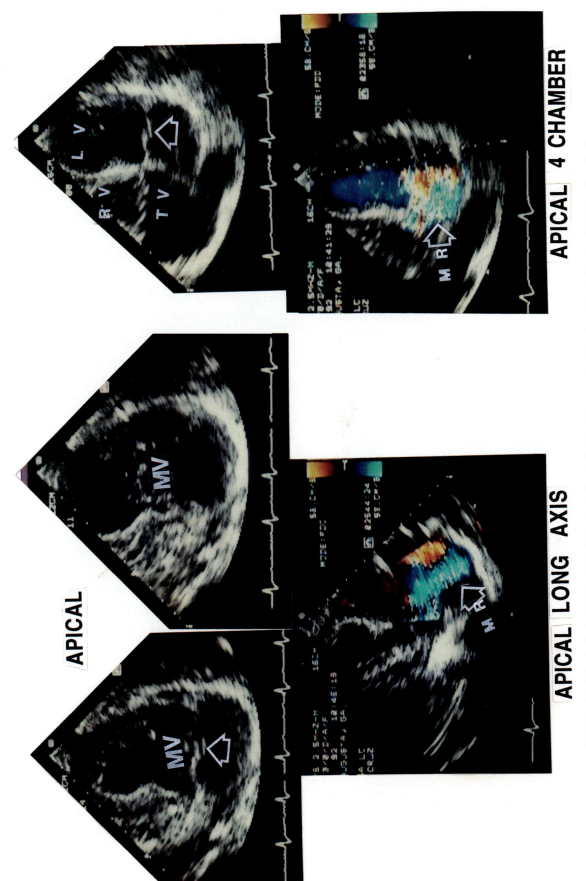

APICAL 4 CHAMBER

APICAL LONG AXIS

APICAL

Figure 11–26. Apical views showing systolic mitral prolapse (arrows) and redundant "floppy" mitral leaflets in diastole (above, center). A large anteromedial MR jet is seen on colorflow Doppler (below). Tricuspid valve prolapse is also present (above, right).

267

PARASTERNAL LONG AXIS

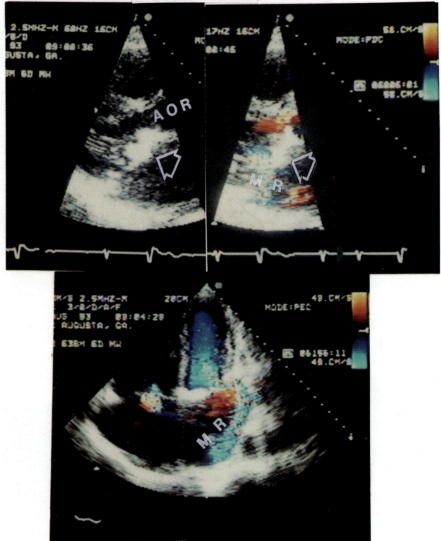

APICAL 4 CHAMBER

Figure 11–27. Parasternal long-axis view (above, left) showing marked thickening and prolapse of the anterior mitral leaflet (arrow). Colorflow Doppler in same plane (above, right) shows posterior mitral regurgitant jet (MR). Apical four-chamber view (below) shows the MR jet along the posterolateral left atrial wall.

valve ring or in fibrosa of the posterior leaflet near its attachment. With further growth, MAC penetrates adjacent myocardium or projects into the posterior submitral angle. In about 3% of patients with MAC, the latter undergoes an unexplained central softening[92] so that a sterile "abscess" containing caseous material forms; to the pathologist it may resemble a tuberculoma or gumma. This unusual variant of MAC is of relatively large size and round shape and is of importance to the echocardiographer because it simulates neoplastic or thrombotic left atrial masses.

Hemodynamic complications of MAC include mitral regurgitation (MR) and stenosis (MS). Severe, extensive MAC is believed to cause MR by (1) deforming and restricting motion of the posterior mitral leaflet, thus interfering with systolic valve closure, and (2) preventing sphincter-like systolic narrowing of the LV myocardium adjacent to the mitral annulus by a "splinting" action of the long rigid MAC bar.[93] MAC is seldom the sole cause of severe MR but is probably often a contributory factor to MR attributable to various valvar or myocardial lesions.

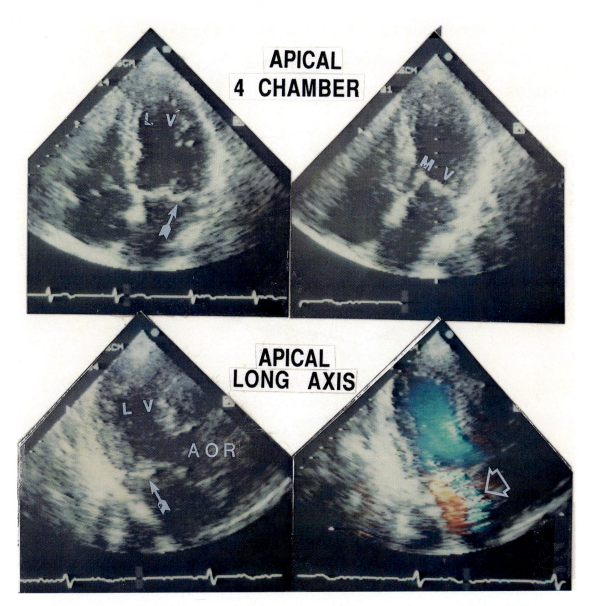

APICAL 4 CHAMBER

APICAL LONG AXIS

Figure 11–28. Apical four-chamber view (above) in systole (left) and diastole (right). The mitral valve (MV) leaflets are thickened and prolapsed (arrow), especially the posterior one, as seen also in the apical long-axis view (below, left). Colorflow Doppler shows an anterior MR jet (open arrow).

MAC causing MS has been documented by cardiac catheterization in a few instances.[94-98] The LV chamber usually has been small and hypertrophied and the MAC massive so that it encroaches considerably on the already small LV inflow area.

In a small percentage of patients with end-stage renal disease on long-term dialysis, gross calcification can occur in both mitral leaflets and progress in a matter of months to MS.[97] This calcification occurs in the annulus region and basal part of the leaflets, sparing the free edges of the latter; this distribution of calcium is useful to the pathologist as well as the echocardiographer in distinguishing it from rheumatic calcific MS. The calcification tends to have distinctive rounded edges and involve the LV myocardium more invasively than the usual MAC of old age. MAC in adults below age 40 is almost invariably associated with chronic renal failure, with hereditary disease such as Marfan's and Hurler's syndromes accounting for a very rare instance.

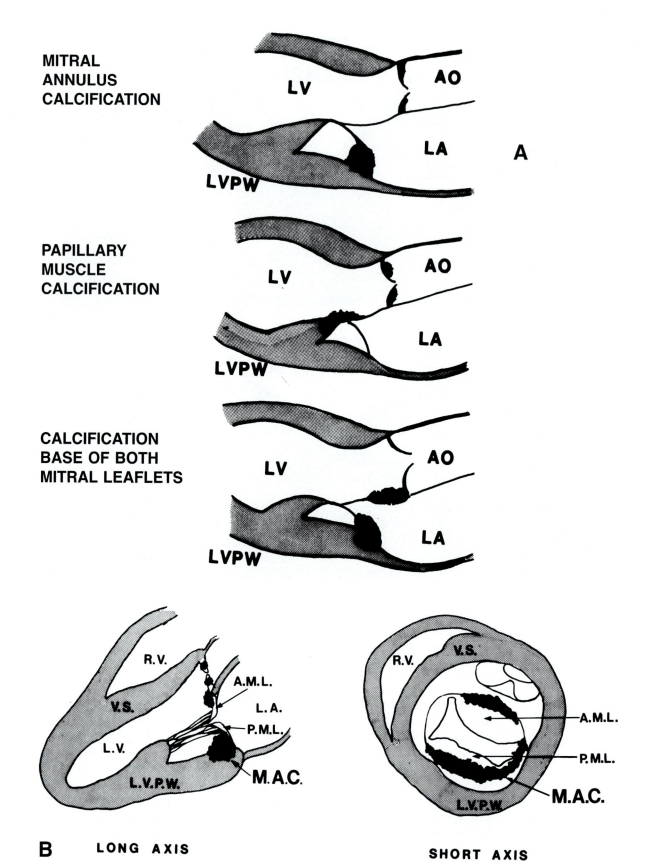

MITRAL
ANNULUS
CALCIFICATION

LV

AO

LVPW

LA

A

PAPILLARY
MUSCLE
CALCIFICATION

LV

AO

LVPW

LA

CALCIFICATION
BASE OF BOTH
MITRAL LEAFLETS

LV

AO

LVPW

LA

B   LONG AXIS

R.V.

V.S.

A.M.L.

L.A.

P.M.L.

L.V.

L.V.P.W.

M.A.C.

SHORT AXIS

R.V.

V.S.

A.M.L.

P.M.L.

L.V.P.W.

M.A.C.

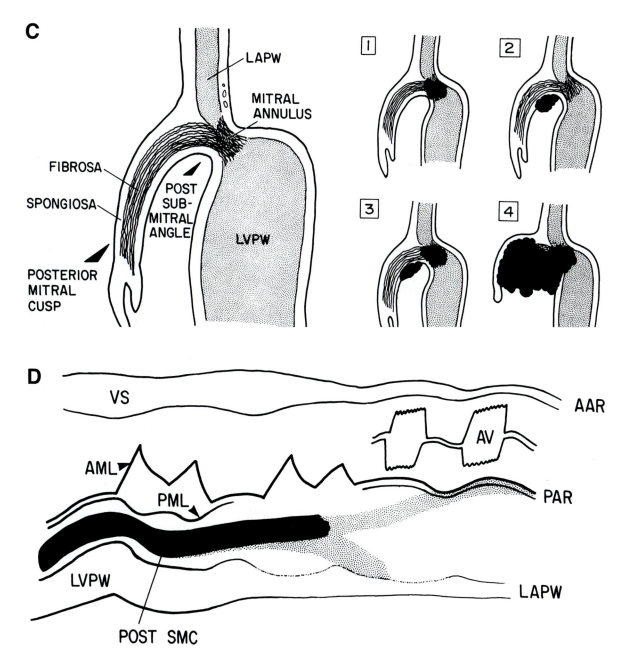

Fig 11–29. (A) Diagram of parasternal long-axis view showing various types of calcification in the mitral apparatus. (Above) Common "mitral annulus calcification" at base of posterior mitral leaflet. (Center) Papillary muscle–chordal calcification. (Below) Calcification of base of both mitral leaflets, sparing the free edges as seen in chronic renal failure or sometimes degenerative calcification of the elderly. (B) Diagrams in long-axis view (left) and short-axis view (right) showing the location of mitral annulus calcification (MAC) at the attachment of the posterior mitral leaflet (PML) to the left ventricular posterior wall (LVPW). Note calcification also at the base of the anterior mitral leaflet (AML). (Reproduced, with permission, from Am J Cardiol 1979[89]). (C) Diagram showing anatomy of the posterior left atrioventricular region, including the posterior mitral cusp. The fibrosa of this cusp is anchored to the fibrosa of the mitral annulus (LAPV and LAPW, left atrial and ventricular posterior wall). At right are shown some variants of mitral annulus calcification. No. 2 is common; no. 4 represents massive MAC seen only in elderly women. (Reproduced, with permission, from Am J Cardiol 1979[89]). (D) Diagram showing M-mode sweep with typical appearances of MAC (posterior submitral calcification). MAC is represented by the thick black band between mitral valve and LV posterior wall. (Reproduced, with permission, from Am J Cardiol 1979[89]).

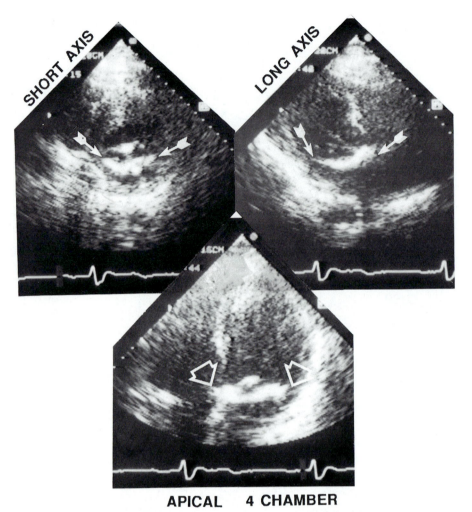

Figure 11–30. Parasternal short-axis view (above, left), modified long-axis view (above, right), and apical four-chamber view (below) showing extensive mitral annulus calcification (arrows). Maximal length of calcification is about 4 cm; width is 1 to 5 cm.

APICAL   4 CHAMBER

Cardiac conduction disturbances at A-V or bundle branch level are more common in patients with MAC than in the age- and sex-matched patient population with no MAC on echocardiography.[98,99] However, the association is not, in most cases, one of direct cause and effect, because the usual posterior LV location of MAC is remote from the anterior site of the His bundle and its main branches. It is only in the uncommon cases of calcification in the central fibrous body or intervalvar fibrosa that direct interruption of the specific conduction pathways is anatomically comprehensible.[100]

Atrial fibrillation often has been present in most series of patients with MAC reported over the last 50 years, but the 12-fold excess of atrial fibrillation in subjects with MAC in the Framingham data over non-MAC controls[87] was surprising. Possible causative factors include LV dilatation (secondary to MR or to associated heart disease) and extension of sclerocalcific MAC pathology into the adjacent LA myocardium.

Echocardiographic Appearances of MAC (Figures 11–29 to 11–36)

As might be expected from the very wide range of extent of MAC, the 2D echo picture can vary from a small nodule or sliver of bright calcification to a massive shelf of MAC filling most of the posterior LV chamber at the basal LV level. In cases of average or moderate severity, in parasternal long-axis view, a bright, dense, round or oval echo is seen at the point of attachment of the posterior mitral leaflet to the posterior LV-LA junction (Figures 11–30 and 11–31). In the parasternal short-axis view, MAC manifests as a curved dense bar between the mitral valve and the LV posterior wall, a location already familiar to M-mode echocardiographers.[102-105] A narrow rim of MAC can be mistaken for poste-

PARASTERNAL SHORT-AXIS

PARASTERNAL LONG-AXIS

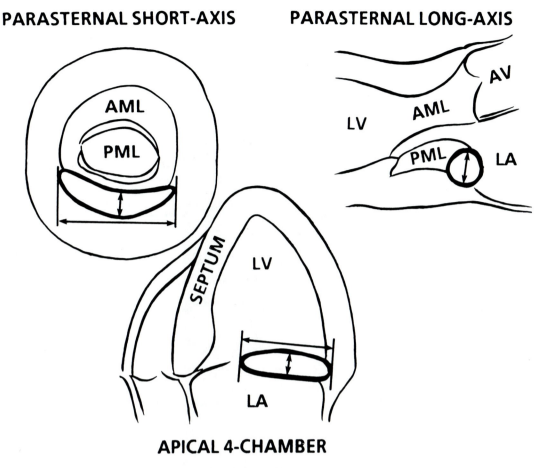

APICAL 4-CHAMBER

Figure 11–31. Diagrams of parasternal short-axis, long-axis, and apical four-chamber views showing location of MAC and how the length and thickness of a mitral annulus calcification are measured.

rior mitral leaflet calcification. On the other hand, a large, thick MAC can obscure the posterior leaflet echocardiographically.

In the apical four-chamber view through the central LV chamber showing the mitral leaflets, MAC is seen as a dense echo at or near the attachment of the posterior leaflet. Tilting the transducer to image a more posterior LV plane may bring into view the full transverse extent of MAC so that it appears as a bright echogenic bar interposed between LA and LV. Not rarely, MAC at the base of the posterior mitral leaflet is accompanied by calcification of the basal part of the anterior mitral leaflet.[106] In such cases it is important to note that the free edges of the leaflets are of normal thickness and mobility, thus distinguishing the valve from a rheumatically stenotic valve. Doppler recordings of forward mitral flow do not reveal significant MS, but colorflow Doppler imaging of the stream flowing into the LV chamber may be somewhat narrower than normal because motion of both leaflets is restricted at their bases.

Grading of the severity of MAC on 2D echo has been attempted on the basis of its maximum width (thickness) in the parasternal view.[99] MAC width less than 5 mm was called *minimal* to *mild,* and width over 5 mm was designated *moderate* to *severe.* This method did not consider the transverse or circumferential extent of MAC. Others have categorized MAC as mild, moderate, or severe according to the length (along the mitral annulus) of the MAC, irrespective of its thickness. A reasonable approach seems to be to

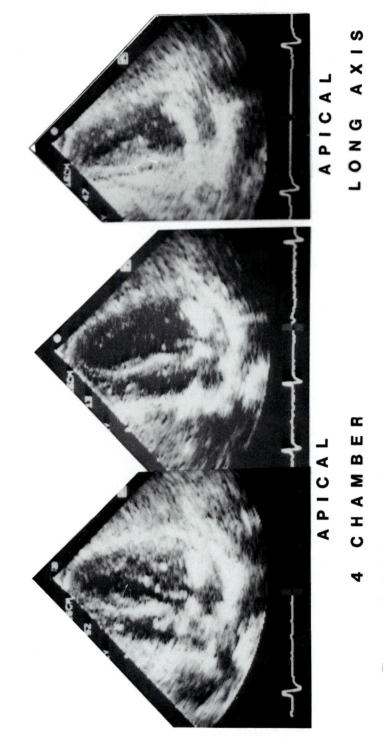

A P I C A L
L O N G   A X I S

A P I C A L
4   C H A M B E R

Figure 11–32. Apical views showing large mitral annulus calcification (arrows). In this patient the calcification appears as a discrete mass, simulating a left atrial mass.

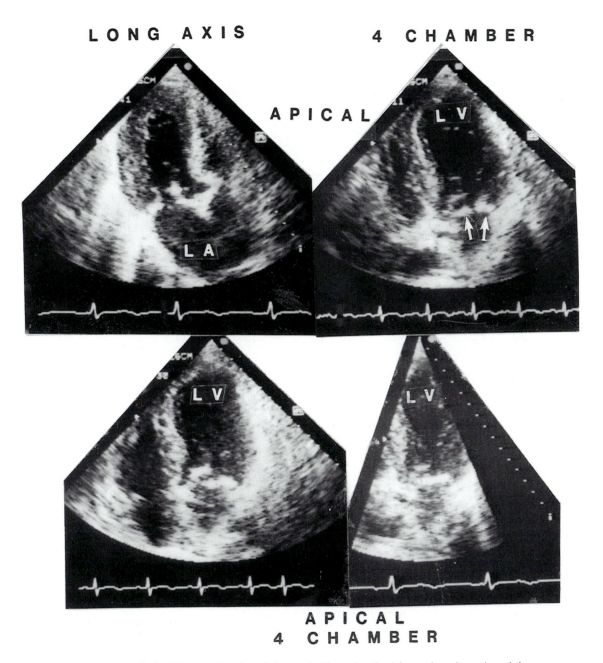

Figure 11–33. Apical long-axis view (above, left) and apical four-chamber view (above, right, and below, left) show calcification of the base of both mitral leaflets (arrows). The free edges of the mitral leaflets are not calcified. In a more posterior plane (below, right), the posterior mitral basal leaflet (mitral annulus) calcification is seen.

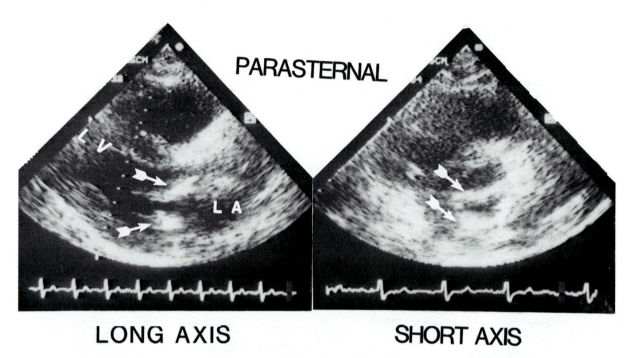

PARASTERNAL

LONG AXIS   SHORT AXIS

Figure 11–34. Parasternal long-axis and short-axis views showing much calcification of the basal part of the anterior and posterior mitral leaflets (arrows). The free edges of the cusps are not calcified. The patient was on long-term hemodialysis for end-stage renal disease.

measure the maximum length and maximum thickness of the MAC (Figure 11–31) in either parasternal short-axis or apical four-chamber view.[107]

Echocardiographers should be aware of the uncommon but important variant of MAC that manifests on 2D echo as a relatively large, round mass rather than a transverse bar (Figure 11-32). A central soft caseation in the mass appears as a sonolucency within it. Such masses have been mistaken on radiography, CT, and echocardiography for calcified granulomas or myxomas, and patients have even been subjected to cardiac surgery on that basis. The very typical location at the attachment of the posterior mitral leaflet and the calcific configuration are the keys to the correct diagnosis.

Another variant of MAC occurs where calcification is located in the basal parts of both leaflets, but the free edges are spared. A mild example of this type is shown in Figure 11-33. More severe and even massive basal calcification of the mitral leaflets is an unusual but characteristic finding in some patients with end-stage renal disease on long-term dialysis (Figures 11-34 and 11-35). Careful imaging in all possible apical and parasternal planes is necessary to visualize the full extent of posterior MAC as well as basal anterior mitral leaflet or intervalvar fibrosa calcification (Figure 11-36).

Papillary Muscle Calcification

This is often associated with MAC (and, like it, is easily identified on 2D echo) in elderly patients (Figures 11-37 to 11-39). There is ample echocardiographic confirmation of Roberts' earlier autopsy observations that such calcification frequently occurs in association with MAC. Both lesions might produce or aggravate MR, but the extent of this role is uncertain. Aortic valve calcification is also often present, the third member of this calcific triad.

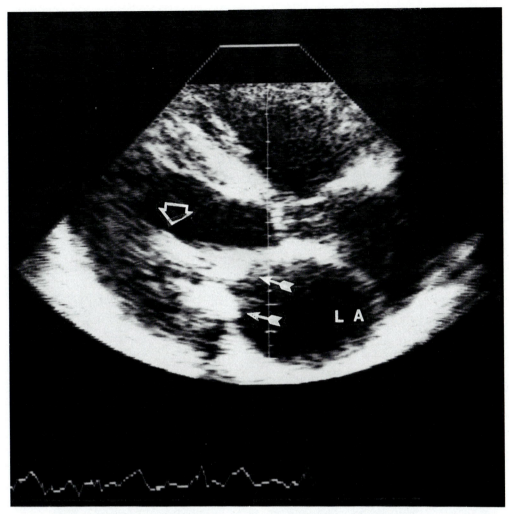

PARASTERNAL   LONG   AXIS

Figure 11–35. Parasternal long-axis view in a patient with end-stage renal disease with massive calcification of both mitral leaflets (thin arrows). The open arrow indicates heavy papillary muscle calcification.

FLAIL MITRAL VALVE

Flail motion of a mitral leaflet or part of a leaflet results from rupture of one or more chordae tendineae or of a papillary muscle. Although the cause of the rupture and the nature of associated cardiac pathology can vary considerably, the echocardiographic manifestations of a flail mitral leaflet have certain features in common over a wide spectrum of chordal or papillary muscle disruption.

Chordae Tendineae Rupture

Bacterial endocarditis[108,109] and myxomatous degeneration[110] are the principal causes. Rarely, trauma or spontaneous rupture of normal chordae is responsible.

In patients with bacterial endocarditis, chordae to the anterior leaflet are affected more commonly than the posterior ones.[111] Usually vegetations are adherent to the valve leaflets or the ruptured chord, and they modify the 2D echo appearances. In patients with myxomatous degeneration, the nonflail part of the mitral valve shows typical contours of MVP.

APICAL
4 CHAMBER   **LONG AXIS**

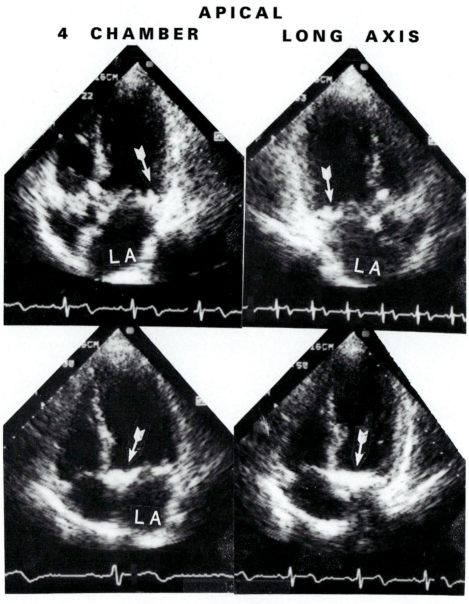

APICAL
4 CHAMBER

Figure 11–36. Apical four-chamber views (above, left) and apical long-axis views (above, right) showing typical mitral annulus calcification (arrows) at the base of the posterior mitral leaflet. Apical four-chamber views in more posterior planes showing the extensive distribution of the calcification (arrows).

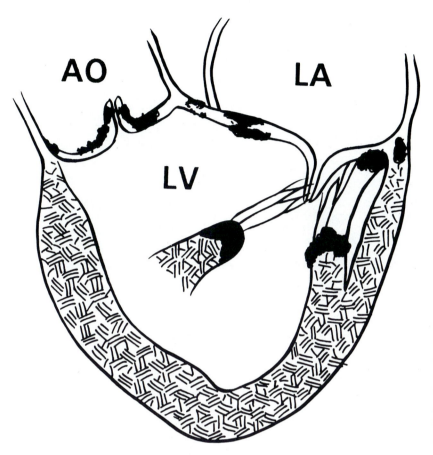

Figure 11–37. Diagram showing common sites of intracardiac calcification in elderly patients. Isolated calcification of one of these sites can occur, but often two or more sites are calcified concomitantly (i.e., MAC, papillary muscle, basal anterior leaflet, intervalvar fibrosa, and aortic valve).

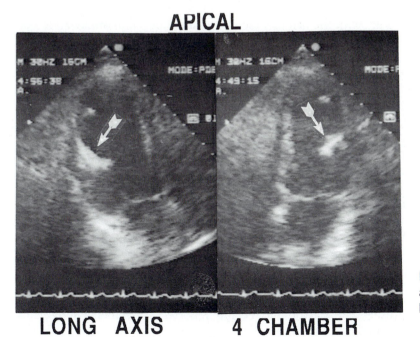

Figure 11–38. Apical long-axis (left) and apical four-chamber views (right) showing heavy papillary muscle calcification (arrows).

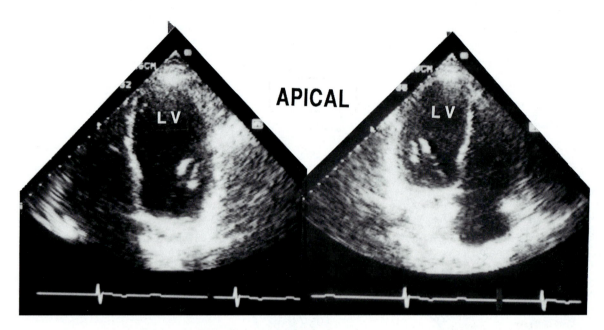

Figure 11–39. Apical modified four-chamber view (left) and long-axis views (right) showing papillary muscle calcification.

On viewing the real-time 2D echo recording, the key finding is selective exaggerated motion of the untethered part of the valve in diastole, while the rest of the valve moves normally. This loose, erratic motion of the flail leaflet segment may be better appreciated in one view than in others. In systole, the typical configuration is nonapposition of the flail leaflet, the free edge of which projects toward the atrium (Figures 11–40 and 11–41). This pathognomonic finding is rapid and easily missed; perhaps only in one frame, perhaps only in a particular plane, it is best visualized in the parasternal long-axis and apical four-chamber planes. In other cases, the flail leaflet component may be conspicuous, producing a "double contour" with the flail part parallel to and 2 or 3 mm on the atrial side of the normal part of the same leaflet. M-mode recordings best document the presence of an irregular diastolic flutter of the flail leaflet.[112-115] Systolic flutter of this leaflet is even more specific for the diagnosis of flail leaflet.[112,114-116]

On colorflow Doppler, the MR jet tends to be very eccentric and in a direction opposite to the flail leaflet (Figures 11–40 and 11–41).

Papillary Muscle Rupture

Although first described nearly 2 centuries ago, this disorder was not diagnosed clinically until 1948.[117] It is said to complicate acute myocardial infarction in 1% to 3% of cases and to account for 5% of infact-related deaths.[118-121] It may complicate either transmural or subendocardial infarction. The posteromedial papillary muscle ruptures four times as often as the anterolateral muscle. In a recent Mayo Clinic series, 21 of 22 patients with papillary muscle rupture had inferior infarction, and the posteromedial muscle was ruptured in all.[122] This striking disparity is attributed to the fact that the posteromedial papillary muscle has a single effective blood supply from the posterior descending artery, whereas the anterolateral one has a dual supply.

In the era before cardiac surgery, 80% of patients died by the first 24 hours; only 6% survived over 2 months.[123] The Mayo Clinic recently reported a perioperative mortality of 27% and 64% 7-year survival for those who survived surgery[122]; 43% of patients in this series had single-vessel coronary disease, commonly right coronary, less frequently circumflex artery.

APICAL
LONG AXIS

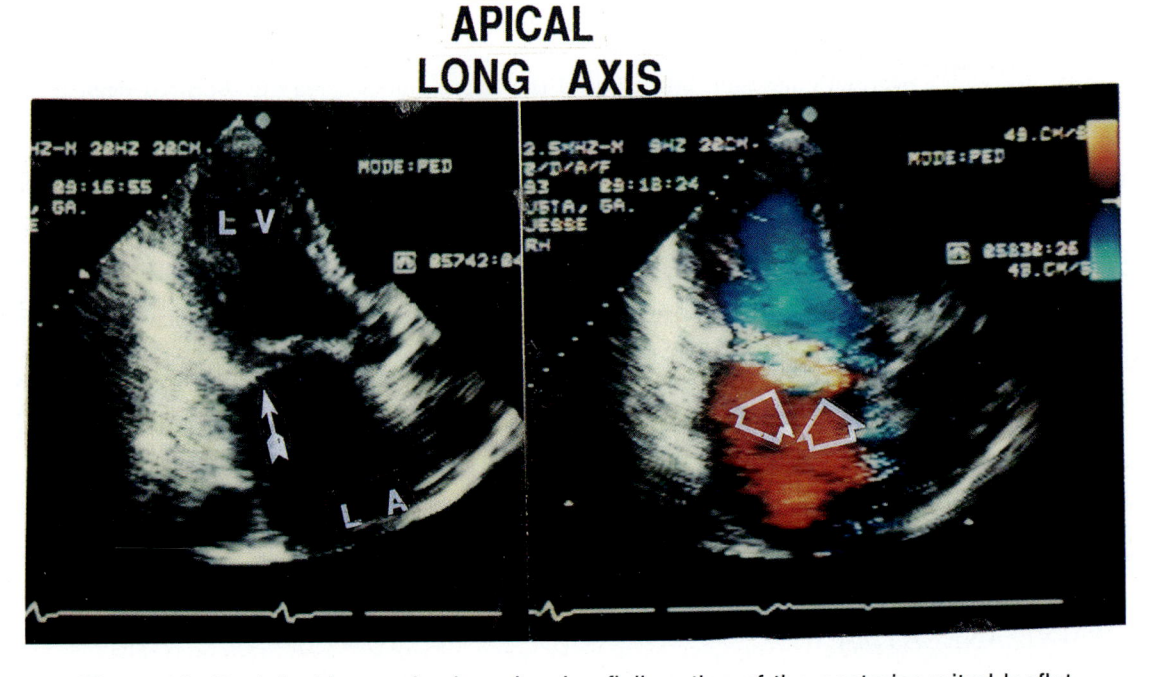

Figure 11–40. Apical long-axis view showing flail motion of the posterior mitral leaflet (left). The leaflets do not coapt. Colorflow Doppler (right) in same view shows a mitral regurgitant jet (arrows) parallel and contiguous to the anterior mitral leaflet.

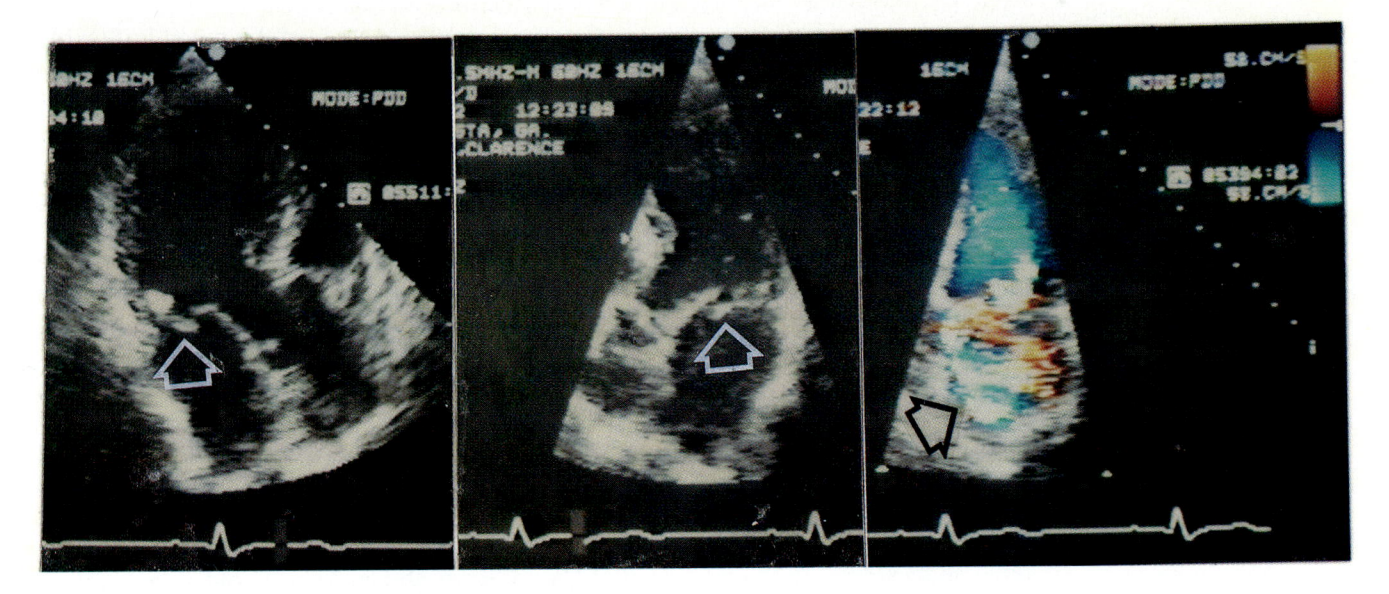

Figure 11–41. Apical long-axis (left) and apical four-chamber views (center) showing flail posterior mitral leaflet motion with lack of proper leaflet coaptation. Colorflow Doppler in apical four-chamber view shows a medial (anterior) mitral regurgitant jet (arrow).

In the same Mayo Clinic series, partial rupture of the main papillary muscle or rupture of one or more of its multiple heads had occurred in 68%, and complete papillary muscle rupture occurred in 32%. The latter manifests with rapid deterioration resulting in pulmonary edema and cardiogenic shock. Partial rupture also commonly results in progressively increasing cardiac failure, though less dramatically than with complete rupture, and may even present as chronic MR.

Papillary muscle rupture nearly always occurs in the first week after onset of myocardial infarction. Infarction of the LV wall underlying the ruptured papillary muscle is often of relatively small size so that the LV ejection fraction is only mildly subnormal. In fact, it has been suggested that good contraction of the noninfarcted LV may contribute to papillary muscle rupture by exerting greater shearing force on the soft, necrotic papillary muscle.[121]

Echocardiography of Papillary Muscle Rupture[123-128]

In the Mayo Clinic series, actual visualization of the ruptured papillary muscle was possible in half the cases by conventional 2D echo.[123] In other cases, flail mitral valve motion was observed, similar to that due to ruptured chordae tendineae. In some instances, the avulsed tip or apex of the papillary muscle can be identified as attached to the flail leaflet with chordae intact. The stump of the affected muscle may also be noted. Rapid, erratic motion of papillary muscle tip, with "loose" chordae and flail leaflet, may provide a spectacular sight in real-time viewing. Initial reports indicate that TEE is very useful in diagnosing papillary muscle rupture when transthoracic 2D echo is equivocal.[123]

MITRAL VALVE ANEURYSM

Autopsy observations on mitral valve aneurysms (MVAs) were made in the mid-nineteenth century by the renowned pathologist Rokitansky (1852), as well as by Habershaw (1855), Ogle (1858), and Pelvet (1867). In nearly all reported instances, the MVA appears to have resulted from local damage of a mitral leaflet in a patient with aortic endocarditis and aortic regurgitation.[129] It has been postulated that the aortic regurgitant jet carries bacteria from the infected aortic valve and implants the infection on the area of anterior mitral leaflet. After endocarditis at this mitral site has weakened the mitral leaflet, the impact of the aortic regurgitant jet and the ventricular systolic pressure then causes the affected area of mitral leaflet to expand or balloon toward the left atrium until it reaches "the size of a walnut," thus forming the MVA. It is possible that in some cases the infection migrates from aortic to mitral valve by contiguous spread (marche descendante of the French). As might be expected, MVAs occur predominantly (but not invariably) on the anterior rather than posterior mitral leaflet.

Prior to the introduction of antibiotics in the 1940s, the pathology of MVA was very different from what it was after bacterial endocarditis was treated by antibiotics. In the pre-antibiotic era, MVAs were actually "false aneurysms"—the "thromboaneurysms" of Ribbert (1924). Apparently, ulceration of a mitral leaflet by infection was sometimes followed by a solid mass of vegetations, thrombi, and necrotic valve tissue being driven into the ulcer crater by intraventricular pressure. Antibiotic therapy allowed longer survival so that true aneurysms of the mitral leaflet developed, conforming to MVAs of the type now encountered at autopsy and on echocardiograms.

In a landmark paper, Saphir and Leroy[130] first gave an excellent description of such postantibiotic MVA in 5 patients, who were a subgroup of 53 fatal cases of subacute bacterial endocarditis. Their description of MVA (slightly abridged here) holds true today:

A well-circumscribed, round, smooth outpouching or ballooning of part of a leaflet of the mitral valve, 0.8 to 1.5 cm in diameter. At first glance it appears a large vegetation; only by gentle compression, its saclike nature becomes evident. A small perforation at the summit of the aneurysm was present in four out of five cases. In four there were small firm vegetations at the periphery (base) of the aneurysm. On the ventricular aspect of the valve, corresponding to the MVA which bulged into the left atrium, the mouth of the MVA man-ifests as a small round defect with smooth but thickened margins. When incised, the MVA contains blood or small loose thrombi.

In subsequent autopsy or surgical descriptions[131-135] of MVA also, perforations of varying size were found in the aneurysmal wall.

How common is MVA as a complication of bacterial endocarditis? In one series of 58 patients operated on for aortic regurgitation due to bacterial endocarditis, the mitral valve showed endocarditis pathology in 10; 2 of these had MVA.

The 2D echo features of MVA have been similar in most reports.[136-140] A localized bulge (saccular aneurysm) of the anterior mitral leaflet, protruding into the left atrium, is the rule during systole. Reid et al.[136] noted that this bulge persisted in diastole in all five of their cases. However, in some other instances, the MVA "collapsed" during dias-tole.[138,139] The patient of Lewis et al.[141] was remarkable in that the posterior mitral leaflet was aneurysmal and adhered in part to the left atrial posterior wall, creating the illusion in some echo views of a septum or accessory chamber within the left atrium.

As it does with other mitral lesions, TEE images MVAs with superior clarity and de-tail, so TEE is useful when MVA cannot be well distinguished from other mitral pathology on conventional 2D echo. Colorflow Doppler is well suited to detection of the presence and size of MVA perforation and the extent of consequent mitral regurgitation.

The 2D echo appearances of MVA bear some resemblance to those of mitral valve prolapse, and in fact, the two can occur in the same valve. The presence of aortic valve vegetations and regurgitation, the local saccular nature of the mitral leaflet protrusion, and detection of perforation in it by colorflow Doppler all favor MVA over mitral valve pro-lapse.

LOCAL MITRAL VALVE TUMOR OR MASSES

Local "mass" lesions situated on or originating from a mitral leaflet are not rare on echocar-diography, and diagnosis of their nature constitutes an important and intriguing diagnos-tic task. One of the common causes is a calcific nodule or small plaque near the edge of the leaflet; another is a vegetation of bacterial or fungal endocarditis.

However, there are many other types of mitral valvar tumors or masses, all of which are rare but should be known to echocardiographers because (1) they may exhibit 2D echo peculiarities that help in identifying their pathologic nature, (2) they may produce clinically important complications, chiefly of systemic embolization, (3) some of them re-quire surgical excision, and (4) echocardiography is either the only or the best means of diagnosing the presence of these valve lesions because physical signs are often absent and other imaging techniques are less informative.

Whereas some of these mitral valve masses are in fact tumors in the sense that they are neoplastic and appear solid on echocardiography, others, such as cysts or aneurysms, are not strictly tumors and tend to have a sonolucent center with a balloon-like border.

Mitral Papillary Fibroelastoma

Next to myxomas, this is probably the most important form of cardiac neoplasm, com-prising about 5% of the latter in Prichard's series[142] of cardiac tumors. Nasser and Parker[143] collected 39 cases reported before 1971. This tumor has been reported under a wide va-riety of names, at least 14,[144] of which *papillary fibroelastoma* (CPFE) is in most common use at present. *Giant Lambl's excrescences* is another term used. The autopsy characteristics of CPFE had been well studied by the third quarter of this century.[142,145-147]

The CPFE is a benign small tumor with multiple papillary fronds. It may be pedun-culated or sessile. Each villus of the papilliferous neoplasm consists of a core of dense fi-brous tissue surrounded by myxomatous tissue (loose cellular elements in a matrix of acid mucopolysaccharide) and lined on its surface by hyperplastic endocardium.

Elastic tissue is present as disorganized masses or well-defined elastic fibrils. Submerged in water, the fronds or villi of the tumor exhibit a typical fine undulation likened to the fine tentacles of a sea anemone.

Diagnosis of CPFE became possible during life only after the advent of cardiac ultrasound, because physical signs are usually absent and the tumor is generally too small to be well imaged by other invasive or noninvasive modalities. Echocardiography is eminently suited to detect CPFE, which it reveals as a small 0.5- to 1.5-cm mass on a valve cusp. The tumor has been thus visualized on each of the four cardiac valves; several examples of mitral CPFE have been well documented during the last decade.[148-152] The chief differential diagnoses include bacterial vegetations and local valvular sclerocalcific lesions of a degenerative nature. Careful scrutiny of the magnified image on real-time viewing may reveal highly diagnostic minute projections exhibiting a rapid undulation or fine surface flutter around a central dense core.[153] In a minority of instances the CPFE is attached to ventricular endocardium rather than to a valve. In a remarkable case, 10 CPFE tumors were present concomitantly, 5 on the subvalvar mitral area and 5 on the LV endocardium.[152] Another similar case has been reported recently.[153a]

The echocardiographic diagnosis of CPFE has gained considerably in clinical significance with the realization that some of the patients reported had experienced TIAs or cerebrovascular accidents (CVAs).[148-150] There is evidence that thrombi tend to form on CPFEs and then embolize.[150] Coronary embolization resulting in angina, myocardial infarction, or sudden death has been reported. TEE is particularly useful in identifying CPFEs by providing better visualization of the unique 2D echo texture and surface undulation of a mitral valve "mass."[152,154]

A CPFE 1.5 cm in size attached to the anterior mitral leaflet caused obstruction to mitral flow resulting in Doppler findings like those of moderate mitral stenosis.[154]

Mitral Valve Myxoma

Atrial myxomas are the most common and important of all cardiac tumors, but mitral valve myxomas are little known to most cardiologists. Meisner et al.[155] found 5 instances of mitral valve myxoma diagnosed by echocardiography by 1993 and added 1 more. In 1934, Jaleski[156] collected reports of 22 valvar myxomas, of which 4 were on the mitral valve. Echocardiographically, a mobile mass was visualized attached to the anterior leaflet[157-159] or the posterior leaflet.[160] One of the 2 cases of Gosse et al.[158] was nonmobile and extended to the anterolateral papillary muscle. Recurrence on the mitral valve of an excised left atrial myxoma has been reported.[160]

Mitral Valve Fibroma

First described by Luschka in 1855, as many as 75 cardiac fibromas had been reported in the English literature until 1988,[161] mostly in children. Fibromas are commonly intramural, embedded within the myocardium, but rare instances of mitral valve involvement by encroachment of a large mural fibroma have been reported.[162]

Other Rare Mitral Valve Tumors

Lipomas of the mitral valve have been reported in children,[163,164] the neoplastic masses were obvious on echocardiography. In the case of Behman et al.,[164] the posterior mitral leaflet was replaced by a sessile lipoma, and another lipoma partially replaced the posteromedial papillary muscle.

Rhabdomyosarcoma of the mitral valve of botryoid shape manifested as a large, mobile polypoid mass attached to the ventricular surface of the anterior mitral leaflet in an 8-year-old boy.[165]

Mitral valve cysts are extremely rare in adults and older children, although small, multiple cysts are frequently found on the cardiac valves in young infants. A 2.5-cm cyst attached to the anterior mitral leaflet was reported by Leatherman et al.[166] It manifested as a filling defect in the contrast-filled chamber on angiocardiography.

BACTERIAL ENDOCARDITIS: GENERAL REMARKS

Detection of bacterial endocarditis is one of the most important indications for echocardiography. Some general remarks on the anatomic aspects of the topic are worth bringing to the attention of echocardiographers.

1. Vegetations commonly occur on the atrial side of mitral and tricuspid valves and on the ventricular side of aortic and pulmonary valves. Vegetations are thought to begin at the line of valve closure, but as they enlarge, they may spread to cover adjacent areas of the leaflet or cusp.

Satellite vegetations sometimes can develop by implantation of bacteria from a primary site to another site by direct contact (so-called kissing lesions) or where a jet from an infected valve strikes an endocardial surface. An example of the latter is endocarditis of the anterior mitral leaflet secondary to aortic valve endocarditis with regurgitation.

2. Focal leaflet damage or destruction can result in ulceration, perforation, or aneurysm. Likewise, chordae tendineae may rupture, rendering the affected part of the leaflet flail. Such destructive valve lesions are usually (but not always) accompanied by vegetations detectable by echocardiography.

3. Valve infection may spread to an adjacent vessel wall or the myocardium. Weakening of the aortic wall results in a sinus of Valsalva aneurysm, which in turn can rupture into any of the four cardiac chambers, usually the right ventricle or atrium. Alternatively, the aortic wall may perforate into the pericardium, causing acute tamponade, or leak into a contained pouchlike space (pseudoaneurysm).

4. *Ring abscess* is a term applied to extension of infection from a valve to part or all of the annulus of that valve. It is most often associated with infected prosthetic valves but also can complicate native valve endocarditis—in decreasing order of frequency, the aortic, mitral, tricuspid, and pulmonic valves. Sometimes infection burrows into myocardium rather than annulus, forming a myocardial abscess and occasionally disrupting the cardiac conduction pathways resulting in atrioventricular or bundle branch block. Ring or myocardial abscesses contain necrotic or infected thrombotic material; being of different texture, the material is sonolucent or partly so on echocardiography.

5. Embolization due to detachment or fragmentation of a vegetation is a dreaded complication, because it can result in infarction of the viscera supplied by the occluded artery and also carry infected thrombus to that area. The target viscera is the lung in right-sided endocarditis with mitral or aortic valve lesions; embolic hazards include infarction of the brain, heart, kidney, bowel, or lower limbs.

6. Between 20% and 40% of proven instances of bacterial endocarditis do not show vegetations on routine (transthoracic) echocardiography because of small size of the vegetations or other technical limitations. Echo evidence of valve destruction or of new severe regurgitation (as compared with previous echo Doppler recordings) is useful diagnostically in such cases. However, with TEE, the echocardiographic diagnostic yield approaches 100%.

The sensitivity and specificity of echocardiography in detection of vegetations is an important issue. The sensitivity of conventional TTE is mentioned in the literature as 30% to 80%, 60% to 70% being a widely quoted statistic. Whether a vegetation is identified as such depends not only on the adequacy of the standard echo "windows" but also on the size and echogenicity of the vegetation, presence of preexisting valve sclerosis or thickening, skill and experience of sonographer and echocardiologist, and quality of the echo equipment. Recent work suggests that whereas two-thirds of vegetations of all sizes taken together are diagnosed by TTE, only a quarter of small vegetations (<5 mm) are so diagnosed. The augmented resolution of TEE has raised the sensitivity for detecting vegetation to between 85% and 100%.

Bacterial endocarditis of the mitral valve has been known to pathologists and clinicians since the early descriptions of Osler,[167] updated by subsequent authors during this century.[168-173] Vegetations of varying size, shape, and number are the most characteristic feature at autopsy, as well as on echocardiography. However, other pathologic changes

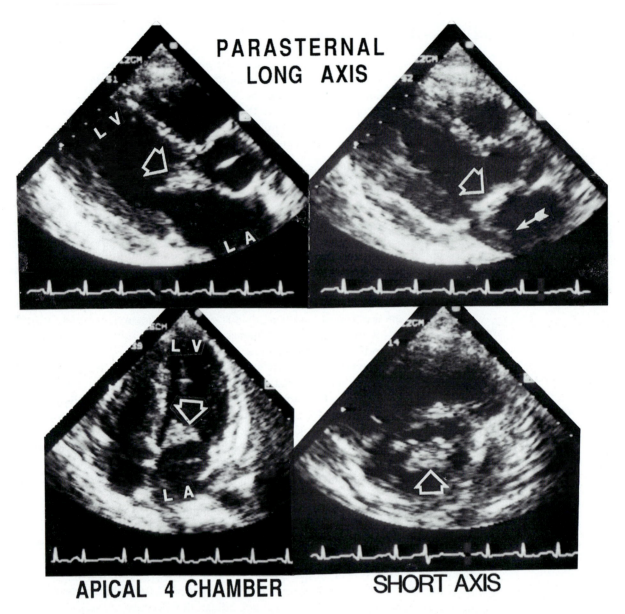

PARASTERNAL
LONG AXIS

APICAL 4 CHAMBER   SHORT AXIS

Figure 11–42. (Above) Parasternal long-axis views in diastole (left) and systole (right) showing a vegetation on the anterior mitral leaflet (open arrows). A ruptured chord (thin arrow) attached to the anterior leaflet is evident in systole (above, right). The vegetation's size and shape can be appreciated in the apical four-chamber view (below, left) and parasternal short-axis view (below, right).

involving destruction of valve tissue and chordae with resulting flail motion or perforation and ring abscess formation are also common at surgery or autopsy and also have their counterparts on 2D echo and Doppler.

Early M-mode descriptions of mitral vegetations aroused much interest and were diagnostically helpful but need not be discussed in detail because they have been superseded by 2D echo findings,[174-178] which can be summarized as follows:

Vegetations are pedunculated or sessile "masses" attached to the atrial surface of a mitral leaflet (Figures 11–42 to 11–47) varying in size from a few millimeters to a few centimeters. Typically, they have a shaggy or fluffy border or even have satellite smaller tags or mobile elements "orbiting" around the main vegetation. As a vegetation heals under chemotherapy, it becomes denser and more defined. Typically, the affected leaflet has a

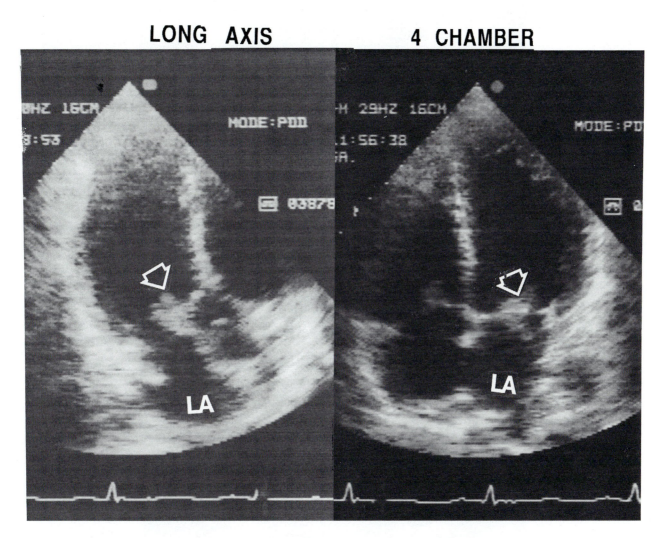

Figure 11–43. Apical long-axis view (left) and four-chamber view (right) in patient L.B. showing a large, complex vegetation on the anterior mitral leaflet.

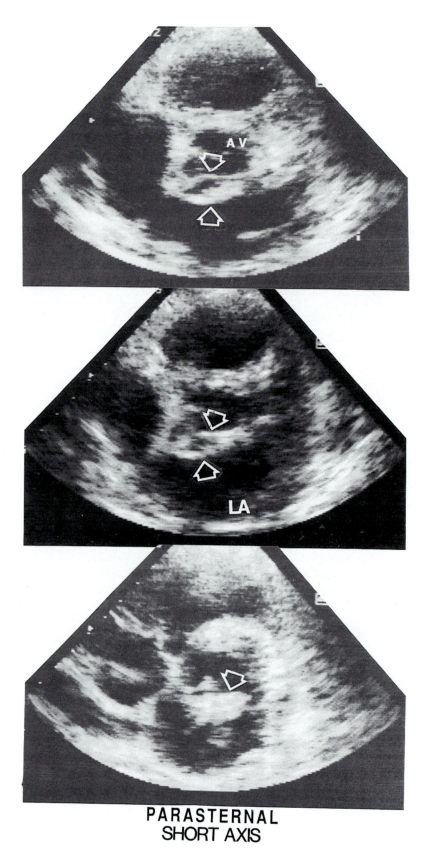

PARASTERNAL
SHORT AXIS

Figure 11–44. Parasternal short-axis views in same patient (L.B.) showing abscess behind aortic root (above) in attachment of anterior mitral leaflet (center) and the vegetation itself on the same leaflet (arrows).

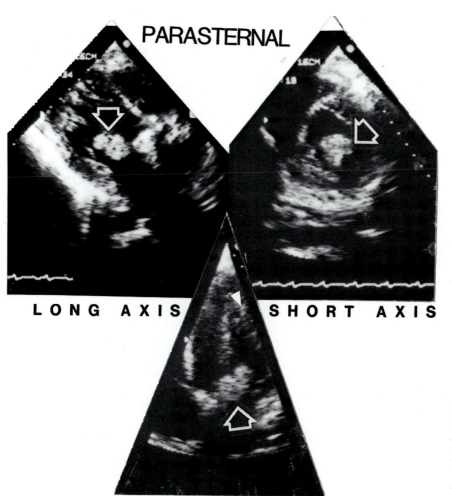

PARASTERNAL

LONG AXIS   SHORT AXIS

APICAL

Figure 11–45. (Above) Parasternal long-axis (left) and short-axis (right) views of patient M.D. as well as apical four-chamber view (below) all show a large vegetation on the anterior mitral valve (arrows).

normal or even exaggerated amplitude of motion during the cardiac cycle. Sometimes endocarditis manifests as a local area of marked thickening (or nodule) *in* rather than *on* the leaflet, in which case it has to be differentiated from sclerocalcific changes of degenerative or old rheumatic etiology.

Chordal rupture results in flail motion of a minor or major part of the leaflet, a spectacular finding if a vegetation is adherent to the flail segment. A paravalvar or ring abscess tends to form in the space between aortic root and left atrium (Figures 11-44, 11-46, and 11-47). In extreme cases, the abscess extends along the mitral annulus, in effect separating the leaflet from its attachment to ventricular wall. Colorflow and pulsed-wave Doppler recordings show the extent of MR and an undue amount of turbulence attributable to the vegetation or flail leaflet agitating or "stirring" the regurgitant stream.

Perforation of a mitral leaflet (usually the anterior) may be suspected if severe regurgitation is present *without* detectable flail motion. The hole in the leaflet may itself be seen on 2D echo,[179] but this was the exception rather than the rule until colorflow Doppler was available to reveal the MR jet emerging from the substance rather than the edge of the mitral leaflet.

Rare instances of vegetations attached to mitral annulus (Figure 11-48) rather than edge or mobile part of leaflet have been reported. Such vegetations appear fixed, with only a barely discernible oscillation.

APICAL

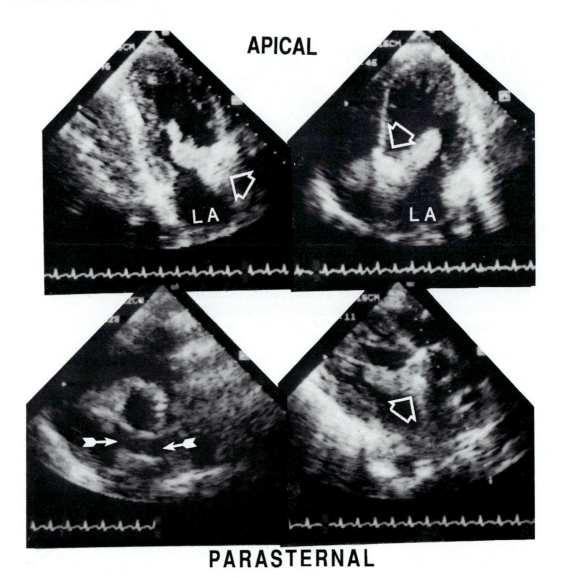

PARASTERNAL

Figure 11–46. (Above) A week later in same patient (M.D.)—apical long-axis and four-chamber views show extension of the infective process (open arrow) from the anterior mitral leaflet to its basal attachment. Parasternal short-axis view (below, left) shows abscess space posterior to the aortic root (thin arrow).

Echo simulators of mitral vegetations include sclerocalcific nodules in elderly patients or those with previous old endocarditis (bacterial or rheumatic), myxomatous redundant mitral valves (thick folds in diastole resembling vegetation), and the rare instances of mitral leaflet aneurysm or neoplasm.

TEE has undoubtedly improved the 2D echo visualization of mitral vegetations.[180-184] Because of higher-frequency transducers and greater proximity of the probe to the lesion, the contour and texture of vegetations are imaged with much greater clarity and definition. Moreover, vegetations are seen that did not appear at all on TTE. Serious complications of mitral endocarditis such as perivalvar abscess tracking through the intervalvar fibrosa (between mitral and aortic valve rings) or fistula formation between the LV, LA, or other chambers or vessels are identified better by TEE.

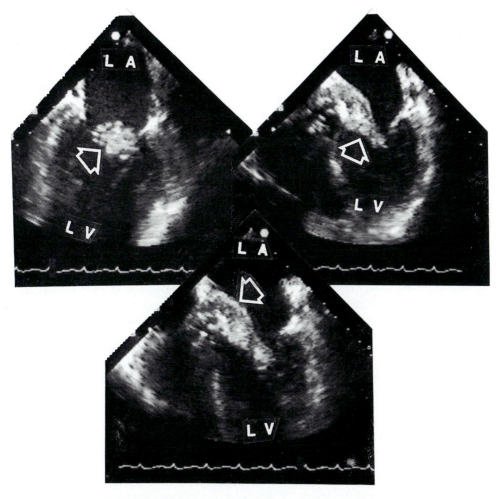

Figure 11–47. TEE in same patient (M.D.) showing the involvement of the anterior mitral leaflet in greater detail, as well as the abscess (lower frame).

LONG AXIS SHORT AXIS APICAL 4-CHAMBER

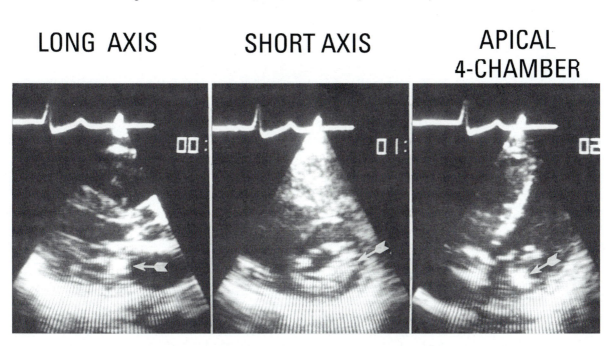

Figure 11–48. Parasternal long-axis view (left) short-axis view (center), and apical four-chamber view (right) in a patient with a staphylococcal vegetation on mitral annulus calcification.

REFERENCES

1. Ranganathan N, Lam JHC, Wigle ED, et al. Morphology of the human mitral valve: II. The valve leaflets. Circulation 1970;41:459.
2. Rusted IE, Scheifley CH, Edwards JE. Studies of the mitral valve: I. Anatomic features of the normal mitral valve and associated structures. Circulation 1952;7:82.
3. Cheichi MA, Lees WM, Thompson R. Functional anatomy of the normal mitral valve. J Thorac Surg 1956;32:378.
4. McAlpine WA. Heart and Coronary Arteries. New York: Springer-Verlag, 1975, p 39.
5. Silver MD. Cardiovascular Pathology, 2d ed. New York: Churchill-Livingstone, 1991, p 27.
6. Barlow JB. Perspectives on the Mitral Valve. Philadelphia: FA Davis, 1987, pp 1-13.
7. Walmsley T (ed). Quain's Anatomy: The Heart, part 3, vol 5, 2d ed. London: Longman, Green, 1929, p 81.
8. Brock RC. The surgical and pathological anatomy of the mitral valve. Br Heart J 1952;14:48.
9. Lam JHC. Morphology of the human mitral valve: I. Chordae tendineae: A new classification. Circulation 1970;41:449.
10. Cheng TO. Some new observations on the syndrome of papillary muscle dysfunction. Am J Med 1969;47:924.
11. Davis PKB, Kinmouth JB. The movements of the annulus of the mitral valve. J Cardiovasc Surg 1963;4:427.
12. Perloff JK, Roberts WC. The mitral apparatus: Functional anatomy of mitral regurgitation. Circulation 1972;46:227.
13. Roberts WC. Morphological features of the normal and abnormal mitral valve. Am J Cardiol 1983;51:1005.
14. Wood P. An appreciation of mitral stenosis. Br Med J 1954;1:1051.
15. Brock RC. The surgical and pathological anatomy of the mitral valve. Br Heart J 1952; 14:489.
16. Hanson TP, Edwards BS, Edwards JE. Pathology of surgically excised mitral valves. Arch Pathol Lab Med 1985;109:823.
17. Silver MD. Cardiovascular Pathology, 2d ed. New York: Churchill-Livingstone, 1991, p 949.
18. Chopra P, Tandon HD, Raizada V, et al. Comparative studies in mitral valves in rheumatic heart disease. Arch Intern Med 1983;143:661.
19. Lachman AS, Roberts WC. Calcific deposits in stenotic mitral valves. Circulation 1978;57:808.
20. Daley R, Mattingly TW, Holt CL, et al. Systemic arterial embolism in rheumatic heart disease. Am Heart J 1951;42:566.
21. MacCallum WG. Rheumatic lesions of the left auricle of the heart. Bull Johns Hopkins Hosp 1924;35:329.
22. Lie JT, Entman ML. "Hole-in-one" sudden death: Mitral stenosis and left atrial thrombus. Am Heart J 1976;91:798.
23. Leder AA, Bosworth WC. Angiokeratoma corporis diffusum universale (Fabry's disease) with mitral stenosis. Am J Med 1965;38:814.
24. Korvetz LJ, Lorincz AE, Schiebler GL. Cardiovascular manifestations of the Hurler syndrome. Circulation 1965;31:132.
25. McAllister HA, Fenglio J. Cardiac involvement in Whipple's disease. Circulation 1975;52:152.
26. Misch KA. Development of heart valve lesions during methysergide therapy. Br Med J 1974;2:365.
26a. Voda J, Glagov S, Brooks H. Mechanism of abnormal motion of the posterior leaflet in mitral stenosis. Cardiology 1982;69:245.
27. Joyner CR, Reid JM, Bond JP. Reflected ultrasound in the assessment of mitral valve disease. Circulation 1963;27:506.
28. Segal BL, Likoff W, Kingsley B. Echocardiography: Clinical application in mitral stenosis. JAMA 1966;193:161.
29. Cope GD, Kisslo JA, Johnson ML. A reassessment of the echocardiogram in mitral stenosis. Circulation 1975;52:664.
30. Fisher ML, Parisi AF, Plotnick GD, et al. Assessment of severity of mitral stenosis of echocardiographic leaflet separation. Arch Intern Med 1979;139:402.
31. Raj MVJ, Bennett DH, Stovin PJI, et al. Echocardiographic assessment of mitral valve calcification. Br Heart J 1967;38:81.

32. Zanolla L, Marino P, Nicolisi GL, et al. Two-dimensional echocardiographic evaluation of mitral valve calcification. Chest 1982;82:154.

33. Wong M, Tei C, Shah PM. Sensitivity and specificity of two-dimensional echocardiography in the detection of valvular calcification. Chest 1983;84:423.

34. Henry WL, Maron MB, Griffith MS. Measurement of mitral orifice area in patients with mitral valve disease by real-time two-dimensional echocardiography. Circulation 1975;51:827.

35. Nichol PM, Gilbert BW, Kisslo JA. Two-dimensional echocardiographic assessment of mitral stenosis. Circulation 1977;55:120.

36. Wann LS, Weyman AE, Feigenbaum H. Determination of mitral valve area by cross-sectional echocardiography. Ann Intern Med 1978;88:337.

37. Glover MU, Warren SE, Vieweg WVR, et al. M-mode and two-dimensional echocardiographic correlation with findings at catheterization and surgery in patients with mitral stenosis. Am Heart J 1983;105:98.

38. Hanson TP, Edwards BS, Edwards JE. Pathology of surgically excised mitral valves. Arch Pathol Lab Med 1985;109:823.

39. Stewart WJ, Currie PJ, Salcedo EE, et al. Evaluation of mitral leaflet motion by echocardiography and jet direction by Doppler color flow mapping to determine the mechanism of mitral regurgitation. J Am Coll Cardiol 1992;20:1353.

40. Carpentier A, Chauvaud S, Fabiani JN, et al. Reconstructive surgery of mitral valve incompetence. J Thorac Cardiovasc Surg 1980;79:338.

41. Yoshida K, Yoshikawa J, Yamaura Y, et al. Value of acceleration flows and regurgitant jet direction by color Doppler flow mapping in the evaluation of mitral valve prolapse. Circulation 1990;81:879.

42. Grayburn PA, Berk MR, Spain MG, et al. Relation of echocardiographic morphology of the mitral apparatus to mitral regurgitation in mitral valve prolapse: Assessment by Doppler color flow imaging. Am Heart J 1990;119:1092.

43. Veyrat C, Kalmanson D, Gourtchigluian C, et al. Flow mapping of regurgitant jets in mitral valve prolapse. Am J Noninvas Cardiol 1987;1:329.

44. Veyrat C, Bas S, Smadja G, et al. Color Doppler assessment of mitral regurgitation in combined lesions. Am J Noninvas Cardiol 1990;4:210.

45. Kaul S, Pearlman JD, Touchstone DA, et al. Prevalence and mechanisms of mitral regurgitation in the absence of intrinsic abnormalities of the mitral leaflets. Am Heart J 1989;118:963.

46. Bulkley BH, Roberts WC. Dilatation of the mitral annulus. Am J Med 1975;59:457.

47. Boltwood CM, Tei C, Wong M, et al. Quantitative echocardiography of the mitral complex in dilated cardiomyopathy: The mechanism of functional mitral regurgitation. Circulation 1983;68:49.

48. Laskey WK, St John Sutton M, Seevi G, et al. Left ventricular mechanics in dilated cardiomyopathy. Am J Cardiol 1984;54:620.

49. White PD. Heart Disease. New York: Macmillan, 1931, p 485.

50. Burch GE, DePascuale NP, Phillips JH. The syndrome of papillary muscle dysfunction. Am Heart J 1968;75:399.

51. Shelbourne JC, Rubenstein D, Gorlin R. A reappraisal of papillary muscle dysfunction. Am J Med 1969;46:862.

51a. Kisanuki A, Otsuji Y, Kuroiwa R, et al. Two-dimensional echocardiographic assessment of papillary muscle contractility in patients with prior myocardial infarction. J Am Coll Cardiol 1993;21:932.

52. Miyatake K, Izumi S, Okamoto M, et al. Semiquantitative grading of severity of mitral regurgitation by real-time two-dimensional Doppler flow imaging technique. J Am Coll Cardiol 1986;7:82.

53. Helmcke F, Nanda NC, Hsiung MC, et al. Color Doppler assessment of mitral regurgitation with orthogonal planes. Circulation 1987;75:175.

54. Spain MG, Smith MD, Grayburn PA, et al. Quantitative assessment of mitral regurgitation by Doppler color flow imaging. J Am Coll Cardiol 1989;13:585.

55. Bolger AF, Eigler NL, Pfaff JM, et al. Computer analysis of Doppler color flow mapping images for quantitative assessment of in vitro fluid jets. J Am Coll Cardiol 1988;12:450.

56. Simpson IA, Valdes-Cruz LM, Sahn DJ, et al. Doppler color flow mapping in simulated in vitro regurgitant jets. J Am Coll Cardiol 1989;13:1195.

57. Thomas JD, Liu CM, Flaschkampf FA, et al. Quantification of jet flow by momentum analysis. Circulation 1990;81:247.

58. Cape EG, Yoganathan AP, Weyman AE, et al. Adjacent solid boundaries after the size of regurgitant jets on Doppler color flow maps. J Am Coll Cardiol 1991;17:1094.

59. Chen C, Thomas JD, Anconina J, et al. Impact of impinging wall jet on color Doppler quantification of mitral regurgitation. Circulation 1991;84:712.

60. Enriquez-Sarano M, Tajik AJ, Bailey KR, et al. Color flow imaging compared with quantitative Doppler assessment of severity of mitral regurgitation: Influence of eccentricity of jet and mechanism of regurgitation. J Am Coll Cardiol 1993;21:1211.

61. Barlow JB, Pocock WA. Mitral leaflet billowing and prolapse, in JB Barlow (ed): Perspectives on the Mitral Valve. Philadelphia: FA Davis, 1987, pp 47, 68.

62. Silver MD. Cardiovascular Pathology, 2d ed. New York: Churchill-Livingstone, 1991, p 963.

63. Bulkley BH, Roberts WC. Dilatation of the mitral annulus. Am J Med 1975;59:457.

64. Goodman D, Kimbiris D, Linhart JW. Chordae tendineae rupture complicating the systolic click–late systolic murmur syndrome. Am J Cardiol 1974;33:681.

65. Marchand P, Barlow JB, duPlessis LA, et al. Mitral regurgitation with rupture of normal chordae tendineae. Br Heart J 1966;28:746.

66. Salazar AE, Edwards JE. Friction lesions of ventricular endocardium: Relation to chordae tendineae of mitral valve. Arch Pathol 1970;90:364.

67. Corrigal D, Popp R. Mitral valve prolapse and infective endocarditis. Am J Med 1977;63:215.

68. McMahon SW, Hickey AJ, Wilcken DEL. Risk of infective endocarditis in mitral valve prolapse with and without systolic murmurs. Am J Cardiol 1987;59:105.

69. Barnett HJM, Boughner DR, Taylor DW, et al. Further evidence relating mitral valve prolapse to cerebral ischemic events. N Engl J Med 1980;302:139.

70. Hanson MR, Conomy JP, Hodgman JR. Brain events associated with mitral valve prolapse. Stroke 1980;11:499.

71. Schnee MA, Bucal AA. Fatal embolism in mitral valve prolapse. Chest 1983;83:235.

72. Gross CM, Nichols FT, VonDohlen TW, et al. Mitral valve prolapse and stroke: Echocardiographic evidence for a missing etiologic link. J Am Soc Echocardiogr 1989;2:94.

73. Pomerance A. Ballooning deformity (mucoid degeneration) of atrioventricular valves. Br Heart J 1969;31:343.

74. Dillon JC, Haine CL, Chang S, et al. Use of echocardiography in patients with prolapsed mitral valve. Circulation 1971;43:503.

75. Kerber RE, Isaeff DM, Hancock EW. Echocardiographic patterns in patients with the syndrome of systolic click and late systolic murmur. N Engl J Med 1971;284:691.

76. Devereux RB, Perloff JK, Reichek N, et al. Mitral valve prolapse. Circulation 1976;54:3.

77. Popp RL, Brown OR, Silverman JF, et al. Echocardiographic abnormalities in the mitral valve prolapse syndrome. Circulation 1974;49:428.

78. Demaria AN, Neumann A, Lee G, et al. Echocardiographic identification of the mitral valve prolapse syndrome. Am J Med 1977;62:819.

79. Gilbert BM, Schatz RA, von Ramm OT, et al. Mitral valve prolapse: Two-dimensional echocardiographic and angiographic correlation. Circulation 1976;54:716.

80. Morganroth J, Mardelli TJ, Naito M, et al. Apical cross-sectional echocardiography: Standard for the diagnosis of idiopathic mitral valve prolapse syndrome. Chest 1984;79:23.

81. Wann LS, Gross CM, Wakefield RJ, et al. Diagnostic precision of echocardiography in mitral valve prolapse. Am Heart J 1985;109:803.

82. Alpert MA, Carney RJ, Flaker GC, et al. Sensitivity and specificity of two-dimensional echocardiographic signs of mitral valve prolapse. Am J Cardiol 1984;54:792.

83. Krivokapich J, Child JS, Dadourian BJ, et al. Reassessment of echocardiographic criteria for diagnosis of mitral valve prolapse. Am J Cardiol 1988;61:131.

83a. Levine RA, Triulzi MO, Harrigan P, et al. The relationship of mitral annular shape to the diagnosis of mitral valve prolapse. Circulation 1987;75:756.

84. Mathey DG, Decoodt PR, Allen HN, et al. The determinants of onset of mitral valve prolapse in the systolic click–late systolic murmur syndrome. Circulation 1976;53:872.

85. Winkle RA, Goodman DJ, Popp RL. Simultaneous echocardiographic, phonocardiographic recordings at rest and during amyl nitrite administration in patients with mitral valve prolapse. Circulation 1975;51:522.

86. Noble LM, Dabestani A, Child JS. Mitral valve prolapse: Cross-sectional and provocative M-mode echocardiography. Chest 1982;82:158.

87. Savage DD, Garrison RJ, Castelli WP, et al. Prevalence of submitral (anular) calcium and its correlates in a general population-bases sample (the Framingham study). Am J Cardiol 1983;51:137.

88. Kirk RS, Russell JGB. Subvalvular calcification of mitral valve. Br Heart J 1969;31:684.

89. D'Cruz I, Panetta F, Cohen H, Glick G. Submitral calcification or sclerosis in elderly patients: M mode and two-dimensional echocardiography "in mitral annulus calcification." Am J Cardiol 1979;44:31.

90. Guthrie J, Fairgreve J. Aortic embolism due to myxoid tumor associated with myocardial infarction. Br Heart J 1963;25:17.

91. Ridolfi RL, Hutchins GM. Spontaneous calcific emboli from calcific mitral annulus fibrosus. Arch Pathol Lab Med 1976;110:117.

92. Silver MD. Cardiovascular Pathology, 2d ed. New York: Churchill-Livingstone, 1991, p 169.

93. Korn D, Desanctis RW, Sell S. Massive calcification of the mitral annulus. N Engl J Med 1962;267:900.

94. Hammer WJ, Roberts WC, deLeon AC. "Mitral stenosis" secondary to combined "massive" mitral annular calcific deposits and small hypertrophic left ventricles. Am J Med 1978;64:371.

95. Ramirez J, Flowers NC. Severe mitral stenosis secondary to massive calcification of the mitral annulus with unusual echocardiographic manifestation. Clin Cardiol 1980;3:284.

96. Osterberger LE, Goldstein S, Khaja F, et al. Functional mitral stenosis in patients with massive mitral annulus calcification. Circulation 1981;64:472.

97. Depace NL, Rohrer AH, Kotler MN, et al. Rapidly progressive, massive mitral annular calcification: occurrence in a patient with chronic renal failure. Arch Intern Med 1981;141:1663.

98. Nair CK, Aronow WS, Sketch MH, et al. Clinical and echocardiographic characteristics of patients with mitral annular calcification. Am J Cardiol 1983;51:992.

99. Mellino M, Salcedo EE, Lever HM, et al. Echocardiographic-quantified severity of mitral annulus calcification: Prognostic correlation to related hemodynamic, valvular rhythm and conduction abnormalities. Am Heart J 1982;103:222.

100. Yater WM, Cornell VH. Heart block due to calcareous lesions of bundle of His. Ann Intern Med 1935;8:777.

101. Nestico PF, DePace NL, Morganroth J, et al. Mitral annular calcification: Clinical, pathophysiological and echocardiographic review. Am Heart J 1984;107:989.

102. Gabor GE, Mohr BD, Goel PC, et al. Echocardiographic and clinical spectrum of mitral annular calcification. Am J Cardiol 1976;38:836.

103. D'Cruz IA, Cohen HC, Prabhu R, et al. Clinical manifestations of mitral annulus calcification with emphasis on its echocardiographic features. Am Heart J 1977;94:367.

104. Dashkoff N, Karakushansky M, Come PC, et al. Echocardiographic features of mitral annulus calcification. Am Heart J 1977;94:585.

105. Curati WL, Petitclerc R, Winsberg F. Ultrasonic features of mitral annulus calcification. Radiology 1973;122:215.

106. D'Cruz IA, Devaraj N, Hirsch LG. Unusual echocardiographic appearances attributable to submitral calcification simulating left ventricular masses. Clin Cardiol 1980;3:260.

107. D'Cruz IA, Vaughan C, Sastry V. Echocardiographic aspects of mitral annulus calcification. Echocardiography (accepted for publication).

108. Roberts WC, Braunwald E, Morrow AG. Acute severe mitral regurgitation secondary to ruptured chordae tendineae. Circulation 1966;33:58.

109. Roman JA, Steelman RB, DeLeon AC, et al. The clinical diagnosis of acute severe mitral insufficiency. Am J Cardiol 1971;27:284.

110. Goodman D, Kimbiris D, Linhart JW. Chordae tendineae rupture complicating the systolic click–late systolic murmur syndrome. Am J Cardiol 1974;33:681.

111. Silver MD. Cardiovascular Pathology, 2d ed. New York: Churchill-Livingstone, 1991, p 977.

112. Child JS, Skorton DJ, Taylor RD, et al. M-mode and cross-sectional echocardiographic features of flail posterior mitral leaflets. Am J Cardiol 1979;44:1383.

113. Humphries WG, Hammer WJ, McDonough MT, et al. Echocardiographic equivalents of a flail mitral leaflet. Am J Cardiol 1977;40:802.

114. Mintz GS, Kotler MN, Segal BL, et al. Two-dimensional echocardiographic recognition of ruptured chordae tendineae. Circulation 1978;57:244.

115. Chandaratna PAN, Aronow WS. Incidence of ruptured chordae tendineae in the mitral valvular prolapse syndrome. Chest 1979;75:334.

116. Sze KC, Nanda NC, Gramiak R. Systolic flutter of the mitral valve. Am Heart J 1978;96:157.

117. Davison S. Spontaneous rupture of a papillary muscle of the heart. J Mt Sinai Hosp 1948;14:941.

118. Sanders RJ, Neuberger KT, Ravin A. Rupture of papillary muscles. Dis Chest 1957;31:316.

119. Cederqvist L, Soderstrom J. Papillary muscle rupture in myocardial infarction. Acta Med Scand 1964;176:287.

120. Vlodaver Z, Edwards JE. Rupture of ventricular septum or papillary muscle complicating myocardial infarction. Circulation 1977;55:815.

121. Nishimura RA, Schaff HV, Shub C, et al. Papillary muscle rupture complicating acute myocardial infarction. Am J Cardiol 1983;51:373.

122. Silver MD. Cardiovascular Pathology, 2d ed. New York: Churchill-Livingstone, 1991, p 979.

123. Kishon Y, Oh JK, Schaff HV, et al. Mitral valve operation in postinfarction rupture of a papillary muscle. Mayo Clin Proc 1992;67:1023.

124. Erbel R, Schweizer P, Bardos P, et al. Two-dimensional echocardiographic diagnosis of papillary muscle rupture. Chest 1981;71:595.

125. Mintz GS, Victor MF, Kotler MN, et al. Two-dimensional echocardiographic identification of surgically correctable complications of acute myocardial infarction. Circulation 1981;64:91.

126. Eisenberg PR, Barzilai B, Perez JE. Noninvasive detection by Doppler echocardiography of combined ventricular septal and mitral regurgitation in acute myocardial infarction. J Am Coll Cardiol 1984;4:617.

127. Patel A, Miller F, Khandheria B, et al. Role of transesophageal echocardiography in the diagnosis of papillary muscle rupture secondary to myocardial infarction. Am Heart J 1989;118:1330.

128. Stoddard MF, Keedy DL, Kupersmith J. Transesophageal echocardiographic diagnosis of papillary muscle rupture complicating acute myocardial infarction. Am Heart J 1990;120:690.

129. Jarco S. Aneurysm of heart valves. Am J Cardiol 1968;22:273.

130. Saphir O, Leroy EP. True aneurysm of the mitral valve in subacute bacterial endocarditis. Am J Pathol 1948;24:83.

131. Maclean N, MacDonald MK. Aneurysm of the mitral valve in subacute bacterial endocarditis. Brit Heart J 1957;19:550.

132. English TAH, Honey M, Cleland WP. Ruptured true aneurysm of mitral valve. Br Heart J 1972;34:434.

133. Hoffman FG, Robinson JJ. Aneurysm of the mitral valve associated with bacterial endocarditis. Am Heart J 1962;63:826.

134. Pocock WA, Lakier JB, Hitchcock JF, et al. Mitral valve aneurysm after infective endocarditis in the billowing mitral valve syndrome. Am J Cardiol 1977;40:130.

135. Gonzalez-Lavin L, Lise M, Ross DN. The importance of the "jet lesion" in bacterial endocarditis involving the left heart. J Thorac Cardiovasc Surg 1970;59:185.

136. Reid CL, Chandaratna PAN, Harrison E, et al. Mitral valve aneurysm: Clinical features, echocardiographic-pathologic correlations. J Am Coll Cardiol 1983;2:460.

137. Enia F, Celona G, Filippone V. Echocardiographic detection of mitral valve aneurysm in patient with infective endocarditis. Br Heart J 1983;49:98.

138. Teskey RJ, Chan KL, Beanlands DS. Diverticulum of the mitral valve complicating bacterial endocarditis: Diagnosis by transesophageal echocardiography. Am Heart J 1989;118:1063.

139. Chua SO, Chiang CW, Lee YS, et al. Perforated aneurysm of the anterior mitral valve. Chest 1990;97:753.

140. Northridge DB, Gnanapragasam JP, Houston AB. Diagnosis of mitral valve aneurysm by transesophageal echocardiography. Br Heart J 1991;65:227.

141. Lewis BS, Colsen PR, Rosenfeld T, et al. An unusual case of mitral valve aneurysm. Am J Cardiol 1982;49:1293.

142. Prichard RW. Tumors of the heart: Review of the subject and report of 150 cases. Arch Pathol Lab Med 1951;51:98.

143. Nasser SGA, Parker JC. Incidental papillary endocardial tumor. Arch Pathol 1971;92:370.

144. Gorton ME, Soltanzadeh H. Mitral valve fibroelastoma. Ann Thorac Surg 1989;47:605.

145. Raeburn C. Papillary fibro-elastic hematomas of the heart valves. J Pathol Bacterial 1953;65:371.

146. Pomerance A. Papillary "tumors" of the heart valves. J Pathol Bacteriol 1961;81:135.

147. Heath D, Best PV, Davis BT. Papilliferous tumors of the heart valves. Br Heart J 1961;23:20.

148. Topol EJ, Biern RP, Reitz BA. Cardiac papillary fibroelastoma and stroke. Am J Med 1986;80:129.

149. Fowles RE, Miller C, Egbert BM, et al. Systemic embolization from a mitral endocardial fibroma detected by two-dimensional echocardiography. Am Heart J 1981;102:128.

150. McFadden PM, Lacy JR. Intracardiac papillary fibroelastoma: An occult cause of embolic neurologic deficit. Ann Thorac Surg 1987;43:667.

151. Shub C, Tajik AJ, Seward JB, et al. Cardiac papillary fibroelastomas. Mayo Clin Proc 1981;56:629.
152. deVirgilio C, Dubrow TJ, Robertson JM, et al. Detection of multiple cardiac papillary fibro-elastomas using transesophageal echocardiography. Ann Thorac Surg 1989;48:119.
153. Richard J, Castello R, Dressler FA, et al. Diagnosis of papillary fibroelastoma of the mitral valve complicated by non-Q-wave infarction with apical thrombus. Am Heart J 1993;126:710.
153a. Lee KS, Topol EJ, Stewart WJ. Atypical presentation of papillary fibroelastoma mimicking multiple vegetations in suspected subacute bacterial endocarditis. Am Heart J 1993;125:1443.
154. Thomas MR, Jayakrishnan AG, Desai J, et al. Transesophageal echocardiography in the detection and surgical management of a papillary fibroelastoma of the mitral valve causing partial mitral valve obstruction. J Am Soc Echocardiogr 1993;6:83.
155. Meisner JS, Daboin NP, Keller PK, et al. Myxoma of the mitral valve detected by trans-esophageal echocardiography. Am Heart J 1993;125:1449.
156. Jaleski TC. Myxoma of the heart valves: Report of a case. Am J Pathol 1934;10:399.
157. Sandrasagra FA, Oliver WA, English TAH. Myxoma of the mitral valve. Br Heart J 1979;42:221.
158. Gosse P, Herpin D, Roudaut R, et al. Myxoma of the mitral valve diagnosed by echocardiography. Am Heart J 1986;111:803.
159. Barold SS, Hicks GL, Nanda NC, et al. Mitral valve myxoma diagnosed by two-dimensional echocardiography. Am J Cardiol 1987;59:182.
160. Read CD, White HY, Murphy ML, et al. The malignant potentiality of left atrial myxoma. J Thorac Cardiovasc Surg 1974;68:857.
161. Kutayli F, Malouf J, Slim M, et al. Cardiac fibroma with tumor involvement of the mitral valve: Diagnosis by cross-sectional echocardiography. Eur Heart J 1988;9:563.
162. Gonzales-Crussi F, Eberts TJ, Mirrin DL. Congenital fibrous hematoma of the heart. Arch Pathol Lab Med 1978;102:491.
163. Barberger-Gateau P, Pacquet M, Desaunifrs D, et al. Fibrolipoma of the mitral valve in a child. Circulation 1978;58:955.
164. Behman R, Williams G, Gerlis L, et al. Lipoma of the mitral valve and papillary muscle. Am J Cardiol 1983;51:1459.
165. Hajar R, Roberts WC, Folger GM. Embryonal botyroid rhabdomyosarcoma of the mitral valve. Am J Cardiol 1986;57:376.
166. Leatherman L, Leachman RD, Hallman GL, et al. Cyst of the mitral valve. Am J Cardiol 1968;21:428.
167. Osler W. Gulstonian lectures on malignant endocarditis. Lancet 1885;1:415.
168. Libman E. Characterization of various forms of endocarditis. JAMA 1923;80:813.
169. Kelson SR, White PD. Notes on 250 cases of subacute bacterial (streptococcal) endocarditis studied and treated between 1927 and 1939. Ann Intern Med 1945;22:40.
170. Lepeschkin E. On the relation between the site of valvular involvement in endocarditis and the blood pressure resting on the valve. Am J Med Sci 1952;224:318.
171. Pelletier LL, Petersdorf RG. Infective endocarditis. Medicine 1977;56:287.
172. Saphir O. Endocarditis (non-rheumatic), in SE Gould (ed): Pathology of the Heart. Springfield, Ill: Charles C Thomas, Publisher, 1960, p 710.
173. Freidberg CK. Subacute bacterial endocarditis. JAMA 1950;144:572.
174. Gilbert BW, Harvey RS, Crawford F, et al. Two-dimensional echocardiographic assessment of vegetative endocarditis. Circulation 1977;55:346.
175. Martin RP, Meltzer RS, Chia BL, et al. Clinical utility of two-dimensional echocardiography in infective endocarditis. Am J Cardiol 1980;46:379.
176. Mintz GS, Kotler MN, Segal BG, et al. Comparison of two-dimensional and M-mode echocardiography in the evaluation of patients with infective endocarditis. Am J Cardiol 1979;65:816.
177. Wann LS, Hallam CC, Dillon JC, et al. Comparison of cross-sectional echocardiography in infective endocarditis. Circulation 1979;60:728.
178. D'Cruz IA, Collison HK, Gerrardo L, et al. Two-dimensional echocardiographic detection of staphyloccal vegetation attached to calcified mitral annulus. Am Heart J 1982;103:298.
179. Matsumoto M, Strom J, Hirose H, et al. Preoperative echocardiographic diagnosis of anterior mitral valve leaflet fenestration associated with infective endocarditis. Am J Cardiol 1979;43:738.

180. Erbel R, Rohmann S, Drexler N, et al. Improved diagnostic value of echocardiography in patients with infective endocarditis by transesophageal approach. Eur Heart J 1988;9:43.

181. Klodas E, Edwards WD, Khandheria BK. Use of transesophageal echocardiography for improving detection of valvular vegetations in subacute bacterial endocarditis. J Am Soc Echocardiogr 1989;2:38.

182. Mugge A, Daniel WG, Frank G, et al. Echocardiography in infective endocarditis. J Am Coll Cardiol 1989;14:631.

183. Tamms MA, Gussenhoven EJ, Bos E, et al. Enhanced morphological diagnosis in infective endocarditis by transesophageal echocardiography. Br Heart J 1990;63:109.

184. Birmingham GD, Rahko PS, Ballantyne F. Improved detection of infective endocarditis with transesophageal echocardiography. Am Heart J 1992;123:774.

12

Left Ventricle: Anatomy and Measurements

The shape of the normal left ventricle is that of a truncated ellipsoid[1]; it also has been described as that of a cone with blunted apex and slightly convex sides. Thus it has a wide base at the mitral annulus and tapers toward a narrow apex. The left ventricle (LV) long axis, the axis of the cone, is directed downward, forward, and to the left. In transverse cross section, the LV is circular or nearly so at its base, midsection, and apex, so the LV chamber is roughly symmetrical in shape, unlike the right ventricle (RV). (Abnormalities of LV shape are consistently associated with various LV disease states, as will be discussed below). Those who are accustomed to viewing angiocardiograms know that the LV chamber appears oval in shape in the left anterior oblique projection, the vertical dimension being slightly larger than the transverse one; in the right anterior oblique projection, the LV has been described as bullet-shaped, its apex or point downward and to the left.

EXTERNAL ANATOMY OF THE LV

The base of the LV, the mitral annulus, is marked externally by the coronary sulcus, in which runs the circumflex branch of the left coronary artery. On the posterior LV aspect, the coronary sinus runs obliquely just above the junction between the left atrium (LA) and LV. Anteriorly and inferiorly, shallow interventricular grooves demarcate the junction of left and right ventricles. The left anterior descending and posterior descending arteries course in these grooves.

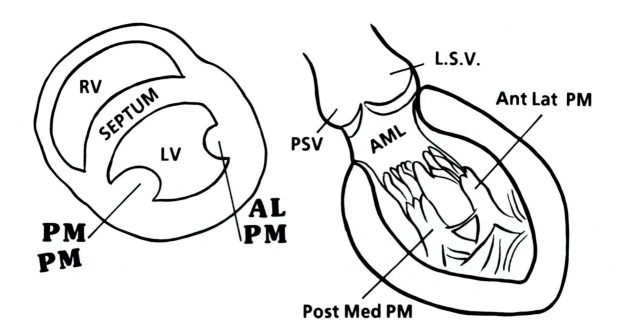

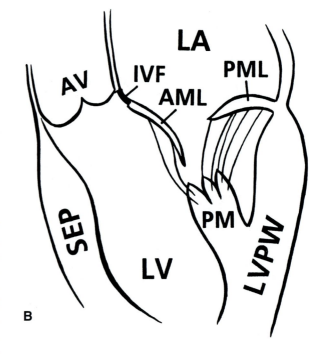

Figure 12–1. (A) Diagram showing LV chamber with posteromedial and anterolateral papillary muscles in short-axis view (left) and in interior of LV chamber with septum removed (right). (B) Diagram showing relationships of mitral valve to aortic valve with connecting intervalvar fibrosa (IVF) (AV, aortic valve; AML and PML, anterior and posterior mitral leaflet; SEP, septum; PM PM, posteromedial papillary muscle and AL PM, anterolateral papillary muscle; LVPW, left ventricular posterior wall); LSV and PSV, left and posterior sinus of valsalva. (C) Diagram showing long-axis view (above) and short-axis view (below) of left ventricular and mitral apparatus anatomy. Normal anatomy is seen at left and various sites of calcification at right. Conventional abbreviations are used (AML and PML, anterior and posterior mitral leaflets; I Val Sept, intervalvar septum or fibrosa; Cal Ao Val, calcification aortic valve; post SMC, posterior submitral calcification, better known as mitral annulus calcification; Ant SMC, anterior submitral calcification, refers to calcification in the intervalvar fibrosa and the base of the anterior mitral leaflet).

300

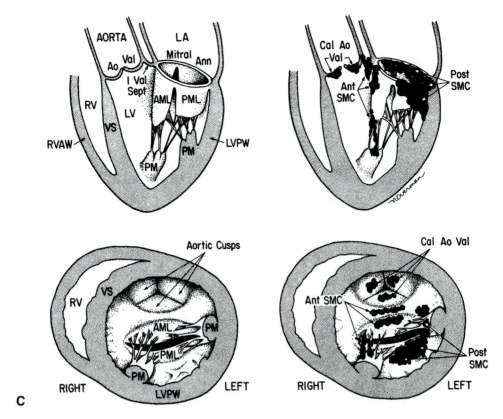

C

Figure 12–1 (*Continued*)

Externally, the LV has five surfaces; however, there is no sharp border or defining line separating these surfaces; instead, there is a smooth, rounded transition from one to the other. The five surfaces are (1) the *anterolateral* surface, facing the anterior chest wall; (2) the *left lateral* surface, facing the left hemithorax; it includes a curvature known as the *obtuse margin* (the acute margin of the heart lies at the junction of the anterior and inferior surfaces of the right ventricle); (3) the *inferior* or *diaphragmatic* surface, which rests on the diaphragmatic part of the pericardial sac; (4) the *true posterior* or *posterobasal* surface, which is a short strip just below the coronary sinus and sulcus posteriorly; it faces directly backward, toward the spine, and is closely related to the esophagus and descending thoracic aorta; and (5) the *anterobasal* surface, which forms the "left shoulder" of the heart, lying just below the left appendage; between the two runs the left main coronary artery.

The *LV length* (long axis) is measured from the LV apex to the mitral annulus or from the LV apex to the aortic valve annulus, a measurement that can be made at autopsy as well as on two-dimensional (2D) echo in apical views. This LV dimension in autopsied adult hearts is an average of 7.5 ± 1 cm.[2]

INTERNAL LV ANATOMY (Figure 12–1)

The various external surfaces of the LV mentioned above are together often referred to as the *LV free wall;* the remainder of the LV is formed by the interventricular (usually abbreviated to ventricular) septum. The ventricular septum is roughly triangular in shape, broad at its base and tapering toward the LV apex. The septum has a transverse curvature, concave to the LV chamber, conforming to the circular cross-sectional LV contour.

In its longitudinal axis (base to apex), the ventricular septum has a more gentle or slight curvature than its transverse curvature; in fact, it may be almost flat in some cases.

Most of the ventricular septum is *muscular* (i.e., myocardial), except for a small oval area of collagenous tissue just below the right coronary and noncoronary cusps of the aortic valve. This *membranous part of the ventricular septum* is thin (1 to 2 mm thick) and continuous with the fibrous support and attachment (annulus) of the aortic valve, reinforced at either side by the right and left fibrous trigones. The membranous ventricular septum on its LV side is situated entirely within the LV chamber. However, on its right side, the upper part of the membranous septum forms part of the right atrium, while the lower part is part of the right ventricle. This important anatomic situation is due to the fact that the tricuspid valve attachment (septal leaflet) is closer to the apex than to the mitral valve attachment, as the tricuspid annulus crosses the membranous ventricular septum obliquely.

The LV chamber is divided into a posterior *inflow tract* leading from the mitral orifice to the LV apex and an anterior *outflow tract* from the apex to the aortic valve. The anterior mitral leaflet hangs like a curtain suspended from the base of the heart and separates the LV inflow from the LV outflow. Thus the inflow tract is bounded by the anterolateral and posteroinferior LV walls, the inferior (posterior) part of the ventricular septum, and the anterior mitral leaflet. The outflow tract is bounded by the anterior LV wall, the anterior part of the ventricular septum, and the anterior mitral leaflet. The long axes of the LV inflow and outflow tracts meet at an acute angle at the LV apex. This angle is about 30 to 45 degrees so that blood streaming into the LV during diastole reverses direction by 135 to 150 degrees to rush out of the aortic valve in systole. The LV outflow just below the aortic valve makes an angle of 30 to 45 degrees with the lower LV outflow tract because the "infundibular" septum angles sharply rightward with reference to the rest of the muscular septum, especially in the elderly, giving the septum a sigmoid shape.[4]

The upper one-half or one-third of the LV outflow tract is smooth,[5] whereas the lower septum has on its surface small irregular trabeculations (trabeculae carneae). The LV free wall is covered with larger and more numerous trabeculations, especially at the LV apex and around the bases of the two papillary muscles. Trabeculations vary in configuration from mere ridges on the endocardium, to bands fixed at both ends but separated from endocardium, to bands crossing the LV chamber from the papillary muscle or LV wall to the septum or from the apical septum to the basal septum. During ventricular contraction, endocordial "folding" takes place in grooves between trabecular ridges; by encroaching on LV internal volume, trabeculations augment systolic emptying of the LV chamber.[6]

WALL THICKNESS

The thickness of the ventricular septum and of the LV wall has been measured in several autopsy studies.[2,7-10] The thicknesses of these structures as measured in postmortem specimens is an average of 1.3 ± 0.2 cm; however, these values are higher than the actual diastolic measurements during life, and systolic thicknesses approximate in vitro systolic measurements because of cardiac rigor mortis. Echocardiographic study of septal and LV wall thickness has been done on an extensive scale and has demonstrated that the range of normal thicknesses of these structures on the M-mode tracing is 7 to 11 mm.

Over the last two decades, M-mode measurement of LV wall thickness and septal thickness (Figure 12–2) have been cited and discussed in textbooks, papers, and routine clinical practice as if the LV free wall and ventricular septum were perfectly uniform in thickness through all their extent. Anyone who has looked closely at 2D echoes or at autopsy hearts knows that this is not so. Thus the ventricular septum is thinnest at the membranous part and thickest near the junction of its middle and basal thirds, where the septal band of the RV crista augments septal thickness. Another site of septal thickness is just

LV MEASUREMENTS

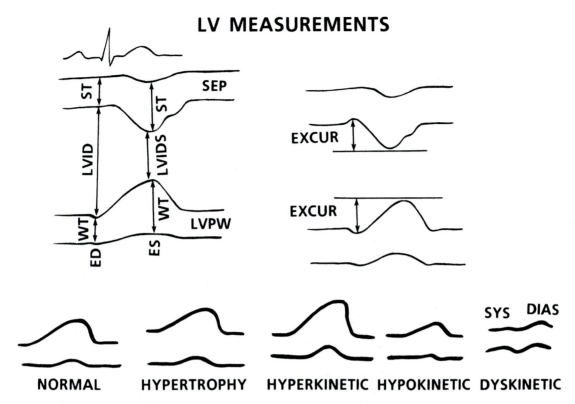

Figure 12–2. Diagram showing how LV measurements are made on the M-mode echo (LVID, left ventricular internal dimension, end-diastole; LVIDS, same at end-systole; ST, septal thickness, end-diastole and end-systole; WT, left ventricular posterior wall thickness, end-diastole, ED, and end-systole, ES; SEP, septum; LVPW, left ventricular posterior wall; EXCUR, systolic excursions of SEP and LVPW). Normal and abnormal contours of LVPW systolic motion and thickening are shown below.

below the aortic valve (proximal septal bulge), especially in elderly persons with sigmoid septum contour.[4]

The LV free wall tends to be thickest at basal level and thinner near the apex; the latter may be only 2 mm thick at its very tip.[12] The LV papillary muscles were discussed in Chapter 11, but will be mentioned here again because these two papillary muscles are very much part of the LV chamber scene (Figures 12-3 and 12-4). They are designated posteromedial and anterolateral with respect to their LV locations (Figure 12-1). However, in the parasternal short-axis view their location appears to be medial and lateral, respectively, so that these designations might be more convenient. The lateral papillary muscle is longer, and its apex extends higher (closer to mitral annulus) than the medial one. The lateral papillary muscle has a simple grooved head in 70% to 85% of cases; the medial one is shorter and divided into two, three, or more heads in 60% to 70% of cases.[13,14]

The two LV papillary muscles are always located on the LV free wall; unlike the RV, there are never any papillary muscles on the septum. Though there is some variation in topography of papillary muscles with reference to the "longitude and latitude" of the LV chamber, the bases of both muscles are rooted in the middle one-third of the LV. Their apices, or heads, point toward the mitral valve and protrude into the basal third of the LV. Extra papillary muscles are not very uncommon, located in between the usual two muscles and perhaps nearer to the LV apex (Figure 12-5). Chorda muscularis (muscular instead of tendinous chord from the papillary muscle to the mitral leaflet attachment) is another anatomic variant recognizable on echocardiography (Figure 12-6).

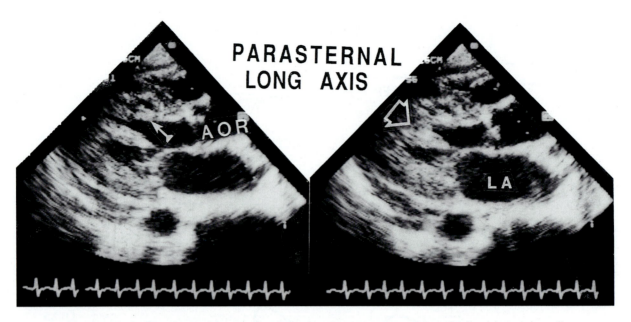

Figure 12–3. Parasternal long-axis view showing parasternal longitudinal band (small arrow). The anterolateral papillary muscle is shown (open arrow).

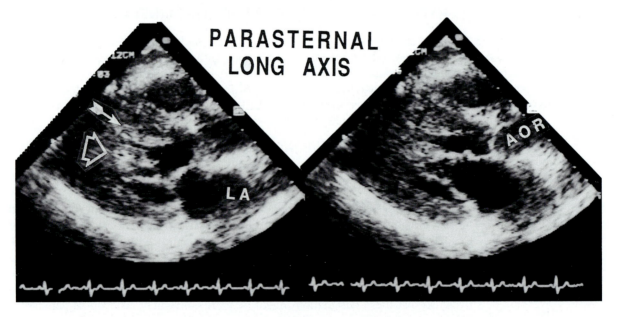

Figure 12–4. Parasternal views showing (left) a longitudinal paraseptal band (thin arrow) and adjacent to it the anterolateral papillary muscle (open arrow). (Right) The chordal connection of the latter to mitral leaflets is well seen; the demarcation of paraseptal band from septum is unclear, creating the illusion of marked septal hypertrophy.

THE LEFT VENTRICLE IN OLD AGE

Heart weight increases with advancing age. Waller and Roberts[15] reported increased heart weight in two-thirds of 40 autopsies of patients over 90 years of age. It is probably not due to hypertrophy of muscle fibers but rather to a greater amount of interstitial collagen, calcific deposits in valve leaflets or the perivalvar region, or increase in subepicardial and

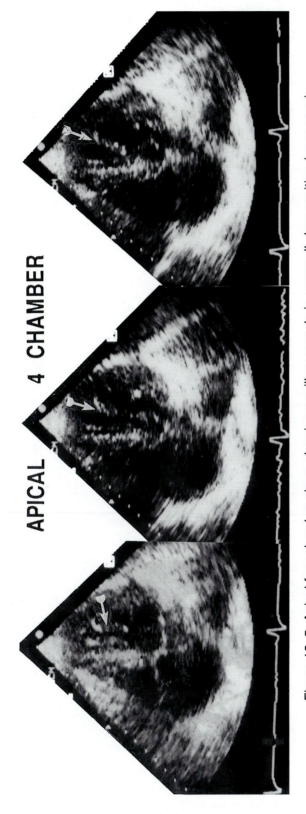

APICAL 4 CHAMBER

Figure 12–5. Apical four-chamber views showing papillary muscle in unusually low position (near apex) with its mitral chordal connections (arrows).

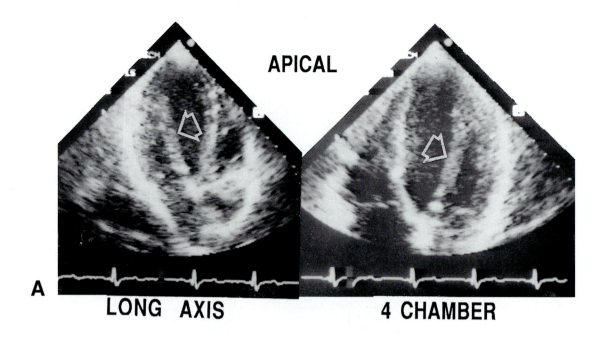

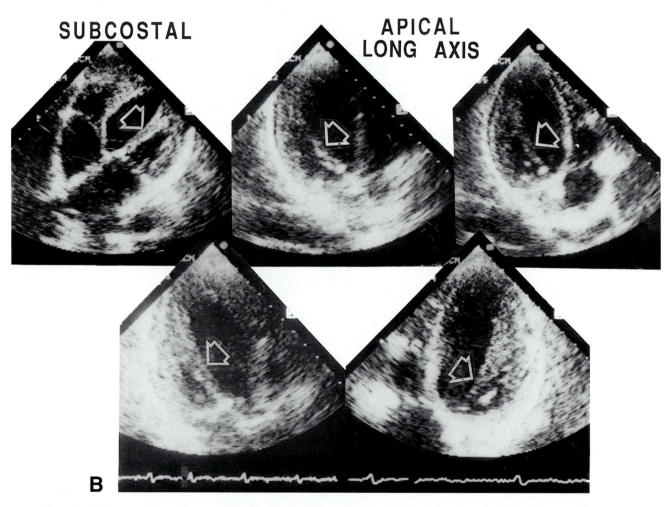

Figure 12–6. (A) Apical four-chamber view (left) and apical long-axis view (right) showing abnormal muscle band arising in papillary muscle and inserting at the site of attachment of the anterior mitral leaflet (chorda muscularis); i.e., chorda tendinea is replaced by myocardium. (B) Subcostal (above, left) and apical long-axis views (above, right, and below, left), and modified apical four-chamber view (below, right) showing chorda muscularis from papillary muscle to base or attachment of anterior mitral leaflet.

interatrial septal fat. Of these three factors, the latter two can be visualized on echocardiography and therefore are relevant to practitioners of cardiac ultrasound.

An increase in the fibrous tissue content of the LV wall, especially in subendocardial and subepicardial regions, begins to appear at about age 60. Lenkiewicz et al.[16] found that collagen content was twice as high in those over age 75 than in those under age 50 (36% versus 17%); muscle tissue decreased from 40% below age 50 to 27% over age 75.[16] This increase in fibrous tissue might explain the reduced compliance and Doppler pattern of mitral flow often encountered in the elderly (*a* peak > *e* peak). LV chamber size and shape alter in the elderly as follows: (1) LV chamber size decreases, (2) the apex-to-base long-axis LV dimension decreases, (3) the basal part of the left ventricle becomes bent or curved, bulging toward the LV outflow tract, and (4) the middle to apical thirds of the septum curve and incline rightward, thus forming the sigmoid septum shape (Figures 12–7 and 12–8) of Goor et al.[17] These authors found that such curvature of the septum in the elderly was more common in those with lighter than heavier hearts.

Echocardiographers commonly encounter the sigmoid septal shape in elderly patients, frequently associated with local anterobasal hypertrophy. There are two points of practical value: First, the basal bulging of the septum, just below the aortic valve (proximal septal bulge), should be recognized as a harmless variant and not mistaken for hypertrophic subaortic stenosis. Second, curvature of the middle to apical septum toward the RV in an apical four-chamber view should not be mistaken for a septal aneurysm; the latter is excluded by normal contraction of the septum.

BANDS AND STRANDS IN THE LV CHAMBER (Figures 12–9 to 12–19)

Normal chordae tendineae are fibrous stringlike structures that originate from one of the two LV papillary muscles and insert on one of the two mitral leaflets. LV structures resembling such chordae in morphology but which arise and/or insert elsewhere are called

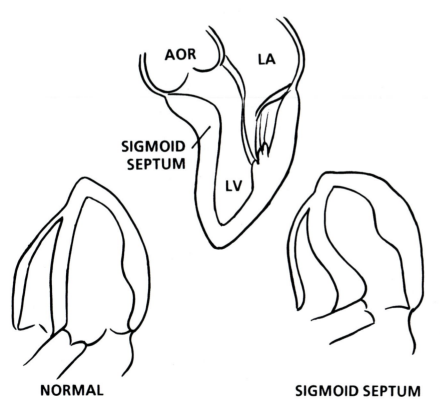

NORMAL   SIGMOID SEPTUM

APICAL 4-CHAMBER VIEW

Figure 12–7. (Above) Diagram of sigmoid septal shape, common variant in elderly individuals. Viewed from the LV side, the basal ventricular septum bulges into the LV outflow tract forming a conspicuous shelf or projection. The apical four-chamber view contour of a normal subject (below, left) and a patient with sigmoid septum (below, right) are shown. The middle to apical septum in the latter may show an enhanced concavity simulating an aneurysm, but it contracts normally.

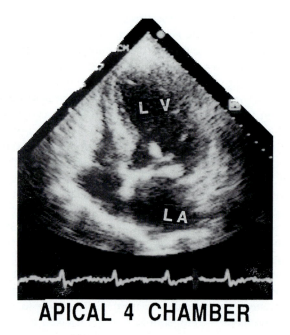

APICAL 4 CHAMBER

Figure 12–8. Apical four-chamber view of an elderly man showing LV shape commonly associated with sigmoid septum. The apical LV is inclined rightward. Calcification in the mitral annulus and papillary muscle is also present.

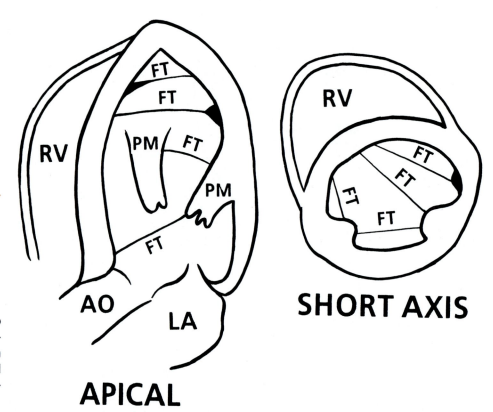

Figure 12–9. Diagram to show various common locations of false tendons (FT) in the LV chamber in apical and short-axis 2D views (PM, papillary muscle).

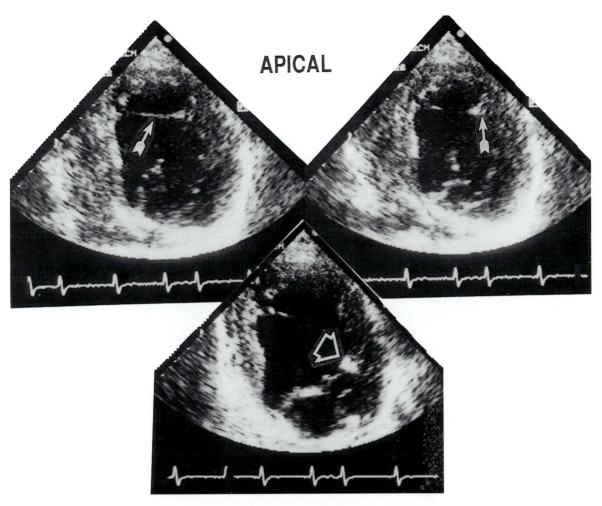

Figure 12–10. The LV chamber is imaged in planes intermediate between apical four-chamber and short-axis views. A false tendon is seen (above, left) as well as a "mini-papillary muscle" at its attachment to the LV wall (above, right). The true papillary muscle and its chordal attachments to the mitral leaflets are seen below (open arrow).

false tendons or *pseudotendons.*[18] These are sometimes grouped together with muscular bands that are also "normal" anatomic variants and can be seen spanning the LV chamber at autopsy and on 2D echo. They were first described by anatomist Sir William Turner a century ago[19] and then apparently were forgotten for three-quarters of a century until Roberts[20] and Pomerance[21] described them again in autopsy hearts. They have been called *anomalous* or *aberrant left ventricular chordae tendineae, chordae,* or *cords* in addition to false tendons. Likewise, the myocardial bands have been named *left ventricular bands, strands* or *moderator bands,* with or without the preceding adjective *aberrant* or *anomalous.*

Initial reports suggested that such LV bands or false tendons are rare, but studies of several large series of postmortem hearts have established that they are common, being present in approximately half the 483 autopsy hearts studied by Boyd et al.[22] and the 686 hearts in the series of Gerlis et al.[23] The latter found the prevalence to be the same in hearts with or without congenital defects.

The LV bands were defined as discrete fibromuscular cordlike structures crossing the LV cavity and having no attachment to the mitral valve leaflets. In the Mayo Clinic material,[22] the false tendons were multiple in 38%; 66% connected the ventricular septum to

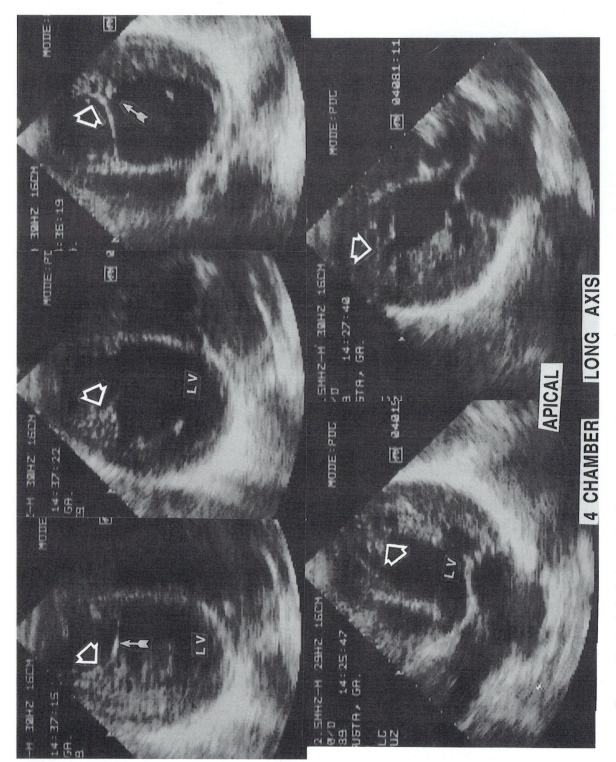

Figure 12–11. Apical views showing transverse false tendon near apex (thin arrow). A "mini-papillary muscle" (open arrow) is present at the attachment of the false tendon to the LV free wall, which can be mistaken for a mural thrombus if the imaging plane does not include the false tendon.

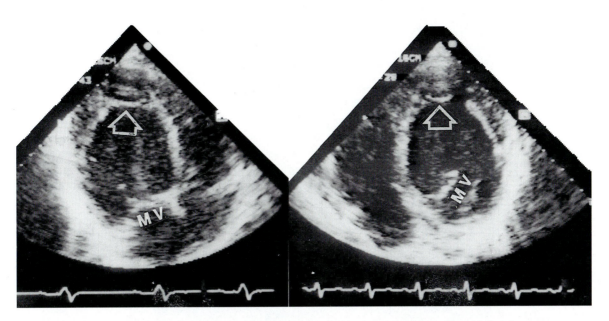

Figure 12–12. Apical long-axis view (left) and apical four-chamber view (right) in a patient with dilated cardiomyopathy (note spheric shape change) showing a prominent apical trabeculation. The latter could be mistaken for the edge of an apical mural thrombus.

the posteromedial papillary muscle, 12% crossed from one papillary muscle to the other, 9% connected the septum and the LV free wall. In the series of Gerlis et al.,[23] nearly all bands were attached at one end to the septum, while the other end was inserted (in descending frequency) on the posteromedial papillary muscle, LV free wall, and anterolateral papillary muscle.

A distinction has been made between false tendons and muscular bands (trabeculations); the former are 2 to 3 mm or less in thickness, and the latter are thicker than that. Some have distinguished between aberrant myocardial bands, which have a free intracavitary course between attachments, and trabeculations, which are in contact with the adjacent LV wall or septum. Others have called the former "prominent" trabeculations and the latter "shallow" trabeculations. Keren et al.[24] distinguished prominent trabeculations into three types: hypertrophic, fibrotic, and combined hypertrophic-fibrotic.

The first 2D echo report, of five instances of false tendons in the LV chamber, by Nishimura et al.,[18] appeared in 1981 and was followed by other large series.[22-26] Linear filamentous or thin bands of echoes are easily visualized when perpendicular to the ultrasound beam (Figures 12–10 and 12–11); in order to depict the entire false tendon, it may be necessary to manipulate the ultrasound probe to image unconventional planes. To differentiate such bands or strands (Figure 12–12) from the reflecting edge of a thrombus, it is important to visualize sonolucent space on both sides of the linear echo; likewise colorflow Doppler will reveal blood flow (color) on either side of the band or false tendon.

The systolic behavior of the band is worth observing closely. Muscular bands shorten and thicken, whereas tendinous ones (false tendons) become loose and curved in systole but taut and straight in diastole. Another caveat: Off-center LV planes transecting the chamber very near the LV wall may show an abundance of trabeculations, often crossing each other in a network-like configuration; this is a normal finding, especially in the vicinity of the LV apex.

Keren et al.,[24] who correlated the 2D echo and anatomic findings in 35 patients whose hearts were removed at transplantation, divided "aberrant" LV bands into three groups

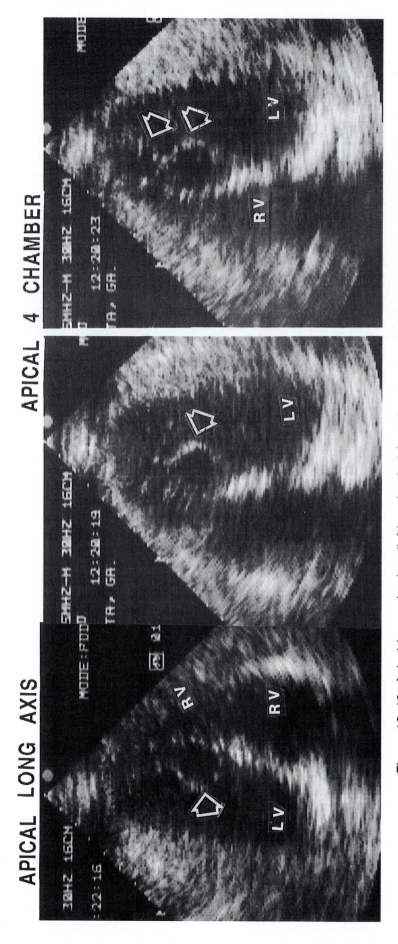

Figure 12–13. Apical long-axis view (left) and apical four-chamber views (center and right) showing unusual aberrant band with multiple mural connections.

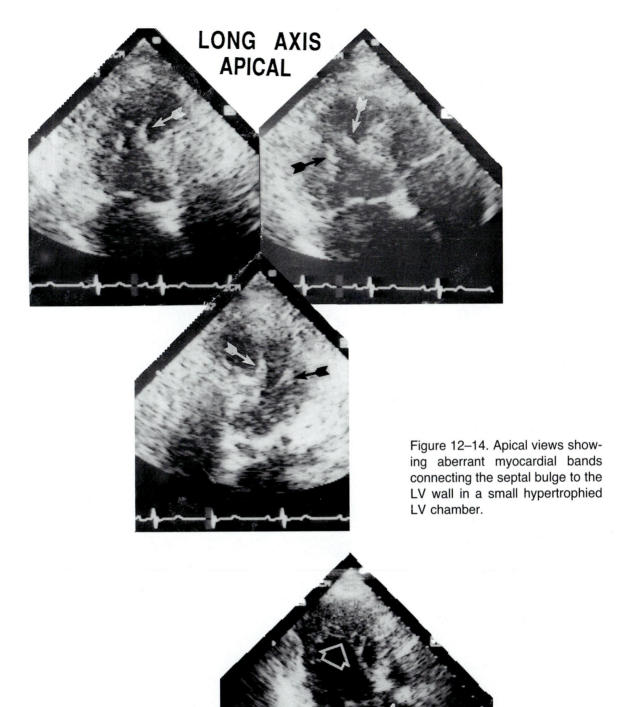

Figure 12–14. Apical views showing aberrant myocardial bands connecting the septal bulge to the LV wall in a small hypertrophied LV chamber.

Figure 12–15. Apical long-axis view showing a complex aberrant band attached proximally to the base of the septum and at the other end to the apical wall by multiple trabeculations (open arrow).

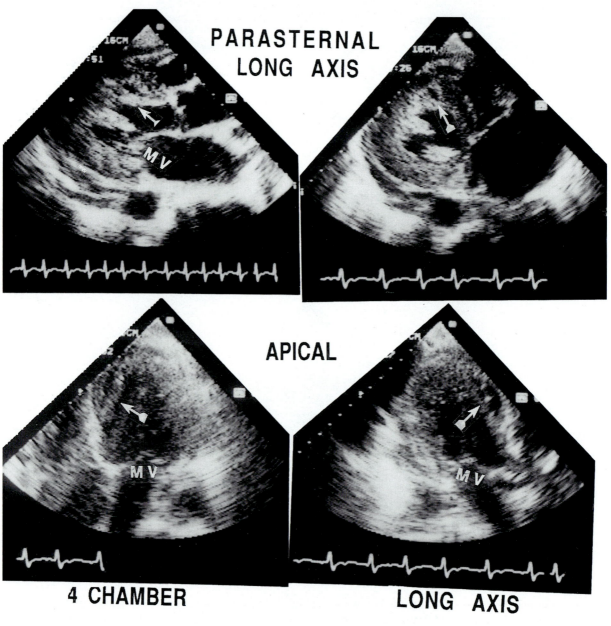

SEPTUM

AORTA

PLB

Figure 12–16. Diagram to show location of very common paraseptal longitudinal muscular band (PLB) or trabeculation. It is attached proximally to the septum just below the aortic valve and distally to the septum near the apex.

PARASTERNAL LONG AXIS

MV

APICAL

MV

MV

4 CHAMBER

LONG AXIS

Figure 12–17. Parasternal views (above) and apical views (below) of same patient as in Figure 12–3 showing aberrant muscular band (arrows).

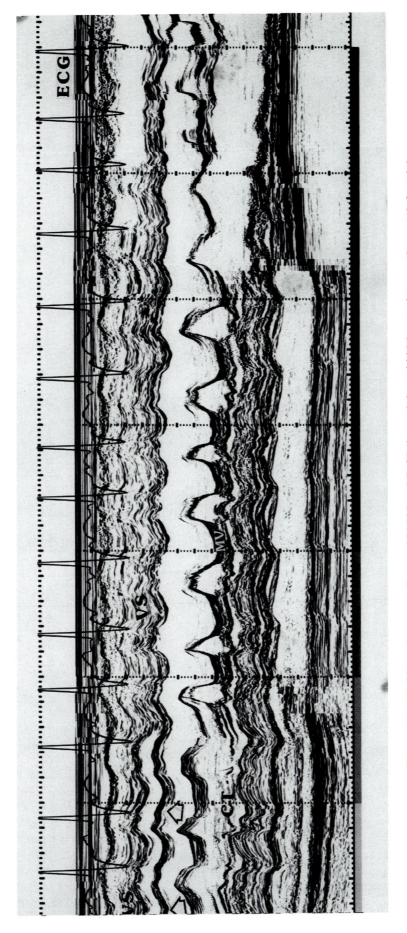

Figure 12–18. M-mode sweep from mid-LV level (left) through basal LV (center) to aortic root–left atrial level (right) showing paraseptal myocardial band (arrow) that merges with the basal septum. The latter appears much thicker than the mid-LV septum.

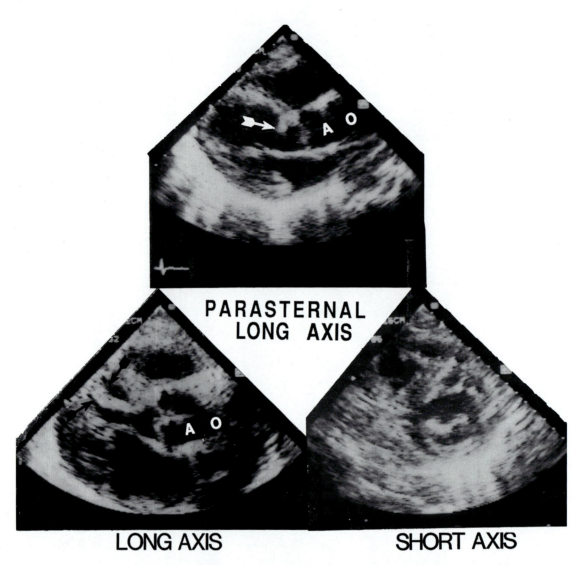

Figure 12–19. Parasternal long-axis view (above) showing unusual local protuberance of the basal septum. In a slightly different plane this is seen to be part of a prominent longitudinal band (below, left). This band is also well seen in parasternal short-axis view.

(transverse, longitudinal, and sagittal) according to their orientation in the LV chamber. Bands that are multiple or complex in contour and connections are not rare (Figures 12–13 to 12–15).

In general, LV bands or strands are not believed to have adverse effects. In a few cases they have been associated with systolic murmurs, ventricular ectopy, or preexcitation, but the connection between the anatomic LV structure and the clinical feature is still tentative and not understood. On the other hand, it is possible that the bands, especially if they are large and muscular, could assist in the efficiency of LV pump action.

To the echocardiographer, these muscular as well as tendinous bands are important because they can sometimes be mistaken for various pathologic structures.[27] For example, the echogenic edge of a *mural thrombus* can mimic a band or false tendon but will have sonolucent space on one side of it and a homogeneous "solid" texture on the thrombus side. Sometimes a small *endocardial elevation* or *protuberance* (see Figures 12–10 and 12–11) marks the attachment of a false tendon to the LV wall, a sort of "mini-papillary muscle." If the latter is imaged but not the false tendon, the endocardial bump could be mistaken for a small mural thrombus, especially if this part of LV is infarcted. Also, *longitudinal muscular bands* or *trabeculations* (Figures 12–16 to 12–19) adjacent to the

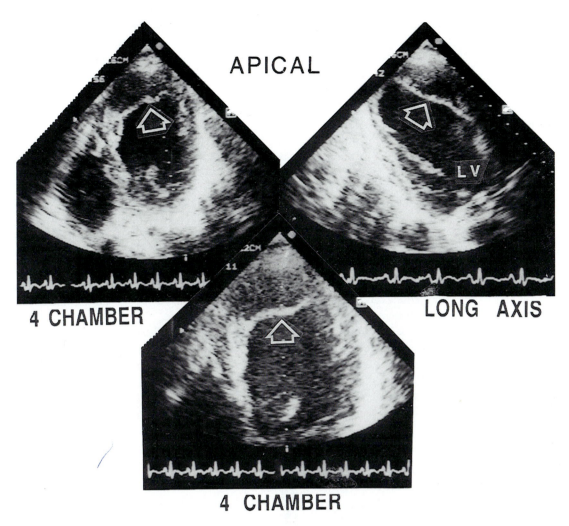

APICAL

4 CHAMBER

LONG AXIS

4 CHAMBER

Figure 12–20. Apical views showing a transverse band echo that simulates an aberrant myocardial band or false tendon. Serial echocardiography in this patient revealed that the band echo represented the residuum of a large apical mural thrombus that had gradually lysed except for the residual band.

septum are very common and best appreciated in the long-axis parasternal view; they can produce the illusion of increased septal thickness, thus raising the possibility of asymmetrical septal hypertrophy (ASH) and hypertrophic cardiomyopathy. Occasionally, the false tendons are so situated as to possibly mimic a *subaortic membrane,* a *flail mitral leaflet,* or *accessory mitral tissue.* Very rarely, partial lysis of a mural thrombus leaves a residual band thrombus (Figure 12–20).

LV OUTFLOW TRACT

The LV outflow tract (LVOT) is that part of the LV chamber that lies immediately below the aortic valve. Some anatomists, notably Walmsley,[28] consider the LVOT as extending all the way from the aortic valve to the LV apex, but in common usage of the term, most angiocardiographers and echocardiographers apply it to the upper part of this region, i.e., to that part of the LV that is bounded posteriorly by the anterior leaflet of the mitral valve.

The interior of the normal LVOT is smooth, with no bands, trabeculations, or papillary muscles. In shape it is like a segment of a cone or a funnel, narrower at the aortic valve level than at its lower end, which widens into the main LV chamber. The anterior and left walls of the LVOT are formed by LV myocardium, except for narrow strips of fibrosa just below the aortic cusps (the right and left fibrous trigones). The right wall of the LVOT is formed by the anterior mitral leaflet, especially its relatively fixed basal portion, and above it the intervalvar fibrosa or trigone that connects it (the basal anterior leaflet) to the aortic valve.

Fixed Subaortic Stenosis

Fixed subaortic stenosis comprises 8% to 10% of all congenital aortic stenoses (valvar, supra- and subvalvar). It is of three anatomic types: (1) discrete membrane, (2) fibromuscular collar, and (3) tunnel or elongated LVOT stenosis. There may be transitional forms that do not fit neatly into one of these categories, and in fact, type 2 may be considered intermediate between types 1 and 3. Fixed subaortic stenosis should not be confused at all with muscular or dynamic subaortic stenosis (hypertrophic cardiomyopathy with LVOT obstruction), which is entirely different in anatomy, physiology, clinical aspects, and therapy.

Type 3 (tunnel) is virtually confined to early childhood. The other two types (membrane and collar types) are encountered in older children and young adults but rarely in older adults. Fixed subaortic stenosis is one of the causes of sudden unexpected death in young male athletes.

Associated intracardiac defects are said to be present in as many as 60% of patients. They include ventricular septal defects, aortic coarctation, pulmonary valve stenosis, and tetralogy of Fallot. Aortic regurgitation is extremely common.

The stenotic lesion is commonly a tough fibroelastic membrane or shelf that projects into the LVOT 1 to 2 cm below the aortic cusps, contiguous to (and often continuous with) the basal part of the anterior mitral leaflet (Figure 12–21). The obstructing mem-

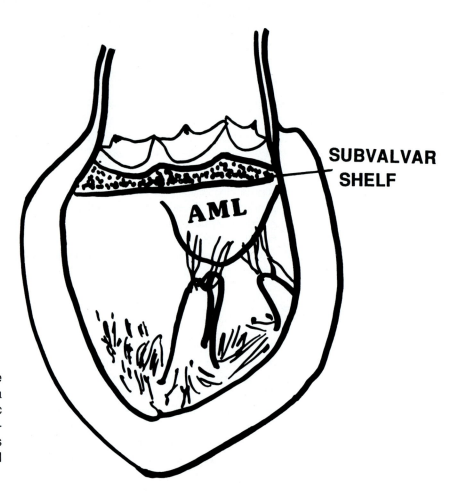

Figure 12–21. Diagram showing the left ventricle open and spread out in a patient with fixed subvalvar aortic stenosis. In actual cases, the subvalvar shelf may not be as extensive as shown here (AML, anterior mitral leaflet).

brane is 2 to 4 mm thick and may be described as one or more transverse bands attached to the membranous ventricular septum. It may appear as a crescentic ridge attached anteriorly to the base of the right coronary cusp of the aortic valve and posteriorly to the base of the anterior mitral leaflet, forming a sort of collar around the inner aspect of the LVOT.

The aortic valve cusps appear thickened and perhaps somewhat deformed by the traumatic impact of the jet emerging from the subvalvar stenosis. This, in turn, (1) leads to aortic regurgitation, which tends to progressively increase with time, and (2) predisposes to bacterial endocarditis, an important complication of this anomaly. It has been suggested that the subvalvar diaphragm might mitigate the complication it was responsible for—aortic regurgitation—by limiting the quantity of regurgitant blood. Unlike valvar aortic stenosis, subvalvar aortic stenosis is not associated with poststenotic aortic root dilatation.

Fixed subaortic stenosis rarely can be due to mitral valve abnormalities, since the anterior mitral leaflet forms the posterior wall of the LVOT. Thus, in endocardial cushion defects of complete or partial types, the attachment of the anterior mitral leaflet is abnormal in such a way that the LVOT is narrower than normal and elongated, forming the "swan-neck" LV deformity well known to angiocardiographers. However, hemodynamically significant LVOT stenosis does not occur in partial or complete atrioventricular (A-V) canal defects. Rare instances of subaortic stenosis due to a malpositioned anterior mitral leaflet and deformation of this leaflet by Carpentier valvoplasty have been reported.

Echocardiography of Fixed (Discrete) Subvalvar Aortic Stenosis (FSAS).

The first echocardiographic sign described as diagnostic of FSAS was not visualization of the obstructing membrane or ridge but of a characteristic M-mode pattern of aortic valve motion.[30-32] One or (rarely) two aortic valve cusps, soon after initial opening in early systole, close abruptly and then flutter through the rest of systole in the "closed" position. This behavior of the cusps is presumed to be due to turbulence or eddies adjacent to the jet emerging from the FSAS.

The site of stenosis (membrane, diaphragm, or collar) is seldom identified on the M-mode echo but usually manifests on 2D echo.[33-38] The parasternal long-axis view is best for this purpose (Figure 12-22), but the apical long-axis view also may be useful.[8] Some authors differentiate between FSAS of thin membrane type and a thicker fibromuscular ridge or collar. The thin linear type can be overlooked easily on a cursory examination. The anterior component of the FSAS (projecting backward from the septal border) is visualized more commonly than the posterior FSAS component (protruding anteriorly from the base of the anterior mitral leaflet).

The anatomic features of the FSAS are depicted in finer clarity and detail by transesophageal echocardiography (TEE) than by conventional 2D echo.[39-41] Thus in a 13-year-old patient the subvalvar membrane ballooned into a cystlike aneurysm in systole but collapsed in diastole[140]; this abnormal tissue was of accessory mitral valve origin. In another child, accessory mitral valve tissue formed a pedunculated mass attached to the base of the anterior mitral leaflet that moved into the aorta in systole but recoiled back into the LVOT in diastole[42]; Doppler showed a gradient of 100 mmHg; the accessory mitral "valve" had chordal attachment to both papillary muscles in this remarkable case. Close anatomic connection and even tethering of the FSAS membrane to the anterior mitral leaflet was demonstrated by TEE in a 44-year-old man by Schwinger and Kronzon.[41]

Colorflow Doppler is useful in FSAS diagnosis by revealing a high-velocity jet emerging from the region of the FSAS membrane rather than from the valve.

LEFT VENTRICULAR INTERNAL DIMENSION (LVID)

This measurement was the only LV measurement performed in the M-mode era, recorded by the single-crystal transducer. At that time, it was presumed to be a true "minor axis" dimension of the LV chamber, from the left (posterior) surface of the ventricular septum

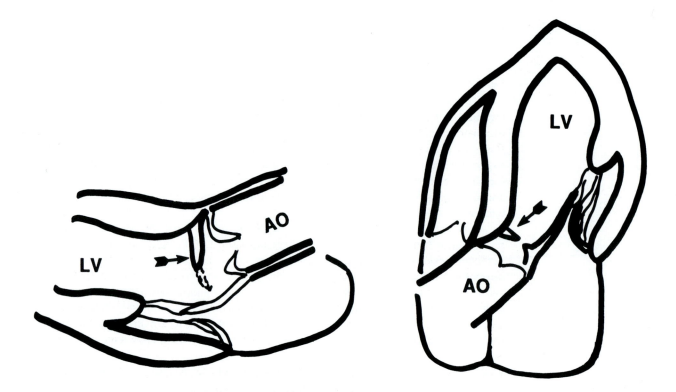

DISCRETE SUBVALVAR

Figure 12–22. Diagram showing parasternal (left) and apical (right) long-axis views in a patient with fixed subvalvar aortic stenosis. The stenosing subvalvar shelf (arrows) is seen to project transversely across the LV outflow tract from the ventricular septum.

to the anterior surface of the LV posterior wall. A rough standardization of the LV level at which the LVID was recorded was attained by ensuring that it was done at mitral chordae tendineae level, i.e., below the level of mitral leaflets but above the level of papillary muscles (see Figure 12–2). Originally it was optimistically believed, at least by some, that this dimension bisected the LV chamber in longitudinal as well as cross-sectional planes, thus representing a true geometric minor axis of a prolate ellipse of rotation.

With the advent of 2D echo, it became evident that such an assumption was not justified, that (1) the M-mode LVID was closer to the LV base than to its apex and (2) that the M-mode LVID could not be relied on to be exactly in the center of the circular LV cross section. The latter is approximated in routine clinical practice by first obtaining a good parasternal short-axis view of the LV chamber, with circular contour, at mitral chordae tendineae level; the M-mode cursor is then positioned so as to bisect this circle by simple inspection.

For a valid LVID, it is important that the long axis of the LV chamber be perpendicular to (or almost so) the ultrasound beam. It is quite frequent, especially in older persons with high diaphragms, that the LV alignment is such that its long axis is oblique rather than perpendicular to the ultrasound beam. The LVID measured in such circumstances would be an overestimate and indicate LV dilatation when the LV is in fact of normal size.

While the LVID can be measured at any point of the cardiac cycle, it is standardized at end diastole, i.e., LVID (D), and end systole, i.e., LVID (S). The end-diastolic LVID is measured at the onset of the inscription of the QRS complex on the ECG. The end-systolic LVID is the smallest dimension obtainable, usually at or very near the most posterior point (nadir) on the septal contour, just before the most anterior point (peak) of the LV posterior wall endocardial contour.

Factors Determining Echocardiographic LVID

The LVID is probably the most important single measurement in routine echocardiography, so the numerous factors causing variation in its magnitude need to be known in detail.

Recording Technique.

The LVID may be overestimated if the LV is tilted or angulated such that its long axis is not parallel to the anterior chest wall but aligned so as to have a more anteriorly directed apex. The LVID also may be overestimated if the short-axis view is not perpendicular to the LV long axis but is in a plane intermediate between the short-axis and apical four-chamber views. Underestimation of the LVID is possible if the M-mode cursor is not in the largest (central) anteroposterior dimension but off to one side of the LV midline, i.e., a chord rather than diameter of the circular LV cross section.

Measuring Technique.

The two commonly used standards for measuring LVID on the M-mode tracing are those of the American Society of Echocardiography (ASE) enunciated by Sahn et al.[42] and the Penn convention described by Devereaux and Reichek[43] in LV mass estimations. Other earlier conventions such as that of the National Institutes of Health (NIH)[64] have been discarded. The ASE method measures the LVID (1) from leading edge (of the posterior septal endocardial echo border) to leading edge (of the LV posterior wall endocardial echo border) and (2) at *onset* of the QRS complex on the ECG. The Penn convention (1) includes the thickness of these two endocardial echo borders in the LVID measurement and (2) measures the LVID at the peak of the R wave.

Heart Rate.

DeMaria et al.[45] reported a 2.7% decrease of LVID, in linear manner, for each 10 beat/min increment in heart rate, by pacing the right atrium to a maximum of 150 beats/min. Abbreviation of diastole with attenuation of LV filling is presumed to cause a smaller LVID. However, Belenkie[46] and Felner et al.[47] did not find changes in LVID with spontaneous (nonpaced) variations in heart rate. It was postulated that reflex factors that increase heart rate also would tend to enhance venous return to the heart.

Respiration.

Brenner et al.[48] noted a 6% decrease in LVID at end-inspiration compared with end-expiration. In addition to a decrease in LV filling during inspiration, movement of the diaphragm may change the imaging plane, but the fluctuations are minimal under normal conditions.

Inter- and Intraobserver Variability.

Interobserver variability is expressed as the mean difference between observers divided by the average measurement. It has been assessed by several groups.[49-51] A mean variability of about 5% for LVID at end diastole was found, and a higher variability was found for end-systolic LVID (7.5%).

Temporal Variability (Reproducibility).[52-55]

This signifies the variability in measurement in serial examinations on the same patient at short intervals (intervals too short to allow the cardiac status to change). This is expressed as the coefficient of variation: the standard deviation of all the measurements in a given case divided by a mean of those measurements. Clark et al.[53] found that a change of 3 mm or more in LVID represented a biologically significant difference.

LV VOLUME

Echocardiography made it possible, for the first time, to noninvasively image the left ventricular (LV) chamber, measure its dimensions, and estimate its volume. Recently, newer imaging modes such as magnetic resonance imaging (MRI) also have been used for this purpose, but the procedures are more expensive and lengthy and less widely available in clinical practice. Since assessment of LV size and function is probably the most common and useful service rendered by the echocardiographer to the clinician, LV chamber size, shape, and geometry need to be discussed in some detail.

Fortunately, LV shape is nearly symmetrical; its shape is usually described as an ellipsoid, i.e., a chamber formed by rotation of an ellipse on its long axis. Fortunately also for echocardiographers, the task of estimating LV volume from its images on film had been addressed earlier by angiocardiographers, in particular Dodge et al.,[56] who had compared angiocardiographic LV volumes with actual volumes of LV chambers from fresh autopsy hearts.

An ellipsoid chamber has a long (major) axis L and two minor (short) axes D_1 and D_2 perpendicular to each other. If the chamber has a circular cross section, $D_1 = D_2$. The volume of an ellipsoid is calculated by the formula

$$\text{LV volume} = \frac{4}{3}\pi \cdot \frac{L}{2} \cdot \frac{D_1}{2} \cdot \frac{D_2}{2}$$

$L/2$ is also known as the *major hemiaxis,* $D_1/2$ and $D_2/2$ are also known as *minor hemiaxes.*

The volume of an ellipsoid chamber also can be calculated from other combinations of measurements[57-65]:

1. The ellipsoid single-plane method (area-length method);

$$\text{LV volume} = \frac{8A^2}{3\pi L}$$

   where the long-axis area A and the long (major) axis L are known.[2]
2. The ellipsoid biplane method[3]:

$$\text{LV volume} = \frac{\pi}{6} \cdot L \left(\frac{4A_1}{\pi D} \right) \cdot \left(\frac{4A_2}{\pi L} \right)$$

   where A_1 and A_2 are areas including the major axis L and minor axis D, respectively.
3. The Simpson rule method. For purposes of measurement, the LV chamber image is "sliced" (manually or electronically) like a loaf of bread into many slices or slabs of equal thickness. Schiller et al.[59] divided the LV into 20 such segments, proceeding from LV base to apex. The volume of each slice is computed as the product of its thickness and its area; the sum of all slices adds up to the total estimated LV volume. The Simpson rule method has the advantage that it is valid even if the LV chamber is asymmetrical or if it deviates from an ellipsoid shape, which often happens in disease states, including ventricular aneurysm, hypertrophic cardiomyopathy, etc. Its disadvantage is that it is more tedious, though digitization of the LV images and appropriate software have facilitated the task.

$$\text{LV volume} = (A_1 + A_2 + A_3 \ldots \text{etc.}) \times H$$

   where H is thickness of each slice and A their respective areas.

In the modified Simpson rule method described by some echocardiographers,[60,61] the LV chamber is "sliced" into only three or four segments obtained by visualizing multiple LV cross sections from parasternal sites at mitral valve level, chordae level, and papillary muscle level either by angulating the 2D probe in different directions, i.e., sweeping toward the LV apex or base, or by sliding the transducer on the chest wall along the LV long axis.

Still other geometric approaches to LV volume estimation have been considered, based on various assumptions about LV shape implicit in the names and formulas of those methods: cylinder + cone, cylinder + hemisphere, bullet-shape, etc. All these LV volume methods require tracing the LV endocardial contour on the videoscreen and suffer from the common practical difficulty that the endocardial border frequently "drops out" in part. Tortoledo et al.[66] attempted to avoid this pitfall by developing a method for estimating ejection fraction from LV volumes computed from a combination of several LV dimensions in parasternal and both apical views. However, the formula was somewhat elaborate and included a visual grading of apical contraction; it has not gained wide acceptance.

Although LV volume estimations by angiocardiography and by 2D echo correlated well in most studies, particularly by the Simpson rule method, it soon became evident that the echocardiographic method consistently underestimates LV volume as compared with angiocardiography, probably due to the following reason: The contrast angiocardiographic image is a shadow or silhouette cast by the x-ray beam on the film and therefore represents the largest LV area in the imaging plane. On the other hand, the 2D echo apical view tends to appear smaller because it is unlikely to capture exactly the true anatomic long-axis plane of largest area; i.e., the 2D echo apical view is probably a little off-center. Comparison of simultaneous 2D echo and contrast angiocardiographic images in a series of patients showed that the 2D echo "apical window" was not precisely at the true LV apex but at a substantial distance from it.

The earliest attempts to estimate LV volume by ultrasound were based on a single measurement, the LV internal dimension (LVID), which was extrapolated to LV volume based on the following assumptions: (1) the LV is ellipsoid in shape, both minor axes D_1 and D_2 being equal, (2) the long (major) axis L is twice the short (minor) axis, and (3) the LVID as obtained in standard parasternal view coincides with the true minor axis of the LV chamber. Then

$$\text{LV volume} = \frac{4}{3}\pi \cdot \frac{D}{2} \cdot \frac{D}{2} \cdot D$$

which approximates D^3, since $\pi = 3.14$. This simplified formula, i.e., LV volume = D^3 = $(\text{LVID})^3$ was shown to have only a fair correlation ($r = 0.64$ to 0.74) with angiocardiographic LV volume. This is not surprising, since all the preceding three assumptions are not strictly true: The LV major axis is consistently less than twice the minor axis; the LV is not perfectly ellipsoidal in shape; and the LVID as obtained by parasternal M-mode does not intersect the center of the major axis but is closer to the LV base (mitral annulus) than it is to the LV apex.

LEFT VENTRICULAR CONFIGURATIONS

The echocardiographer needs to recognize certain atypical LV contours that vary with respect to chamber size, shape, and septal and/or LV wall thickness. Figures 12-23 and 12-24 depict these in long-axis and four-chamber views. Most of them will be discussed and illustrated again in other chapters dealing with specific entities.

CARDIAC SKELETON

Whereas most of the heart consists of myocardium, there is a certain amount of collagenous tissue in the central part of the heart, to which are attached the heart valves and the ventricular and atrial musculature. This fibrous "skeleton" consists of the valve rings (annuli) of the mitral, tricuspid, and aortic valves, bound together by collagenous bands or "ligaments" known by terms such as *right* and *left fibrous trigones, central fibrous body,* and *intervalvar fibrosa* (Figures 12-25 and 12-26). The membranous ventricular septum may be regarded as a component or extension of the cardiac skeleton. Although the cardiac skeleton itself cannot be identified by echocardiography or other imaging as a sepa-

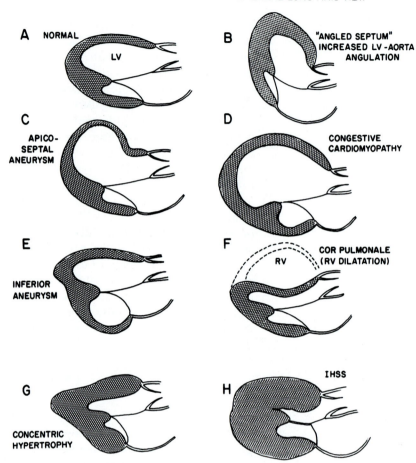

LEFT VENTRICULAR PROFILES IN PARASTERNAL LONG-AXIS VIEW

A NORMAL

B "ANGLED SEPTUM" INCREASED LV-AORTA ANGULATION

C APICO-SEPTAL ANEURYSM

D CONGESTIVE CARDIOMYOPATHY

E INFERIOR ANEURYSM

F COR PULMONALE (RV DILATATION)

G CONCENTRIC HYPERTROPHY

H IHSS

Figure 12–23. Diagram showing various LV configurations, in long axis, commonly encountered in clinical practice. They vary in chamber size, chamber shape, and LV wall/septal thickness.

rate structure or structures, it is important to the cardiologist or sonographer for certain reasons:

1. Infection tends to spread into and along these fibrous rings and "ligaments" from infected valves, resulting in paravalvar ring abscess and subsequently (in some cases) LV pseudoaneurysms or fistulous tracks.

2. Increasing sclerosis and even calcification of the collagenous cardiac skeleton is common in the elderly, sometimes referred to as *Lev's disease,* after Dr. Maurice Lev of Chicago, who studied the pathology several decades ago. Calcification in the region of the fibrous trigones is responsible for unusual dense, well-defined echoes apparently in the LV outflow tract. An example of such calcification, infrequent but not excessively rare, is shown in Figure 12-27. There is never Doppler evidence of LV outflow obstruction; in this respect and in its longitudinal (rather than transverse) alignment in the LV outflow tract, it differs from fixed subvalvar aortic stenosis.

3. Occasionally, such calcification is associated with ECG changes of atrioventricular block, needing pacemaker therapy; however, this is a rare cause of heart block, perhaps unexpectedly so considering that the bundle of His passes through a narrow canal or opening in the central fibrous body.

LEFT VENTRICULAR CONTOURS IN APICAL 4 CHAMBER VIEW

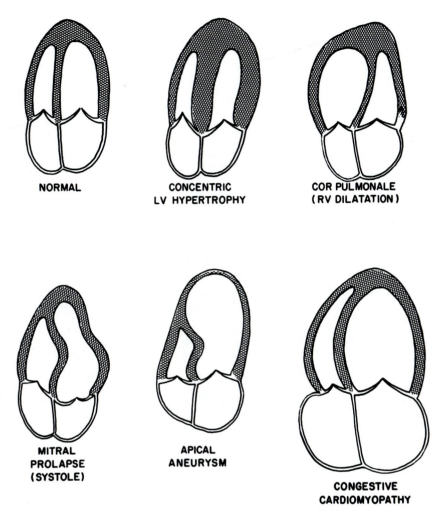

Figure 12–24. Diagram showing some common LV configurations in the apical four-chamber view. The three variables are chamber size and shape and wall thickness.

VENTRICULAR SEPTUM

This structure, of great interest to echocardiographers since the early years of cardiac ultrasound, was mentioned earlier in this chapter. Its abnormal anatomy in hypertrophic cardiomyopathy is dealt with in Chapter 13 and its infarction and rupture in Chapter 14. Congenital ventricular septal defects (VSDs) can occur in various locations (Figure 12-28), identifiable on 2D echo and by colorflow Doppler, which images the high-velocity jet crossing the septal defect. Figure 12-29 illustrates the different locations of the common membranous type of VSD and acquired (post-myocardial infarction) VSD.

The topic of ventricular interdependence was mentioned earlier. Although essentially an issue of pathophysiology, its anatomic basis is abnormal curvature of the septum toward the RV or LV. In extreme spheric dilatation of the LV chambers, the septum bulges conspicuously into the RV chamber; the reverse is true for extreme RV dilatation. In some patients with pericardial constriction, the ventricular septum bulges toward the LV even though the RV is not dilated (Figure 12-30).

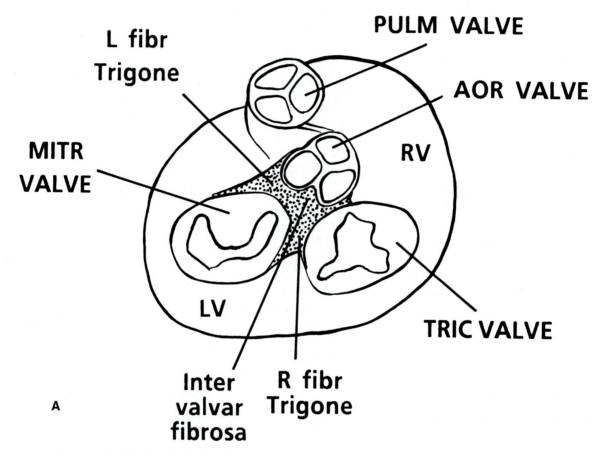

A

Figure 12–25. (A) Diagram showing view of heart from above after removal of both atria, aorta, and pulmonary trunk to show anatomic relationships of the four valves and of the fibrous cardiac skeleton (stippled area) binding the mitral, tricuspid, and aortic valve rings together. (B) Diagrams to show anatomy of the aortic root–septal-mitral-tricuspid junction in longitudinal planes (AR, aortic root; RA, right atrium; STL, septal tricuspid leaflet; RV, right ventricle; LV, left ventricle; AML, anterior mitral leaflet; PER, pericardial reflection). The stippled area below is bare of pericardium. Arrow indicates intervalvar fibrosa.

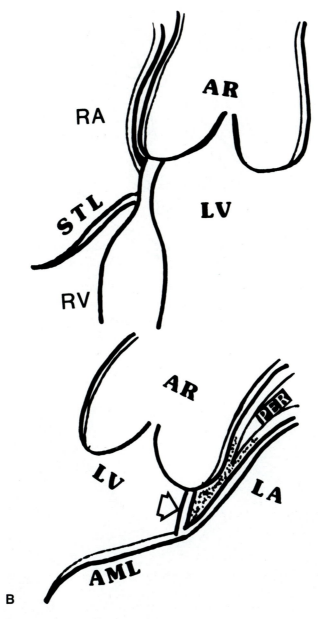

B

Figure 12-25 (*Continued*)

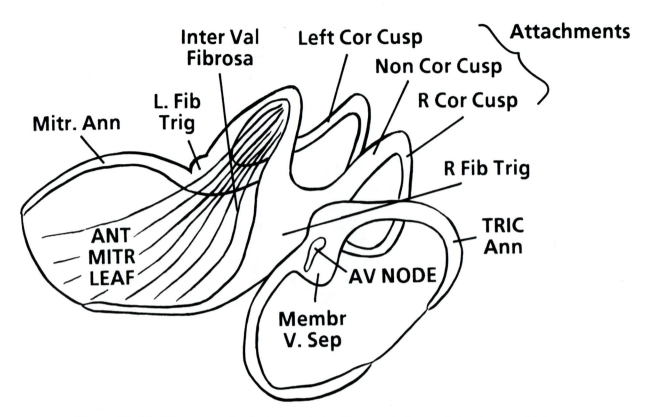

Figure 12–26. Diagrammatic depiction of the fibrous skeleton of the heart, which includes the mitral, tricuspid, and aortic valve rings, as well as the right and left fibrous trigones and intervalvar fibrosa connecting aortic annulus to anterior mitral leaflet.

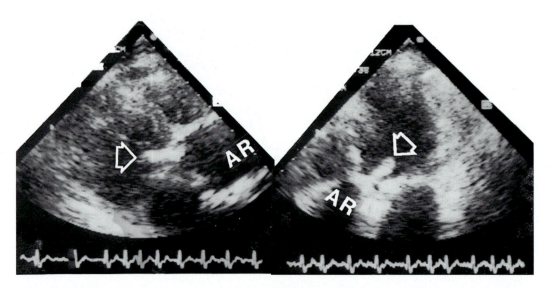

Figure 12–27. Parasternal long-axis view (left) and apical four-chamber view (right) showing uncommon longitudinal calcification in the vicinity of LV outflow tract (arrows). No LV outflow obstruction was detectable by pulsed-wave Doppler.

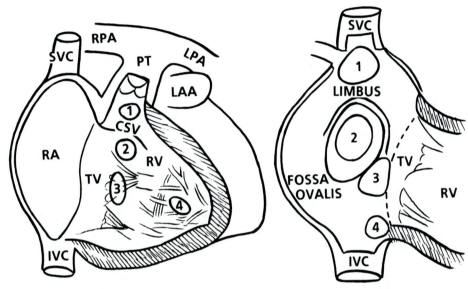

SITES OF VENTRICULAR SEPTAL DEFECT FROM RV SIDE

1- SUPRACRISTAL   2- INFRACRISTAL

3- POSTERIOR   4- MUSCULAR

SITES OF ATRIAL SEPTAL DEFECTS FROM RA SIDE

1- SINUS VENOSUS TYPE

2- OSTIUM SECUNDUM TYPE

3- OSTIUM PRIMUM TYPE

4- CORONARY SINUS TYPE

Figure 12–28. Diagram showing sites of different varieties of ventricular septal defects (left) and atrial septal defects (right).

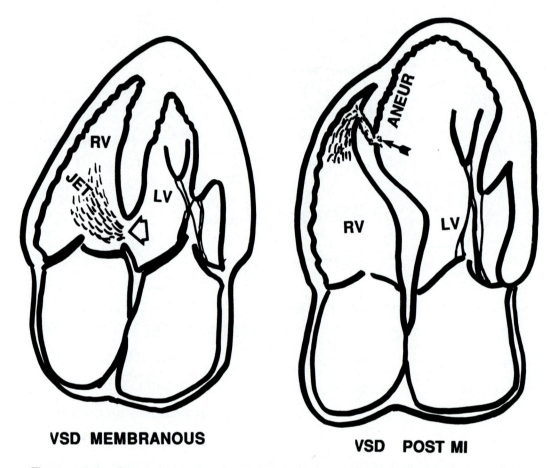

VSD MEMBRANOUS   **VSD   POST MI**

Figure 12–29. Diagram of apical four-chamber view in congenital membranous type ventricular septal defect (left) and postmyocardial infarction variety (right).

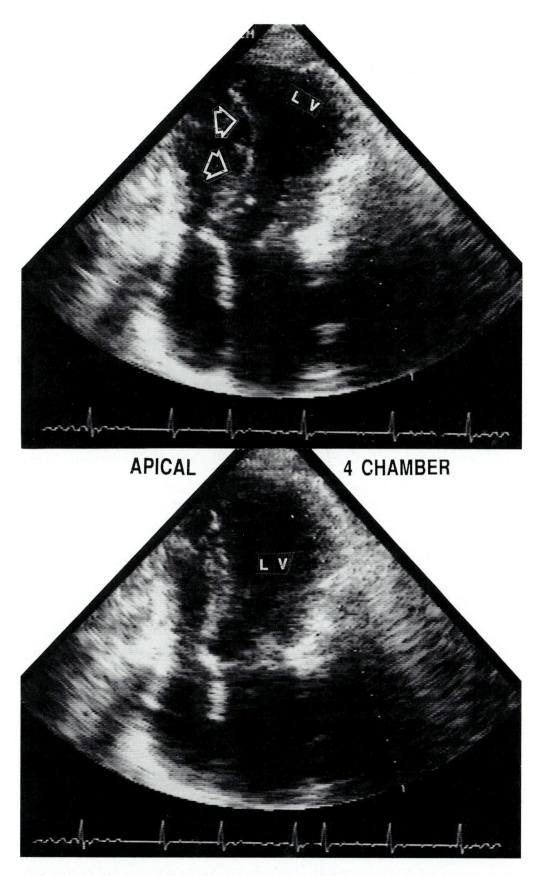

APICAL   4 CHAMBER

Figure 12–30. Apical four-chamber view showing abnormal convexity of ventricular septum toward the LV more prominent in early diastole (above) than in systole (below). This patient had constrictive pericarditis and exhibited an early diastolic "septal bounce" on real-time viewing.

REFERENCES

1. Geiser EA, Bove KE. Calculation of left ventricular mass and relative wall thickness. Arch Pathol 1974;97:13.
2. Eckner FAO, Brown BW, Davidson DL, et al. Dimensions of normal human hearts. Arch Pathol 1969;88:497.
3. Applied anatomy of the heart, in ER Giuliani (ed): Cardiology: Fundamentals and Practice. St. Louis: Mosby–Year Book, 1991, p 77.
4. Goor D, Lillehei CW, Edwards JE. The "sigmoid septum": Variation in the contour of the left ventricular outlet. AJR 1969;107:366.
5. Rosenquist GC, Sweeney LJ. The membranous ventricular septum in the normal heart. Johns Hopkins Med J 1974;135:9.
6. Rushmer RF, Cardiovascular Dynamics. WB Saunders, Philadelphia, 1970.
7. Hutchins GM, Anaya OA. Measurements of cardiac size, chamber volumes and valve orifices at autopsy. Johns Hopkins Med J 1973;133:96.
8. Hutchins GM, Bulkley BH, Moore GW, et al. Shape of the human cardiac ventricles. Am J Cardiol 1978;41:646.
9. Kitzman DW, Scholz DG, Hagen PT, et al. Age-related changes in normal human hearts during the first 10 decades of life. Mayo Clin Proc 1988;63:126.
10. Maron BJ, Henry WL, Roberts WC, et al. Comparison of echocardiographic and necropsy measurements of ventricular wall thickness in patients with or without disproportionate septal thickening. Circulation 1977;55:341.
11. Belenkie I, MacDonald RPR, Smith ER. Localized septal hypertrophy. Am Heart J 1988;115:385.
12. Bradfield JWB, Beck G, Vecht RJ. Left ventricular apical thin point. Br Heart J 1977;39:806.
13. Roberts WG, Cohen LS. Left ventricular papillary muscles. Circulation 1972;46:138.
14. Chiechi MA, Lees WM, Thompson R. Functional anatomy of the normal mitral valve. J Thorac Surg 1956;32:378.
15. Waller BF, Roberts WC. Cardiovascular disease in the very elderly. Am J Cardiol 1983;51:403.
16. Lenkiewicz JE, Davies MJ, Rosen D. Collagen in human myocardium as a function of age. Cardiovasc Res 1972;62:549.
17. Goor D, Lillehei CW, Edwards JE. The "sigmoid septum": Variation in the contour of the left ventricular outlet. AJR 1969;107:366.
18. Nishimura T, Kondo M, Umadome H, et al. Echocardiographic features of false tendons in the left ventricle. Am J Cardiol 1981;48:177.
19. Turner W. Heart with moderate band in left ventricle. J Anat Physiol 1893;27:373.
20. Roberts WC. Anomalous left ventricular band. Am J Cardiol 1969;23:735.
21. Pomerance A. Rarities and miscellaneous endocardial abnormalities, in A Pomerance, MJ Davies (eds): The Pathology of the Heart. Oxford, England: Blackwell Scientific, 1975, p 483.
22. Boyd MT, Seward JB, Tajik AJ, et al. Frequency and location of prominent left ventricular trabeculations at autopsy in 474 normal human hearts. J Am Coll Cardiol 1987;9:323.
23. Gerlis LM, Wright HM, Wilson N, et al. Left ventricular bands: A normal anatomic feature. Br Heart J 1984;52:641.
24. Keren A, Billingham ME, Popp RL. Echocardiographic recognition and implications of ventricular hypertrophic trabeculations and aberrant bands. Circulation 1984;70:836.
25. Vered Z, Meltzer RS, Benjamin P, et al. Prevalence and significance of false tendons in the left ventricle as determined by echocardiography. Am J Cardiol 1984;53:330.
26. Luetmer PH, Edwards WD, Seward JB, et al. Incidence and distribution of left ventricular false tendons. J Am Coll Cardiol 1987;9:323.
27. Choo MH, Chia BL, Wu DC, et al. Anomalous chordae tendineae: A source of echocardiographic confusion. Angiology 1982;33:756.
28. Walmsley R. Anatomy of the left ventricular outflow tract. Br Heart J 1979;41:263.
29. Davis RH, Feigenbaum H, Chang S, et al. Echocardiographic manifestations of discrete subvalvar aortic stenosis. Am J Cardiol 1974;33:277.
30. Popp RL, Silverman JF, French JW, et al. Echocardiographic findings in discrete subvalvar aortic stenosis. Circulation 1974;49:226.
31. Krueger SK, French JW, Forker AD, et al. Echocardiography in discrete subaortic stenosis. Circulation 1979;59:506.
32. Weyman AE, Feigenbaum H, Hurwitz RA, et al. Cross-sectional echocardiography in evaluating patients with discrete subaortic stenosis. Am J Cardiol 1976;37:358.

33. Shore DF, Smallhorn J, Stark J, et al. Left ventricular outflow tract obstruction coexisting with ventricular septal defect. Br Heart J 1982;48:421.

34. Motro M, Schneeweiss A, Shem-Tov A, et al. Two-dimensional echocardiography in discrete subaortic stenosis. Am J Cardiol 1984;53:896.

35. Wilcox WD, Seward JB, Hagler DJ, et al. Discrete subaortic stenosis. Mayo Clin Proc 1980;55:425.

36. Disessa TG, Hagan AD, Isabel-Jones JB, et al. Two-dimensional echocardiographic evaluation of discrete subaortic stenosis from the apical long axis view. Am Heart J 1981;101:774.

37. Tencate FJ, Van Dorp WG, Hugenholtz PG, et al. Fixed subaortic stenosis: Value of echocardiography for diagnosis and differentiation between various types. Br Heart J 1979;41:159.

38. Gnanapragasam JP, Houston AB, Doig WB, et al. Transesophageal echocardiographic assessment of fixed subaortic obstruction in children. Br Heart J 1991;66:281.

39. Mugge A, Daniel WG, Wolpers HG, et al. Improved visualization of discrete subvalvular aortic stenosis by transesophageal color-coded Doppler echocardiography. Am Heart J 1989;117:474.

40. Schwinger ME, Kronzon I. Improved evaluation of left ventricular outflow tract obstruction of transesophageal echocardiography. J Am Soc Echocardiogr 1989;2:191.

41. Ascuitto RJ, Ross-Ascuitto NT, Kopf GS, et al. Accessory mitral valve tissue causing left ventricular outflow obstruction. Ann Thorac Surg 1986;42:581.

42. Sahn DJ, DeMaria A, Kisslo J, et al. Recommendations regarding quantitation in M-mode echocardiography: Results of a survey of echocardiographic methods. Circulation 1978;58:1072.

43. Devereaux RB, Reichek N. Echocardiographic determination of left ventricular mass in man. Circulation 1977;55:613.

44. Henry WL, Clark CE, Epstein SE. Asymmetric septal hypertrophy. Circulation 1973;47:225.

45. DeMaria AN, Neumann A, Schubart PJ, et al. Systematic correlation of cardiac chamber size and ventricular performance determined with echocardiography and alterations in heart rate in normal persons. Am J Cardiol 1979;43:1.

46. Belenkie I. Beat to beat variability of echocardiographic measurements of left ventricular end-diastolic diameter and performance. J Clin Ultrasound 1979;7:263.

47. Felner JM, Blumenstein BA, Schlant RC, et al. Sources in variability of echocardiographic measurements. Am J Cardiol 1980;45:995.

48. Brenner JI, Wangh RA. Effect of phasic respiration on left ventricular dimension and performance in a normal population. Circulation 1978;57:122.

49. Vignola PA, Bloch A, Kaplan AD, et al. Interobserver variability in echocardiography. J Clin Ultrasound 1977;5:238.

50. Monoson PA, O'Rourke RA, Crawford MH, et al. Measurement of left ventricular wall thickness and systolic thickening by M-mode echocardiography: Interobserver and intrapatient echocardiography. J Clin Ultrasound 1978;6:252.

51. Pollick C, Fitzgerald PJ, Popp RL. Variability of digitalized echocardiography: Size, source and means of reduction. Am J Cardiol 1983;51:576.

52. Bett JHN, Dryburgh LG. Beat to beat variation in echocardiographic measurements of left ventricular dimensions and function. J Clin Ultrasound 1981;9:119.

53. Clark RD, Viorcuska K, Cohn K. Serial echocardiographic evaluation of left ventricular function in valvular disease, including reproducibility guidelines for serial studies. Circulation 1980;62:564.

54. Pietro DA, Voelkel GA, Ray BJ, et al. Reproducibility of echocardiography: A study evaluating the variability of serial echocardiographic measurements. Chest 1981;79:29.

55. Lapido GOA, Dunn FG, Pringle TH, et al. Serial measurements of left ventricular dimensions by echocardiography. Br Heart J 1980;44:284.

56. Dodge HT, Sandler H, Ballew DW, et al. Use of biplane angiocardiography for the measurement of left ventricular volume in man. Am Heart J 1960;60:762.

57. Kan G, Visser CA, Lie KI, et al. Left ventricular volumes and ejection fraction by single plane two-dimensional apex echocardiography. Eur Heart J 1981;2:337.

58. Carr KW, Engler RL, Forsythe JR, et al. Measurement of left ventricular ejection fraction by mechanical cross-sectional echocardiography. Circulation 1979;59:1196.

59. Schiller NB, Acquatella H, Ports TA, et al. Left ventricular volume from paired biplane two-dimensional echocardiography. Circulation 1979;60:547.

60. Erbel R, Schweizer P, Meyer J, et al. Left ventricular volume and ejection fraction determination by cross-sectional echocardiography in patients with coronary artery disease. Clin Cardiol 1980;3:377.

61. Quinones MA, Waggoner AD, Reduto LA, et al. A new, simplified and accurate method for determining ejection fraction with two-dimensional echocardiography. Circulation 1981;64:744.

62. Folland ED, Parisi AF, Moynihan PF, et al. Assessment of left ventricular ejection fraction and volumes by real-time, two-dimensional echocardiography. Circulation 1979;60:760.

63. Mercier JC, Disessa TG, Jarmarani JM, et al. Two-dimensional echocardiographic assessment of left ventricular volume and ejection fraction in children. Circulation 1982;65:962.

64. Wyatt HL, Heng MK, Meerbaum S, et al. Cross-sectional echocardiography: I. Analysis of mathematical models for quantifying mass of the left ventricle in dogs. Circulation 1979;60:1164.

65. Schiller NB, Shah PM, Crawford M, et al. Recommendations for quantitation of the left ventricle by two-dimensional echocardiography. J Am Soc Echocardiogr 1989;2:358.

66. Tortoledo FA, Quinones MA, Fernandez GC, et al. Quantification of left ventricular volumes by two-dimensional echocardiography. Circulation 1983;67:579.

13

Left Ventricular Hypertrophy and Hypertrophic Cardiomyopathy

Early attempts to diagnose left ventricular (LV) hypertrophy were based on M-mode measurements of thickness of the LV wall and ventricular septum (Figure 13-1).[1-3] The range, mean, and standard deviation of normal values were obtained from recordings of normal populations (subjects with no detectable heart disease). Autopsy validation of LV wall thickness measurements is not suitable for corresponding values during life, because postmortem hearts tend to be in a contracted state (cardiac rigor mortis). Autopsy measurements of septal or LV wall thickness correlate better with end-systolic rather than end-diastolic measurements during life.[4] Initial studies of M-mode LV wall thickness in hypertensive patients established the superiority of echocardiography to electrocardiography in diagnosing LV hypertrophy.

Normal adult values for septal thickness and LV posterior wall thickness (mean 9 mm, range 6 to 11 mm in both) were published two decades ago, have been very widely accepted, and are still quoted.[5] Measurements are made at end-diastole (onset of QRS complex or R peak) in parasternal view at mitral chordae level.

Normal LV wall thickness increases gradually with age from a mean of 7.7 mm in the third decade to 8.9 mm in the fifth decade.[6] Septal thickness likewise increases from a mean of 7.6 mm in normal young adults to 9.3 mm in normal middle-aged adults.

Gaasch[7] called attention to the fact that the ratio of end-diastolic LV radius to LV wall thickness (*R/Th* ratio) has a constant relationship to LV systolic pressure in normal children and adults, as well as in the "physiologic hypertrophy of athletes and those with

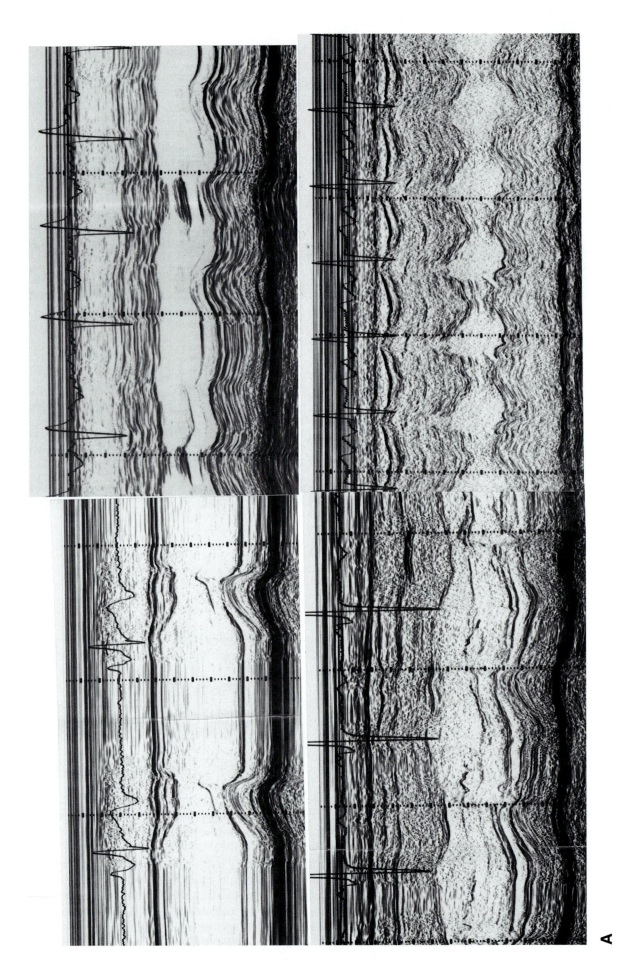

A

Figure 13–1. (See legend on following page.)

M MODE ECHO

2-D ECHO

LONG AXIS

SHORT AXIS

NORMAL

LONG AXIS

SHORT AXIS

ASH

B

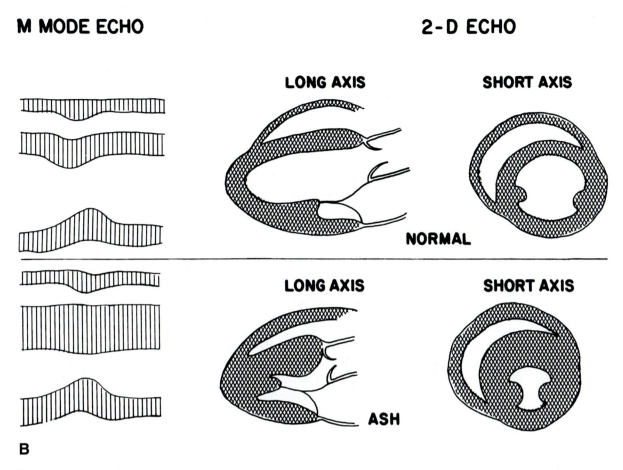

Figure 13–1. (A) M-mode of normal (above, left), mild to moderate concentric LVH (below, left), severe LVH (below, right), and amyloid heart (above, right). (B) Diagram of M-mode (left) and 2D (right) echo in normal (above) and asymmetrical septal hypertrophy (ASH).

compensated chronic aortic regurgitation."[7] Gaasch found this *R/Th* ratio in normal individuals to be 3.0 ± 0.7. Abnormally high values of this ratio signify "inadequate hypertrophy" in disease states such as dilated cardiomyopathy or volume overload; an abnormally low value of the *R/Th* ratio is the rule in compensated severe hypertension or aortic stenosis.

If left ventricular internal dimension (LVID), wall thickness, and peak systolic pressure (approximated by cuff systolic blood pressure) are known, a simplified formula for LV wall stress is *P(R/Th)*, where *P* is the systolic blood pressure. More elaborate formulas are available for estimating meridional and circumferential LV wall stress. For a detailed description and discussion of the methodology of M-mode LV measurements pertaining to criteria for LV hypertrophy, the reader is referred to the publications of Devereux et al.,[8] Levy et al.,[9] and Liebson et al.[10]

LEFT VENTRICULAR MASS

The detection and quantification of LV hypertrophy (LVH) are of much interest to physicians caring for hypertensive patients. For decades the electrocardiogram (ECG) was the only indicator available for this purpose, but the ECG has been amply demonstrated to be very insensitive for LVH; ECG criteria of LVH are satisfied only when LVH is severe.

LVH can be diagnosed in the presence of an abnormally thick ventricular septum and LV posterior wall (>11 mm). Better quantitation of LVH was obtained by estimating LV mass, first derived from the M-mode echo by various groups in the early 1970s.[11-13] This is done by estimating the volume of the LV myocardial "shell," which is the difference between the external volume of the LV and the LV chamber volume. LV mass is then obtained by multiplying the estimated LV myocardial volume by 1.04, the specific gravity of myocardium. Formulas such as that of Troy et al.[11] were used widely in early LV mass studies but not validated by anatomic correlation. Devereux and Reichek[14] were the first to correlate echocardiographic LV mass estimates with LV specimens of the same hearts at autopsy. They tested various geometric formulas and different methods of measuring wall thickness and LVID and found that anatomic LV mass correlated best with LV measurements by the Penn convention ($r = 0.96$) using the following empirical equation:

$$LV \text{ mass} = 1.04[(IVST + LVID + PWT)^3 - LVID^3] - 13.6 \text{ g}$$

where IVST is interventricular septal thickness, PWT is LV posterior wall thickness, and LVID is LV internal dimension (end-diastole).

Devereux et al.[15] confirmed the validity of this method in a further study ($r = 0.92$). Using the American Society of Echocardiography (ASE) method of measuring septal and LV wall thicknesses, Devereux[17] (in 52 patients) and Woythaler et al.[16] (in 50 patients) found a good correlation between echocardiographic and anatomic LV mass ($r = 0.90$ and 0.81, respectively) but a tendency for echocardiographic LV mass to consistently overestimate the actual LV mass by about 20%. This error can be corrected by the formula LV mass = 0.80 • LV mass ASE + 0.6 g.

Combining Devereux's 1977 and 1986 studies of LV mass by the Penn convention, this method was proved quite reliable, with 97% sensitivity and 89% specificity, using 215 g as the cutoff value between normal and increased LV mass.

Devereux et al.[15] also assessed the extent to which the echo-estimated LV mass deviated from the actual anatomic LV mass. In the studies quoted above, by Penn convention or ASE method of measurement, the standard deviation varied from 29 to 47 g. A higher standard deviation can be expected in patients with asymmetrical abnormal LV shapes (LV infarction with or without aneurysm, or right ventricular dilatation[18]).

The standard deviation for repeat LV mass estimations, in individuals with stable cardiac status, is quoted as 30 g or less,[17] a fact of some significance to clinicians as well as those studying various interventions or natural history of hypertensives. The standard deviation of mean LV mass in groups of patients being compared during an investigative study is as low as 20 g for some small groups and 10 g for large groups.

Studies examining the normal limits for LV mass in populations categorized by sex, age, body surface area, and other factors have been performed by Valdez et al.,[19] Gardin et al.,[20] Henry et al.,[21] and Devereux et al.[8] It appears that body surface area correlates best with estimated LV mass. However, men have greater LV mass even after normalizing for body surface area, e.g., 6% or 7% higher in Gardin's series. In Devereux's series, LV wall mass was 89 ± 21 g/m^2 in normal men and 69 ± 19 g/m^2 in normal women. Devereux suggests a cutoff value of 134 g/m^2 in men and 110 g/m^2 in women as the levels above which LV hypertrophy should be diagnosed (97th percentile). LV mass also has been standardized by patient height; thus LV mass index (g/m) > 143 for men and 102 for women is sometimes used as criterion for LV hypertrophy using Penn Convention measurements.[9]

Echocardiography has been established as and remains the method of choice for diagnosing LV hypertrophy, being much more sensitive than ECG. Correlation of the latter with LV mass (estimated by echo or angio) is on the order of (r value) 0.4 to 0.7 using different sets of ECG criteria of LVH or combinations of them or even body surface mapping.

LV HYPERTROPHY IN HYPERTENSION

In four studies comparing estimated echocardiographic LV mass in hypertensive patients versus normal subjects using identical methods and one cutoff level for all individuals, LVH was present in 23% to 48% of hypertensive subjects and 0% to 10% of normal subjects.[22]

Sex

When sex-specific criteria for abnormally high LV mass are used (135 g in men and 110 g in women), a higher proportion of female than male hypertensive patients shows LVH, 43% to 61% versus 81% to 41%, respectively.[23]

Race

Hammond et al.[23] found no difference between whites and blacks in normal populations. However, black patients with essential hypertension have a greater degree of LVH than white patients with a similar level of clinically measured blood pressure.

Age

Increasing age and duration of hypertension were surprisingly not associated with a higher prevalence of LVH on echocardiography. However, there is a small subgroup of elderly hypertensive patients with symptoms of LV failure who have LVH, varying from mild to severe, and hyperdynamic LV contraction on echocardiography. Topol et al.[24] in 1985 described a group of 21 such patients under the term *hypertensive hypertrophic cardiomyopathy.*

The regression of increased LV mass (LVH) in hypertensives after administration of antihypertensive drugs[25] has led to large-scale serial echocardiographic studies in patients undergoing clinical trials of these drugs, as well as requests for echo follow-up of hypertensives under therapy. ACE inhibitors such as captopril and enalapril and sympatholytics such as methyldopa and calcium blockers have all been shown to result in LVH regression. On the other hand, arteriolar vasodilators such as hydralazine and minoxidil do not result in regression of LVH; conflicting data have accumulated with respect to diuretics and beta blockers.

The presence and severity of LV hypertrophy in hypertensive patients are of great importance because it has been amply demonstrated that the prognosis and incidence of cardiac complications correlate better with LV hypertrophy than with any other factor in a hypertensive population. The physician's choice of therapeutic measures, i.e., incremental use of drugs or drug combinations to reduce blood pressure to normal levels, depends on the echo diagnosis of LV hypertrophy.

In a study of 844 mildly hypertensive subjects (average blood pressure 140/91 mmHg), Liebson et al.[10] found that 15.4% had LV hypertrophy by the criteria of 134 g/m^2 for men and 110 g/m^2 for women; by the LV mass index criteria of 143 g/m^2 for men and 102 g/m^2 for women, 32.2% had LV hypertrophy.

LV Shape

It has long been known that patients with moderate to severe LV pressure overload (systemic arterial hypertension or aortic valve stenosis) have heavier left ventricles with thicker walls, as well as alteration in LV chamber shape. These LV cavities are narrower (Figure 13-2) than normal (more elliptic) or in more extreme cases almost tubular in shape. This is not true for patients with low ejection fractions, in whom the LV is normal or even wide (tendency to spheric) in shape (Figure 13-3).

In recent years an attempt has been made to classify LV anatomic features in hypertensives, as assessed by two-dimensional (2D) echo, into subcategories based on LV size, LV mass, and relative LV wall thickness. Unfortunately, the different groups[10,26,27] who have done excellent work on this important topic have not all used the same descriptive terminology.

In the series of Ganau et al.,[27] 165 patients with untreated essential hypertension (mean blood pressure at the time of echocardiography of 152/100 mmHg) were compared with 125 age- and gender-matched normal adults (mean BP 124/77). Of the hypertensives, 52% had a normal LV mass index as well as relative wall thickness (<0.44, which was the 99th percentile value in normal individuals); 13% had normal LV mass but increased relative wall thickness, i.e., *concentric remodeling;* 27% had increased LV mass with normal LV wall thickness, i.e., *eccentric hypertrophy;* and only 8% had *typical concentric hyper-*

APICAL 4 CHAMBER

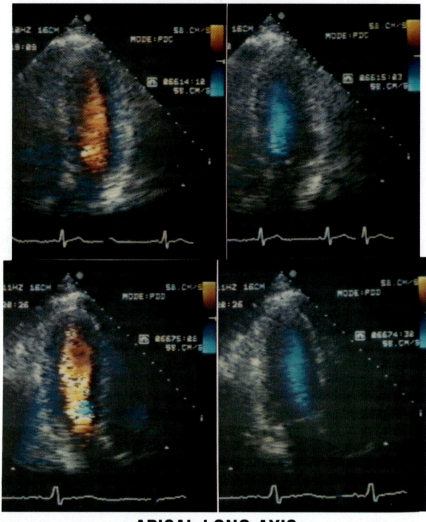

APICAL LONG AXIS

A

Figure 13–2. (A) Apical four-chamber view (above) and apical long-axis view (below) showing narrow elliptical LV chamber. The patient had concentric hypertrophy due to essential hypertension. Compared with the diastolic frames (left), the late systolic frames (right) show some narrowing, but not obliteration, of the LV cavity. (B) 2D echo in parasternal views in diastole and systole showing concentric LV hypertrophy.

trophy with an increase in both LV mass and relative wall thickness. Figure 13-4 is based on these concepts of Ganau et al.[27] and in part modified from their graphic representation.

Instead of concentric LV remodeling, Liebson et al.[10] used the term *eccentric nondilated LV hypertrophy,* and Strauer used the term *irregular LV hypertrophy.* Liebson et al.[10] add an extra category of LV hypertrophy, *disproportionate septal hypertrophy,* wherein septal thickness is 1.5 greater than LV wall thickness.

In the large body of literature that has accumulated around the theme of LV hypertrophy in hypertensive patients, it is generally assumed or implied that the entire LV chamber is surrounded by a wall of uniform thickness or at most that the septum and LV free wall are each of the same thickness in all their extent. The truth is that some parts of the LV are often more hypertrophied than the rest. Thus Lewis and Maron,[28] using 2D echo to study the location of LV hypertrophy in 102 hypertensive patients who had LV wall

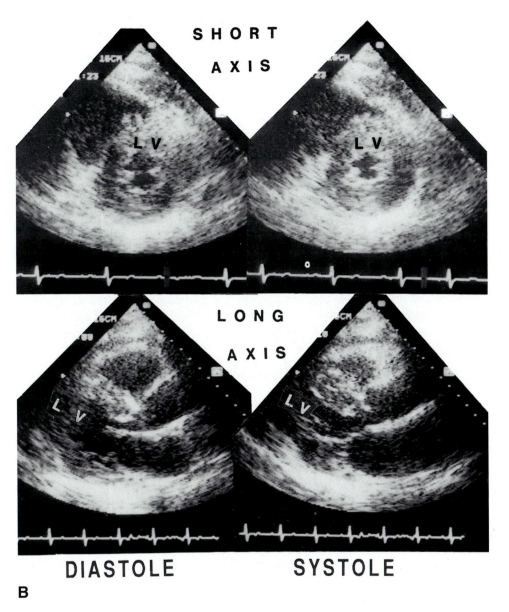

PARASTERNAL

SHORT AXIS

LV

LV

LONG AXIS

LV

LV

DIASTOLE

SYSTOLE

B

Figure 13–2. *(Continued)*

thicknesses greater than 15 mm, found an unexpected diversity of LV hypertrophy patterns. In one-third of patients the hypertrophy pattern was asymmetrical and nonuniform so that at least one segment of the LV was at least 1.5 times the thickness of any other. The ventricular septum alone was unduly hypertrophied in 27; only the anterior septum was hypertrophied in 11; and undue hypertrophy of some parts of septum as well as LV wall was seen in 16. The remaining 67 patients had concentric symmetrical LV hypertrophy.

HYPERTROPHIC CARDIOMYOPATHY (HCM)

It is generally accepted that this term refers to a hypertrophied nondilated left ventricle, in the absence of a cardiac or systemic disease[29,30]—such as aortic valve disease or systemic hypertension—which can itself produce LV hypertrophy. Epstein and Maron[29] quote

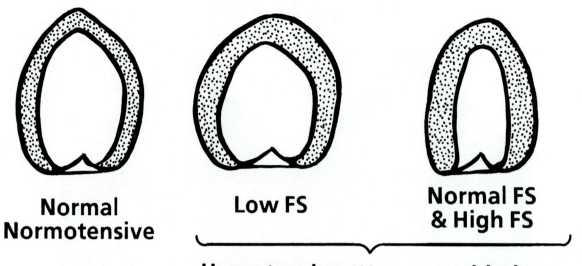

Normal Normotensive   **Low FS**   **Normal FS & High FS**

Hypertensive Hypertrophied Hearts

Figure 13–3. Diagram showing typical LV configurations in normal individuals (left), LV hypertrophy with subnormal ejection fraction, LV dilatation and spherical shape (center), LV hypertrophy with small LV chamber and normal to increased ejection fraction (right).

over 50 names that have been used for this entity over the last 35 years. To the preceding basic definition may be added the additional common features (1) hypertrophy of the ventricular septum exceeding that of the LV wall, (2) a hyperdynamic LV with unduly high ejection fraction (this is due to very vigorous LV wall contraction, whereas the very thick septum is in fact akinetic or hypokinetic), and (3) the frequent presence of LV outflow tract obstruction. The latter was thought initially to be an essential component of HCM, so the disorder was known formerly as *idiopathic hypertrophic subaortic stenosis* (IHSS) in America and *hypertrophic obstructive cardiomyopathy* (HOCM) in Europe. It later became evident that LV outflow obstruction often was absent, so the term *hypertrophic cardiomyopathy* (HCM) has been very widely accepted in recent years, often qualified by the phrase that LV outflow obstruction is or is not present in a particular patient.

At autopsy, heart weight is increased; this is due to considerable myocardial hypertrophy, and the LV chamber is unduly small. In a typical case, a longitudinal section through the LV shows conspicuous thickening of the ventricular septum, which bulges into the LV chamber, reducing the latter to a narrow, curved slit. Hypertrophied papillary muscles encroach further on LV chamber space. During systole, the dynamic juxtaposition of bulging septum and thick papillary muscles may be responsible for causing dynamic muscular intraventricular obstruction (Figure 13-5).

An important echocardiographic feature of HCM is systolic anterior motion (SAM) of the anterior mitral leaflet. The anatomic basis of this finding is systolic buckling of the edge of this leaflet where the chordae tendineae are attached, such that it protrudes into the LV outflow and may impact the ventricular septum in the latter half of systole. A contact lesion—a mural plaque or patch—is often manifest on the left septal surface at this site and constitutes good autopsy evidence that LV outflow obstruction and SAM had been present during life. The repetitive trauma of such mitral-septal contact is probably responsible also for local thickening of the anterior mitral leaflet. Bacterial endocarditis is known to occur at this location in HCM patients.[31]

At autopsy, as well as on echocardiography, severe or even massive hypertrophy of the ventricular septum is the most striking feature of the HCM heart. It was the prime feature in the original anatomic description of HCM by Teare,[32] a British forensic pathologist who encountered it in several cases of sudden death in young individuals. The ventricu-

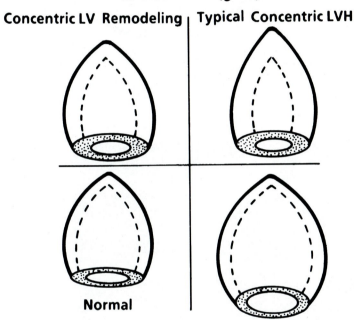

Figure 13–4. Diagram depicting four varieties of anatomic left ventricles in patients with systemic hypertension. (Above) Relative LV wall thickness is plotted against LV mass index. The vertical line (cutoff) separating increased LV mass from normal LV mass was 106 g/m² for women and 111 g/m² for men in this study. (Below) The differences in size, shape, and wall thickness of the four varieties of LV chamber are shown diagrammatically.

lar septum is usually 1.6 cm or more in thickness and may be as much as 4 cm thick; by contrast, the LV free wall shows only mild hypertrophy (12 to 14 mm). In 2% to 20% of HCM patients (in various series), LV hypertrophy is symmetrical (concentric), with equal thickness of the septum and LV wall.

Shape of the Hypertrophied Septum

Viewed from the LV side, the normal ventricular septum is concave longitudinally (from base to apex) and also concave in transverse section. It was shown in postmortem hearts,[33] as well as on 2D echo,[34] that in HCM the ventricular septum is of abnormal catenoid shape; i.e., from the LV side, the septum remains concave in transverse planes but is convex from base to apex. A *catenoid* object is a curved surface with the property of zero curvature at all points.[35] Tension within a structure of zero curvature produces no pressure on the surrounding fluid; the catenoid septum of HCM therefore plays little or no part in normal LV "squeeze" or pump function. It has been suggested that the inordinate septal hypertrophy in HCM and even the typical histologic finding (muscle fiber disarray) might arise from the unique abnormal mechanics of a catenoid-shaped septum.[34] In HCM,

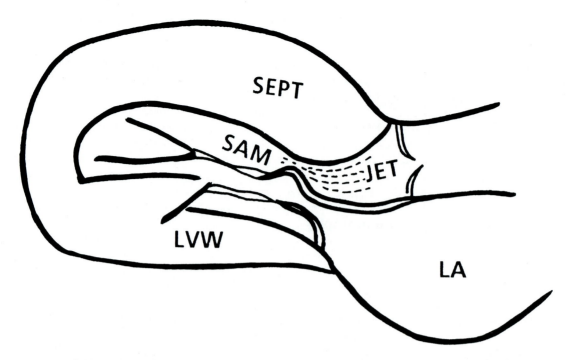

HYPERTROPHIC CARDIOMYOPATHY

A

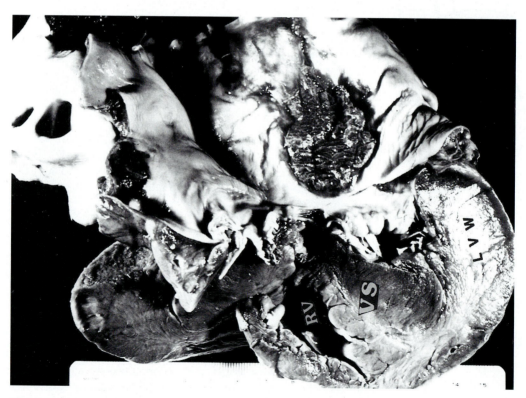

B

Figure 13–5. (A) Salient anatomic and echo features of HCM: thick bulging ventricular septum (SEPT), more hypertrophied than LV wall (LVW), small LV chamber, left atrial (LA) enlargement, abnormal systolic anterior motion (SAM) with LV outflow obstruction causing high-velocity jet. (B) Autopsy specimen of HCM showing massive septal hypertrophy (VS), less LV wall (LVW) hypertrophy, small LV chamber, and left atrial thrombus (arrows), the latter an unusual complication.

the LV free wall contracts hyperdynamically, which may be an attempt to compensate for the akinetic septum or may be an integral element of the myocardial abnormality.

The small size and narrow conical shape of the LV chamber in HCM are familiar to angiocardiographers and pathologists. Typically, in longitudinal section, LV shape is crescentic, or that of a thin, curved wedge, as a result of the reversed curvature (bulging) of the ventricular septum into the LV cavity. While this LV shape is the rule in younger patients, it may be somewhat different in the elderly. Lever et al.[36] observed that the distinctive crescentic or curved wedge shape was present in 75% of patients below age 40; in patients over age 65, septal curvature was normal, but a common finding was a proximal septal bulge, i.e., a local septal protuberance just below the aortic valve, and LV shape was described as ovoid.

Maron et al.[37] studied variations in the location of LV hypertrophy in 125 patients with HCM and classified them into four types. Their type II was the most common pattern (52%), in which hypertrophy involved "substantial portions of both the ventricular septum and the LV free wall." In type I (10%), hypertrophy was restricted to the anterior basal septum, forming a mound or protuberance in long-axis views just below the aortic valve. In type III (20%), the anterior as well as posterior basal septum was hypertrophied, but the LV free wall was unaffected. In type IV, comprising the remaining 18%, hypertrophy was limited to unusual sites, either the posterior septum, anterolateral wall, or apical region.

The relative frequencies of various LV hypertrophy patterns have been considerably different in reports from different centers. Dissimilar criteria for categorization into different patterns have added to the apparent discrepancies. The Toronto group,[38] also with extensive HCM experience, classified their LV hypertrophy patterns into ventricular septal (90%), symmetrical (concentric) LV hypertrophy (5%), apical (3%), midventricular (1%), and posteroseptal and/or lateral wall (1%).

Although uncommon, some of these HCM subvarieties deserve special comment because their diagnosis rests mainly on 2D echo Doppler:

Apical HCM (Figures 13-6 and 13-7) was originally described in Japan; it is for unknown reasons relatively common there and in Israel.[39,40] However, it also occurs in North America. There seem to be two types of apical HCM: The first is the type originally reported in Japanese patients. The LV chamber has a distinctive shape resembling an ace-of-spades configuration. The ECG shows giant inverted T waves in precordial leads. No intraventricular gradient can be demonstrated. In the second type, a small poorly contractile apical LV segment is visualized that communicates with the basal LV chamber through a very narrow midventricular channel.[41] Giant negative T waves are not the rule; catheterization or Doppler (pulsed wave or colorflow) reveals a mid-LV gradient.

Midventricular obstruction was described as an HCM variant in 1975.[42] Further ex-

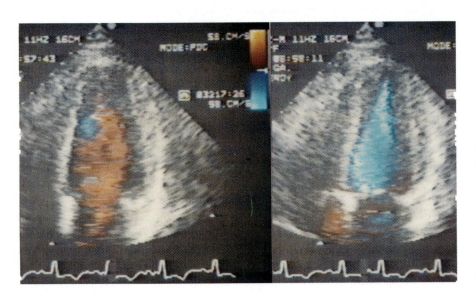

Figure 13–6. Apical four-chamber views at end-diastole (left) and systole (right). The LV chamber is outlined by colorflow Doppler. Note undue hypertrophy of the LV apical region causing an unusually pointed LV chamber apex. Giant T waves were present in V_4 to V_6.

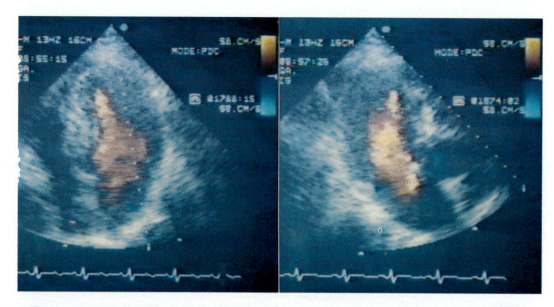

Figure 13–7. Apical four-chamber view (left) and long-axis view (right) with conspicuous hypertrophy of the apical half of the LV. LV chamber shape (depicted by colorflow Doppler) is unusual, with undue narrowing of the apex. The diagnostic "ace-of-spades" shape is seen at left.

amples were added by others, and there is some overlap with apical HCM, as mentioned above.[43] Severe dynamic LV obstruction is rare, but minor systolic gradients (up to 25 mmHg) are not uncommonly detected by Doppler techniques in narrow, hypertrophied LV chambers.

Hypertensive hypertrophic cardiomyopathy was described as a "new" entity by Topol et al.[44] in 1985. Their patients were mostly hypertensive elderly women who had hyperdynamic hypertrophied LV chambers on 2D echo. Such patients are not excessively rare in practice, but whether they should be labeled as a subgroup of HCM, as having hypertensive heart disease, or as having a separate syndrome has not been resolved.

A mild *proximal septal bulge* (local anterobasal septal hypertrophy) is so common in elderly patients that it may be considered a "normal variant" (Figures 13–8 to 13–12). It is frequently associated with the sigmoid septal contour[45] and a decreased angle between aortic root–LV long axis. Doppler does not reveal any LV outflow gradient. The patients reported by Belenkie et al.[46] probably belong in this category; however, by using the criterion that the hypertrophied basal septal segment should equal or exceed 1.7 times the thickness of the adjacent septum, these authors seem to have selected only the most pronounced or extreme examples of proximal septal bulge. This septal variant is more common in hypertensives (Figure 13–13) than normotensives.[46a] It should not be confused with HCM type I of Epstein and Maron,[29] in which the septal hypertrophy is usually more severe and SAM may be present, although exceptionally the sigmoid septum may coexist with HCM.[47] Thus a proximal septal bulge is usually *not* HCM.

Louie and Maron[48] described a subset of 34 HCM patients with extremely thick LV walls (20 to 30 mm thick in three-quarters of this group). Septal thickness also was extreme, even for HCM (30 to 50 mm). Despite such massive hypertrophy, two-thirds of the series had mild symptoms or none; 24 of the 34 (71%) had no evidence of LV outflow obstruction.

Asymmetrical Septal Hypertrophy

In the M-mode era, septal thickness exceeding LV posterior wall thickness by ratios greater than 1.3 and preferably 1.5 was considered a cardinal feature of HCM diagnosis. It soon became evident that septal thickness greater than LV posterior wall thickness could be observed on the M-mode tracing in a variety of circumstances. These included artefacts due to oblique intersection of the septum by the ultrasound beam and fallacious inclusion

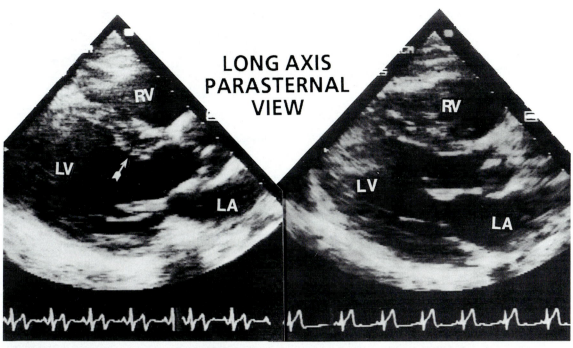

PROXIMAL SEPTAL BULGE   NORMAL

Figure 13–8. Parasternal long-axis views in a normal patient (right) and one with proximal septal bulge (left). The basal septum (arrow) is twice as thick as the midseptum.

of extraseptal echoes due to pacemaker wires, tricuspid chordae, or RV papillary muscles when measuring septal thickness. Even when the ventricular septum is measured correctly, easily done by 2D echo in multiple views, septal/LV wall ratios exceeding 1 and even 1.3 can be encountered in a number of situations[49] other than HCM:

1. Normal individuals—elderly, athletes
2. Conditions provoking LV hypertrophy, such as systemic hypertension,[50,51] aortic stenosis, or end-stage renal disease[52]

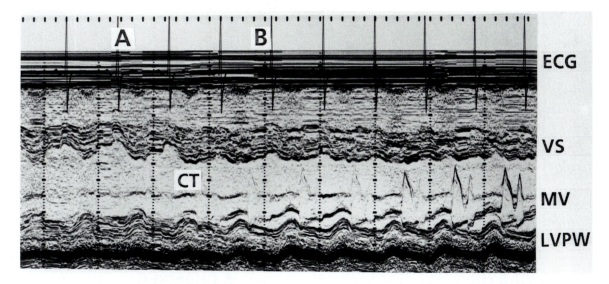

Figure 13–9. M-mode sweep from LV at chordae tendineae (CT) level to mitral valve level. Note that septal thickness increases from former to latter level because of the proximal septal bulge in latter. LV mass estimations would vary considerably depending on whether measurements are made at the first 4 beats (A) or next 4 beats (B).

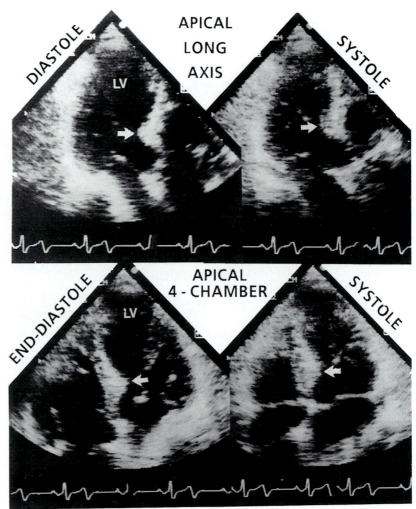

APICAL
LONG
AXIS

PROXIMAL SEPTAL BULGE

Figure 13–10. Apical long-axis view (above) and four-chamber view (below) showing proximal septal bulge (arrows) in diastole (left) and systole (right).

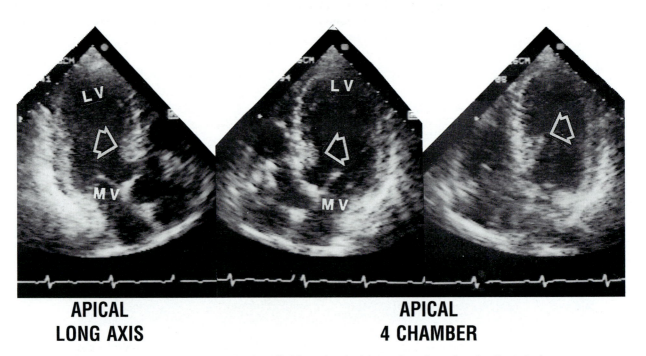

APICAL
LONG AXIS

APICAL
4 CHAMBER

Figure 13–11. Apical long-axis view (left) and apical four-chamber view in diastole (center) and systole (right). A conspicuous proximal septal bulge is evident (arrow) that is accentuated in systole (LV, left ventricle; MV, mitral valve).

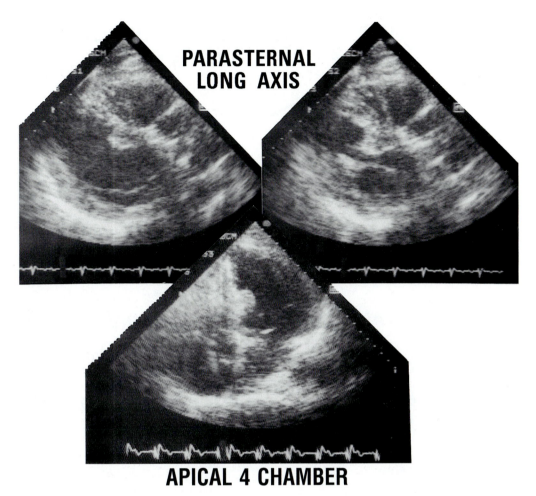

PARASTERNAL LONG AXIS

APICAL 4 CHAMBER

Figure 13–12. (Above) Parasternal long-axis view in diastole (left) and systole (right) showing a proximal septal bulge that is even more prominent in systole. (Below) Apical four-chamber view in another patient showing a local rounded septal prominence that could be mistaken for a thrombus or tumor.

3. Conditions provoking RV hypertrophy, including pulmonary hypertension or pulmonary stenosis[53]
4. Inferior wall infarction resulting in a thin akinetic wall (the septum may undergo compensatory hypertrophy)[54]
5. True hypertrophy of the septum simulated on the echocardiogram by unusual nonmyocardial material augmenting apparent septal size (this applied to a mural thrombus on the septum,[55] to septal infiltration by a lymphoma,[56] or even atypical unusual instances of cardiac amyloidosis[57])

Asymmetrical septal hypertrophy (ASH), with a septal/LV posterior wall ratio greater than 1.5 and a septal thickness greater than 15 mm, was at one time thought virtually diagnostic of HCM. It has since been shown to occur not only in normal athletes[58] but also in the various clinical conditions enumerated above (1 to 4) and, very importantly, in systemic hypertension.[51,59] The term *disproportionate septal hypertrophy* was applied to these instances of ASH if there was no evidence of HCM,[53,59,60] a useful custom to avoid the pitfall of equating ASH with HCM.

It was generally assumed that the anatomic LV hypertrophy pattern in hypertensive patients is usually symmetrical or concentric. Lewis and Maron,[28] who used 2D echo to study the distribution of hypertrophy in 102 hypertensive patients who had LV wall thickness of over 15 mm, observed that the distribution of hypertrophy in the 34 patients who

POSSIBLE EXPLANATION FOR PROXIMAL SEPTAL BULGE IN HYPERTENSIVES

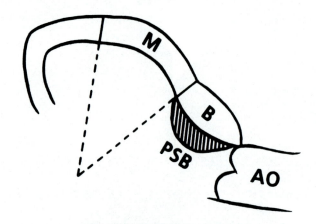

SEPTAL SEGMENT M IS MORE CURVED THAN SEGMENT B.
CONSEQUENTLY, WALL STRESS IS GREATER IN B THAN IN M.
THEREFORE PREFERENTIAL HYPERTROPHY OF B OCCURS, FORMING PROXIMAL SEPTAL BULGE (PSB)

Figure 13–13. Diagram depicting a possible explanation for the proximal septal bulge in hypertensive patients.

did not have concentric LV hypertrophy resembled the variants in LV hypertrophy patterns in HCM.

Mitral Regurgitation in HCM

Mitral regurgitation (MR) is very common in HCM. It was demonstrated in 11 of an early series of 12 HCM patients reported by Braunwald et al.[61] in 1960. Tunick et al.[62] found MR in three-fourths of 116 HCM patients in a more recent series using contemporary Doppler techniques. They found a strong relation between the degree of LV outflow obstruction and the severity of MR. Of 68 patients with little or no outflow obstruction, only 12% had moderate MR, and none had severe MR; moderate to severe MR was present in 55% of the others with severe resting LV outflow gradients.

It is postulated that abnormal systolic leaflet coaptation resulting from abnormal systolic anterior motion (SAM) of the anterior mitral leaflet[63] causes MR (Figure 13-14). However, some believe that this mechanism alone cannot account for MR in all cases; in other cases (perhaps about 20%),[64] anterior leaflet sclerosis secondary to contact trauma or associated mitral annulus calcification[65] is responsible. On colorflow Doppler, MR jets were commonly directed posteriorly in 18 of 20 patients studied by Rakowski et al.[66]

Dynamic Intraventricular Obstruction in HCM

Although this book deals with normal and abnormal cardiac anatomy rather than physiology, the pathophysiology of obstructive HCM is so closely related to anatomy that it needs to be discussed briefly here so that the echocardiographer can understand the M-mode, 2D, and Doppler aspects of this entity.

Originally thought to be an essential feature of HCM, LV outflow obstruction is now

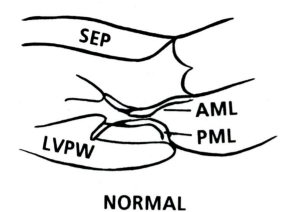

NORMAL

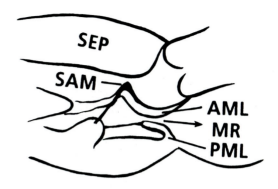

**HCM with SAM
ABNORMAL MITRAL
COAPTATION
and MR**

HCM

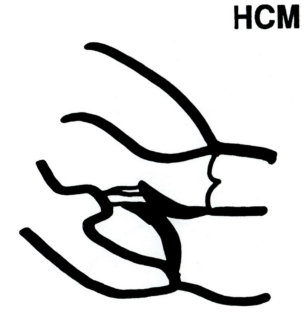

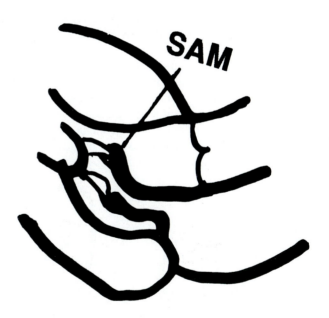

EARLY SYSTOLE

LATE SYSTOLE

Figure 13–14. Diagrams in parasternal long-axis view. (Left) Normal apposition of mitral leaflets. (Right) Abnormal apposition in HCM. The free edge of the anterior mitral leaflet beyond the site of apposition buckles anteriorly (SAM), and improper mitral leaflet apposition permits mitral regurgitation (MR). (Below) The mitral leaflet position changes from early to late systole.

estimated to be present in only 25% of all patients with HCM[67]; three types of obstruction within the LV chamber have been described in HCM[68,69]: (1) LV outflow tract obstruction at the site of anterior mitral leaflet–septal contact, (2) mid-LV obstruction, and (3) LV cavity obliteration (Figure 13–15).

LV outflow tract obstruction is by far the most common in obstructive HCM. On M-mode as well as 2D echo, the anterior mitral leaflet shows an abnormal rapid anterior motion that results in it abutting the septum (or in milder cases, closely approaching it) so that mitral-septal contact exists for a variable duration of middle to late systole. According to Wigle and Rakowski, "mitral leaflet systolic anterior motion could result from Venturi forces acting on the mitral leaflets, due to the rapid, nonobstructed early systolic ejection jet passing closer to the mitral leaflet than is normal, as a result of the outflow tract being narrowed by the ventricular septal hypertrophy."[66]

HCM patients with early-onset and prolonged mitral-septal contact (SAM) always have subaortic pressure gradients. Patients with no SAM or only mild incomplete SAM have little or no LV outflow gradient.[69-71] Pulsed-wave Doppler and colorflow Doppler can localize the site of dynamic obstruction precisely to the level of mitral-septal contact; high-velocity turbulent flow is demonstrated downstream from this site, and jet acceleration may be detected just upstream from the site of obstruction (Figures 13–16 and 13–17).

It should be added that some believe that the LV outflow gradient and SAM leaflet motion do not result from an actual stenosis but rather from rapid and excessive early emptying of a hypercontractile powerful LV chamber. They suggest that the abnormal mitral motion (SAM) results from abnormal papillary muscle anatomy in HCM.

Recently, Klues et al.[72-74] have focused attention on enlargement and elongation of mitral leaflets (especially the anterior) as the primary cause of SAM and the LV outflow gradient. A study of nearly 100 mitral valves excised at surgery or autopsy from HCM patients showed that in 60% there was an increase in mitral leaflet area. It is thought that increased mitral leaflet size, in association with reduced LV outflow tract caliber and the thick, bulging septum, contributes to the subaortic pressure gradient. The echocardiographic recognition of markedly increased mitral leaflet size is not merely of esoteric interest but also influences the type of surgical procedure used in such patients. Thus mitral leaflet plication or even mitral valve replacement may be options.

It was concluded, from a study of mitral valve specimens in 43 patients with HCM and known LV outflow tract obstruction, that two types of anatomy existed in these pa-

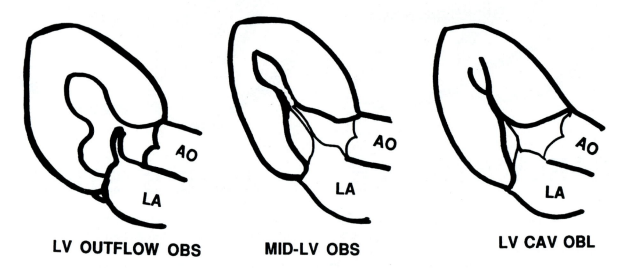

LV OUTFLOW OBS   MID-LV OBS   LV CAV OBL

Figure 13–15. Diagrams in long-axis view in systole in three different varieties of HCM. (Left) LV outflow obstruction with SAM. (Center) Mid-LV obstruction between small apical part and outflow part of LV chamber. (Right) Obliteration of distal half to two-thirds of LV cavity.

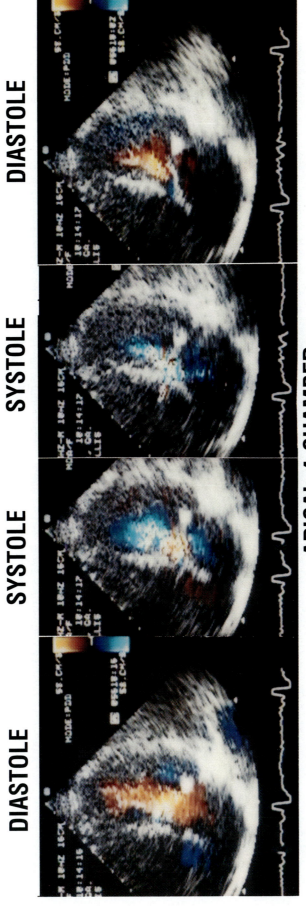

DIASTOLE **SYSTOLE** **SYSTOLE** **DIASTOLE**

APICAL 4 CHAMBER

Figure 13–16. Apical four-chamber view in an HCM patient (W.G.) showing successive frames from the same cardiac cycle (left to right): end-diastole, early systole, late systole, early diastole. Note impressive systolic thickening of the hypertrophied LV wall with marked LV cavity narrowing in systole and LV outflow turbulence in systole.

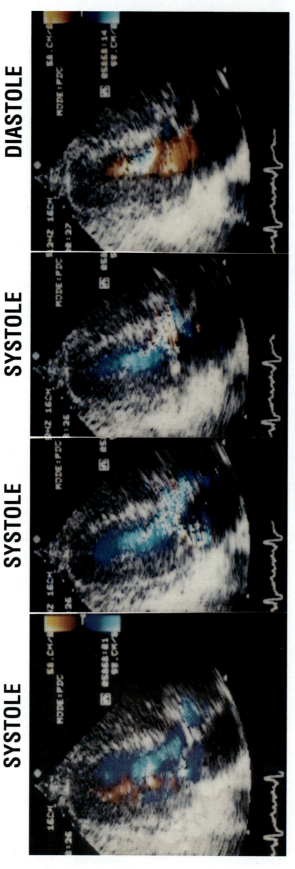

APICAL LONG AXIS

Figure 13–17. Apical long-axis view in same patient (W.G., Figure 13–16) showing successive frames (left to right) at onset of systole, midsystole, late systole, and early diastole. The LV wall thickens markedly in systole, the LV cavity narrows, and turbulence occurs in the LV outflow tract.

tients: (1) The mitral leaflets are abnormally large and situated more posteriorly in a relatively large LV outflow tract. SAM is of large amplitude with a distinctive sharp angle bend; the central and distal parts of the anterior leaflet are free of fibrous thickening. (2) In contrast, the mitral leaflets are of normal size and situated more anteriorly in the LV. The LV outflow tract is narrower, and the anterior mitral leaflet is diffusely thickened secondary to greater mitral-septal contact.

Abnormal coaptation of the mitral leaflets in obstructive HCM was clearly described by Shah et al.[63] as far back as 1981 in 19 patients with HCM who had SAM. This pattern, which was not present in 16 patients with nonobstructive SAM nor in 10 normal individuals, consisted of systolic coaptation of the posterior mitral leaflet with the *middle* anterior leaflet so that the distal anterior leaflet (near its free edge) angulates sharply toward the septum, forming SAM. In normal individuals and those with nonobstructive HCM, the two mitral leaflets coapt at their distal ends (leaflet edges).

Recently, Grigg et al.[75] have observed the same features of abnormal mitral leaflet coaptation from the perspective of transesophageal echocardiography (TEE). They found that the mitral coaptation point in 32 obstructive HCM patients was a mean of 9 mm from the anterior leaflet tip; in a normal control group, the coaptation point was 3 mm or less from the leaflet tip. These authors confirmed the findings of Klues et al.[72-74] of mitral leaflet elongation and systolic anterior angulation of the distal anterior leaflet beyond the coaptation point. Moreover, they noted that the distal edges of the mitral leaflets, instead of forming a watertight seal in systole, formed a funnel that permitted a posteriorly directed MR jet.[75]

Midventricular Obstruction.

Falicov et al.[42] described two patients with HCM in whom an unusual mid-LV site of obstruction was identified on angiocardiography. Autopsy in one of these patients showed displacement of the anterior papillary muscle toward the base of the heart. The authors postulated that systolic obstruction of the mid-LV might result from approximation of the hypertrophied papillary muscle to the bulging septum.

In addition, other varieties of dynamic mid-LV obstruction have been reported; thus it may be part of an apical HCM syndrome.[69] One case of this type was reported by Blazer et al.,[43] who also had another patient with a peculiar membranous mid-LV band with a superimposed dynamic stenotic element provoked by the Valsalva maneuver or sublingual nitroglycerin. They had a third patient with dynamic mid-LV obstruction, in whom they attributed the latter to the coming together of the two hypertrophied papillary muscles.

Mild mid-LV obstruction in HCM is not uncommon, but a severe gradient is rare. The site of mid-LV obstruction may be detectable on 2D echo (Figure 13–18) but colorflow Doppler confirms the diagnosis by demonstrating a high-velocity turbulence in the mid-LV (Figures 13–19 and 13–20). In early diastole, colorflow Doppler may show high-velocity flow into the apical LV, presumably due to enhanced rapid relaxation (Figure 13–21).

Anomalous Insertion of the Papillary Muscle Directly into the Mitral Leaflet in HCM.

In this rare variant, found to occur by Klues et al.[76] in 1% of normal hearts, the papillary muscle itself inserts directly on the mitral leaflet without intervening chordae tendineae. In a series of 75 mitral valves excised from patients with HCM, 10 had anomalous insertion of one or both papillary muscles into the anterior mitral leaflet. Such insertion occurred primarily at one or the other commissure (or both), extending to adjacent areas of the leaflets themselves. This papillary muscle anomaly complicating HCM had been described earlier by Wigle et al.[77]

Klues et al.[76] reported that these HCM patients had a distinctive LV geometry with greatly exaggerated anterior displacement of the papillary muscles and strikingly narrowed LV outflow tract. Subaortic obstruction was attributed to systolic proximity of the hypertrophied papillary muscle to the septum at mid-LV level, forming a long, stenotic mid-cavity segment. The anomalous papillary muscle attachment to the mitral leaflet apparently prevents SAM.

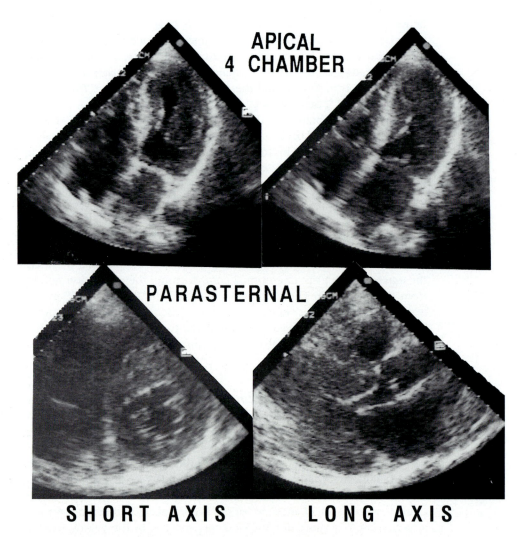

Figure 13–18. Hypertrophic cardiomyopathy showing LV hypertrophy with small LV chamber in patient W.A. In apical four-chamber view (above), the LV chamber is very narrow, especially at mid-LV level, at midsystole (left). The distal two-thirds of the LV chamber obliterates at end-systole (right). (Below) Systolic LV chamber obliteration with impressive systolic thickening of the LV wall.

On 2D echo the muscular chord or papillary muscle inserting on the anterior mitral leaflet can be identified as such but may have to be distinguished from other masses such as large vegetations, thrombus, or tumor. It is easily overlooked, as in 9 of the preoperative echocardiograms of Klues et al.[76] Preoperative recognition of this unusual papillary muscle anomaly in HCM is important because in such patients mitral valve replacement rather than septal myectomy/myotomy appears to be the effective surgical therapy.

Systolic cavity obliteration is considered by some to be a variety of intra-LV obstruction. Entrapment of the catheter tip in an obliterated LV cavity has intriguing implications pertaining to the interpretation of pressure tracings. To the echocardiographer, however, 2D echo visualization of obliteration of the distal (apical) half of the LV cavity manifests as the septum and LV free wall coming into firm contact with each other in late systole with no colorflow in between (Figure 13-23). This appearance is convincing evidence of abnormally hyperdynamic LV contraction. The basal one-half to one-third of the LV chamber just below the aortic and mitral valves can become abnormally narrow in these patients but does not obliterate. At the other end of the colorflow Doppler spectrum, turbulence can occur at a proximal septal bulge without LV outflow obstruction (Figure 13-23).

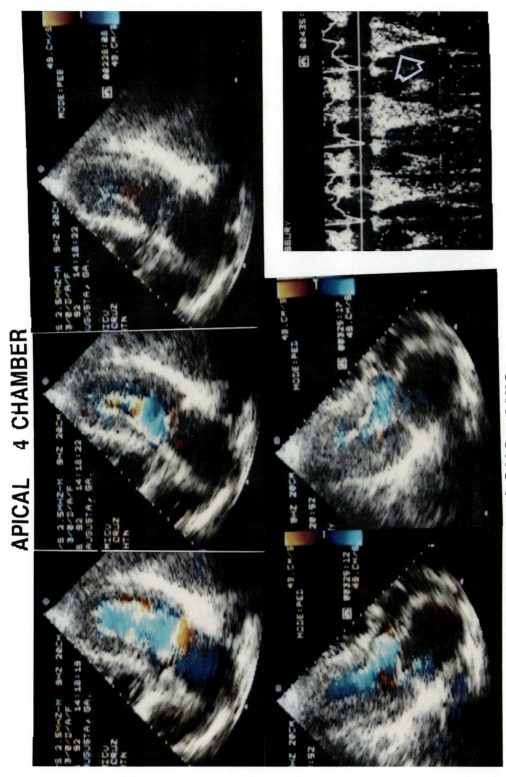

APICAL 4 CHAMBER

APICAL LONG AXIS

Figure 13–19. Apical four-chamber view (above) and apical long-axis view (below) in same patient W.A. with HCM. The LV chamber size and shape are well appreciated by colorflow Doppler. (Above) Early, middle, and late systolic frames show progressive systolic obliteration of the LV chamber. (Below) Systolic near-obliteration of the LV chamber. Doppler recording (below, right) shows dynamic mild mid-LV obstruction.

APICAL 4 CHAMBER

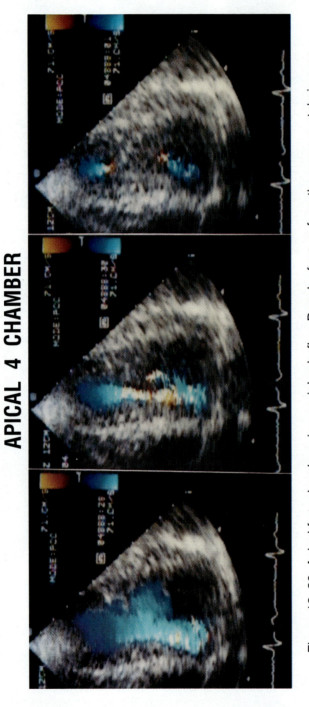

Figure 13–20. Apical four-chamber view serial colorflow Doppler frames from the same systole in a patient with end-stage renal disease and hyperdynamic hypertrophied LV. (Left) Early systole. (Center and right) Marked systolic LV narrowing with tendency to midventricular constriction, i.e., dividing the LV into proximal and distal components.

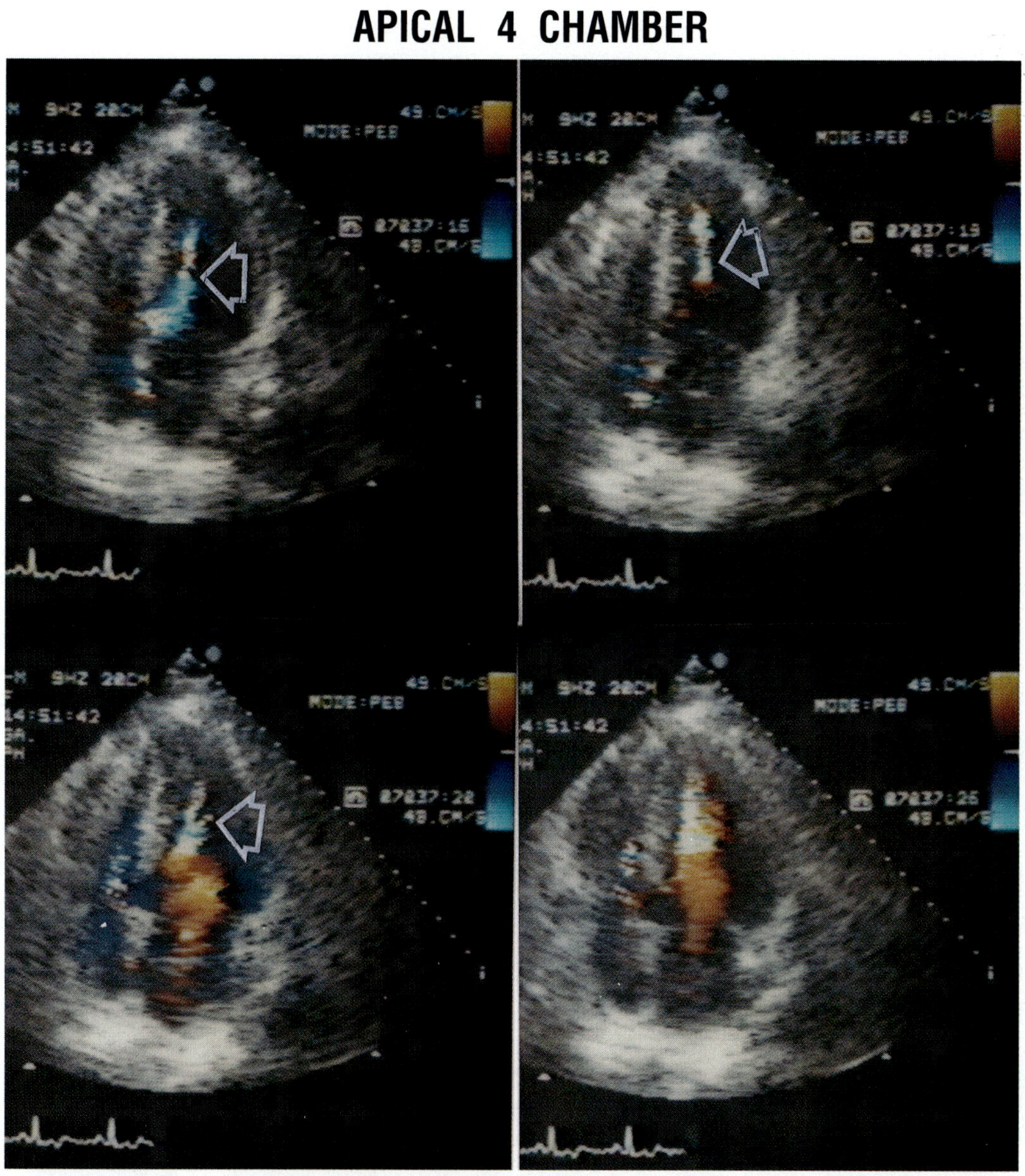

APICAL 4 CHAMBER

Figure 13–21. Apical four-chamber views showing four successive frames in the same cardiac cycle in a patient with HCM. There is near-obliteration of the LV cavity at end-systole (above, left) and then rapid flow into the narrow apical LV cavity (arrow) at the onset of diastole (above, right), which continues as mitral inflow commences (below, left). Finally, the whole LV chamber fills later in diastole (below, right).

Relation of Anatomic/Echocardiographic Features of HCM to Prognosis

The attrition rate, once HCM is diagnosed, is said to be about 4% per year. However, in any particular patient, the outlook is extremely variable. Surprisingly, the severity of myocardial hypertrophy and even the presence or absence of intracardiac systolic obstruction have no strong correlation with longevity.

Sudden death is common in HCM patients, particularly in certain afflicted families, but there is no echocardiographic finding or parameter that is known to predict a high risk for sudden death. Unsuspected HCM is the most commonly found abnormality at autopsy in young competitive athletes who die suddenly.[78] Echocardiography is therefore often used as a screening procedure in those embarking on competitive sports; it is certainly indicated in athletes who have murmurs, abnormal electrocardiograms, or cardiac symptoms while competing.

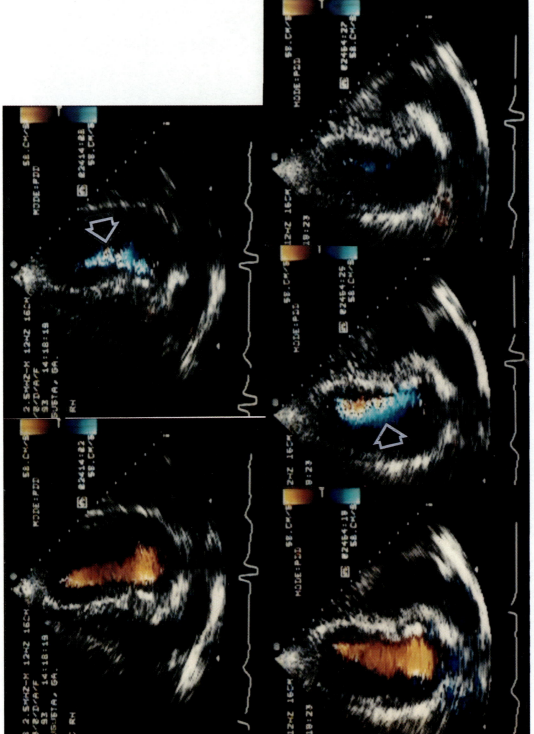

APICAL 4 CHAMBER

DIASTOLE   SYSTOLE

APICAL LONG AXIS

DIASTOLE   SYSTOLE

Figure 13–22. Apical four-chamber view (above). Colorflow Doppler depicts blood flow into the narrow LV chamber at end-diastole (left) and near-obliteration of the cavity in systole (right). Apical long-axis view (below). Colorflow Doppler shows conical-shaped LV chamber at end-diastole (left); the LV cavity (arrows) narrows in midsystole (center) and obliterates at end-systole (right).

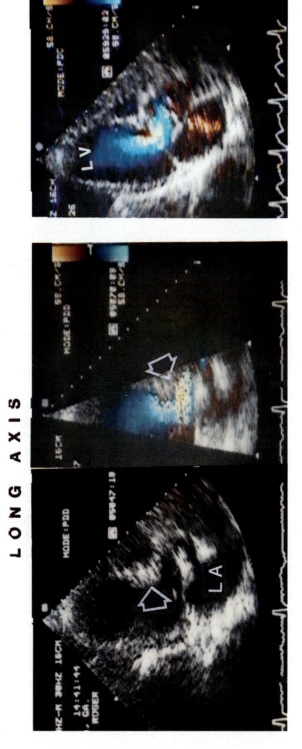

Figure 13–23. (Left) Apical long-axis view in a patient with proximal septal bulge (arrow). Colorflow Doppler (center) shows turbulent flow in LV outflow tract caused by projection of the septal bulge into the stream of systolic flow. (Right) Similar LV outflow turbulence of lesser degree in another patient with sigmoid septum.

The extent of LV hypertrophy, including septal thickness, and of the LV outflow gradient in obstructive HCM remains stable over years, although there are occasional exceptions. The response to drug therapy, such as beta blockers or verapamil, can be assessed by serial Doppler 2D echograms in obstructive HCM.

A small percentage of patients with typical HCM progresses to LV dilatation with deteriorating LV contractility.[79,80] Thus HCM evolves into DCM (dilated cardiomyopathy). Some of these cases have followed surgical resection of septal myocardium; others have followed myocardial infarction.[81] Infarction in HCM is different from the usual MI in non-HCM patients; in HCM, the large epicardial coronary arteries may not be occluded; it is the small intramyocardial arteries that have been blamed, and extensive scarring of the myocardium with LV dilatation may be encountered in these exceptional HCM patients.[82]

REFERENCES

1. Abbasi AS, McAlpin RN, Eber L, et al. Left ventricular hypertrophy diagnosed by echocardiography. N Engl J Med 1973;289:118.
2. Browne PF, Desser KB, Benchimol A, et al. The echocardiographic correlates of left ventricular hypertrophy diagnosed by echocardiography. J Electrocardiol 1977;10:105.
3. Savage DD, Drayer JIM, Henry WL, et al. Echocardiographic assessment of cardiac anatomy and function in hypertensive subjects. Circulation 1979;59:623.
4. Maron BJ, Henry WL, Roberts WC, et al. Comparison of echocardiographic and necropsy measurements of left ventricular thickness in patients with and without disproportionate septal thickening. Circulation 1977;55:341.
5. Feigenbaum H. Echocardiography, 5th ed. Philadelphia: Lea & Febiger, 1994, pp 157, 658.
6. Vandewerf F, Geboers J, Kestleloot H, et al. The mechanism of disappearance of the physiologic third heart sound with age. Circulation 1986;73:877.
7. Gaasch WH. Left ventricular radius to wall thickness ratio. Am J Cardiol 1979;43:1189.
8. Devereux RB, Lutas EM, Casale RN, et al. Standardization of M-mode echocardiographic left ventricular anatomic measurements. J Am Coll Cardiol 1984;4:1222.
9. Levy D, Savage DD, Garrison RJ, et al. Echocardiographic criteria for left ventricular hypertrophy: The Framingham Heart Study. Am J Cardiol 1987;59:956.
10. Liebson PR, Grandits G, Prineas R, et al. Echocardiographic correlates of left ventricular structure among 844 mildly hypertensive men and women in the treatment of mild hypertension study (TOMHS). Circulation 1993;87:476.
11. Troy BL, Pombo J, Rackley CE. Measurement of left ventricular wall thickness and mass by echocardiography. Circulation 1972;45:602.
12. Murray JA, Johnston W, Reid JM. Echocardiographic determination of left ventricular dimensions, volumes and performance. Am J Cardiol 1972;30:252.
13. Bennett DH, Evans DW, Raj MVJ. Echocardiographic left ventricular dimensions in pressure and volume overload. Br Heart J 1975;37:971.
14. Devereux RB, Reichek N. Echocardiographic determination of left ventricular mass in man: Anatomic validation of the method. Circulation 1977;55:613.
15. Devereux RB, Alonso DR, Lutas DM, et al. Echocardiographic assessment of left ventricular hypertrophy: Comparison to necropsy findings. Am J Cardiol 1986;57:450.
16. Woythaler JN, Singer SL, Kwan OL, et al. Accuracy of echocardiography versus electrocardiography in detecting left ventricular hypertrophy: Comparison with postmortem mass measurements. J Am Coll Cardiol 1983;2:305.
17. Devereux RB. Detection of left ventricular hypertrophy by M-mode echocardiography. Hypertension 1987(suppl II);9:19.
18. Reichek N, Helak J, Plappert T, et al. Anatomic validation of left ventricular mass estimates from clinical two-dimensional echocardiography. Circulation 1983;67:348.
19. Valdez RS, Motta JA, London E, et al. Evaluation of the echocardiogram as an epidemiological tool in an asymptomatic population. Circulation 1979;60:921.
20. Gardin JM, Henry WL, Savage DD, et al. Echocardiographic measurements in normal subjects. J Clin Ultrasound 1979;7:439.
21. Henry WL, Gardin JM, Ware JH. Echocardiographic measurements in normal subjects from infancy to old age. Circulation 1980;62:1054.
22. Devereux RB, Pickering TG, Alderman MH, et al. Left ventricular hypertrophy in hyperten-

sion: Prevalence and relationship to pathophysiologic variables. Hypertension 1987(suppl II);9:53–59.

23. Hammond IW, Alderman MH, Devereux RB, et al. The prevalence and correlates of echocardiographic left ventricular hypertrophy among employed patients with uncomplicated hypertension. J Am Coll Cardiol 1986;7:639.

24. Topol EJ, Traill TA, Fortuin NJ. Hypertensive hypertrophic cardiomyopathy of the elderly. N Engl J Med 1985;312:277.

25. Fouad-Tarazi FM, Liebson PR. Echocardiographic studies of regression of left ventricular hypertrophy in hypertension. Hypertension 1987(suppl II);9:65.

26. Strauer BE. Structural and functional adaptation of the chronically overloaded heart in arterial hypertension. Am Heart J 1987;114:948.

27. Ganau A, Devereux RB, Roman MJ, et al. Patterns of left ventricular hypertrophy and geometric remodelling in essential hypertension. J Am Coll Cardiol 1992;19:1550.

28. Lewis JF, Maron BJ. Diversity of patterns of hypertrophy in patients with systemic hypertension and marked left ventricular wall thickening. Am J Cardiol 1990;65:874.

29. Epstein SE, Maron BJ. Hypertrophic cardiomyopathy: An overview, in M Kaltenbach, SE Epstein (eds): Hypertrophic Cardiomyopathy. New York: Springer-Verlag, 1982, pp 5–17.

30. Braunwald E. Heart Disease. Philadelphia: WB Saunders, 1991, pp 1418–1430.

31. LeJemtel TH, Factor SM, Koenigsberg M, et al. Mural vegetations of endocardial trauma in infective endocarditis complicating idiopathic subaortic stenosis. Am J Cardiol 1979;44:569.

32. Teare RD. Asymmetrical hypertrophy of the heart in young adults. Br Heart J 1958;20:1.

33. Hutchins GM, Bulkley BH. Catenoid shape of the interventricular septum: Possible cause of idiopathic hypertrophic subaortic stenosis. Circulation 1978;58:392.

34. Silverman KJ, Hutchins GM, Weiss JL, et al. Catenoid shape of the interventricular septum in idiopathic hypertrophic stenosis: Two-dimensional echocardiographic confirmation. Am J Cardiol 1982;49:27.

35. Thompson AW. On Growth and Form, 2d ed. New York: Macmillan, 1942, p 365.

36. Lever HM, Karam RF, Currie PJ, et al. Hypertrophic cardiomyopathy in the elderly: Distinctions from young based on cardiac shape. Circulation 1989;79:580.

37. Maron BJ, Gottdiener JS, Epstein SE. Patterns and significance of the distribution of left ventricular hypertrophy in hypertrophic cardiomyopathy. Am J Cardiol 1981;48:418.

38. Wigle ED, Sasson Z, Henderson MA, et al. Hypertrophic cardiomyopathy: The importance of the site and extent of hypertrophy. Progr Cardiovasc Dis 1985;28:1.

39. Yamaguchi H, Ishimura T, Nishiyama S, et al. Hypertrophic nonobstructive cardiomyopathy with giant negative T waves (apical hypertrophy). Am J Cardiol 1979;44:401.

40. Keren G, Belhassen B, Sherez J, et al. Apical hypertrophic cardiomyopathy: Evaluation by noninvasive and invasive techniques in 23 patients. Circulation 1985;71:45.

41. Zoghbi WA, Haichin RN, Quinones MA. Mid cavity obstruction in apical hypertrophy. Am Heart J 1988;116:1469.

42. Falicov RE, Resnekov L, Bharati S, et al. Midventricular obstruction: A variant of obstructive cardiomyopathy. Am J Cardiol 1976;37:432.

43. Blazer D, Kotler MN, Parry WR. Noninvasive evaluation of midventricular obstruction by two-dimensional and Doppler echocardiography and colorflow Doppler echocardiography. Am Heart J 1987;114:1162.

44. Topol EJ, Traill TA, Fortuin NJ. Hypertensive hypertrophic cardiomyopathy of the elderly. N Engl J Med 1985;312:227.

45. Goor D, Lillehei CW, Edwards JE. The "sigmoid septum": Variation in the contour of the left ventricular outlet. AJR 1969;107:366.

46. Belenkie I, MacDonald RPR, Smith ER. Localized septal hypertrophy. Am Heart J 1988;115:385.

46a. Carr AA, D'Cruz IA, Davis M, et al. Proximal septal bulge more frequent in hypertensive than in normotensive men (abstract). Am J Hypertens 1990;3(part 2):7.

47. Dalldorf FG, Willis PW. Angled aorta ("sigmoid septum") as a cause of hypertrophic subaortic stenosis. Hum Pathol 1985;16:457.

48. Louie EK, Maron BJ. Hypertrophic cardiomyopathy with extreme increase in left ventricular wall thickness. J Am Coll Cardiol 1986;8:57.

49. Movsowitz HD, Movsowitz C, Jacobs MN, et al. Pitfalls in the echo-Doppler diagnosis of hypertrophic cardiomyopathy. Echocardiography 1993;10:167.

50. Kotler MN, Segal BL, Mintz G, et al. Pitfalls and limitations of M-mode echocardiography. Am Heart J 1977;94:227.

51. Lewis JF, Maron BJ. Diversity of patterns of hypertrophy in patients with systemic hypertension and marked left ventricular wall thickening. Am J Cardiol 1990;65:874.

52. Hess OM, Schneider J, Turina M, et al. Asymmetric septal hypertrophy in patients with aortic stenosis. J Am Coll Cardiol 1983;1:783.

53. Maron BJ, Clark CE, Henry WL, et al. Prevalence and characteristics of disproportionate ventricular septal thickening in patients with acquired or congenital heart disease. Circulation 1977;55:489.

54. Stern A, Kessler KM, Hammer WJ, et al. Septal-free wall disproportion in inferior infarction. Circulation 1978;58:700.

55. Pollick C, Koipillai C, Howard R, et al. Left ventricular thrombus demonstrating canalization and mimicking asymmetric septal hypertrophy on echocardiographic study. Am Heart J 1982;104:641.

56. Cabin HS, Costello RM, Vasudevan C, et al. Cardiac lymphoma mimicking hypertrophic cardiomyopathy. Am Heart J 1981;102:466.

57. Oh JK, Tajik AJ, Edwards WD, et al. Dynamic left ventricular outflow tract obstruction in cardiac amyloidosis detected by continuous-wave Doppler echocardiography. Am J Cardiol 1987;59:1008.

58. Pellicia A, Maron BJ, Spataro A, et al. The upper limit of physiologic cardiac hypertrophy in highly trained athletes. N Engl J Med 1991;324:295.

59. Maron BJ, Edwards JE, Epstein SE. Prevalence and characteristics of disproportionate ventricular septal thickening in patients with systemic hypertension. Chest 1978;73:466.

60. Maron BJ, Savage DD, Clark CE, et al. Prevalence and characteristics of disproportionate septal thickening in patients with coronary artery disease. Circulation 1978;57:250.

61. Braunwald E, Morow AG, Cornell WP, et al. Idiopathic hypertrophic subaortic stenosis. Am J Med 1960;29:924.

62. Tunick PA, Lampert R, Perez JL, et al. Effect of mitral regurgitation on the left ventricular outflow pressure gradient in obstructive hypertrophic cardiomyopathy. Am J Cardiol 1990;66:1271.

63. Shah PM, Taylor RD, Wong M. Abnormal mitral valve coaptation in hypertrophic obstructive cardiomyopathy. Am J Cardiol 1981;48:258.

64. Sasson Z, Rakowski H, Wigle ED, et al. Echocardiographic and Doppler studies in hypertrophic cardiomyopathy. Cardiol Clin 1990;8:217.

65. Nair CK, Kudesia V, Hansen D, et al. Echocardiographic and electrocardiographic characteristics of patients with hypertrophic cardiomyopathy with and without mitral annular calcium. Am J Cardiol 1987;59:1428.

66. Rakowski H, Sasson Z, Wigle ED. Echocardiographic and Doppler assessment of hypertrophic cardiomyopathy. J Am Soc Echocardiogr 1987;1:31.

67. Maron BJ, Bonow RO, Canon RD, et al. Hypertrophic cardiomyopathy. N Engl J Med 1987;316:780.

68. Goodwin JF. The frontiers of cardiomyopathy. Br Heart J 1982;48:1.

69. Maze SS, Kotler MN, Parry WR. Dynamic intracavitary left ventricular obstruction. Am J Noninvas Cardiol 1990;4:76.

70. Wigle ED. Hypertrophic cardiomyopathy (editorial). Circulation 1987;75:311.

71. Jiang L, Levine RA, King ME, et al. An integrated mechanism for systolic anterior motion of the mitral valve in hypertrophic cardiomyopathy based on echocardiographic observations. Am Heart J 1987;113:633.

72. Klues HG, Maron BJ, Dollar AL, et al. Diversity of structural mitral valve alterations in hypertrophic cardiomyopathy. Circulation 1992;85:1651.

73. Klues HG, Roberts WC, Maron BJ. Morphologic determinants of echocardiographic patterns of mitral valve systolic anterior motion in obstructive hypertrophic cardiomyopathy. Circulation 1993;87:1570.

74. Klues HG, Proschan MA, Dollar AL, et al. Echocardiographic assessment of mitral valve size in obstructive hypertrophic cardiomyopathy. Circulation 1993;88:548.

75. Grigg LE, Wigle ED, Williams WG, et al. Transesophageal Doppler echocardiography: Clarification of pathophysiology and importance in intraoperative decision making. J Am Coll Cardiol 1992;20:42.

76. Klues HG, Roberts WC, Maron BJ. Anomalous insertion of papillary muscle directly into anterior mitral leaflet in hypertrophic cardiomyopathy. Circulation 1991;84:1188.

77. Wigle ED, Adelman AG, Auger P, et al. Mitral regurgitation in muscular subaortic stenosis. Am J Cardiol 1969;24:698.

78. Maron BJ, Epstein SE, Roberts WC. Causes of sudden death in competitive athletes. J Am Coll Cardiol 1986;7:204.

79. Yutani C, Imakita M, Ishibashi-Ueda H, et al. Three autopsy cases of progression to left ventricular dilatation in patients with hypertrophic cardiomyopathy. Am Heart J 1985;109:545.

80. Spirito P, Maron BJ, Bonow RO, et al. Occurrence and significance of progressive left ventricular wall thinning and relative cavity dilatation in patients with hypertrophic cardiomyopathy. Am J Cardiol 1987;59:123.

81. Waller BF, Maron BJ, Epstein SE, et al. Transmural myocardial infarction in hypertrophic cardiomyopathy. Chest 1981;79:461.

82. Sutton MStJ, Tajik AJ, Smith HC, et al. Angina in idiopathic hypertrophic subaortic stenosis. Circulation 1980;61:561.

14

Ischemic Heart Disease

From the immense volume of published work on the effects of ischemia on the myocardium, and myocardial infarction in particular, only those aspects essential to the echocardiographer's understanding of the anatomy of myocardial infarction (MI) and its complications will be mentioned here.

The earliest "naked eye" changes in left ventricular (LV) myocardium are seen 15 hours after coronary artery occlusion, and the earliest histologic changes are seen in 6 hours; subsequently, a definite sequence of gross and microscopic changes evolves over the ensuing days and weeks. However, regional LV contraction changes (echocardiographically perceived as LV wall motion abnormalities) begin within a few minutes, even preceding typical electrocardiographic (ECG) changes. There is therefore a diagnostic role for two-dimensional (2D) echo in assessing patients presenting with acute chest pain of very recent onset, especially if no previous MI has occurred and/or the LV is known to have contracted normally by a previous echo- or angiocardiogram.

Three weeks after the onset of MI, scar tissue has started forming, and LV wall thickness at the infarction site has decreased. Over the next 2 months, scar tissue continues to become firmer and denser; an old MI appears unduly dense, echogenic, and akinetic on the M-mode and 2D echocardiogram.

Whereas the general distribution of infarction (and therefore of impaired LV wall motion) usually correlates with the respective major coronary artery occluded, the actual extent or area of affected myocardium is very variable depending on (1) whether the right or left coronary artery is dominant in that particular heart, (2) collateral circulation, and (3) the presence and severity of stenosis of other coronary arteries. Schlesinger's work of over 50 years ago showed that a right-dominant coronary system was present in 48%, left-dominant system in 18%, and a balanced right-left coronary artery distribution in 34%. If the jeopardized myocardium gets substantial blood flow through small arteries from other normal or less stenotic coronary arteries, this tends to minimize the size of infarction. Occlusion of one coronary artery can cause "infarction at a distance" by cutting off collateral blood supply to a "remote" area of myocardium, which, deprived of its own blood supply by an old occlusion, was precariously dependent on another coronary artery through collaterals. Thus the echocardiographic manifestations of a given coronary occlusion can vary over a wide spectrum from a small area of mild hypokinesis to an extensive LV dyskinetic or akinetic area or even an LV aneurysm.

Occlusion of the left anterior descending (LAD) coronary artery produces infarction of the anterior ventricular septum and anterior LV wall; more often than not, the LV apex is also involved. Occlusion of the circumflex artery causes infarction of the LV posterior, inferior, and lateral walls. Occlusion of the right coronary artery (RCA) results in infarction of the posteroinferior wall and posterior septum.

LV WALL MOTION ABNORMALITIES

Local or regional wall motion abnormalities are the hallmark of myocardial ischemia—either infarction or severe ischemia. LV wall motion thus can be graded on a scale: hyperkinetic, normal, hypokinetic, akinetic, dyskinetic. Hypokinesis may be further differentiated into mild and severe. Ischemia or infarction does not directly cause hyperkinesis, but compensatory increased contraction of the nonischemic LV wall or septum is often seen opposite the area of hypokinesis or akinesis.

LV wall motion abnormalities need to be described with reference to LV anatomy. Unfortunately, there has been no uniformity or generally accepted convention as to the precise numbers and topography of myocardial segments, which have varied from 9 to 14 in different studies.[1-6] Common to most of these mapping schemes is first a division of the LV longitudinally into basal, middle, and juxta-apical annular bands, with the LV apex itself at the top of the cone. Each of the three annular segments was then divided into four to five parts, such as anterior, posteroinferior, medial or septal, and lateral.

Another practical difficulty is that in actual experience, wall motion abnormalities (1) may not conform exactly to arbitrary myocardial segments (they may in fact involve part of one segment and part of the adjacent segment) and (2) may gradually increase in severity from one segment to adjoining ones so that it is difficult to designate sharply the hypokinetic, akinetic, and dyskinetic areas.

Another source of unnecessary confusion is lack of standardization of wall scoring, i.e., indicating severity of wall motion impairment by numbers 1+, 2+, 3+, etc., normality as 0 or 1+, hyperkinetic motion as 1 or 0, etc. The Gorlin and Herman system scores hyperkinesis as 0, normal as 1, hypokinesis as 2, akinesis as 3, dyskinesis as 4, and aneurysm as 5.

WALL THICKENING

Systolic LV wall thickening is the difference (in millimeters) between end-systolic and end-diastolic thickness of that particular wall segment. Wall thickening has been used as an index of regional wall contraction (and therefore indirectly of the presence of ischemia or infarction) because it is easy to measure directly. On the other hand, LV wall motion is a qualitative assessment, a subjective call depending on the experience and skill of the observer.

Systolic wall thickness can be measured accurately on the M-mode tracing, but only with respect to the small area of ventricular septum and LV posteroinferior wall that can be recorded by the "icepick" M-mode beam. 2D echo measurements of wall thickening, though less precise (because of suboptimal definition of endocardium and epicardium) than the M-mode measurements, can be done on any part of the LV wall.

Systolic thinning of the infarcted area has been noted in some patients with acute infarction; systolic wall thickness is actually less than diastolic thickness due to stretching or expansion of the infarct.

Echocardiographic visualization of a specific extent of LV wall motion abnormality does not always mean infarction of that exact area for several reasons: (1) Severe ischemia or occlusion by thrombus which soon recanalizes (perhaps after thrombolytic therapy) may cause hypokinesis or akinesis because of myocardial stunning, but the myocardium remains viable and begins to contract again if its perfusion somehow improves. (2) Infarcted muscle fibers may act as a "parallel mechanical resistor" and impede contraction in an adjacent nonischemic segment. (3) "Ischemia at a distance" may be occurring. This refers to the situation where coronary artery occlusion can cause infarction or severe ischemia of an LV segment outside its "territory" by cutting off flow in collateral vessels to that territory already in jeopardy due to a previous occlusion. Deducing which coronary arteries are obstructed from observations on which LV segments are hypokinetic, akinetic, or dyskinetic is not only an exercise in cardiac anatomy but also vital to prognosis and further management.

CORONARY SUPPLY OF LV WALL AND SEPTUM (Figure 14–1)

In parasternal short-axis view, the circular configuration of the LV cross section includes territories of all three main coronary arteries. The LAD coronary artery supplies the anterior half of the circle, i.e., the anterior half of the ventricular septum and the anterolateral LV wall. The posterior half of the circle is divided into circumflex artery territory left of the midline and right coronary artery (RCA) right of the midline, the latter including the posterior part of the ventricular septum.

In the long-axis parasternal view, the part of septum visualized (basal and middle thirds) is in LAD territory, and the part of the LV posterior wall visualized is in circumflex artery territory. In the apical long-axis view, the entire length of the posteroinferior wall is visualized, its supply shared by the RCA and circumflex artery to varying extent. The anteroseptal wall and apex are in LAD territory. In the apical four-chamber view, showing the LV inflow tract from the mitral annulus to the apex, the LAD supplies the midseptum and apical septum, as well as the apex itself; the circumflex artery supplies the posterolateral LV wall; and the basal one-third of septum is most often in RCA territory.

ECHOCARDIOGRAPHY OF LV INFARCTION

It has long been known that infarcts are characterized by a hypokinetic, akinetic, or dyskinetic echo-dense appearance of the affected LV segment on M-mode (Figure 14-2) or 2D echo (Figure 14-3). Abnormal segmental thinning may be evident (Figure 14-4), especially if the adjacent noninfarcted segment is hypertrophied (Figure 14-5).

Infarct Expansion and LV Remodeling

Infarct expansion was recognized as a common event in the natural history of MI in the late 1970s by pathologists and echocardiographers at Johns Hopkins.[6-9] The important distinction between infarct extension and expansion was made by Hutchins and Bulkley,[6] who studied 76 acute recent MIs at autopsy. MI extension, recognized histologically as more recent foci of necrosis (more recent than the original MI), was present in only 17% of the series. MI expansion, characterized by acute dilatation and thinning of the area of infarction not explained by additional myocardial necrosis, was detected in as many as 59% of cases.

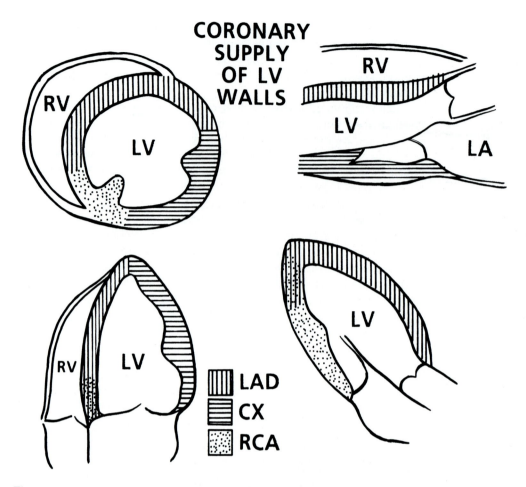

Figure 14–1. Diagram showing parasternal views (above) and apical views (below) with common distribution pattern of coronary arterial supply to the LV walls: left anterior descending (LAD), vertical shading; circumflex (CX), horizontal shading; right coronary (RCA), stippled shading. Considerable variation from this pattern can exist depending on which artery is unduly dominant.

Infarct expansion is a detrimental change or complication of MI of much clinical significance. First, it predisposes to cardiac rupture. In a series of 110 autopsied MI patients, 23 of 56 (43%) with MI expansion showed LV rupture in the zone of expansion, whereas only 1 of 56 (2%) without infarct expansion had rupture. Moreover, rupture was more frequent in those with the most severe MI expansion; expanded MI LV thickness was less than in the noninfarcted LV wall and even less in those showing rupture. Second, infarct expansion leads to aneurysm formation and eventually often also to overall LV dilatation.

Infarct expansion occurring within 3 weeks of transmural MI is the main factor in LV dilatation.[10] As healing progresses, connective-tissue cells connect disrupted myocyte fibers of the "soft" MI and strengthen the LV wall, resisting further stretching.

Noninfarcted myocardium also takes part in the process of post-MI remodeling. There are dilatation and sometimes hypertrophy of noninfarct LV wall areas, which contribute to the LV dilatation.[11] Thus not only is early LV shape change (at the infarction site) an important predictor of early mortality after anterior MI[12] but so also is a generalized LV size increase and change toward a spherical shape[13] in patients with lowest ejection fractions and manifestations of congestive failure. McKay et al.[11] showed that the magnitude of the remodeling process is directly proportional to infarct size as assessed by LV wall motion abnormality during the acute MI phase.

Over the last decade, the natural history of MI expansion, LV dilatation, and remodeling has been studied extensively, mainly by 2D echo. This has happened because of in-

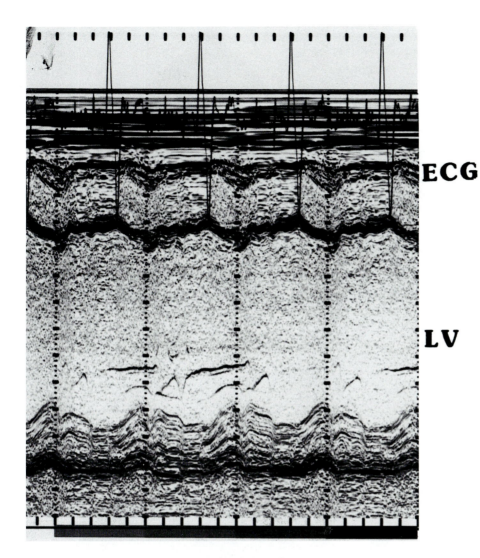

ECG

LV

Figure 14–2. M-mode echocardiogram of a patient with septal infarction. The LV chamber is dilated (LVID 70 mm). The septum is thin (8 mm) and densely echogenic, with echo texture very different from the LV posterior wall, which is 13 mm thick.

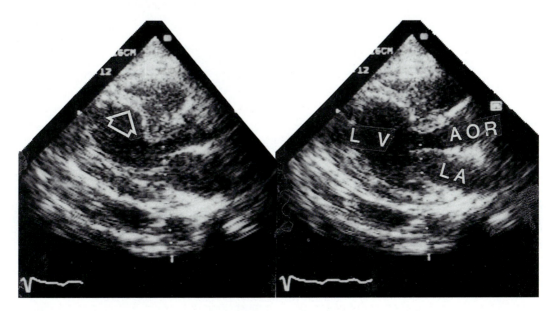

Figure 14–3. Parasternal long-axis views in systole (left) and diastole (right). The midseptum is akinetic (arrow), while the basal septum and LV posteroinferior wall contract.

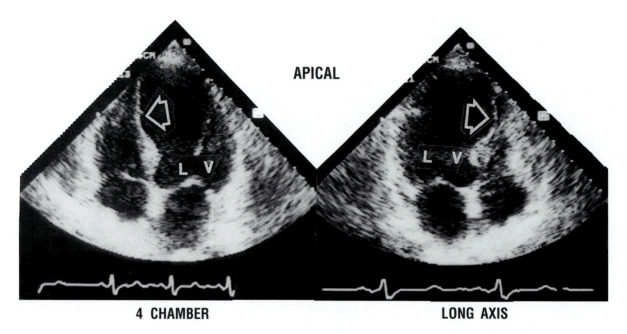

Figure 14–4. Apical four-chamber view (left) and long-axis view (right) showing abnormally thin infarcted septal segment.

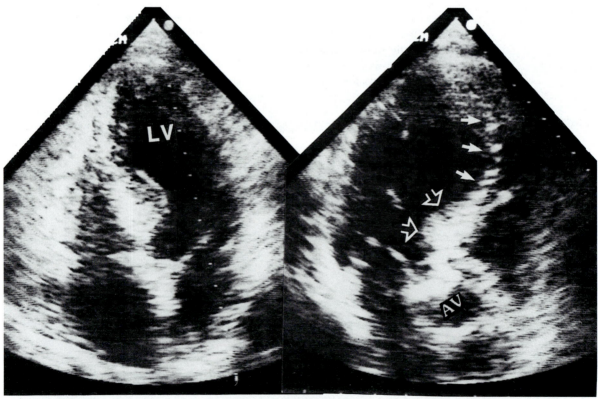

Figure 14–5. Apical four-chamber view (left) and apical long-axis view (right) of a patient with septal infarction. The middle to apical septum is thin and bulges into the right ventricle, but the basal segment of septum is hypertrophied, forming a prominent bulge.

tense interest in the possible prevention or attenuation of these deleterious LV changes by various therapeutic interventions such as early reperfusion of occluded coronary arteries by thrombolytic agents and drugs such as nitroglycerin, captopril, and enalapril. A review of these numerous widely publicized studies is beyond the scope of this book, but they have served to make clinicians aware of the changes in LV volume and shape that follow MI, as well as their assessment by 2D echo.

VENTRICULAR ANEURYSM

This is a common complication of transmural (full-thickness) MI, occurring with a frequency of 5% to 40% in different series. To the pathologist, an LV aneurysm is an area of LV outpouching, the wall of which is formed entirely or mainly by fibrous replacement of myocardium.[14,15] However, to the angiocardiographer or echocardiographer, an LV aneurysm is regional dilatation or bulging that persists in diastole as well as systole. There is thus a convex distortion of LV shape affecting part of the chamber beyond the range of normal contour.

LV aneurysms develop within the first 2 to 4 weeks of infarction. Thereafter, there may be little change in some cases, whereas in others a diffuse LV dilatation slowly evolves.

About 80% of LV aneurysms involve the LV apex. In some of these the aneurysm manifests as no more than a small protrusion at the very tip of the apex, but more often the adjacent ventricular septum and/or the LV free wall are also part of the aneurysm. In extreme cases, the whole apical half of the LV chamber balloons out into a huge aneurysm with only the basal LV contractile, resembling a lightbulb. Other less common sites of LV aneurysm include the inferior wall and posterobasal wall (between the mitral annulus and the posteromedial papillary muscle). Septal aneurysms may affect only the juxta-apical septum, only the basal septum, or virtually the entire septum; the aneurysmal septal segment bulges into the right ventricular (RV) chamber.

LV aneurysms cause deterioration of cardiac status and worsen prognosis in three ways: (1) by predisposing to thrombus formation and thereby to systemic thromboembolism, (2) by further impairing LV pump function, in addition to the adverse effect of the infarction itself, by producing a ventricular "dead space" that absorbs wasteful contractile LV energy, and (3) by leading to ventricular tachycardia or fibrillation, the arrhythmogenic myocardium being not the fibrous aneurysmal sac itself but rather the electrically abnormal myocardium at the aneurysmal rim.

Hochman et al.,[16] who studied 34 LV aneurysms at autopsy and another 45 after surgical resection, differentiated LV aneurysms into two types. In type I, with extensive fibroelastosis, the endocardium undergoes a progressive thickening, with new elastic fibrils appearing within 3 to 4 weeks after onset of MI. Lamellar organization of elastic fibers occurs gradually over a year, morphologically similar to the aorta, the so-called aorticization of Hutchins and Bannayan.[17] This type I LV aneurysm seldom contains thrombus but does somehow predispose to ventricular tachycardia. Type II aneurysms have little or no fibroelastosis but often do have thrombus layered on the internal surface; they are less prone to ventricular arrhythmia.

On 2D echo,[18-22] LV aneurysms manifest as a regional or local bulge, the wall motion in this area being characterized as akinetic or dyskinetic. There is an important distinction between LV aneurysm and LV dyskinesis. In the former, the convex deformation of shape persists throughout the cardiac cycle; in the latter, the affected LV segment bulges outward in systole (in contrast to the inward "squeezing down" motion of the rest of the LV), but LV shape returns to normal in diastole (Figures 14-6 and 14-7). The latter (dyskinesis) is often loosely referred to as an aneurysm, especially by angiocardiographers; such semantic discrepancies are possibly responsible for the apparently large range in incidence of LV aneurysm complicating MI from one center to another or for differences in angiocardiographic and echocardiographic reports on the same patient.

In some patients, the demarcation between normally contractile and aneurysmal LV

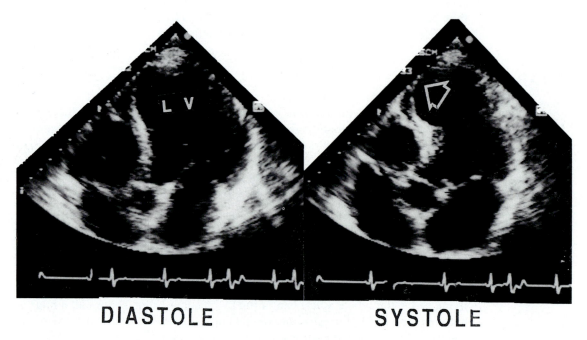

Figure 14–6. Apical four-chamber view showing dyskinesis of the distal (apical) septum, with conspicuous bulging in systole but not diastole.

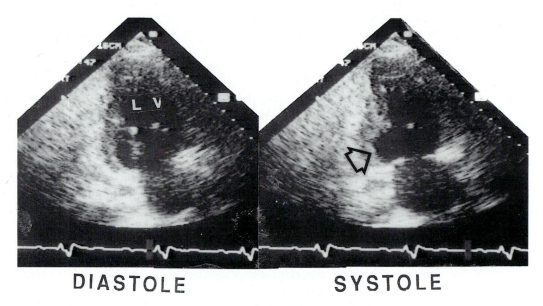

Figure 14–7. Apical long-axis view showing dyskinesis of the posterobasal wall, which bulges prominently in systole but only slightly in diastole.

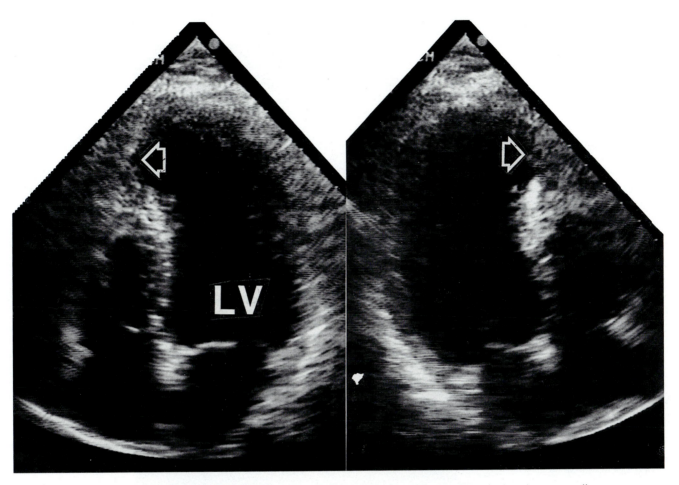

Figure 14–8. Apical four-chamber view (left) and long-axis view (right) showing a small local LV aneurysm (arrow) at junction of septum with apex.

wall—the so-called hinge point—is sharp and easily identified as the recording is viewed in real time. In other patients, there is a gradual transition from hypokinetic to akinetic or dyskinetic aneurysmal wall; these patients usually have very dysfunctional LV chambers and may evolve eventually into "ischemic" cardiomyopathy.

Apical aneurysms do not necessarily appear as local protrusions (Figure 14–8) but are in fact often seen as a widening of the normal tapered apical contour (Figure 14-9). Normally, the LV chamber always narrows from mid-LV toward the apex; a failure to so narrow or a tendency to apical expansion (relative to the mid-LV) should be called an *aneurysm.*

It is often necessary to scan the LV chamber along multiple meridians in apical views to best appreciate the aneurysmal distortion of LV shape. Unconventional off-center planes may have to be imaged for the same purpose.

In patients with LV aneurysms being considered for possible coronary bypass surgery or aneurysmectomy, the extent and contractility of the nonaneurysmal LV wall and septum are important considerations. The size and function of the residual LV chamber (excluding the aneurysm) have been studied by echocardiographers[21] because of the vital bearing they may have on aneurysm resectability and survival with medical therapy. Barrett et al.[21] devised a simple though arbitrary method of estimating an index of residual myocardium based on the percentage of LV contour long axis in apical views that belongs to normal LV wall versus aneurysm. Good surgical results after aneurysmectomy were obtained in those with an index of 0.42 or more.

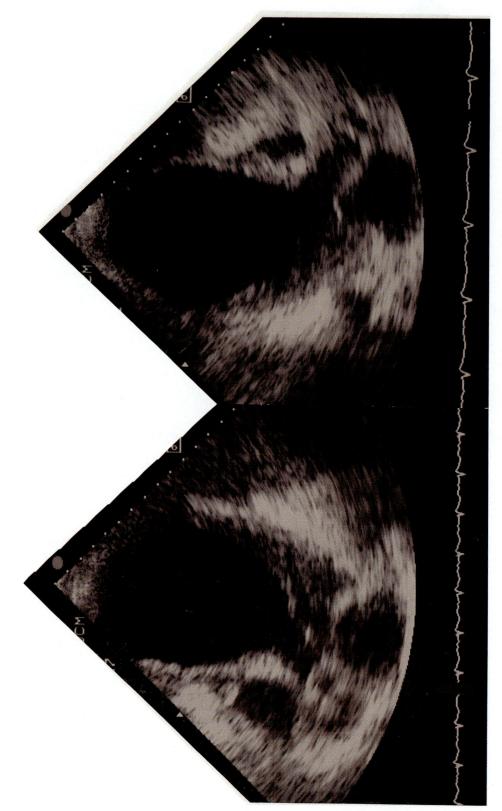

Figure 14–9. Most of this severely dilated LV chamber was akinetic (huge apical aneurysm) except for some contractility in its basal one-third. The ejection fraction by MUGA was 8%.

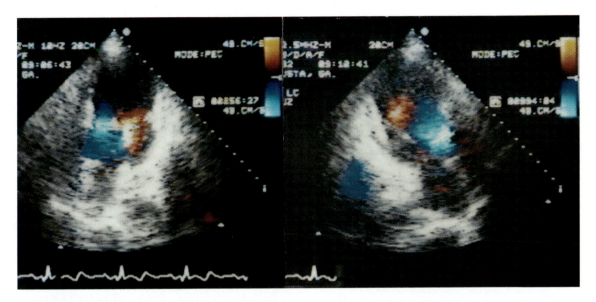

Figure 14–10. Apical long-axis view (left) and four-chamber view (right) of a patient with a large apical aneurysm (arrows). Stasis of blood in the aneurysm manifests as darker color and partial absence of color.

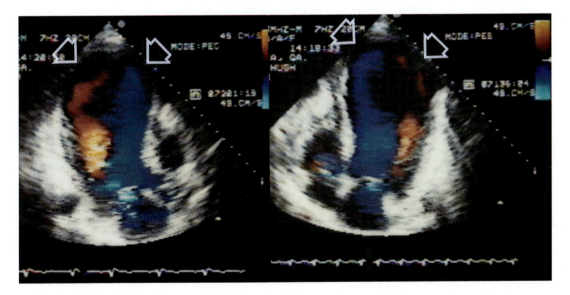

Figure 14–11. Apical four-chamber view (left) and long-axis view (right) showing absence of colorflow Doppler signals in the apical one-third of the left ventricle. This patient had a large apical aneurysm with such sluggish flow in it that it did not register on colorflow Doppler.

Figure 14–12. (A) Diagram in parasternal view comparing normal appearance (above) with small (center) and large (below) posterobasal aneurysm. The latter needs to be distinguished from a pseudoaneurysm. (B) Parasternal long-axis view (left) apical four-chamber view in diastole (center) and in systole (right). An aneurysm (arrows) of the posterobasal wall, involving also the basal posterolateral wall, causes a regional distortion of normal LV shape in this patient (B.W.). Note systolic expansion of aneurysm.

Relative stasis of blood flow is the rule in large apical aneurysms, evident on color-flow Doppler as absence of color in the aneurysm (Figure 14-10) or fragmentation and darkening of color (Figure 14-11).

Posterobasal or inferior wall aneurysms (Figure 14-12A) are much less common than anteroseptal-apical aneurysms. Posterobasal aneurysms are restricted to the segment between the mitral annulus and the posteromedial papillary muscle and are usually only a shallow bulge. However, occasionally they can be quite large (Figures 14-12 to 14-15), exhibit stasis within (Figure 14-13), and even develop a mural thrombus (Figure 14-15).

Inferior wall aneurysms comprise less than 10% of postinfarction LV aneurysms. Those limited to the posterobasal wall (between the mitral annulus and the posteromedial papillary muscle) produce a typical abnormal bulge on the long-axis view and widening of the normal distance between attachment of posterior mitral leaflet to mitral annulus and the papillary muscle (Figures 14-14 and 14-15). Exceptionally, such a posterobasal aneurysm can be of huge size[22a] and involve also the adjacent posterobasal ventricular septum so that it encroaches massively into the RV chamber (Figures 14-16 and 14-17).

Rarely, LV aneurysms can occur in unusual sites, unrelated to MI. One such site is that part of the membranous ventricular septum which separates the LV chamber from the RA (the so-called atrioventricular septum). Transesophageal echocardiography (TEE) in such a case may show a sonolucent space projecting into the RA chamber and communicating through a narrow opening with the LV chamber.[22b]

Another variety, first described in the African Bantu, occurs in the submitral valve area. It was later reported from other countries but is rare in the United States. Congenital diverticula of the LV are protrusions at the LV apex or elsewhere in the LV wall and contain actively contracting myocardium in their walls. Therefore, during systole, blood flows from the diverticulum to the LV chamber, distinguishing it from LV pseudoaneurysm, in which systolic flow is in the reverse direction.[22c]

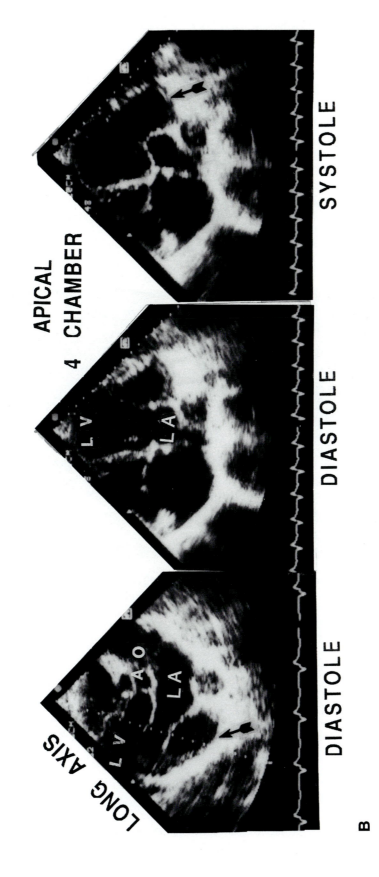

Figure 14–12. (Continued)

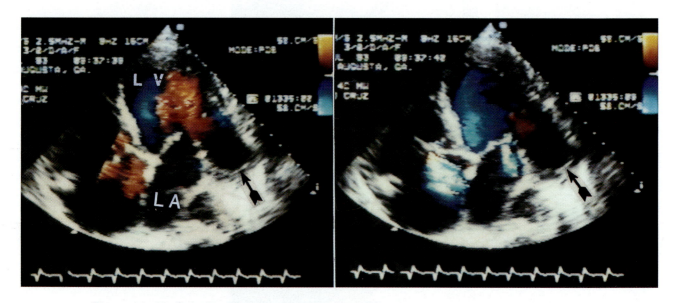

Figure 14–13. Colorflow Doppler, in apical four-chamber view in diastole (left) and systole (right) in the same patient (B.W.) showing stasis (absence of color) in the region of the posterobasal LV aneurysm (arrows).

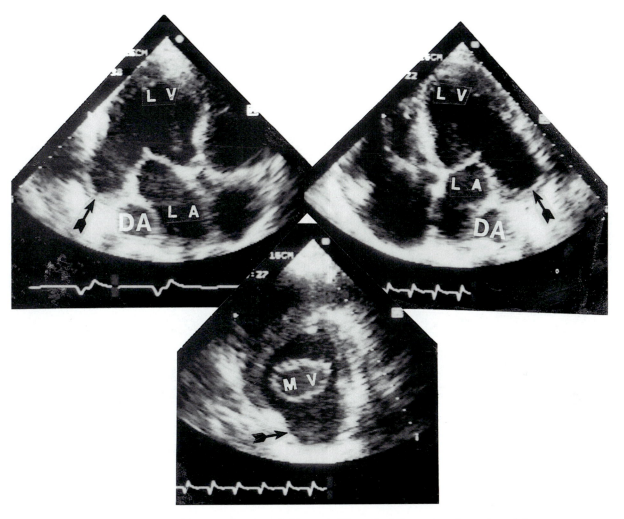

Figure 14–14. Apical long-axis view (above, left), apical four-chamber view (above, right), and parasternal short-axis view (below) of same patient (B.W.). Conspicuous local distortion of LV shape by an aneurysm of this size is an uncommon complication of posterobasal infarction.

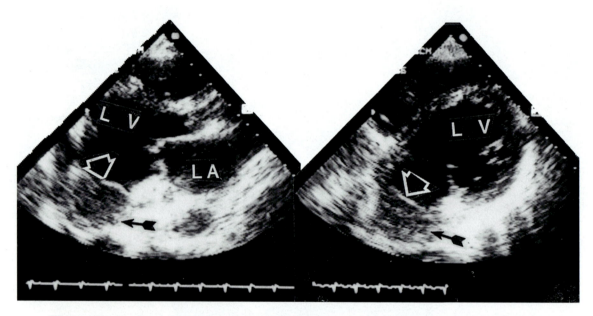

Figure 14–15. Parasternal long-axis view (left) and short-axis view (right) of a very large posteromedial inferior LV aneurysm that is partly filled by a thrombus (small thin arrows). The interface between blood in the LV chamber and thrombus is echogenic (open arrow).

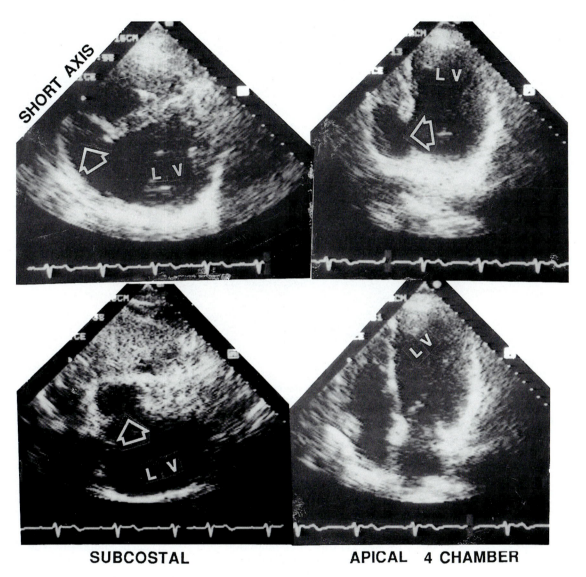

Figure 14–16. Unusual LV aneurysm of the basal posterior septum is seen in the two upper frames and left lower frame (arrows) but not in the standard apical four-chamber view (below, right).

PARASTERNAL
SHORT AXIS

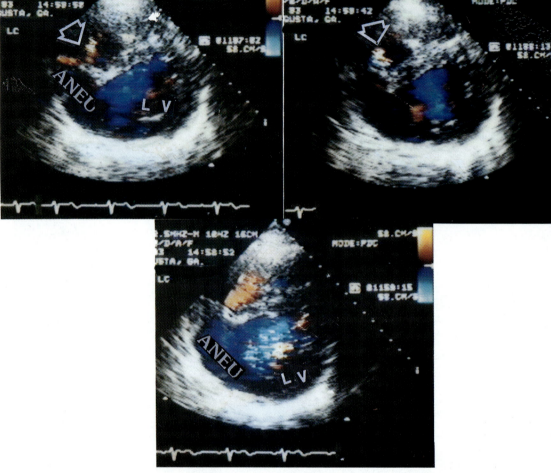

Figure 14–17. Colorflow Doppler in short-axis view of same patient showing posterior septal aneurysm with a small high-velocity jet (arrows) emerging from the apex of the aneurysm.

LV PSEUDOANEURYSM (Figure 14–18)

Sometimes LV wall rupture after infarction does not result in tamponade and death because the pericardial hematoma is limited by local adhesions. A large cavity is formed that communicates through a narrow "neck"—the site of LV rupture—with the main LV chamber.[23] Blood flows from the LV to the pseudoaneurysm in systole and in the reverse direction in diastole. LV pseudoaneurysms differ from true LV aneurysms in three important respects: (1) the wall of a pseudoaneurysm contains no myocardium, consisting instead of organized clot and pericardial adhesions; true LV aneurysms have walls of infarcted myocardium; (2) pseudoaneurysms have a strong tendency to rupture sooner or later, and so, once diagnosed, need to be surgically repaired; true aneurysms virtually never rupture once the acute phase (first week or two) is past; and (3) true LV aneurysms never have a narrow neck, the aneurysm always being wider where it joins normal LV wall than it is in its bulged or protruded convexity. LV pseudoaneurysms, on the other hand, invariably have a narrow neck or mouth, while the false aneurysm itself is usually large, sometimes larger than the LV chamber itself.

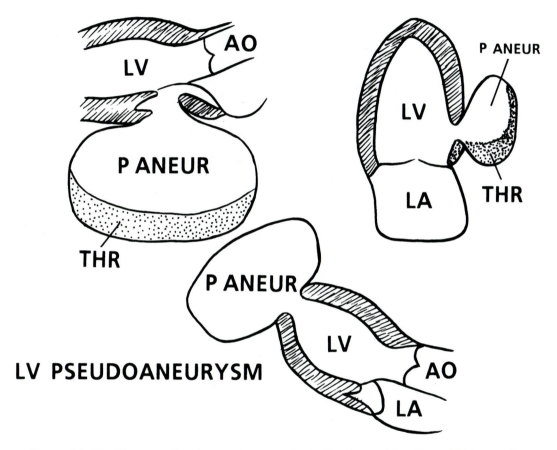

Figure 14–18. Diagram showing common variants in size and location of LV pseudo-aneurysms. (Above, left) Very large pseudoaneurysm following rupture of the poster-obasal LV wall. (Above, right) Smaller pseudoaneurysm of the posterolateral wall. (Below) Apical pseudoaneurysm. Note narrow neck, rounded shape of pseudo-aneurysm, and thrombus within it.

Echocardiography of LV Pseudoaneurysms (Figures 14–19 to 14–21)

The 2D echo features of LV pseudoaneurysm are highly diagnostic[24-26]: (1) an abrupt break or gap in LV wall continuity, where the sonolucency of the LV chamber communicates with the sonolucent space representing the pseudoaneurysm, (2) a spherical or ellipsoidal shape and usually large size, (3) a neck or mouth that is narrow, a small fraction of the maximum diameter of the pseudoaneurysm itself, (4) conspicuous expansion in systole, (5) obvious displacement or distortion of adjacent cardiac chambers (RV or LA), depending on the location and size of the pseudoaneurysm, (6) on pulsed-wave or color-flow Doppler, flow into the pseudoaneurysm from the LV chamber in early systole and in the reverse direction in early diastole, and (7) layered or mobile thrombus in the pseudoaneurysm. Using TEE, an LV pseudoaneurysm has been better visualized by a transgastric approach than by other views.[26a]

An LV pseudoaneurysm can be simulated by a partly lysed apical LV thrombus such that it intervenes between an apical pocket or aneurysm and the main LV chamber. The residual thrombus is then mistaken for the apical LV wall and the LV apex is mistaken for pseudoaneurysm.[26b]

POST-MYOCARDIAL INFARCTION RUPTURE OF THE VENTRICULAR SEPTUM

This complication occurs in about 1% of cases of myocardial infarction and accounts for 5% of all deaths from MI; 25% of patients with acquired ventricular septal defect (AVSD), of which MI is virtually the sole cause, die within the first 24 hours in cardiogenic shock; 90% die by the end of 2 months if the defect is not surgically repaired.

The crucial finding on 2D echo is visualization of the defect in the muscular ventricular septum.[27-32] The apical four-chamber and subcostal views are the best for this purpose. The septal discontinuity is a clean-cut gap in only a minority of cases; more often it is an oblique jagged or sinuous defect that may require unorthodox or off-center views to show it up best. The defect is better seen in systole than in diastole.

Contrast echocardiography to opacify the right ventricle, so as to demonstrate the AVSD shunt as a nonopacified stream, has been used as an adjunct to 2D echo. However, colorflow Doppler and pulsed-wave Doppler have proven even more useful and convenient to reveal the site as well as approximate size of the left-to-right shunt across the AVSD[31-39]; a turbulent flow is seen on the RV side of the defect. An uncommon variant of AVSD is perforation of the apex of a postinfarction septal aneurysm (See Figures 14–15 and 14–16).

Almost all patients with AVSD have a septal aneurysm surrounding the site of septal rupture. Sometimes the AVSD cannot be visualized on 2D echo, perhaps due to its ragged edges or tortuous track or to overlying thrombus, but the Doppler manifestations are detectable. Colorflow Doppler picks up a high-velocity jet usually directed anteriorly, reflecting the LV-RV systolic pressure gradient; this Doppler signal may be detected even when no AVSD can be visualized on 2D echo.

AVSD can complicate anterior as well as posterior MIs. Rupture occasionally can be shown by colorflow Doppler to have occurred at more than one site in the septal infarct. Rarely, a blood track dissects or burrows through the septum longitudinally, with an entry tear on the LV side and one or more sites on the RV side.

Both 2D echo and colorflow Doppler are very valuable in the noninvasive differential diagnosis of AVSD from severe mitral regurgitation due to papillary muscle rupture or "dysfunction"; both complications of acute MI manifest with rapid deterioration of cardiac status and a new systolic murmur. Echocardiography also provides information about associated LV or RV wall motion abnormalities; the more extensive these are, the worse is the prognosis; on the other hand, the nonischemic LV wall tends to compensate with

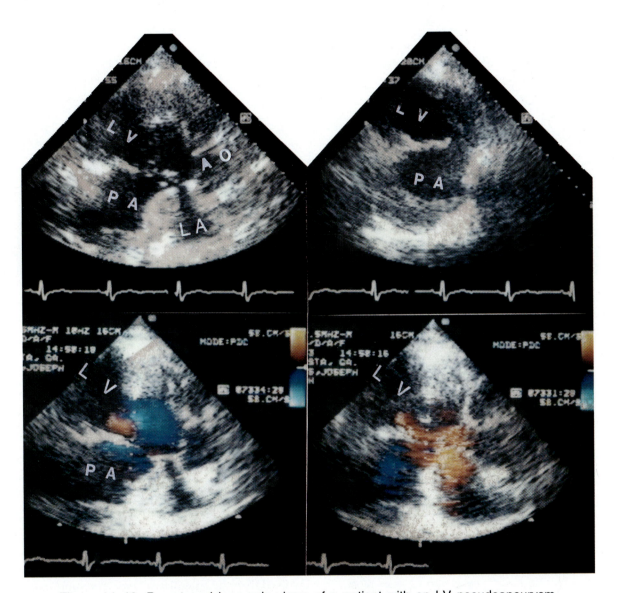

Figure 14–19. Parasternal long-axis views of a patient with an LV pseudoaneurysm (PA) following rupture of the LV posterobasal wall. The pseudoaneurysm has caused gross distortion of the posterior LV-LA junction simulating an LA mass (above, left). A thrombus is seen in the pseudoaneurysm (above, right). Colorflow Doppler shows systolic flow into the pseudoaneurysm from LV (below, left) and in the reverse direction in diastole (below, right).

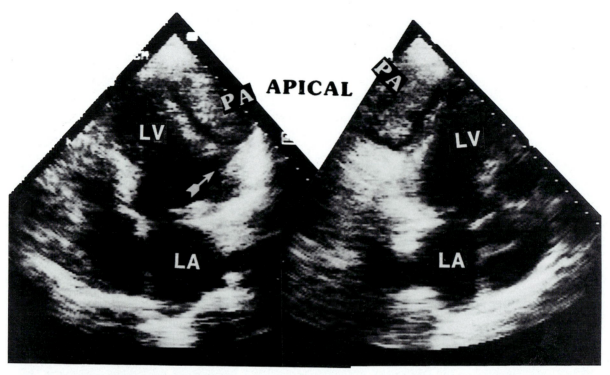

Figure 14–20. Apical four-chamber view (left) and apical long-axis view (right) of a patient (F.P.) with a pseudoaneurysm (PA) that communicated with the LV chamber through a narrow neck (arrow) at the basal posterolateral wall. The pseudoaneurysm contained a thrombus that embolized soon after this echocardiogram, causing a stroke.

hyperkinetic motion. TEE has proven superior to transthoracic 2D echo in detecting AVSD, especially when dissection of the septum is part of the septal pathology.[39a,39b]

PAPILLARY MUSCLE RUPTURE

Like septal rupture, this is a rare complication occurring during the first week of MI (about 1% of cases), accompanied by a new systolic murmur and abrupt rapid deterioration of cardiac status. It is fatal within 2 weeks in 80% of cases. The posteromedial papillary muscle is 6 to 12 times more often involved than the anterolateral one. The rupture may sever the papillary muscle entirely from the LV wall, or only one of the heads may rupture. The break can occur at the base, middle, or apex of the papillary muscle; in the latter case it may appear to be a chordal rather than myocardial rupture.

On 2D echo, the normal continuity of papillary muscle–chord–mitral leaflets, in long-axis views, is replaced by only the stump (base) of the papillary muscle, with flail motion of one or both mitral leaflets.[40,41] The severed apical portion of the ruptured papillary muscle is attached to and moves with the flail leaflet and chords, a striking and unusual motion pattern that may mimic a vegetation. Mitral regurgitation is severe. These echocardiographic findings can be appreciated in finer detail by TEE, as reported by Sakai et al.,[42] who also reported another instance of papillary muscle rupture caused by trauma (motorcycle accident) in a 17-year-old.

Partial papillary muscle rupture has been identified by 2D echo in at least three reports.[40,42a,42b] The ruptured fragment is not loose but remains attached to the LV wall by

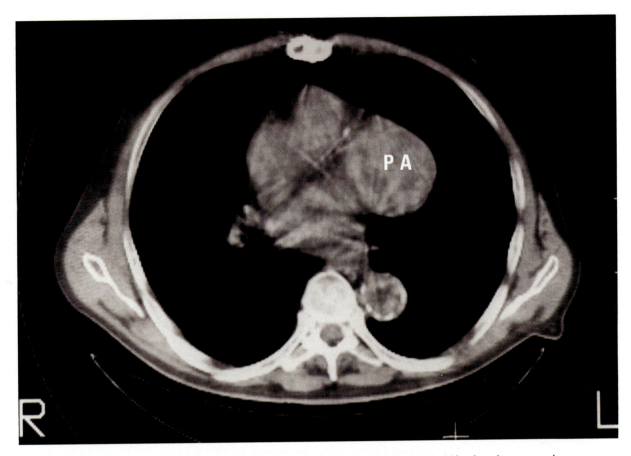

Figure 14–21. CT of thorax in same patient (F.P, Figure 14–20) showing pseudo-aneurysm.

a thin shred of myocardium; the patient may not be in serious decompensation at this stage, but later complete rupture results in catastrophic failure.[40,42a,42b]

PAPILLARY MUSCLE DYSFUNCTION WITHOUT RUPTURE

Papillary muscle dysfunction is an ill-defined entity invoked when mitral regurgitation is encountered in a patient with inferior infarction. The concept of papillary muscle dysfunction was introduced 30 years ago by Burch et al.[43] in the pre-echocardiographic era. Subsequently, different authors have claimed to have observed various 2D echo findings that would explain mitral regurgitation.[43a,44,45] These include (1) fibrosis of papillary muscles as part of the inferior wall infarction, the LV size and shape being normal, (2) LV dilatation or posteroinferior aneurysm, with altered alignment of the papillary muscles and chordae with respect to LV mitral annulus and leaflets such that the mechanics of mitral leaflet apposition in systole are rendered abnormal, causing mitral regurgitation, and (3) restraint or retraction of one of the mitral leaflets toward the apex with lack of normal closing motion so that mitral leaflet apposition is incomplete.

Whether these hypotheses are in fact true and valid has been questioned. Dense sclerosis or calcification of the posteromedial (much less often the anterolateral) papillary muscle[46] is common, but mitral regurgitation on colorflow Doppler may be absent or slight in some cases, casting doubt on its direct causal role for mitral regurgitation. Nonapposition of mitral leaflets is seldom clearly seen on 2D echo, even when mitral regurgitation is severe.

LV WALL RUPTURE[47-54]

Morgagni collected 10 cases of cardiac rupture in 1765 and referred to the first description by William Harvey in 1647. By 1925, 654 cases had been reported, and soon ventricular rupture became recognized as a major cause of death from MI. An incidence of 3% to 13% was mentioned in several autopsy series of MI, except for one series of 87 cases of cardiac rupture comprising 24% of MI fatalities.

This catastrophic complication occurs within 2 weeks of the onset of MI in over 90% of cases, in the first week in 70%, and in the first 24 hours in 22%.

Nearly always it is an acute transmural (full-thickness) MI that ruptures. Generally, the MI is large, but in one series it was less than 3 cm in size in one-fourth of cases. Histologically, myocardial necrosis with or without hemorrhage is always seen. Rupture of an old infarct is excessively rare and, in the very few cases described, occurred in a ventricular aneurysm.

LV free wall rupture can occur at any LV location, but common sites include (1) near the septal attachment, either anteriorly or posteriorly, (2) at the LV apex, and (3) between the basal attachments of the two LV papillary muscles. At autopsy, there is evidence of acute coronary artery occlusion in 75% of LV rupture, usually by a fresh thrombus.

An obvious LV wall tear is noted at autopsy in four-fifths of cases; in the rest, the pathology has been described as a "hemorrhagic dissection." Whereas death is literally sudden in most instances, within a matter of minutes, in other cases there is a more gradual "giving way" of the necrotic LV wall with slow leak of blood into the pericardial sac.[53] Most patients with post-MI rupture are between 50 and 70 years of age. Hypertension is a frequent predisposing condition.[52]

Subacute Ventricular Wall Rupture

Rupture of the LV free wall, a major recognized complication of acute MI, can result in (1) *sudden death* due to hemopericardium and "hyperacute" cardiac tamponade, (2) *pseudoaneurysm* of the LV, the hematoma being walled off by blood clot and pericardial adhesions, thus forming a chamber or space containing blood that communicates with the true LV chamber, and (3) *subacute LV wall rupture.* This entity has emerged as a result of clinicopathologic series from many centers in the 1970s and 1980s. The patient survives for several hours or even days, permitting lifesaving surgical repair if the diagnosis is made in time. In this emergency situation, echocardiography has a vital role to play, and hence this situation merits special attention.[55-60]

Lopes-Sendon et al.[60] in 1992 collected 128 patients, documented in 40 reports, and added 18 cases of their own. They estimate that the total incidence of LV free wall rupture in acute MI is about 5% and that subacute LV wall rupture comprises about one-third of these.

The echocardiographic features are as follows: (1) Generally, there is pericardial effusion, which tends to be of moderate size and localized solely or predominantly to the vicinity of the rupture site. However, it must be kept in mind that a small pericardial effusion is common (6% to 37% of patients) in acute MI.[8] It is the combination of unexpected hypotension or cardiogenic shock with a pericardial effusion on 2D echo that suggests subacute LV wall rupture. (2) The pericardial space is not entirely sonolucent, as it is usually in effusions, but contains "solid" or even dense echoes. This has been a very consistent finding in many reported series, and similar echo appearances have been produced experimentally in dogs by introduction of blood into the pericardial sac.[61] (3) There are echo signs of tamponade. RV wall compression has been found particularly useful in this situation by several groups. (4) Surprisingly, an actual LV wall tear or gap is seldom visualized. Local akinesis, wall thinning, and altered density or texture have been described at what is later found (at surgery or autopsy) to be the site of egress of blood. However, similar echo changes are often seen if the LV wall is infarcted but not ruptured.

LV wall rupture that is not immediately fatal is presumed to be due to a slow leak of blood into the pericardial sac, which in turn leads to development of tamponade over hours. Possible reasons why hemorrhage into the pericardium is gradual or intermittent include (1) a small tortuous or serpiginous myocardial tear, (2) formation of clots within a tear, thus plugging it, at least temporarily, and (3) rise in intrapericardial pressure, which also retards the cardiac leak.

Pericarditis

In autopsy series of MI, the incidence of pericarditis is about 13% to 45%, as manifested by local epicardial thickening and organizing fibrinous exudate. The pericarditis is essentially "dry" in half the cases and accompanied by a small pericardial effusion in the others.[62] However, in patients receiving anticoagulant therapy, hemopericardium can be a serious complication, even causing tamponade.

REFERENCES

1. Heger JJ, Weyman AE, Wann LS, et al. Cross-sectional echocardiographic analysis of the extent of left ventricular asynergy in acute myocardial infarction. Circulation 1980;61:1113.
2. Weiss JL, Bulkley BH, Hutchins GM, et al. Two-dimensional echocardiographic recognition of myocardial injury in man: Comparison with postmortem studies. Circulation 1981;63:401.
3. Visser CA, Lie KI, Kan G. Detection and quantification of acute, isolated myocardial infarction by two-dimensional echocardiography. Am J Cardiol 1981;47:1020.
4. Gibson RS, Bishop HL, Stamm RB, et al. Value of two-dimensional echocardiography in patients with acute myocardial infarction. Am J Cardiol 1982;49:1110.
5. Jaarsma W, Visser Ca, Eenige MJ, et al. Predictive value of two-dimensional echocardiographic and hemodynamic measurements on admission with acute myocardial infarction. J Am Soc Echocardiogr 1988;1:187.
6. Hutchins GM, Bulkley BH. Infarct expansion versus extension. Am J Cardiol 1978;41:127.
7. Schuster EH, Bulkley BH. Expansion of transmural myocardial infarction: A pathophysiological factor in cardiac rupture. Circulation 1979;60:1532.
8. Bulkley BH. Site and sequelae of myocardial infarction (editorial). N Engl J Med 1981;305:337.
9. Eaton LW, Weiss JL, Bulkley BL, et al. Regional cardiac dilatation after acute myocardial infarction: Recognition by two-dimensional echocardiography. N Engl J Med 1979;300:57.
10. Erlebacher JA, Weiss JL, Eaton LW, et al. Late effects of acute infarct dilatation on heart size. Am J Cardiol 1982;49:1120.
11. McKay RG, Pfeffer MA, Pasternak RC, et al. Left ventricular remodeling after myocardial infarction: A corollary to infarct expansion. Circulation 1986;74:693.
12. Meizlish JL, Berger HJ, Plankey M, et al. Functional left ventricular aneurysm formation after acute anterior transmural myocardial infarction. N Engl J Med 1984;311:1001.
13. D'Cruz IA, Aboulatta H, Killam H, et al. Quantitative two-dimensional echocardiographic assessment of left ventricle shape in ischemic heart disease. J Clin Ultrasound 1989;8:569.
14. Schlicter J, Hellerstein HK, Katz LN. Aneurysm of the heart: A correlative study of 102 proved cases. Medicine 1954;33:43.
15. Cabin HS, Roberts WC. True left ventricular aneurysm and healed myocardial infarction. Am J Cardiol 1980;46:754.
16. Hochman JS, Platia EF, Bulkley BH. Endocardial abnormalities in left ventricular aneurysms. Ann Intern Med 1984;100:29.
17. Hutchins GM, Bannayan GA. Development of endocardial fibroelastosis following myocardial infarction. Arch Pathol 1971;91:113.
18. Weyman AE, Peskoe SM, Williams ES, et al. Detection of left ventricular aneurysms by cross-sectional echocardiography. Circulation 1976;54:936.
19. Visser CA, Kan G, David GK, et al. Echocardiographic-cineangiographic correlation in detecting left ventricular aneurysm. Am J Cardiol 1982;50:337.
20. Arvan S, Badillo P. Contractile properties of the left ventricle with aneurysm. Am J Cardiol 1985;55:338.
21. Barrett MJ, Charuzi Y, Corday E. Ventricular aneurysm: Cross-sectional echocardiographic approach. Am J Cardiol 1980;46:1133.
22. Baur HR, Daniel JA, Nelson RR. Detection of left ventricular aneurysm on two-dimensional echocardiography. Am J Cardiol 1982;50:191.

22a. DePace NL, Dowinsky S, Untereker W, et al. Giant inferior wall left ventricular aneurysm. Am Heart J 1990;119:400.

22b. Lin L-J, Chen J-H, Yang Y-J, et al. Aneurysm of the atrioventricular septum between the left ventricle and right atrium without atrial septal defect. Am Heart J 1993;126:735.

22c. Weyman AE. Principles and Practice of Echocardiography, 2d ed. Philadelphia: Lea & Febiger, 1994, p 673.

23. Roberts WC, Morrow AG. Pseudoaneurysm of the left ventricle. Am J Med 1967;43:639.

24. Catherwood E, Mintz GS, Kotler MN, et al. Two-dimensional echocardiographic recognition of left ventricular pseudoaneurysm. Circulation 1980;62:294.

25. Gatewood RP, Nanda NC. Differentiation of left ventricular pseudoaneurysm by pulsed Doppler with two-dimensional echocardiography. Am J Cardiol 1980;46:869.

26. Loperfido F, Pennestri F, Mazzari M, et al. Diagnosis of left ventricular pseudoaneurysm by pulsed Doppler echocardiography. Am Heart J 1981;110:1291.

26a. Stoddard MF, Dawkins PR, Longaker RA, et al. Transesophageal echocardiography in the detection of left ventricular pseudoaneurysm. Am Heart J 1993;125:534.

26b. Badano L, Piazza R, Bisignani G, et al. A large left ventricular thrombus evolving toward canalization and mimicking a left ventricular pseudoaneurysm. J Am Soc Echocardiogr 1993;6:446.

27. Scanlan JG, Seward JB, Tajik AJ. Visualization of ventricular septal rupture utilizing wide angle two-dimensional echocardiography. Mayo Clin Proc 1979;54:381.

28. Farcot JC, Boisante L, Rigand M, et al. Two-dimensional echo sector angiographic diagnosis of ventricular septal defect after acute anterior myocardial infarction. Am J Cardiol 1980;45:370.

29. Rogers EW, Glassman RD, Feigenbaum H, et al. Aneurysms of the posterior interventricular septum with postinfarction ventricular septal defect. Chest 1980;78:741.

30. Bishop HL, Gibson RS, Stamm RB, et al. Role of two-dimensional echocardiography in the evaluation of patients with ventricular septal rupture post myocardial infarction. Am Heart J 1981;102:965.

31. Pandis IP, Mintz GS, Goel I, et al. Acquired ventricular septal defect after myocardial infarction: Detection by combined two-dimensional and Doppler echocardiography. Am Heart J 1986;111:427.

32. Recusani F, Raisaro A, Sgalambro A, et al. Ventricular septal rupture after myocardial infarction: Diagnosis by two-dimensional and pulsed Doppler echocardiography. Am J Cardiol 1984;54:277.

33. Eisenberg PR, Barzilai B, Perez JE. Noninvasive detection by Doppler echocardiography of combined ventricular septal rupture and mitral regurgitation. J Am Coll Cardiol 1984;4:617.

34. Keren G, Sherez J, Roth A, et al. Diagnosis from acute myocardial infarction by combined two-dimensional and pulsed Doppler echocardiography. Am J Cardiol 1984;53:1202.

35. Come PC. Doppler detection of acquired ventricular septal defect. Am J Cardiol 1985;55:586.

36. Drobac M, Gilbert B, Howard R, et al. Ventricular septal defect after myocardial infarction: Diagnosis by two-dimensional contrast echocardiography. Circulation 1983;67:335.

37. Miyatake K, Okamoto M, Kinoshita N, et al. Doppler echocardiographic feature of ventricular septal rupture in myocardial infarction. J Am Coll Cardiol 1985;5:182.

38. Fortuin DF, Sheikh KH, Kisslo J. The utility of echocardiography in the diagnostic strategy of postinfarction ventricular septal rupture. Am Heart J 1991;121:25.

39. Amico A, Iliceto S, Rizzo A, et al. Color Doppler findings in ventricular septal dissection following myocardial infarction. Am Heart J 1989;117:195.

39a. Koenig K, Kasper W, Hofmann T, et al. Transesophageal echocardiography for diagnosis of rupture of the ventricular septum or papillary muscle during acute myocardial infarction. Am J Cardiol 1987;59:362.

39b. Ballal RS, Sanyal RS, Nanda NC, et al. Usefulness of transesophageal echocardiography in the diagnosis of ventricular septal rupture secondary to acute myocardial infarction. Am J Cardiol 1993;71:366.

40. Come PC, Riley MF, Weintraub R, et al. Echocardiographic detection of complete and partial papillary muscle rupture during acute myocardial infarction. Am J Cardiol 1985;56:787.

41. Pandian NG, Isner JM, McInerney KP, et al. Noninvasive assessment of the complicated myocardial infarction: Use of Doppler and two-dimensional echocardiography to differentiate ventricular septal rupture from rupture of mitral apparatus. Echocardiography 1985;2:329.

42. Sakai K, Nakamura K, Hosoda S. Transesophageal echocardiographic findings of papillary muscle rupture. Am J Cardiol 1991;68:561.

42a. Nishimura RA, Shub C, Tajik AJ. Two-dimensional echocardiographic diagnosis of partial papillary muscle rupture. Br Heart J 1982;48:598.

42b. Hanlon JT, Conrad AK, Combs DT, et al. Echocardiographic recognition of partial papillary muscle rupture. J Am Soc Echocardiogr 1993;6:101.

43. Burch GE, Depascuale NP, Phillips JH. Clinical manifestations of papillary muscle dysfunction. Arch Intern Med 1963;12:112.

43a. Tallary VK, Depasculae NP, Burch GE. The echocardiogram in papillary muscle dysfunction. Am Heart J 1972;83:12.

44. Ogawa S, Hubbard FE, Mardelli TJ, et al. Cross-sectional echocardiographic spectrum of papillary muscle dysfunction. Am Heart J 1979;97:312.

45. Godley RV, Wann LS, Rogers EW. Incomplete mitral leaflet closure in patients with papillary muscle dysfunction. Circulation 1981;63:565.

46. Chandaratna PAN, Ulene R, Nimalasuriya A, et al. Differentiation between acute and healed myocardial infarction by signal averaging and color encoding two-dimensional echocardiography. Am J Cardiol 1985;56:381.

47. London RE, London SB. Rupture of the heart. Circulation 1965;31:202.

48. Bjork G, Mogensen L, Nyquist O, et al. Studies of myocardial rupture with cardiac tamponade in acute myocardial infarction. Chest 1972;61:4.

49. Sweet SE, Sterung R, McCormick JR, et al. Left ventricular false aneurysm after coronary bypass surgery. Am J Cardiol 1979;43:154.

50. Eisenmann B, Bareiss P, Pacifico AD, et al. Anatomic, clinical and therapeutic features of acute cardiac rupture. J Thorac Cardiovasc Surg 1978;76:78.

51. Fox AC, Glassman E, Isom OW. Surgically remediable complications of myocardial infarction. Progr Cardiovasc Dis 1979;21:461.

52. Edmondson HA, Hozie HJ. Hypertension and cardiac rupture. Am Heart J 1943;24:719.

53. Coma-Canella I, Lopez-Sendon J, Gonzalez LN, et al. Subacute left ventricular free wall rupture following acute myocardial infarction. Am Heart J 1983;106:278.

54. Feneley MP, Chang VP, O'Rourke M. Myocardial rupture after acute myocardial infarction. Br Heart J 1983;49:550.

55. DeSoutter P, Halphen C, Haiat R. Two-dimensional echocardiographic visualization of free ventricular wall rupture in acute anterior myocardial infarction. Am Heart J 1984;108:1360.

56. Garcia-Fernandez MA, Moreno M, Rossi PN, et al. Echocardiographic features of hemopericardium. Am Heart J 1984;107:1035.

57. Hermoni H, Engel PJ. Two-dimensional echocardiography in cardiac rupture. Am J Cardiol 1986;57:180.

58. Knopf WD, Talley JD, Murphy DA. An echo-dense mass in the pericardial space as a sign of left ventricular free wall rupture during acute myocardial infarction. Am J Cardiol 1987;59:1202.

59. Papas PJ, Cernaianu AC, Baldino WA, et al. Ventricular free wall rupture after myocardial infarction. Chest 1991;99:892.

60. Lopez-Sendon J, Gonzalez A, Desa EL. Diagnosis of subacute ventricular wall rupture after acute myocardial infarction: Sensitivity and specificity of clinical, hemodynamic and echocardiographic criteria. J Am Coll Cardiol 1992;19:1145.

61. Lopez-Sendon J, Garcia-Fernandez MA, Coma-Canella I, et al. Identification of blood in the pericardial cavity in dogs by two-dimensional echocardiography. Am J Cardiol 1984;53:1194.

62. Galve E, Garcia del Castillo H, Evangelista A, et al. Pericardial effusion in the course of myocardial infarction. Circulation 1986;73:294.

15

Cardiomyopathy

The term *cardiomyopathy* was introduced in the 1950s by Brigden[1] to refer collectively to primary myocardial disease; by strict definition, myocardial hypertrophy, dilatation, or damage secondary to congenital, rheumatic, coronary, or hypertensive heart disease is excluded. Over 30 years ago, Goodwin et al.[2] classified cardiomyopathies into three categories: congestive, hypertrophic, and restrictive. This classification is still valid and widely used. Congestive (dilated) cardiomyopathy is very common; hypertrophic cardiomyopathy is less common but an important entity for cardiologists as well as echocardiographers (see Chapter 13); and restrictive cardiomyopathy is an uncommon hemodynamic entity that can result from diverse etiologies. Although dilated cardiomyopathy (DCM) and hypertrophic cardiomyopathy (HCM) both present with symptoms of congestive heart failure and carry the risk of sudden death, they are exact opposites in many aspects of anatomy (and echocardiographic appearance).

In DCM, the left ventricular (LV) chamber is dilated and diffusely hypocontractile, with little or no LV wall or septal hypertrophy. In HCM, the LV chamber is small with hypertrophied and hypercontractile LV walls; more often than not, the ventricular septum is more severely hypertrophied and hypokinetic, with dynamic systolic narrowing of the LV outflow tract.

DILATED (CONGESTIVE) CARDIOMYOPATHY

The original adjective *congestive* used by Goodwin et al.[2] was thought to be vague and was gradually replaced by *dilated*.[3] DCM is the end result of any of a long list of over 100 causes, which can be grouped into the following categories:

1. Infective (bacterial, viral, protozoan)
2. Nutritional and metabolic
3. Autoimmune (collagen disease)
4. Inborn errors of metabolism
5. Familial neurologic, neuromuscular, and myopathic
6. Drugs and chemicals

In this country, certain clinical varieties of DCM are important, the foremost being alcoholic, with others such as peripartum cardiomyopathy and the toxic effects of cancer chemotherapy also not uncommon. In a large percentage of cases, no etiologic factor is obvious, and the label *idiopathic DCM* is used; many believe that these are "burnt out" cases of viral (possibly Coxsackie) myocarditis.

At autopsy, the ventricles are dilated, and heart weights are considerably increased: 400 to 940 g (mean 632 g) in men and 360 to 860 g (mean 551 g) in women in the large, well-studied series of Roberts et al.[3a] Longer survival since diagnosis results in heavier hearts. The typical DCM heart is large, flabby, and pale, with all four chambers obviously dilated.[3-6] The LV wall thickness is normal to slightly increased; the thicker the wall, the better is the prognosis in terms of longevity.[6]

Histologically, the cut surface of LV myocardium shows small areas of fibrosis, especially subendocardially. Grossly visible scarring was noted in 14% of DCM hearts in the series of Roberts et al.[3] Patchy endocardial thickening, especially at the LV apex, is common and may be the site of thrombus formation. Conversely, mural apical thrombi can organize and eventually evolve into endocardial plaques.

In the description of Roberts et al.,[3] rigorous criteria were used for diagnosing DCM at autopsy, including dilatation of both ventricles and anatomically normal valves and pericardium, with coronary artery stenosis absent or of insignificant degree. However, a pervasive trend has developed to use the term *ischemic cardiomyopathy* for patients with diffuse LV hypokinesis who have severe extensive coronary artery stenosis. These patients have had multiple MIs and probably ischemia of the intervening noninfarcted myocardium.

ECHOCARDIOGRAPHY OF DCM

Soon after *M-mode echo* examination of the chamber became possible, it became evident that certain very consistent abnormalities[7-9] were the rule in DCM (Figure 15-1):

1. Increased LV internal dimension at end-diastole (57 to 80 mm or more) as well as end-systole
2. Decreased systolic shortening fraction of the LV dimension, from 27% down to 10% or less
3. Hypokinesis (diminished systolic excursion) of the ventricular septum as well as LV posterior wall, less than 4 and 9 mm, respectively. Corya et al.[7] found that the sum of the excursions of septum and LV posterior wall was usually less than 13 mm in patients with DCM but usually 13 mm or more in patients with coronary heart disease. Caveats: (a) "ischemic cardiomyopathy" will behave like primary DCM, and (b) septal akinesis or paradoxical motion occurs in a minority of DCM patients due to massive tricuspid regurgitation with gross RV volume overload or secondary to left bundle branch block.
4. The mitral valve M-mode echo has a typical double-diamond configuration, situated in the posterior half of the LV chambers, so that an abnormally

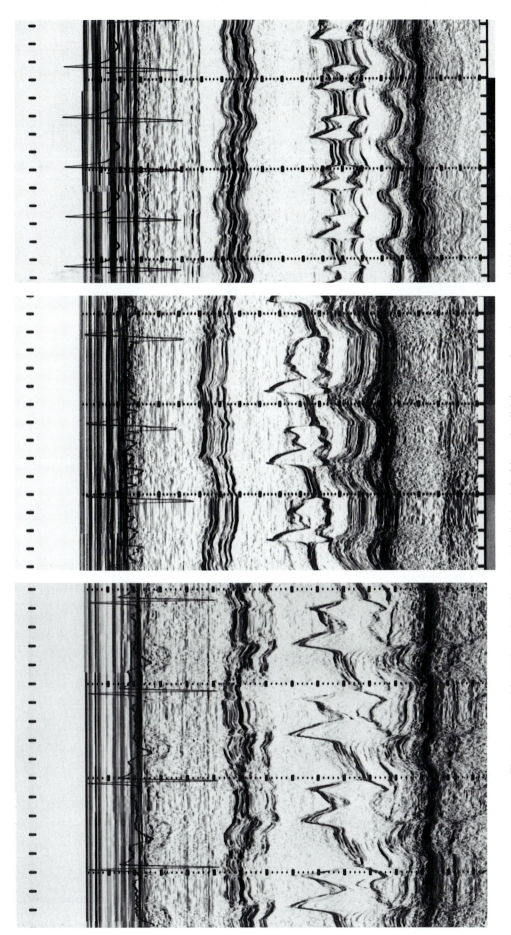

Figure 15–1. M-mode echo of normal individual (left) and mild (center) and severe (right) dilated cardiomyopathy. Note increased LV size, different mitral valve contour, increased E point–septal separation (EPSS), and hypokinesis of septum as well as LV posterior wall in the cardiomyopathic hearts. Scale more compressed at center and right.

397

MITRAL E POINT – SEPTAL SEPARATION

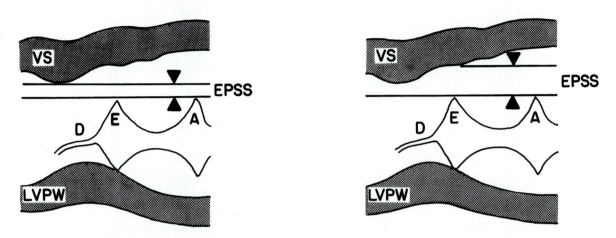

Figure 15–2. Two different ways of measuring EPSS on M-mode echo: Upper normal limit is 5 mm by method on left (Massie et al.) and 10 mm by method at right (D'Cruz et al.). Both methods are used widely.

wide separation is noted between the ventricular septum and mitral E peak,[10,11] exceeding 10 mm (Figure 15-2).

5. Mild to moderate left atrial dilatation is the rule.

On *two-dimensional (2D) echo* the main findings are (Figures 15-3 and 15-4):

1. Diffuse LV wall hypokinesis. Although there may sometimes be minor disparities in different LV regions[12], there is no LV segment that contracts normally.[13,14]
2. Large chamber size
3. Abnormal LV shape, becoming more globular (spheric)

Because of the word *dilated* in the name itself and by its traditional definition since

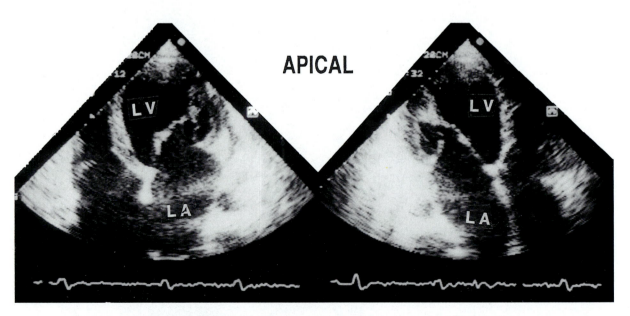

Figure 15–3. Apical long-axis view (right) and apical four-chamber view (left) in a man with alcoholic cardiomyopathy. LV shape is spheric.

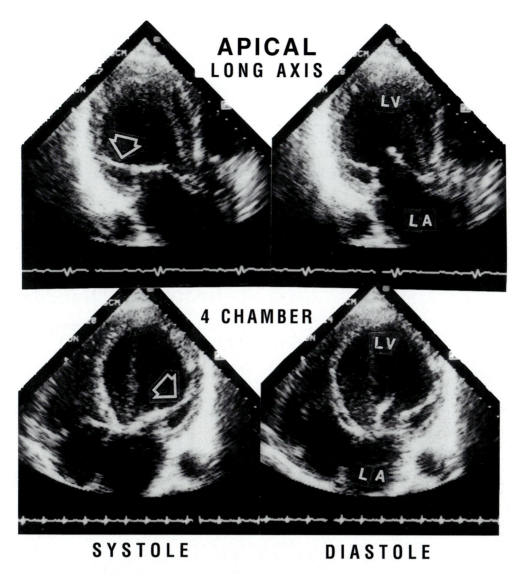

APICAL LONG AXIS

4 CHAMBER

SYSTOLE   DIASTOLE

Figure 15–4. Apical four-chamber views (below) and long-axis views (above) in a patient with dilated cardiomyopathy. Alignment of the papillary muscles with the mitral valve is abnormal (arrows), the former being displaced toward the basal posterolateral wall. Note poor LV contraction; the systolic LV size (left) is only slightly smaller than the diastolic LV size (right).

1961, it has long been considered essential to the diagnosis of DCM that the LV chamber be dilated. On M-mode, this means that the end-diastolic LV internal dimension must exceed 56 mm, widely accepted as the upper normal limit.

In a series of intriguing papers, Keren et al.[15-17] described an entity they call "mildly dilated congestive cardiomyopathy" (Figures 15-5 and 15-6); their patients all had cardiac failure, low ejection fractions (<30%), but normal to marginally increased LVID. Subsequently, groups of similar cases of "mildly dilated" or even "nondilated" congestive cardiomyopathy have been reported by D'Cruz et al.,[18] Gavazzi et al.,[19] Zimmerman et al.,[20] and Kurozumi et al.[21]

Left Ventricular Shape

In 1823, Laennec[22] observed that when ventricles were dilated, "the augmentation of the cavity seems to be more in its breadth than length." He noted that "when both ventricles were dilated, the heart assumes a rounded shape, being nearly as wide at the apex as at the base."

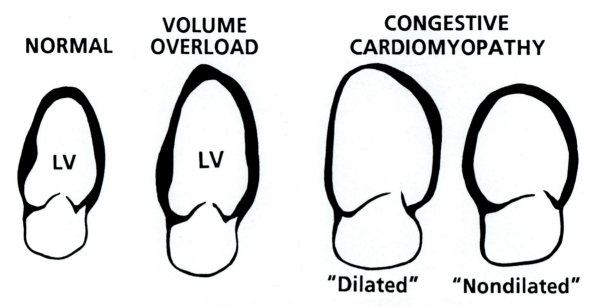

NORMAL **VOLUME OVERLOAD** **CONGESTIVE CARDIOMYOPATHY**

"Dilated" "Nondilated"

Figure 15–5. Diagram comparing LV size and shape in normal individuals, volume overload (MR or AI), dilated cardiomyopathy, and "nondilated" cardiomyopathy. LV shape tends to the spheric in the latter two.

However, until two decades ago, scant scientific attention was directed toward LV shape as an attribute of LV anatomy. Hutchins et al.[23] considered the basic relationships between LV shape and function in normal and abnormal hearts. They pointed out that a spherical shape would be ideal for the receiving chamber of a pump, because a sphere can accommodate the maximum volume per unit wall area. On the other hand, an ejection pump chamber working against resistance functions most efficiently when it is a narrow cylinder or cone. Since the LV chamber serves the dual purpose of receiving and ejecting blood, the actual LV shape (prolate ellipsoid) is a compromise between a sphere and a cylinder (or cone).

Deterioration of LV systolic performance has long been known to be associated with a change in LV shape toward the spheric or globular, first to pathologists at autopsy, then to radiologists viewing chest radiographs, later to angiocardiographers, and recently to those imaging the heart noninvasively by cardiac ultrasound, computed tomography (CT), or magnetic resonance imaging (MRI). Shape analysis based on autopsy cardiac measurements was reported by various authors, notably Janicki et al.[24] Over the last 20 years, several groups have expressed LV shape as a simple ratio of LV long axis (also called *major axis* or *length L*) to LV short axis (also called *minor axis, width,* or *diameter D*) or the reciprocal of this ratio, i.e., *L/D* or *D/L*. These measurements of L and D were made on cineangiograms[25,26] or on 2D echocardiograms.[27,28]

D'Cruz et al.[18,29,30] studied LV shape in normal individuals as well as DCM patients in apical views not only by long-axis/short-axis ratios but also by measuring the LV area/L^2 ratio and the ratio of $(D_1 + D_2 + D_3)/3L$, where D_1, D_2, and D_3 are three transverse LV dimensions such that they are perpendicular to LV length L and divide L into four equal parts. These ratios LV area/L^2 and $(D_1 + D_2 + D_3)/3L$ are perhaps better suited to assessing LV shape than a simple *L/D* ratio because the former takes into account that the LV chamber is not a perfect ellipsoid with its widest transverse dimension precisely bisecting the LV length; in fact, the widest LV transverse dimension is substantially closer to the LV base than to its apex.

D'Cruz et al.[18,30] as well as those who had studied LV shape by *L/D* ratios on angiocardiograms and 2D echo, have found that the LV chamber in DCM is consistently more spheric than normal. Laskey et al.,[26] on angiocardiographic data, reported *L/D* ratios of 1.5 to 2.22 (mean 1.8) in normal individuals and 1.2 to 1.6 (mean 1.4) in DCM patients.

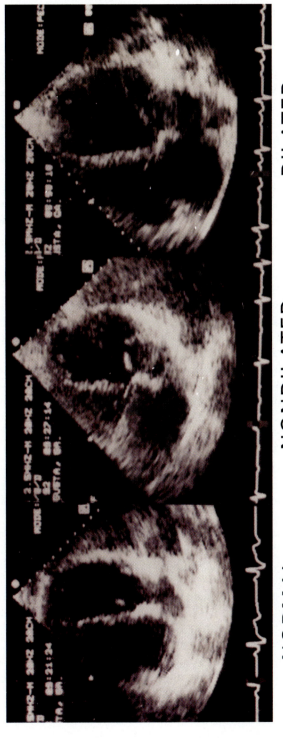

NORMAL   NONDILATED   DILATED
          CARDIOMYOPATHY   CARDIOMYOPATHY

Figure 15–6. Typical examples in apical four-chamber views of three individuals: normal, "nondilated" cardiomyopathy, and dilated cardiomyopathy. Note wider (spheric) shape in the latter two patients.

Borow et al.[27] found a similar *L/D* ratio in normal individuals (1.7); in DCM patients it was 1.49 in those with "appropriate" hypertrophy but even more spheric (1.22) in those with lack of LV hypertrophy. Douglas et al.[28] related LV shape to prognosis in a series of DCM patients and found that improved survival was associated with a left ventricular internal dimension (LVID) of <76 mm and a *D/L* ratio of <0.76 (i.e., *L/D* ratio of 1.316).

D'Cruz et al. found mean normal values of *D/L* ratio to be 0.55 ± 0.06, which is equivalent to a mean *L/D* ratio of 1.82. Mean normal value for the LV shape descriptor LV area/D^2 ratio was 0.50 ± 0.05 and for the shape descriptor $(D_1 + D_2 + D^3)/3L$ ratio was 0.52 ± 0.05.[18] Surprisingly, the more dilated cardiomyopathic LV chambers did not have more spheric shapes than those with lesser LV dilatation. One explanation for this finding is that LV shape change occurs early in the process of myocardial function deterioration, subsequent to which dilatation continues but with little further change in LV shape.[29] In this study it was found that LV dilatation comparable with that in DCM but due to volume overload (aortic and/or mitral regurgitation) is associated with close to normal LV shape, significantly different from LV shape in DCM.[18]

Another intriguing finding in the study by D'Cruz et al. comparing LV shape in patients with dilated congestive cardiomyopathy (LVID > 56 mm) with LV shape in patients with nondilated or borderline dilated congestive cardiomyopathy was that LV shape in the latter was abnormal (tendency to spheric), thus resembling LV shape in "classic" DCM but significantly more spheric than normal LV shape.

LV Thrombi in Dilated Cardiomyopathy

One-third to one-half of patients with DCM have mural LV thrombi at autopsy.[31-34] 2D echo in a large series of 123 DCM patients revealed LV thrombi in 36%.[35] Follow-up data in 96 of these patients, over a mean 2-year period, showed that systemic emboli occurred in 11% but were not more frequent in patients with 2D evidence of LV thrombi. LV thrombi were as frequent in ischemic as in idiopathic DCM in the series of Gottdiener et al.[35] These authors noted that serial echocardiograms over many months in DCM showed persistence of LV thrombi with little change, whereas LV mural thrombi developing in acute myocardial infarctions usually show partial or complete regression on follow-up.

Echocardiographic Features of DCM Correlating with Prognosis[36–39]

It might be expected that the more impaired LV systolic function is (reflected in LVID systolic shortening fraction or ejection fraction), the worse is the prognosis. This is in fact what was reported by some,[36-38] but others did not find the LV ejection fraction a strong predictor of survival.[28,39]

Douglas et al.[28] related LV size by echocardiography to prognosis by comparing data from 16 survivors followed for 52 months (mean) with data from 20 who died in 11 months (mean). They found that improved survival was associated with end-diastolic dimension of less than 76 mm.

Another item of LV anatomy that can be measured echocardiographically, which has some bearing on prognosis in DCM, is the presence and degree of LV hypertrophy.[40,41] Benjamin et al.[6] reported that long-surviving patients with DCM had greater LV wall thickness and larger heart weights than those with shorter life spans, even though both groups had similar LV chamber sizes and ejection fractions. The degree of LV hypertrophy in DCM also can be expressed as a relationship between echocardiographically estimated LV mass and volume. The larger the ratio of LV mass to LV volume or of LV wall thickness to LVID, the better is the prognosis.[38a]

RV Dilatation

Pathologic descriptions of DCM usually state that it is characterized by dilatation of all four chambers. However, from the echocardiographer's perspective, this is not always so. Lewis et al.[39] found that of 67 consecutive patients with DCM, 38 had an approximately equal degree of RV and LV dilatation (diastolic LV area < 2.0 times RV area, in apical four-

APICAL 4 CHAMBER

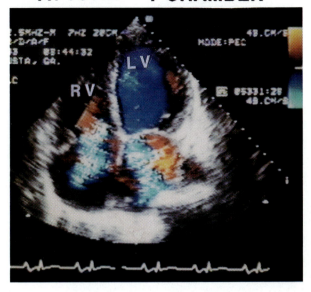

Figure 15–7. Apical four-chamber view of a patient with dilated cardiomyopathy. All four chambers are dilated, with both ventricles unduly wide. 3+ MR and TR are present.

chamber view), but in the other 29, LV dilatation dominated over RV size. Patients in the latter group without obvious RV dilatation had better survival and less severe mitral and tricuspid regurgitation than the DCM patients with obvious RV dilatation.

Mitral regurgitation is extremely common in DCM (Figures 15-7 to 15-9) and often of severe degree.[42-45] Its mechanism is complex and controversial. Dilatation of the mitral annulus is probably the most important single factor,[45] another being papillary muscle "dysfunction" either by inadequate contraction or by altered alignment of the papillary muscle–chordae tendineae apparatus. LV free wall dysfunction also may have a role in mitral regurgitation (MR) causation, though this is not thoroughly understood.

Likewise, *tricuspid valve regurgitation* is very common (Figure 15-7), often moderate and occasional massive in severity, in DCM.[46] As with MR, its mechanisms are somewhat uncertain and presumed to be due to tricuspid annulus dilatation or to displacement of papillary muscles away from their normal optimal position for systolic valve closure.[47,48]

PATTERNS OF FLOW IN THE LV CHAMBER

The cyclic pattern of blood flow within the normal LV chamber differs from that in the dilated hypocontractile LV chamber of DCM, in diastole as well as systole, a finding that has been revealed only recently by pulsed-wave or colorflow Doppler in apical views.

In normal individuals, a broad central stream flows through the mitral valve toward the LV apex during rapid early diastolic LV filling and again with left atrial contraction. In systole, a dominant outflow stream normally proceeds from apex to aortic valve, with no flow in the opposite direction.[49] In dilated dysfunctioning LV chambers of idiopathic or ischemic DCM, the transmitral diastolic stream courses along the posterolateral LV wall and then turns at the apex to flow away from the apex along the septum.[45,50-53] In systole, the stream from apex along the septum to the aortic valve is narrow, and another simultaneous stream moves laterally toward the apex. Thus an abnormal flow persists in the apical half of the LV during much or even all of systole (Figures 15-8 and 15-9). Another way to describe this phenomenon is to view the LV chamber as comprising two compartments functionally, a medial one in which flow proceeds normally from apex to base in systole and a lateral one in which a slow abnormal stream continues toward the LV apex.

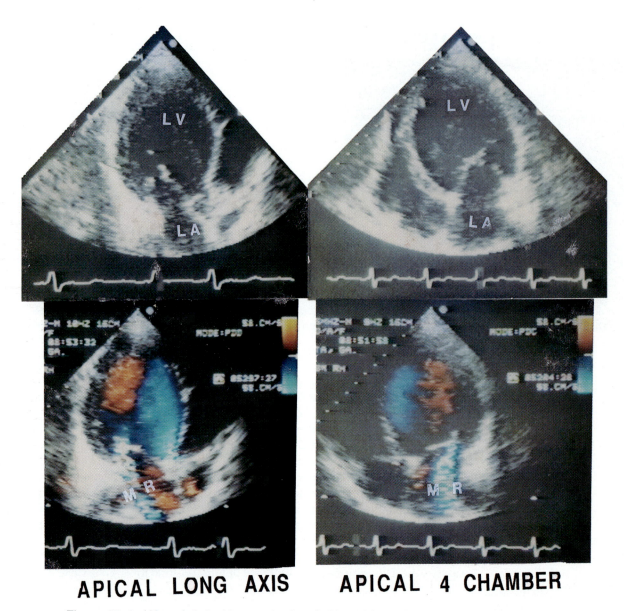

APICAL LONG AXIS   APICAL 4 CHAMBER

Figure 15–8. (Above) Apical long-axis view (left) and four-chamber view (right) at end-diastole of a patient with dilated cardiomyopathy. Note increased LV width, i.e., tendency to spheric shape, with bulging of the septum into the RV chamber. In fact, chambers other than LV are not dilated. (Below) Colorflow Doppler demonstrates a posterior MR jet. Note abnormal persistence of red color in lateral part of LV chamber even at end-systole, signifying abnormal stream toward apex.

The mechanisms leading to such profound alteration in flow patterns in DCM are uncertain; our own work (unpublished) indicates a correlation between the presence and degree of this colorflow Doppler abnormality and (1) severity of impairment of LV systolic function and (2) width of LV chamber, i.e., more pronounced abnormality of intraventricular flow in wider LV chambers.

RESTRICTIVE CARDIOMYOPATHY

This category of myocardial disease is uncommon and of diverse etiologies, all of which have in common infiltration of the myocardium by an abnormal substance or tissue. The

APICAL 4 CHAMBER

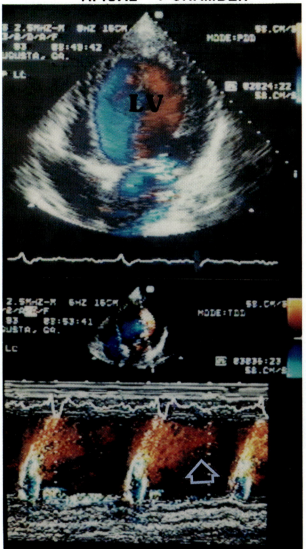

Figure 15–9. (Above) Apical four-chamber view in a patient with dilated cardiomyopathy showing a wide (spheric) LV chamber. Colorflow Doppler in late systole shows MR and abnormal persistence of flow toward the apex (red color) in the lateral part of the LV chamber. The latter is also demonstrated (arrows) on the M-mode colorflow Doppler (below).

best known and most prevalent variety of this syndrome is cardiac amyloidosis, often regarded as the prototype of restrictive or infiltrative cardiomyopathy. Other forms of interstitial myocardial deposition known to have presented with the clinical-hemodynamic features of restrictive cardiomyopathy (RCM) include hemachromatosis, glycogen storage disease, mucopolysaccharidosis, cardiac lymphoma, and a small percentage of cases of cardiac sarcoidosis and scleroderma. In certain tropical countries, notably in East Africa, endomyocardial fibrosis (EMF) is common and may in fact be the dominant cause of heart failure. Somewhat similar is a peculiar form of severe endocardial thickening accompanying chronic eosinophilia in the blood (Loeffler's eosinophilic endomyocardial disease).

Amyloid Cardiomyopathy

Autopsy findings have been well described,[54-56] particularly by Roberts et al.,[54,55] from whose accounts some salient features are briefly mentioned here: The heart weight is mildly to severely increased (300 to 900 g; mean 554 g), yet the ventricular chambers are not dilated in 80% of cases. Both atria are always dilated.

Minute quantities of amyloid are common in hearts of the elderly,[57] so it is not merely the detection of amyloid but its presence in excessive amount that is diagnostic of the amyloid heart. Amyloid is deposited in between muscle fibers, which may in places undergo secondary atrophy. In some cases, larger macroscopic accumulations of amyloid may possibly account for the infarction-like ECG patterns occasionally encountered.

The most consistent anatomic change at autopsy is a firm, rubbery, "stiff" myocardium on palpation so that the excised empty heart retains its shape rather than "collapsing" by gravity as normal or DCM hearts do. This lack of compliance, resisting normal diastolic filling, is the basic physiologic abnormality causing progressive heart failure. The ability of the ventricles to contract may or may not be impaired, which is reflected in the echocardiographic appearances. Amyloid deposits occur in various other parts of the heart as follows: (1) in cardiac valves, causing nonspecific thickening or flat, "waxy," glistening small

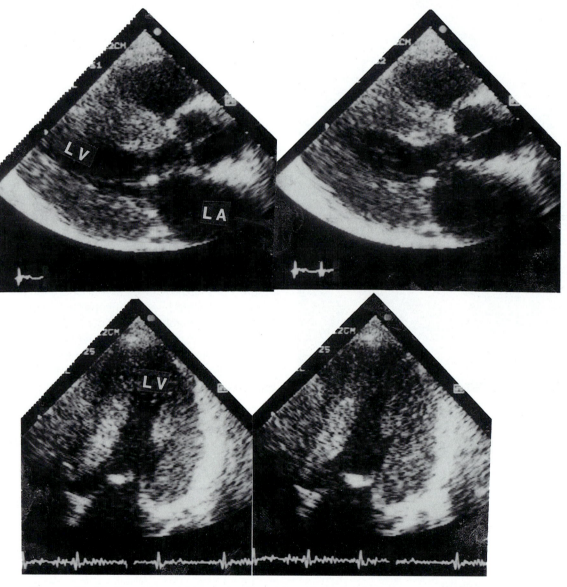

Figure 15–10. Parasternal long-axis view (above) and apical four-chamber view (below). There is considerable "hypertrophy" of the septum as well as LV free wall, with a "sparkling" texture. There is little change in LV size (which is normal) between diastole (left) and systole (right). This patient (D.K.) was an elderly man with severe refractory congestive heart failure that proved fatal over a 14-month period of observation.

plaques (rarely verrucous nodules), (2) heavy papillary muscle amyloid involvement, (3) tan, "waxy," focal endocardial deposits (these may be sites for mural thrombi), (4) focal deposits of amyloid on the visceral pericardium, and (5) consistent involvement of the walls of intramyocardial coronary arteries but not the larger epicardial coronary arteries.

Echocardiography of RCM (Figures 15–10 to 15–12)

The M-mode features of RCM were useful enough to suspect the entity,[58-60] particularly in conjunction with the clinical findings (congestive heart failure in an elderly patient without hypertension): (1) symmetrically increased thickness of LV wall and ventricular septum, (2) small to normal LV chamber size, (3) hypokinesis and decreased systolic thickening of LV wall and septum, and (4) a small pericardial effusion.

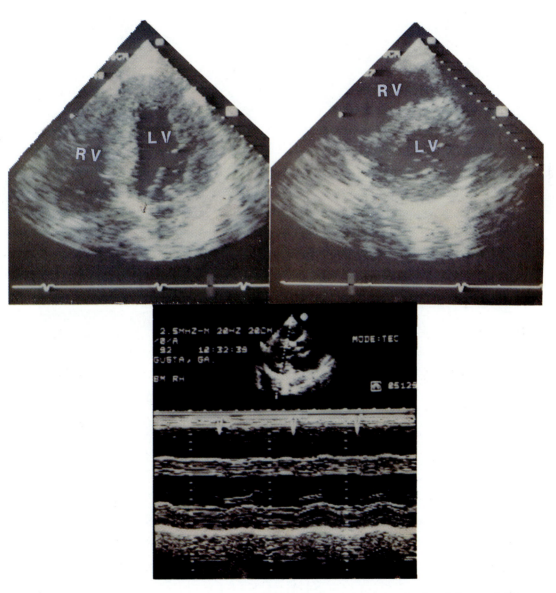

Figure 15–11. Apical four-chamber view (left), parasternal short-axis view (above, right), and M-mode of LV (below, right) in an elderly patient with amyloid heart. Note nondilated thick-walled LV chamber with diffuse LV hypokinesis. The LV myocardium has a bright speckled texture.

LONG AXIS

4 CHAMBER

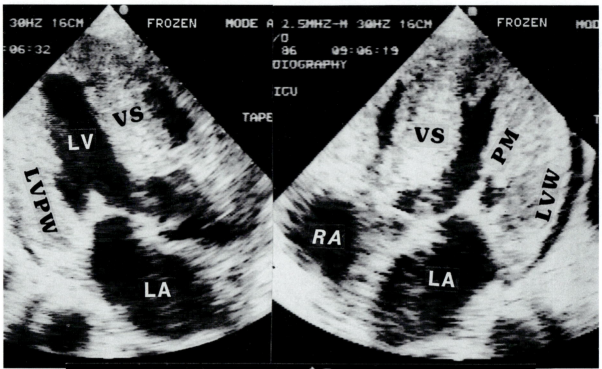

SUBCOSTAL

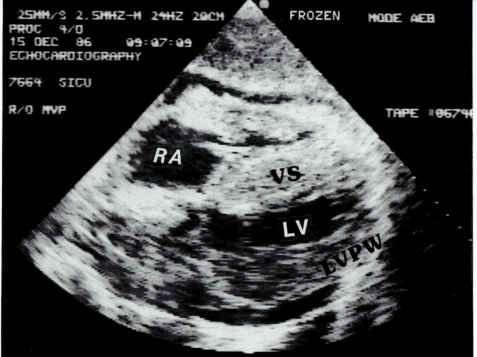

Figure 15–12. Apical long-axis view (above, left), four-chamber view (above, right), and subcostal view (below) of a patient (U.W.) with amyloid heart showing small LV chamber, very thick walls with a bright sparkling texture, and a small pericardial effusion.

These four features can be visualized also on 2D echo.[61-65] LV systolic performance is usually, though not always, subnormal in a diffuse or global manner. Occasionally, the ventricular septum is 1.5 or more times thicker than the LV wall, thus simulating hypertrophic cardiomyopathy. ECG voltage tends to be low in amyloid cardiomyopathy, distinguishing it from true myocardial hypertrophy due to HCM or hypertensive heart disease, which manifests with high ECG voltage.[65]

A "sparkling" diffuse appearance of the myocardium on 2D echo, also termed *highly refractile echo* texture, is noted commonly in patients with amyloid RCM and was hailed initially as a valuable diagnostic sign,[60-63] but later it was considered a nonspecific finding seen also in HCM and end-stage renal disease.[62,66]

Brief mention is made below of various forms of RCM other than amyloid:

1. In *idiopathic hemochromatosis* or that following a large number of blood transfusions for chronic refractory anemia, the LV walls are thickened and stiff, but the LV chamber is usually dilated.[67-69]

2. In *idiopathic eosinophilia,* the LV cavity is of normal or increased size, rarely small. It is regarded as a form of RCM[70] because hemodynamically the main abnormality is a noncompliant LV with normal contractile ability and ejection fraction. There is conspicuous endocardial thickening and stiffness and frequent mural thrombi. Borer's series of 19 patients with RCM included 10 with idiopathic eosinophilia and 5 with hemachromatosis following 100 transfusions or more.[59]

3. Finally, one must be aware of patients who present with congestive heart failure, have the hemodynamic profile of RCM as well as an echocardiographic picture compatible with RCM,[71] yet do not show infiltration by any abnormal material on microscopic examination. The four patients with *idiopathic restrictive cardiomyopathy* reported by Siegal et al.[72] were of this type.

REFERENCES

1. Brigden W. Uncommon myocardial diseases: The non-coronary cardiomyopathies. Lancet 1957;273:1179.
2. Goodwin JF, Gordon H, Hollman A, et al. Clinical aspects of cardiomyopathy. Br Med J 1961;1:69.
3. Roberts WC, Ferran VJ. Pathological anatomy of the cardiomyopathies. Hum Pathol 1975;6:287.
3a. Roberts WC, Siegel RJ, McManus BM. Idiopathic dilated cardiomyopathy. Am J Cardiol 1987;60:1340.
4. Johnson RA, Palacios I. Dilated cardiomyopathies of the adult. N Engl J Med 1982;307:1051.
5. Feild BJ, Baxley WA, Russell RO. Left ventricular function and hypertrophy in cardiomyopathy with depressed ejection fraction. Circulation 1973;47:1022.
6. Benjamin IJ, Schuster EH, Bulkley BH. Cardiac hypertrophy in idiopathic dilated cardiomyopathy. Circulation 1981;64:442.
7. Corya BC, Feigenbaum H, Rasmussen S, et al. Echocardiographic features of congestive cardiomyopathy compared with normal subjects and patients with coronary artery disease. Circulation 1974;49:1153.
8. Ghafour AS, Gutgesell HP. Echocardiographic evaluation of left ventricular function in children with congestive cardiomyopathy. Am J Cardiol 1979;44:1332.
9. Fortuin NJ, Pawsey CGK. The evaluation of left ventricular function by echocardiography. Am J Med 1977;63:1.
10. Massie BM, Schiller NB, Ratshin RA, et al. Mitral-septal separation: New echocardiographic index of left ventricular function. Am J Cardiol 1977;39:1008.
11. D'Cruz IA, Lalmalani GG, Sambasivan V, et al. The superiority of mitral E point–ventricular septal separation to other echocardiographic indicators of left ventricular performance. Clin Cardiol 1979;2:140.

12. D'Cruz IA, Lalmalani GG, Vaidya PV. Cardiac failure and infarction ECG pattern in a chronic alcoholic. Arch Intern Med 1980;140:391.

13. Chandaratna PAN, Aronow WS. Mitral valve ring in normal versus dilated left ventricle: Cross-sectional echocardiographic study. Chest 1981;79:151.

14. Goldberg SJ, Valdes-Cruz LM, Sahn DJ, et al. Two-dimensional echocardiographic evaluation of dilated cardiomyopathy in children. Am J Cardiol 1983;52:1244.

15. Keren A, Billingham ME, Weintraub D, et al. Mildly dilated congestive cardiomyopathy. Circulation 1985;72:302.

16. Keren A, Billingham ME, Popp RL. Features of mildly dilated congestive cardiomyopathy compared with idiopathic restrictive cardiomyopathy and typical dilated cardiomyopathy. J Am Soc Echocardiogr 1988;1:78.

17. Keren A, Gottlieb S, Tzivoni I, et al. Mildly dilated congestive cardiomyopathy. Circulation 1990;81:506.

18. D'Cruz IA, Daly DP, Hand RC. Left ventricular shape in idiopathic dilated cardiomyopathy and cardiomyopathy with or without only mild ventricular dilatation. Am J Cardiol 1992;69:1499.

19. Gavazzi A, DeMaria R, Renosto G, et al. The spectrum of left ventricular size in dilated cardiomyopathy. Am Heart J 1993;125:410.

20. Zimmerman E, Chwojnik A, Lerman J. Idiopathic dilated cardiomyopathy with or without mild dilatation of the cardiac ventricles in multiple family members. Am J Cardiol 1992;69:972.

21. Kurozumi H, Hayakawa M, Kajiya T, et al. Clinical evaluation of observations in poorly contracting and nondilated left ventricles (nondilated cardiomyopathy). Am J Cardiol 1992;69:1367.

22. Laennec RTH (trans by J Forbes). A Treatise on Diseases of the Chest. Philadelphia: Webster, 1823, p 346.

23. Hutchins GM, Bulkley BH, More GW, et al. Shape of the human cardiac ventricles. Am J Cardiol 1978;41:646.

24. Janicki JS, Weber KT, Shroff S. Regional and global shape and size of the intact myocardium. Fed Proc 1981;40:2017.

25. Gould KL, Lipscomb K, Hamilton GW, et al. Relation of left ventricular shape, function, and wall stress in man. Am J Cardiol 1974;34:627.

26. Laskey WK, St John-Sutton M, Zeevi G, et al. Left ventricular mechanics in dilated cardiomyopathy. Am J Cardiol 1984;54:620.

27. Borow KW, Lang RM, Neumann A, et al. Physiologic mechanisms governing hemodynamic responses to positive inotropic therapy in patients with dilated cardiomyopathy. Circulation 1988;77:625.

28. Douglas PS, Morrow R, Ioli A, et al. Left ventricular shape, afterload, and survival in idiopathic dilated cardiomyopathy. J Am Coll Cardiol 1989;13:311.

29. D'Cruz IA, Shroff SG, Janicki JS, et al. Differences in the shape of the normal, cardiomyopathic, and volume overloaded human left ventricle. J Am Soc Echocardiogr 1989;2:408.

30. D'Cruz IA, Daly DP, Shroff SG. Left ventricular shape and size in dilated cardiomyopathy: Quantitative echocardiographic assessment. Echocardiography 1991;8:187.

31. Taliercio CP, Seward JB, Driscoll DJ, et al. Idiopathic dilated cardiomyopathy in the young. J Am Coll Cardiol 1985;5:1126.

32. Falk RH, Foster E, Coats MH. Ventricular thrombi and thromboembolism in dilated cardiomyopathy. Am Heart J 1992;123:136.

33. Segal JP, Stapleton JF, McClellan JR, et al. Idiopathic cardiomyopathy. Curr Prob Cardiol 1978;3:1.

34. Hatle L, Orjavik O, Storstein O. Chronic myocardial disease. Acta Med Scand 1976;199:399.

35. Gottdiener JS, Gay JA, Van Voorhees L, et al. Frequency and embolic potential of left ventricular thrombus in dilated cardiomyopathy. Am J Cardiol 1983;52:1281.

36. Unverferth DV, Magioren RD, Moeschberger ML, et al. Factors influencing the one-year mortality of dilated cardiomyopathy. Am J Cardiol 1984;54:147.

37. Schwartz F, Mall G, Zebe H, et al. Determinants of survival in patients with congestive cardiomyopathy. Circulation 1984;70:923.

38. Baker BJ, Leddy C, Galie N, et al. Predictive value of M-mode echocardiography in patients with congestive heart failure. Am Heart J 1986;111:697.

38a. Ortiz J, Matsumoto AY, Ghefter CGM, et al. Prognosis in dilated myocardial disease. Echocardiography 1993;10:247.

39. Lewis JF, Webber JD, Sutton LL, et al. Discordance in degree of right and left ventricular dilatation in patients with dilated cardiomyopathy. J Am Coll Cardiol 1993;21:649.

40. Feild BJ, Baxley WA, Russell RO, et al. Left ventricular function and hypertrophy in cardiomyopathy with depressed ejection fraction. Circulation 1973;67:1022.

41. Gaasch WH, Zile MR. Evaluation of myocardial function in cardiomyopathic states. Prog Cardiovasc Dis 1984;27:115.

42. Dickerman SA, Rubler S. Mitral and tricuspid valve regurgitation in dilated cardiomyopathy. Am J Cardiol 1989;63:629.

43. Ballester M, Jajoo J, Rees S, et al. The mechanism of mitral regurgitation in dilated left ventricle. Clin Cardiol 1983;6:333.

44. Meese RB, Adams D, Kisslo J. Assessment of valvular regurgitation by conventional and color flow Doppler in dilated cardiomyopathy. Echocardiography 1986;3:505.

45. Maze SS, Kotler MN, Parry WR, et al. An echocardiographic and Doppler study of the mechanisms of mitral regurgitation in left ventricular dilatation. Am J Noninvas Cardiol 1988;2:313.

46. Gupta MK, Sasson Z. The mechanisms and importance of tricuspid regurgitation and hepatic pulsations in dilated cardiomyopathy. Echocardiography 1991;8:195.

47. Mikami T, Kudo T, Sakurai N, et al. Mechanisms for development of functional tricuspid regurgitation determined by pulsed Doppler and two-dimensional echocardiography. Am J Cardiol 1984;53:160.

48. Waller BF, Moriarty AT, Eble JN, et al. Etiology of pure tricuspid regurgitation based on annular circumference and leaflet area. J Am Coll Cardiol 1986;7:1063.

49. Wittlich N, Erbel R, Drexler M, et al. Color-Doppler flow mapping of the heart in normal subjects. Echocardiography 1988;5:157.

50. Delemarre BJ, Bot H, Visser CA, et al. Pulsed Doppler echocardiographic description of a circular flow pattern in spontaneous left ventricular contrast. J Am Soc Echocardiogr 1988;1:114.

51. D'Cruz IA, Sharaf IS. Patterns of flow within the dilated cardiomyopathic left ventricle. Echocardiography 1991;8:227.

52. Pennestri F, Biasucci LM, Rinelli G, et al. Abnormal intraventricular flow patterns in left ventricular dysfunction determined by Color Doppler study. Am Heart J 1992;124:966.

53. Egeblad H, Nolsoe C. Piston engine and paddle wheel heart: Color-coded Doppler ventriculography in primary myocardial disease with good and poor pump function. Am J Noninvas Cardiol 1993;7:89.

54. Buja LM, Khoi NB, Roberts WC. Clinically significant cardiac amyloidosis. Am J Cardiol 1970;26:394.

55. Roberts WC, Waller BF. Cardiac amyloidosis causing cardiac dysfunction: Analysis of 54 necropsy patients. Am J Cardiol 1983;52:137.

56. Schroeder JS, Billingham ME, Rider AK. Cardiac amyloidosis. Am J Med 1975;59:269.

57. Waller BF, Roberts WC. Cardiovascular disease in the very elderly. Am J Cardiol 1983;51:403.

58. Child JS, Leviman JA, Abbasi AS, et al. Echocardiographic manifestations of infiltrative cardiomyopathy. Chest 1976;70:726.

59. Borer JS, Henry WL, Epstein SE. Echocardiographic observations in patients with systemic infiltrative disease involving the heart. Am J Cardiol 1977;39:184.

60. Siqueira-Filho AG, Cunha CLP, Tajik AJ, et al. M-mode and two-dimensional echocardiographic features in cardiac amyloidosis. Circulation 1981;63:188.

61. Cueto-Garcia L, Reeder GS, Kyle RA, et al. Echocardiographic findings in systemic amyloidosis. J Am Coll Cardiol 1985;6:737.

62. Falk RH, Plehn JF, Deering T, et al. Sensitivity and specificity of the echocardiographic features of cardiac amyloidosis. Am J Cardiol 1987;59:418.

63. Nicolisi GL, Pavan D, Lestuzzi C, et al. Prospective identification of patients with amyloid heart disease by two-dimensional echocardiography. Circulation 1984;70:432.

64. Chiaramada SA, Goldman MA, Zema MJ, et al. Real-time cross-sectional echocardiographic diagnosis of infiltrative cardiomyopathy due to amyloid. J Clin Ultrasound 1980;8:58.

65. Carroll JD, Gaasch WH, McAdam PWJ. Amyloid cardiomyopathy: Characterization by a distinctive voltage-mass relation. Am J Cardiol 1982;49:9.

66. Bhandari AK, Nanda NC. Myocardial texture characterization by two-dimensional echocardiography. J Am Coll Cardiol 1983;51:817.

67. Finch SC, Finch CA. Idiopathic hemachromatosis: An iron storage disease. Medicine 1955;34:381.

68. Buja LM, Roberts WC. Iron in the heart. Am J Med 1971;51:209.

69. Cutler DJ, Isner JM, Bracey AW, et al. Hemachromatosis heart disease: An unemphasized cause of potentially reversible restrictive cardiomyopathy. Am J Med 1980;69:923.
70. Roberts WC, Liegler DG, Carbone PP. Endomyocardial disease and eosinophilia. Am J Med 1969;46:28.
71. Chew CYC, Ziady GM, Raphael MJ, et al. Primary restrictive cardiomyopathy. Br Heart J 1977;39:399.
72. Siegel RJ, Shah PK, Fishbein MC. Idiopathic restrictive cardiomyopathy. Circulation 1984;70:165.

16

Left Ventricular Thrombus
and other "Masses"

Thrombi often develop in the left ventricular (LV) chamber in patients after myocardial infarction, with or without aneurysm formation.[1-6] Pseudoaneurysms are also common sites of clot formation. Thrombi virtually never occur in normally contracting ventricles; the very rare exceptions occur in people who have had hypercoagulable states.[7]

Postmortem studies published three to five decades ago described a high prevalence of thrombi in infarcted left ventricles, as high as half to two-thirds of cases. The main factors predisposing to formation of thrombi are blood stasis and endocardial damage. Both these factors come into play at and near the LV apex in acute myocardial infarction (MI) and in post-MI LV aneurysms. Colorflow Doppler commonly reveals little or no flow (absence or fragmentation of color) in this region in large apical or anteroseptal-apical aneurysms.

About half the patients with LV mural thrombus at autopsy have postmortem evidence of systemic emboli. Cerebral emboli are the most common (and clinically important). Infarction of kidney and spleen is common but often symptomatically silent; also common are occlusion of the aortic bifurcation (Leriche syndrome) and iliac or femoral arteries. Rarer is mesenteric artery occlusion.

Almost all post-MI thrombi are located at or very near the LV apex.[1-6] Extensive mural thrombi, overlying correspondingly large MIs, may extend from the apex to several centimeters along the ventricular septum or the adjacent LV free wall. Thrombi restricted to the basal septum or free LV wall are extremely uncommon.

413

LV thrombi vary considerably in size, shape, consistency, and tenacity of adherence to the subjacent myocardium. Flat mural thrombi, often laminated, are firmly adherent to the ventricular wall; they do not detach and embolize, but fresh thrombotic material (which can embolize) may form on the surface of the old, dense thrombus. Sometimes the thrombus is large, conical, and fills the apical one-third of the LV chamber. This latter type might even serve a useful purpose in "closing off" much of the LV dead space in LV aneurysms, thus avoiding wasteful pumping of blood into a large, blind aneurysmal sac.

Thrombi that protrude into the LV chamber are believed to be at a higher risk for embolization; ie., a projecting piece may break off. Mobile, pedunculated thrombi are uncommon but are the most prone to embolize.

Small pea- or marble-sized thrombi are often found at autopsy enmeshed in LV trabeculations near the LV apex. "Soft," newly formed thrombi are important clinically because they may be easily swept away in the bloodstream yet may not be distinctly seen on echocardiography because they do not reflect ultrasound well.

LV THROMBI ECHOCARDIOGRAPHY (Figures 16–1 to 16–6)

A few reports of LV thrombi appeared during the M-mode era, but M-mode had serious limitations in thrombus detection because (1) an echo mass within the LV chamber due to thrombus could not be differentiated easily from other LV structures, normal or abnormal, and (2) the LV apex, by far the most common location for thrombi, is not visualized on M-mode.

The two-dimensional (2D) echo characteristics of an LV thrombus[8-15a] are as follows: (1) a clearly delineated echo-dense intracavitary mass (2) adjacent to but distinct from the endocardium (3) in an LV region that is hypokinetic, akinetic, dyskinetic, or aneurysmal. In addition, (4) the mass is usually located at or near the LV apex and (5) is visualized in two or more views through all the cardiac cycle. According to data from several different centers, thrombi are said to occur in 32% to 56% of new anterior MIs but only 0% to 4% of acute inferior MIs. Most thrombi can be visualized within the first 5 days of onset of the MI and even earlier (24 to 48 hours) in extensive apical-anteroseptal infarcts (in which case a high mortality is predicted). Surgeons find a very high incidence of thrombi in aneurysms they operate on (48% to 95%).

Artefacts, very commonly present in the general apical area in apical 2D echo views, should not be mistaken for thrombi. They usually represent reverberations from the plastic transducer casing or the chest wall and consist of an aggregation of parallel lines. Manipulation or rotation of the transducer shows that the artefactual echoes extend beyond the LV chamber endocardial boundary and do not "move" with the LV endocardium image.

Certain normal components or variants of LV anatomy are often mistaken for thrombi by less experienced operators. (1) *Papillary muscles* in normal location should not be a source of fallacy, but an accessory papillary muscle near the apex could mimic a thrombus, especially if that part of the LV is infarcted. (2) *Trabeculations,* which are normally more numerous and prominent near the apex than elsewhere, can be mistaken for small mural thrombi. When the underlying area of LV myocardium is infarcted, these trabeculations become scarred and more echogenic than usual, which makes them even more difficult to distinguish from small mural thrombi. Trabeculations and muscular bands spanning the LV chamber near its apex are usually identifiable by their morphology and contractile nature, but occasionally, a partly resolved thrombus can form a band or arch not very different in appearance.

Another pitfall is that of overlooking a thin, flat mural thrombus that lines the thin wall of an infarction or aneurysm. The combined thickness of thin LV wall and thrombus may be on the same order as expected LV wall thickness. In such situations, the edge of the thrombus might be detectable as a small lip or ridge distinct from the subjacent endocardium (Figure 16–3).

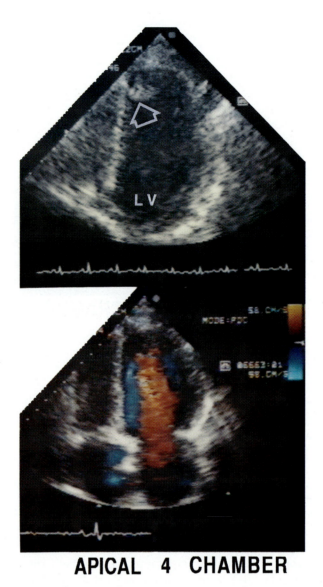

APICAL 4 CHAMBER

Figure 16–1. (Above) Apical view showing a small thrombus at the junction of septum and apex (arrow). (Below) Apical four-chamber view. In this plane the thrombus is not visible, but colorflow Doppler shows absence of color at the junction of the septum and apex, indicating local stasis.

The sensitivity of 2D echo for detecting LV thrombi is quoted at 77% to 95% and its specificity as 86% to 93%.[16] Echocardiography is used widely as the method of choice for diagnosing intracardiac masses, and LV thrombi in particular.

The natural history of LV thrombi and quantitative assessment of the risk of embolization were virtually unknown until elucidated by serial 2D echo studies during the last decade.[11-22] The usual trend is for the thrombus to gradually decrease in size over weeks or months and eventually disappear or at least shrink to a small, dense linear or irregular density or apparent thickening of apical endocardium. In one series, serial 2D echoes of 109 consecutive patients with acute anterior MI revealed LV thrombi in 59; interestingly, 9 of these changed from flat mural to protruding shape, and 15 of protruding type evolved to mural thrombi over time.

Several large studies have indicated that the incidence of clinically manifest systemic embolism is less than 5% after acute MI, although the autopsy incidence is higher, many embolic events being symptomatically "silent." However, when echocardiography has re-

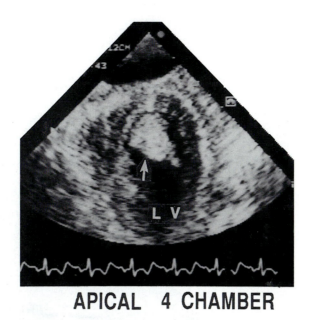

APICAL 4 CHAMBER

Figure 16–2. Apical view showing a dense apical thrombus, about 3 × 2 cm, protruding into the LV chamber.

vealed an LV thrombus in an acute MI patient, the incidence of embolization is about one-fifth to one-fourth of cases.[11,20] Other reports suggest a wider range from 6% to 35%. Embolization is most common within the first month of MI and virtually always in the first 6 months.

The shape and mobility (or lack of it) of the thrombus on 2D echo are very important in predicting the risk of embolization. Comparing patients with LV thrombi who embolized with those who did not, those with a thrombus protruding into the LV chamber had a 5-fold higher incidence of emboli than those with a flat mural LV thrombus.[11] Conspicuous mobility of part or most of the thrombus predicted a 20-fold high incidence of embolization. A pedunculated, freely mobile thrombus has such a high probability of breaking off that there are anecdotal reports of surgical intervention to remove them. Haugland et al.[20] believed that thrombi with a central lucency were twice as likely to embolize as homogeneous, solid thrombi.

Hitherto transesophageal echocardiography (TEE) has been used extensively for achieving better imaging of posterior cardiac structures, but not of the LV apical region, because of the latter's anterior location. However, it has been demonstrated recently that TEE can attain improved visualization of the LV apex and is therefore helpful in identifying apical LV thrombi when conventional transthoracic apical views are equivocal.[23] Thus thrombi were diagnosed in 19 of 36 patients with suspected apical thrombi so studied. Twelve of the 36 patients were found to have "heavy trabeculation or extremely high echo reflection" at the LV apex by TEE,[23] a common and often difficult differential diagnosis of apical thrombi.

Regional stasis of blood in large LV apical aneurysms manifests on 2D echo as an echo cloud of smokelike, swirling, indistinct opacity (dynamic intracavitary echoes).[24] Similar appearances also can be seen within an LV pseudoaneurysm.[25] It is now generally acknowledged that this echo appearance in a cardiac chamber probably results from the aggregation or clumping of red blood cells secondary to abnormally sluggish flow of blood at the affected site and that it often heralds formation of thrombi.

Although initially detected in the left atrium in patients with a stenotic or prosthetic mitral valve, spontaneous echo contrast is also noted occasionally in dilated, poorly contracting LV chambers.[26] Left atrial "smoke" of this type has been reported in one-third of patients with dilated cardiomyopathy, on TEE.[27]

4 CHAMBER

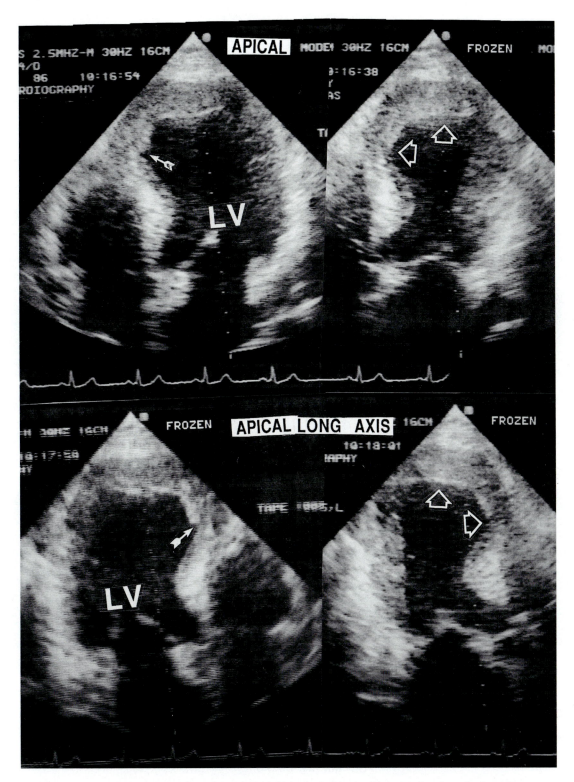

Figure 16–3. Apical four-chamber view (above) and apical long-axis view (below) in a patient with recent large anteroseptal-apical infarction. A flat mural thrombus (large open arrows) lines most of the aneurysmal infarction. Identification is facilitated by detection of the thrombus edge (small arrow).

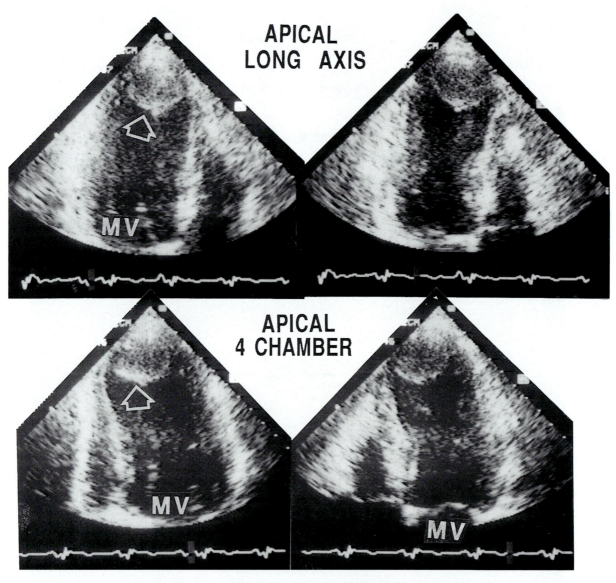

Figure 16–4. Apical four-chamber view (below) and apical long-axis view (above) in diastole (left) and systole (right) showing a large apical aneurysm that contains a large spherical thrombus (arrows). The edge of the thrombus is more echogenic than the rest of the thrombus.

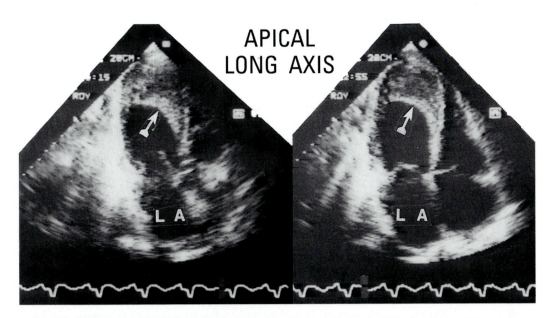

Figure 16–5. Apical long-axis view (diastole, left; systole, right) of patient with a large apical thrombus occupying almost half the LV chamber. The edge of the thrombus is more echogenic than the rest of it; note change in its contour in systole.

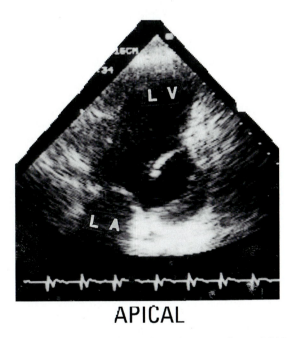

Figure 16–6. Apical view showing a large basal posterolateral LV aneurysm containing a thrombus. The papillary muscle is calcified.

LEFT VENTRICULAR TUMOR

Neoplastic LV masses are all very rare, especially in comparison with LV thrombi. However, echocardiographers need to be aware of them because they enter into the differential diagnosis of thrombi, especially when LV wall motion is normal. Only a very few instances of *LV myxoma* have been reported.[28,29] In one such patient, a 32-year-old man, a mobile mass was visualized in the LV chamber that was pushed anterior to the mitral valve in diastole by mitral flow and moved into the LV outflow tract in systole.[29]

LV lipomas can be subepicardial, intramyocardial, or subendocardial.[30] The latter are sessile and fixed, in contrast to LV myxomas, which are mobile and less densely echogenic. In two cases with 2D echo visualization, the lipomas were large masses originating in the LV apex and protruding toward the LV outflow tract. Both these patients, aged 57 and 67 years, presented with syncope or presyncope.[31,32] It is presumed that the bulky tumor mass somehow seriously impeded LV emptying.

Papillary fibroelastomas are small benign masses that usually occur on the mitral or aortic valve, but exceptionally, they may be attached to the LV wall endocardium. In such a patient, a 71-year-old woman with seven cerebrovascular accidents over the previous 7 years, 2D echo showed a mass 16 × 14 mm attached to the LV wall near a papillary muscle by a short stalk.[33] As with valvar tumors of this type, careful 2D observation can reveal a typical structure: a dense central core with a "gelatinous" outer part and finely undulating, tiny fronds.[33]

Other benign LV tumors include rhabdomyomas, fibromas, and hemangiomas. The first are found exclusively and the second predominantly in infants and children and can be intramural or intracavitary, the latter fixed or mobile. They vary in size; hemangiomas are usually less than 3 cm in size, whereas fibromas are 3 to 10 cm. Ninety percent of rhabdomyomas are multiple.

Malignant primary tumors comprise 25% of all primary cardiac neoplasms. They are sarcomas of various histologic types, depending on origin from myocardial, vascular, fibrous, or lymphoid tissue. Rapid invasive growth of the tumor is the rule, into a cardiac chamber or pericardium or both.

Metastatic neoplastic tumors of the heart are said to be 20 to 40 times as common as primary tumor. In patients who have died of metastatic malignancies, 1.5% to 20% show cardiac metastases at autopsy. Pericardial involvement is the most common; next is myocardial involvement; and intracavitary spread (including valve tissue) is least common. Carcinomas of the lung and breast are the most frequent sites of primary malignancy. Sarcomas and malignant melanomas have a predilection for implantation on the endocardium, thus producing intracavitary masses. On 2D echo, these masses are easier to detect than myocardial or pericardial metastases. Studies describing 2D echo findings in patients with metastatic involvement of the heart reflect a wide spectrum with pericardial effusions or infiltrative thickening, undue local thickening of the LV wall or septum by intramyocardial metastases, or protrusion of the latter type of tumor into the ventricular cavity.[34-36]

PAPILLARY MUSCLE ABNORMALITIES

Normal papillary muscles and some of their pathologic alterations were described in Chapter 11 on the mitral valve and Chapter 12 on LV anatomy. However, it is worth drawing attention to this topic again with regard to masses in the LV chamber because (1) unusually low (apical) origin of a papillary muscle (Figures 16–7 and 16–8) could simulate a protruding or pedunculated thrombus, (2) very exceptionally, a calcified papillary muscle can be the site of formation of a pedunculated LV thrombus (Figure 16–9), and (3) much more commonly, papillary muscle calcification presents as a dense, well-defined echo in the LV chamber. It is not widely known that the 2D echo appearances of this entity can

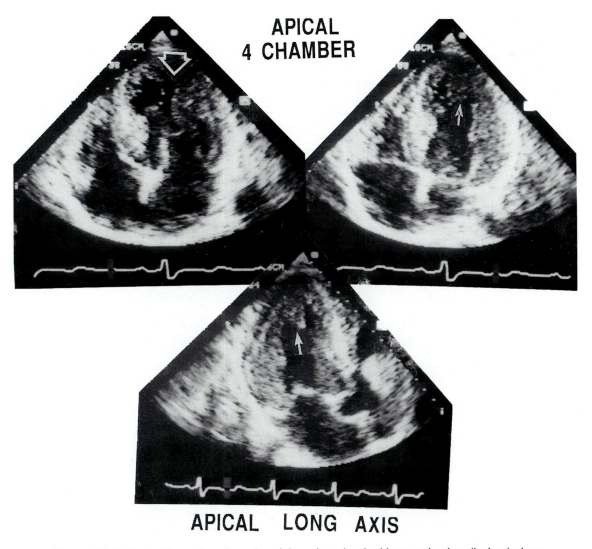

Figure 16–7. Apical four-chamber view (above) and apical long-axis view (below) showing unusual location of a papillary muscle near the LV apex and its chordal connections to mitral leaflets and septum, which could be mistaken for an LV thrombus.

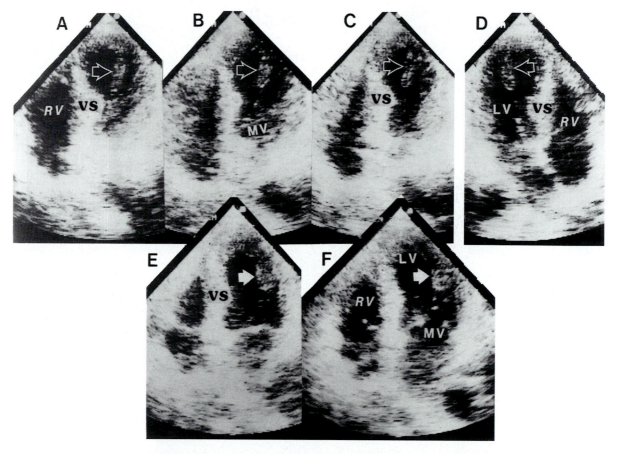

Figure 16–8. (Above) Apical views in different planes showing an accessory papillary muscle taking origin near the LV apex (open arrows). (Below) Apical four-chamber views in same patient showing normal papillary muscle (solid arrows).

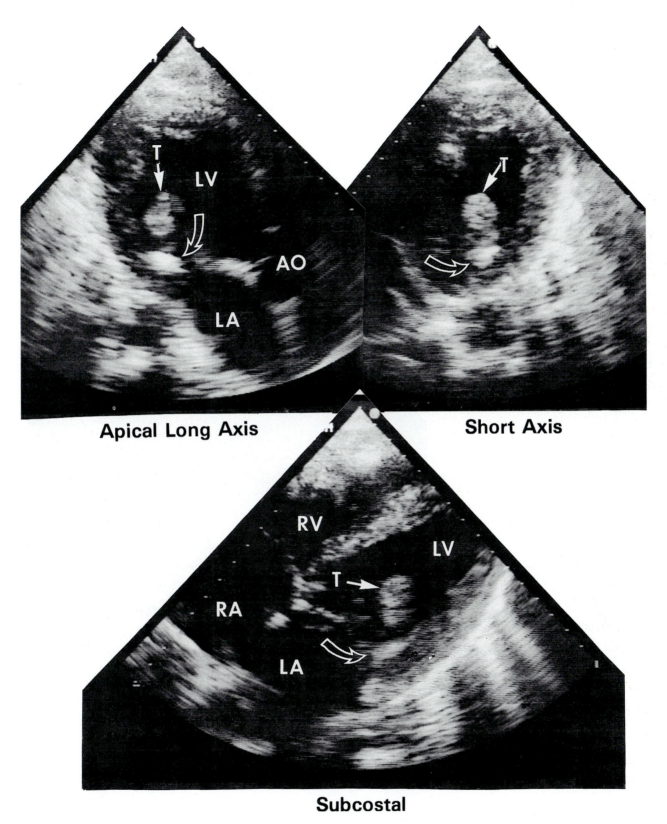

Apical Long Axis   **Short Axis**

Subcostal

Figure 16–9. Apical long-axis view (above, left), modified short-axis view (above, right), and subcostal view (below) showing a pedunculated mobile thrombus (T) attached to papillary muscle calcification (open arrow).

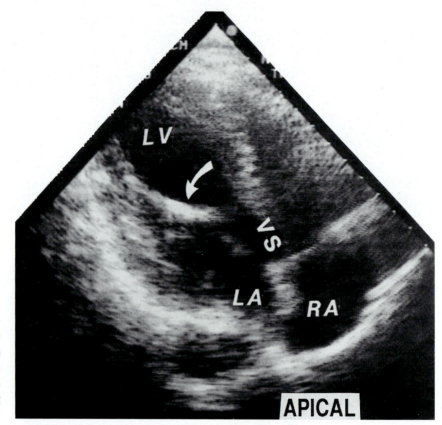

Figure 16–10. Unconventional modified long-axis view. Calcified papillary muscle (arrow) protruding into the LV chamber; it should not be mistaken for a thrombus (VS, ventricular septum; LA, left atrium; RA, right atrium).

APICAL 4-CHAMBER

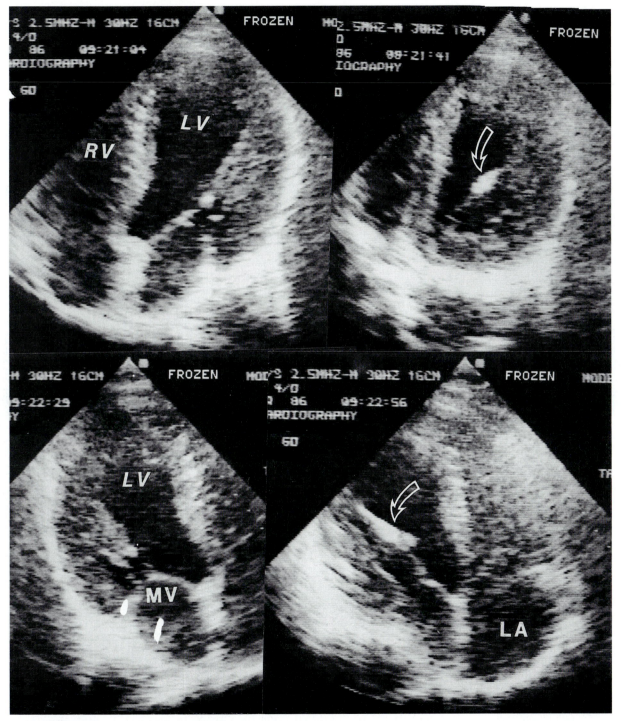

APICAL LONG AXIS

Figure 16–11. Apical views showing localized nature of papillary muscle calcification. Calcification is not seen in planes at left but is visualized (arrows) in planes imaged at right.

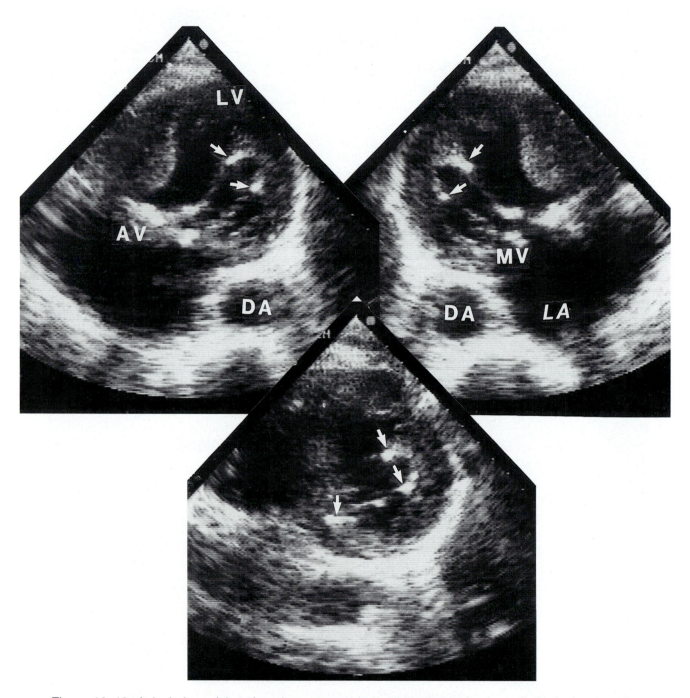

Figure 16–12. Apical views (above) and parasternal long- and short-axis views (below) showing discrete calcification in two separate heads of the same papillary muscle (arrows). The other papillary muscle also shows calcification.

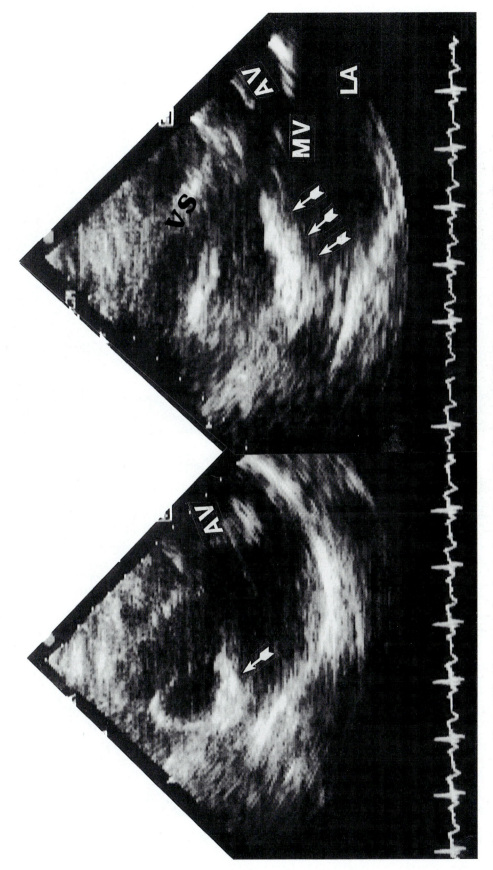

Figure 16–13. Long-axis views of a patient with inferior wall infarction showing massive calcification of the posterior papillary muscle (arrows) as part of infarct calcification.

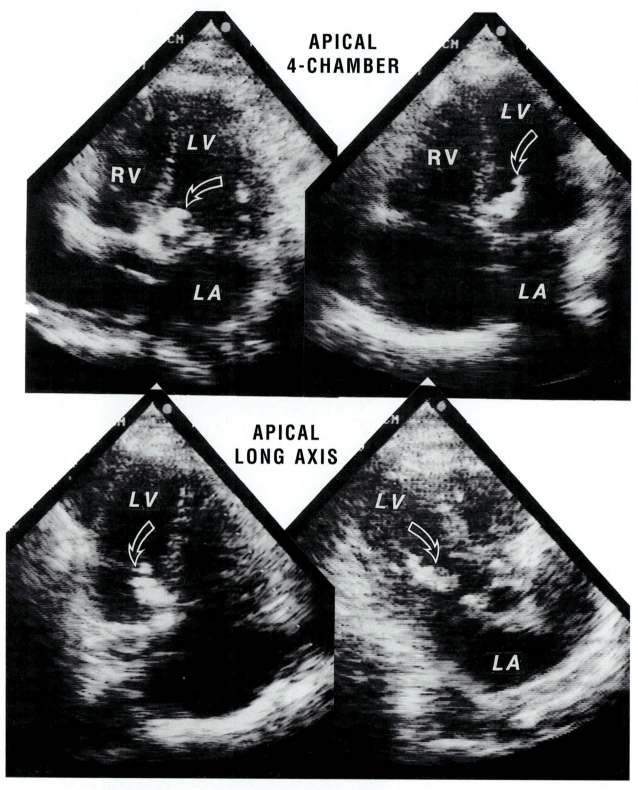

Figure 16–14. Apical four-chamber views (above) and long-axis views (below) show-ing unusual calcification (arrows) in an anomalous false tendon or band running from the papillary muscle to the region of attachment of the anterior mitral leaflet.

cover a wide morphologic spectrum (Figures 16–10 to 16–14). Calcification may occur only at the papillary muscle tip, along its entire length, or even more extensively as inferior infarct calcification, of which papillary muscle calcification is only a part (Figure 16–13). A somewhat bizarre variant is calcification of an anomalous band that is attached at one end to a papillary muscle and at the other end to the attachment of the anterior mitral leaflet (Figure 16–14).

In the practice of clinical echocardiography, these papillary muscle abnormalities are more common (yet seldom written about or illustrated) than the various rare LV neoplasms mentioned earlier.

REFERENCES

1. Parkinson J, Bedford DE. Cardiac infarction and coronary thrombis. Lancet 1928;1:4.
2. Bean BW. Infarction of the heart: Clinical course and morphological findings. Ann Intern Med 1938;12:71.
3. Jordan RA, Miller RD, Edwards JE, et al. Thromboembolism in acute and healed myocardial infarction: Intracardiac mural thrombosis. Circulation 1952;6:1.
4. Hellerstein HK, Martin JW. Incidence of thromboembolic lesions accompanying myocardial infarction. Am Heart J 1947;33:443.5.
5. Abrams DL, Edelist A, Luria ML, et al. Ventricular aneurysm: A reappraisal based on 65 consecutive autopsied cases. Circulation 1963;27:164.
6. Graber JD, Oakley CM, Pickering JF, et al. Ventricular aneurysm and appraisal of diagnosis and surgical therapy. Br Heart J 1972;34:830.
7. DeGroat TS, Parameswaran R, Popper PM, et al. Left ventricular thrombi in association with normal left ventricular wall motion in patients with malignancy. Am J Cardiol 1985;56:827.
8. Asinger RW, Mikell FL, Sharma B, et al. Observations on detecting left ventricular thrombus with two-dimensional echocardiography. Am J Cardiol 1981;47:145.
9. Reeder GS, Tajik AJ, Seward JB. Left ventricular mural thrombus: Two-dimensional echocardiographic diagnosis. Mayo Clin Proc 1981;56:82.
10. Stratton JR, Lighty GW, Pearlman AS, et al. Detection of left ventricular thrombus by two-dimensional echocardiography. Circulation 1982;66:156.
11. Visser CA, Kan G, Meltzer RS, et al. Embolic potential of left ventricular thrombus after myocardial infarction: A two-dimensional echocardiographic study of 119 patients. J Am Coll Cardiol 1985;5:1276.
12. Friedman MJ, Carlso K, Marcus FI, et al. Clinical correlations in patients with acute myocardial infarction and left ventricular thrombus detected by two-dimensional echocardiography. Am J Med 1982;72:894.
13. Spirito P, Chiarella F, Domenicucci S, et al. Prognostic significance and natural history of left ventricular thrombi in patients with acute anterior myocardial infarction. Circulation 1985;72:774.
14. Jugdutt BI, Sivaram CA. Prospective two-dimensional echocardiographic evaluation of left ventricular thrombus and embolism after acute myocardial infarction. Circulation 1985;72:774.
15. Keren A, Goldberg S, Gottlieb S, et al. Natural history of left ventricular thrombi. J Am Coll Cardiol 1990;15:790.
15a. Vandenberg BF, Kerber RE. Left ventricular thrombi in acute and chronic coronary artery disease, in RE Kerber (ed): Echocardiography in Coronary Artery Disease. Mt Kisco, NY: Futura Publishing, 1988, pp 53–63.
16. Asinger RW, Mikell FL, Elsperger J, et al. Incidence of left ventricular thrombosis after acute myocardial infarction: Serial evaluation by two-dimensional echocardiography. N Engl J Med 1981;305:297.
17. Keating EC, Gross SA, Schlamowijz RA, et al. Mural thrombi in myocardial infarction: Prospective study by two-dimensional echocardiography. Am J Med 1983;74:989.
18. Weinreich DJ, Burke JF, Pauletto FJ. Left ventricular mural thrombi complicating acute myocardial: Long-term follow-up with serial echocardiography. Ann Intern Med 1984;100:789.
19. Spirito P, Belloti P, Chiarella F, et al. Spontaneous morphologic changes in left ventricular thrombi: A prospective two-dimensional echocardiographic study. Circulation 1987;75:737.
20. Haugland JM, Asinger RW, Mikell FL, et al. Embolic potential of left ventricular thrombi detected by two-dimensional echocardiography. Circulation 1984;70:588.

21. Gloret RL, Cortada X, Bradford J, et al. Classification of left ventricular thrombi by their history of systemic embolization using pattern recognition of two-dimensional echocardiograms. Am Heart J 1985;110:761.

22. Stratton JR, Resnick AD. Increased embolic risk in patients with left ventricular thrombi. Circulation 1982;66:755.

23. Chen C, Koschyk KD, Hamm C, et al. Usefulness of transesophageal echocardiography in identifying small left ventricular apical thrombus. J Am Coll Cardiol 1993;21:208.

24. Mikell FL, Asinger RW, Elsperger KJ, et al. Regional stasis of blood in the dysfunctional left ventricle: Echocardiographic detection and differentiation from early thrombosis. Circulation 1982;66:755.

25. D'Cruz IA, Jain M, Jain A. Dynamic intracavitary echoes in left ventricular pseudoaneurysm. Am Heart J 1986;112:418.

26. Doud DN, Jacobs WR, Moran JF, et al. The natural history of left ventricular spontaneous contrast. J Am Soc Echocardiogr 1990;3:465.

27. Siostrzonek P, Koppensteiner R, Gossinger H, et al. Hemodynamic and hemorrheologic determinants of left atrial spontaneous echo contrast and thrombus formation in patients with idiopathic dilated cardiomyopathy. Am Heart J 1993;125:430.

28. Bjork VO, Bjork L. Left ventricular myxoma. Thorax 1965;20:534.

29. Mazer MS, Harringan PR. Left ventricular myxoma: M-mode and two-dimensional echocardiographic features. Am Heart J 1982;104:875.

30. Heath D. Pathology of cardiac tumors. Am J Cardiol 1968;21:315.

31. Alam M, Silverman N. Apical left ventricular lipoma presenting as syncope. Am Heart J 1993;125:1788.

32. Weyman AE. Principles and Practice of Echocardiography, 2d ed. Philadelphia: Lea & Febiger, 1994, p 1143.

33. Ong LS, Nanda NC, Barold SS. Two-dimensional echocardiographic detection and diagnostic features of left ventricular papillary fibroelastoma. Am Heart J 1982;103:917.

34. Kutalek SP, Panidis IP, Kotler MN, et al. Metastatic tumors of the heart detected by two-dimensional echocardiography. Am Heart J 1985;109:343.

35. Grenadier E, Lima CO, Barron JV, et al. Two-dimensional echocardiography for evaluation of metastatic cardiac tumors in pediatric patients. Am Heart J 1984;107:122.

36. Lestuzzi C, Biasi S, Nicolosi GL, et al. Secondary neoplastic infiltration of the myocardium diagnosed by two-dimensional echocardiography in seven cases with anatomic confirmation. Am J Cardiol 1987;9:439.

17

Aortic Valve

NORMAL ANATOMY

Interposed between the left ventricular (LV) outflow tract and the aorta, the aortic valve faces upward and rightward, but only slightly anteriorly. It is anterosuperior and slightly to the right of the mitral annulus.

The aortic valve has three cusps, usually of equal size, each of which consists of a thin but tough central layer (lamina fibrosa) lined on the aortic as well as LV aspects by glistening endocardium. Each cusp is relatively thick at its attachment to the aorta, which is U-shaped, and markedly concave toward the aorta. At the center of the free edge of each cusp is a small triangular or pyramidal thickening (nodule of Arantius), from which delicate strands of collagen radiate to the basal attachment of the cusp. The free border of the cusp on either side of the nodule of Arantius is unduly thin and called the *lunule*. The latter is demarcated from the rest of cusp by a thin line, the linea alba, which also represents the line of apposition to the adjacent cusp. The nodules of Arantius may have collagenous "tails" or prolongations on either side along the lunules (Figure 17-1). The lunular region is frequently fenestrated, but deficiencies in the appositional parts of the cusps do not cause regurgitation. Lambl's excrescences (small filaments of fibrinous material) are common on the nodules of Arantius and linea alba. Each cusp is 15 to 22 mm tall at its middle.

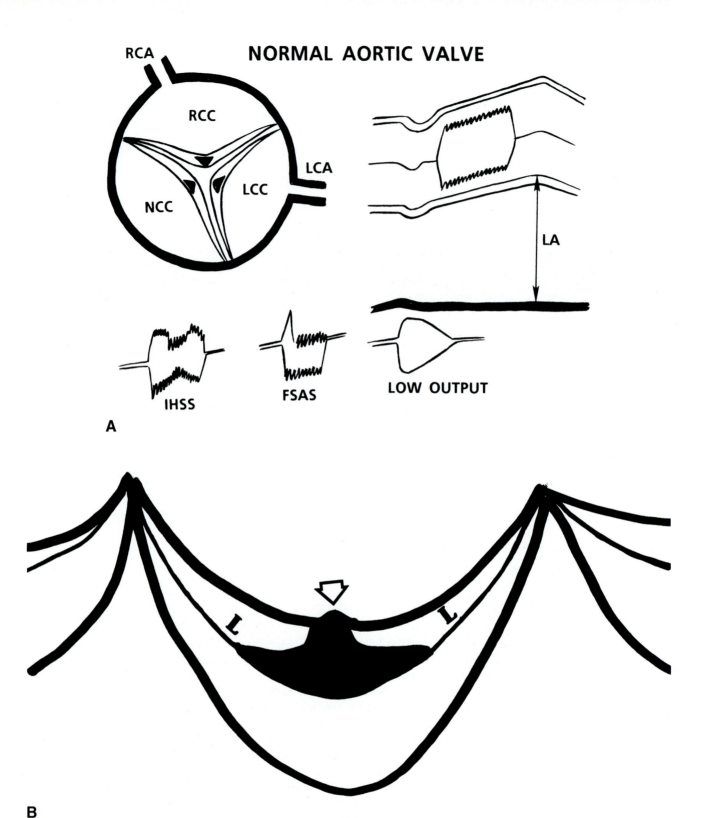

NORMAL AORTIC VALVE

RCA

RCC

LCA

NCC · LCC

LA

IHSS

FSAS

LOW OUTPUT

A

L · L

B

Figure 17–1. (A) Diagram showing anatomy of normal aortic valve in parasternal short-axis view (above, left) (RCC, LCC, NCC, right, left, and noncoronary aortic cusps, respectively; RCA and LCA, right and left coronary arteries, respectively). (Above, right) M-mode of normal aortic root and valve and left atrium (LA). (Below) Abnormal aortic valve motion patterns seen in idiopathic hypertrophic subaortic stenosis (IHSS), fixed subaortic stenosis (FSAS), and low output states, respectively. (B) Diagram of normal aortic cusp showing nodule of Arantius (arrow). The lunule (L) is at the edge of the cusp.

The aortic annulus is not a simple ring as the name might imply. It is a more complex structure that might be described as a coronet-like cylinder with three symmetrical rounded crests. The latter also have been called *scallops* or *crenations;* each of these separates one cusp from the adjacent cusp. The lowest part of each scallop is thickened and even sometimes calcified in the elderly. The U-shaped spaces between the cusp attachments are filled in by fibrous tissue, which is continuous with contiguous components of the "cardiac skeleton" such as the membranous interventricular septum and the fibrosa connecting the base of the anterior mitral leaflet to the aortic valve and root. In circumference, the aortic valve is 60 to 85 mm in men and 57 to 79 mm in women.

One of the three cusps of the aortic valve is anterior; the other two, posterior. At present, most clinicians and pathologists identify the cusps according to coronary artery origin from the respective sinuses of Valsalva; when closed or nearly closed, each cusp and its sinus of Valsalva form a cup or hemispheric shape with concavity upward. Thus the anterior cusp is called the *right coronary cusp;* the left posterior cusp, the *left coronary cusp;* and the right posterior cusp, the *noncoronary cusp.*

The zone between any two adjacent cusps is sometimes known as a *commissure;* however, unlike the mitral valve, there is no continuity of cusp tissue at this point. The cusps may be considered as being inserted on the "annulus" at the commissures, and the wall is locally thickened at these three sites (so-called commissural mound), an occasional site of calcification in the elderly. The free edge of each cusp is longer than a straight line joining its two corners. This extra length permits the free edge of the cusp to meet the other two cusps in the midpoint of the valve circle in diastole and in systole to move back against the aortic valve, provided the cusps are supple and mobile. The nodules of Arantius of each cusp meet in the center of the valve in diastole, thus ensuring complete leak-proof sealing off of the blood in the aorta in diastole.

ECHOCARDIOGRAPHY OF THE NORMAL AORTIC VALVE

M-mode in the parasternal view at aortic valve level shows a typical "box pattern"; i.e., a rectangle or parallelogram contour interrupts the linear echo that represents the apposed cusps in diastole. Normally, the aortic valve opens abruptly, the open cusps remain equidistant (parallel) or almost so during LV ejection, and then they close abruptly as systole ends. Cusp separation in normal individuals is 15 to 25 mm, with 20 mm as an average. In patients with poor LV function and low cardiac output, the cusps do not close abruptly but tend to drift gradually toward each other.

The anterior cusp on the M-mode tracing is the right coronary cusp; the posterior one is the noncoronary cusp. The normal left coronary cusp does not appear in the M-mode image, but if it is sclerotic and restricted in mobility, it may project into the central aortic valve area in systole, appearing as an abnormal thick central linear echo in the middle of the aortic root.

On two-dimensional (2D) echo in the parasternal long-axis view, the anterior (right coronary) and posterior (noncoronary) cusps are seen as thin echoes meeting in the center of the aortic root at its origin. The two cusps are of equal size and bulge gently toward the LV chamber. In the short-axis parasternal view, a typical triradiate configuration of the closed aortic valve (Figure 17-2), an inverted-Y configuration, is seen, especially if the valve is mildly thickened (Figure 17-3). In systole the valve opens widely, each cusp forming a side of an equilateral triangle; each side of the "triangle" may be convex outward rather than straight. However, because of the very thin structure and low echogenecity of normal aortic cusps, it is very often difficult in actual practice to delineate the complete orifice of the open aortic valve (unlike the open mitral valve).

Fenestrations of the Aortic Cusps

Small defects in the aortic valve cusps near their free edge (lunules) are very frequent but cause no aortic regurgitation because they are above the line of closure (linea alba).[1] Foxe[2] noted that such fenestrations increase in prevalence with age from infancy to age 40.

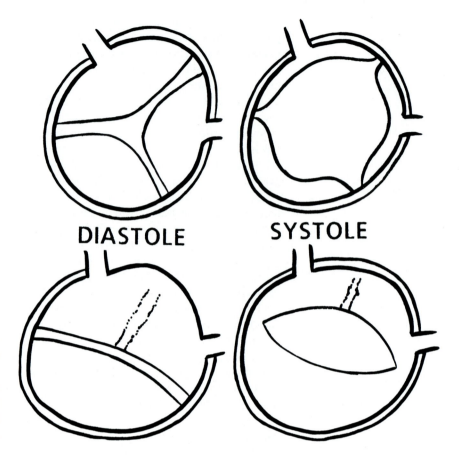

Figure 17–2. Diagram showing normal three-cusp aortic valve (above) and bicuspid aortic valve (below). Position of cusps in diastole is shown at left and in systole at right. Bicuspid valve cusps cannot fully open, and so project into the LV outflow stream.

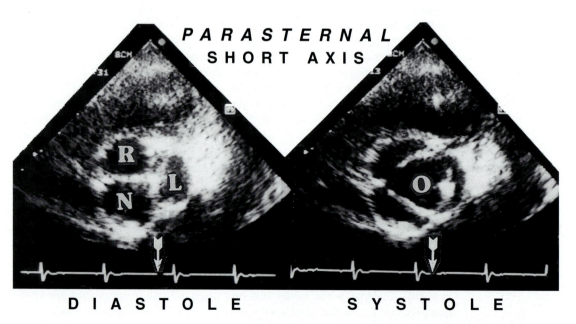

Figure 17–3. Parasternal short-axis view to show a slightly thickened aortic valve closed in diastole (left) and open in systole (right) (O, valve orifice; R, L, and N indicate the right, left, and noncoronary cusps, respectively; small arrows indicate point in cardiac cycle on the ECG).

Friedman and Hathaway[1] suggested that dilatation of the aortic ring may stretch the cusps and thereby elevate the line of cusp apposition, thus drawing the fenestration from the appositional to the area where the fenestration could cause a regurgitant jet. Rare instances of congenital fenestrations causing severe aortic regurgitation have been reported.[3] Bacterial endocarditis and trauma can cause acquired aortic cusp fenestration. Fenestrations of an aortic valve cusp, if multiple, can weaken the structure and result in spontaneous rupture under the stress of diastolic aortic blood pressure, producing abrupt catastrophic regurgitation.

BICUSPID AORTIC VALVE

The bicuspid aortic valve (BAV) was described by renowned nineteenth-century physicians including Paget (1844), Peacock (1866), and Osler (1886),[4] who were aware that the BAV tended to become sclerotic and stenotic with advancing age. BAV is the most common of all congenital cardiac anomalies, occurring in about 1% to 2% of the population. In subjects with coarctation of the aorta, BAV is much more prevalent and may approach 50%; there is an association also with bicuspid pulmonary valve.

Autopsy studies indicate that BAV is congenital in etiology. Histologic studies do not support the view that some cases of BAV are due to rheumatic adhesions between the adjacent edges of two cusps. BAVs are believed to have little or no stenosis at birth or during childhood but to develop stiffness and sclerocalcific changes causing pressure gradients during adult life. Calcification is said to be invariable over age 60. Excellent autopsy descriptions of BAV have been published by Bacon and Matthews,[5] Roberts,[6] Edwards,[7] and Waller et al.[8]

Usually one of the two cusps of the BAV is larger than the other; the larger one is called the *conjoined cusp,* formed by lack of separation of two cusps; the smaller cusp is called the *single cusp.* The conjoined cusp commonly shows a ridge or raphe on its aortic surface, which begins at the cusp attachment and may or may not extend all the way to its free edge.

The common configuration is that the two cusps of a BAV are oriented in anteroposterior relationship (Figures 17–2 and 17–4), the larger anterior cusp replacing the right and left coronary cusps; both coronary arteries arise from this large sinus of Valsalva. The smaller posterior cusp is the usual noncoronary cusp.

In a minority of cases the BAV is such that the two cusps have a right-left orienta-

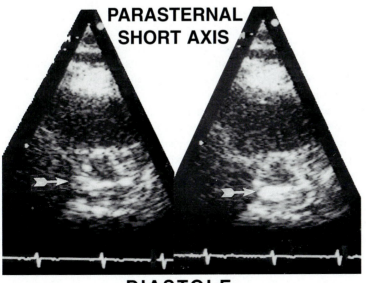

PARASTERNAL SHORT AXIS

DIASTOLE

Figure 17–4. Parasternal short-axis view showing thickening of a bicuspid aortic valve (arrows). Both frames are in diastole.

tion. One coronary artery arises above each cusp. When the cusps have an anteroposterior relationship, the line of apposition is transverse; with a right-left relationship, the line of apposition runs from front to back.

Hemodynamic Complications of BAV

Of Roberts' 85 cases of BAV, aortic stenosis was present in 61, of which all but 2 showed calcific changes.[6] Only 13 of the 85 functioned normally. Aortic regurgitation was frequently present concomitantly with stenosis. Calcification was absent or minimal in BAV with pure isolated aortic regurgitation or with normal valve function. It has long been recognized that a BAV is at a mechanical disadvantage in the sense that such a valve cannot open fully because the cusps project into the aortic lumen, unlike the normal three-cusp aortic valve, which opens widely to permit a large triangular stream of flow during systole. It has been observed that the larger cusp of a BAV is often somewhat redundant with respect to the smaller cusp, thus overlapping it during LV ejection. An oblique ejection stream results.

As a rule, stenotic BAVs are dome-shaped during systole with a small orifice at the summit of the dome; the severity of the stenosis depends on the area of this orifice. In adolescents and young adults, the cusp dome may be only slightly thickened and not calcified, whereas the stenosis can be mild, moderate, or severe in accord with decreasing size of the effective aortic valve orifice.

The BAV is prone to bacterial endocarditis. It was present in 25% of patients with BAV in the series of Bacon and Matthews.[5] Roberts[6] stated that this complication was often responsible for aortic regurgitation in patients with BAV. It is tragic when a potentially lethal complication afflicts an asymptomatic young individual who has what is commonly regarded as a minor cardiac abnormality with little or no clinical manifestations or physical signs. It is all the more important that the echocardiographer should be alert at diagnosing BAV so that such persons can be given antibiotic prophylaxis at the time of dental procedures, endoscopy, etc. The aortic valve should be scrutinized particularly for BAV structure in patients with aortic coarctation because BAV may be associated in as much as half of such patients, as in a series of 36 patients of Scovil et al.[9]

Echocardiography of Bicuspid Aortic Valve[7–15]

In the M-mode era of the 1970s, the echocardiographic diagnosis of BAV was described chiefly on the basis of an eccentric line of diastolic closure on the M-mode tracing of the aortic root.[7–9] An *eccentricity index*—the ratio of aortic root radius (half the aortic root diameter) to the smallest distance between the line of diastolic closure and the nearest aortic wall—of more than 1.5[7] or 1.3[8] was thought to indicate a BAV. Normal three-cusp aortic valves usually show a line of diastolic closure that is central, or almost so, within the aortic root M-mode recording. However, the eccentricity index was not found to be highly specific or highly sensitive for BAV. Another rather nonspecific abnormality described as suggestive of BAV on M-mode is an aggregation of multiple parallel lines (rather than one sharp line) representing the closed aortic valve.[7]

Fowles et al.[13] demonstrated the superiority of 2D to M-mode echo in identifying BAV. In the parasternal long-axis view, a gross inequality in size of the anterior and posterior aortic valve cusps during diastolic closure is suggestive of BAV, but the diagnostic 2D echo appearances of BAV are evident in the short-axis parasternal view of the aortic root (Figure 17–4). In this view, the normal triradiate pattern in diastole is replaced by a single line (usually transverse). Viewed in real-time, motion of the cusps helps confirm the distinction between a two-cusp and three-cusp aortic valve. BAV is often difficult to distinguish from a three-cusp valve with a very small rudimentary left coronary cusp.

Heavy irregular aortic valve calcification may obscure cusp margins on the 2D echo and hence impede diagnosis of BAV. Extensive calcification does not prevent BAV identification if the cusps are uniformly sclerotic and retain their contour. On the other hand, normal cusps are so thin that their margins may be difficult to ascertain, especially if the echo window is suboptimal. The ideal aortic valve for assessing cusp pattern or number is one that is mildly thickened with well-delineated margins.

QUADRICUSPID AORTIC VALVE[16–20]

This rare anomaly is less than one-tenth as frequent as the quadricuspid pulmonary valve. Hurwitz and Roberts[16] in 1973 collected 13 cases of quadricuspid aortic valve from the literature and added 2 of their own (out of 6000 autopsies). The common pattern of a four-cusp aortic valve is three equal cusps plus a fourth hypoplastic cusp.[17,18] Other variants are three equal cusps and one larger cusp and four equal cusps.[19] In the majority of cases of a four-cusp aortic valve, the valve has been competent, but about a quarter have shown regurgitation.[16]

AORTIC VALVE CALCIFICATION AND STENOSIS[21–28]

Aortic valve stenosis is the most common fatal valve lesion. In children and young adults, stenosis can exist without calcification, but in later life, significant aortic valve stenosis is regularly accompanied by some degree of calcification. On the other hand, aortic valve calcification with little or no stenosis is extremely common in the elderly (Figure 17-5); such persons have systolic aortic murmurs, but only a slight pressure gradient is revealed by Doppler or invasive studies.

One-fifth of all individuals over age 65 have macroscopic calcification of the aortic valve at autopsy. The process of calcification begins as minute specks in the fibrosa of the aortic valve cusp and grows into calcific nodules or rocklike masses. Calcification commonly appears first at the bases (attachments) of the cusps, presumably because mechanical stress and hinge action are maximal at this region of the cusp. Another frequent early site of calcification is the nodule of Arantius (Figure 17-5). Calcification may progress more or less equally among the three cusps, and this is usually true in really stenotic valves. However, it is very common to find heavy calcification in one cusp but very little in the other two. It has long been known, as a general rule, that if one cusp retains good mobility and freedom from sclerocalcific change, that aortic valve will never be severely stenotic, however severe the calcification in the other two cusps.

Calcification is at first contained within the cusp fibrosa but may enlarge to extend beyond this layer and form large, chalky, hard masses. Progressive diffuse sclerocalcific change of the aortic valve is accompanied by increasing limitation of mobility, resulting in hemodynamically important stenosis. However, the severity of stenosis depends on the area of the effective valve orifice and need not be proportional to the degree of calcification. In other words, cusps are often very stiff and unyielding but only slightly calcified.

The etiopathology of aortic valve stenosis falls into one of three main categories: (1) "Senile" degenerative calcification of the elderly accounts for most patients over 70 years of age. The edges of the cusps are well preserved with no commissural adhesions or distortions. (2) In rheumatic scarring, the cusps become adherent at their edges to a varying degree. With age, the valve becomes progressively more fibrotic and calcified. The mitral valve also may show similar changes; the presence of concomitant mitral stenosis makes it extremely likely that aortic stenosis is rheumatic. (3) Congenitally bicuspid aortic valves are believed to be nonstenotic in childhood but to get stiffer and calcified in adult life, especially in the region of the raphe of the conjoined (larger) cusp. Severe aortic valve stenosis in infancy is usually due to a unicuspid valve; some unicuspid valves can present with aortic valve stenosis in the second or third decades. First described by Edwards[26] in 1958, this anomaly resembles bicuspid aortic valve stenosis in that the valve is dome-shaped with severity of stenosis depending on the size of the orifice at the summit of the dome and in the tendency for the stenosis to inevitably become more severe because of sclerosis and calcification with advancing age.

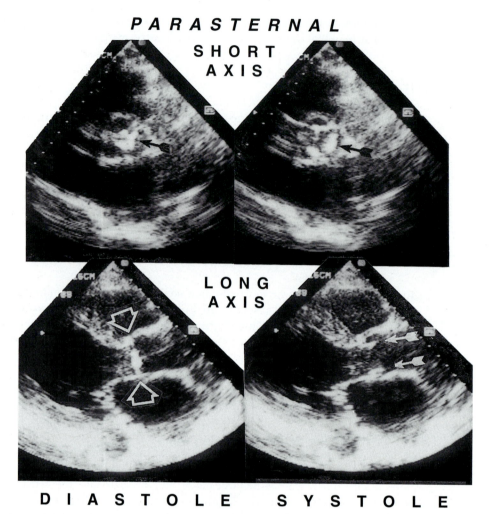

PARASTERNAL

SHORT AXIS

LONG AXIS

DIASTOLE   SYSTOLE

Figure 17–5. Parasternal short-axis view (above) and long-axis view (below) in a patient with nodular sclerocalcific changes in the aortic valve but no stenosis. The valve is closed in diastole (left) and opens well in diastole (right). Arrows indicate the location of aortic valve cusps.

The relative proportions of the three main types of aortic valve stenosis vary widely in the autopsy literature, depending on when the study was done and also on the age profile and geographic location of the population. The main reason for the disparities is the rapidly falling incidence of rheumatic fever in Western countries over the last four decades so that "new" cases of rheumatic aortic stenosis are now uncommon in most of the United States, Canada, and Europe. Rheumatic valve disease has continued to be prevalent in the developing countries and therefore in immigrant populations in North America. Moreover, we do still continue to encounter elderly patients who suffered rheumatic carditis and then valvar involvement in the 1930–1950 period. Roberts and Perloff[24] found that 90% of calcified stenotic aortic valves after age 62 were three-cusp valves; only 10% were bicuspid.

Other rare causes of aortic valve stenosis include systemic lupus erythematosus (SLE),[29] especially after steroid therapy, ochronosis, Fabry's disease, postradiation valve damage, tumors, and large vegetations of the aortic valve.

In severe aortic valve stenosis, the LV shows concentric hypertrophy with uniformly thick walls and small cavity; papillary muscles and trabeculations are also hypertrophied. Heart weights in the 600- to 800-g or even 1000-g range are common. The septum is as thick as or slightly thicker than the LV free wall. If the LV fails, the LV chamber may not be unduly small, but it rarely exceeds the upper normal limit in size. In elderly symptomatic patients with severe aortic valve stenosis, the LV wall may show only mild hypertrophy. This may be explained by (1) dilatation accompanying LV decompensation, (2) ischemic heart disease, or (3) some other unknown factor limiting the development of hypertrophy.

The natural history of aortic valve stenosis is characterized by a slow progression of severity in some, but in others (particularly mild stenosis) there is no change.

Poststenotic dilatation of the ascending aorta is common in patients with aortic stenosis. It is not proportional to the severity of stenosis. Turbulence of blood flow above the aortic valve and ensuing vibration of the aortic wall somehow induce a weakening of the latter, which dilates in response to the pulsatile aortic pressure. The ascending aorta is mildly and diffusely dilated, but sometimes the dilatation is asymmetrical. Aortic valve stenosis predisposes to aortic dissection, particularly in patients with bicuspid or unicuspid aortic valve stenosis.[30]

Echocardiography of Aortic Valve Stenosis[31–34]

The parasternal long-axis view is the best for detecting aortic valve stenosis. The normal aortic cusps fly apart at onset of systole and may be identified as thin lines parallel to the aortic walls. Aortic valve stenosis is characterized by systolic doming, the stenotic orifice being at the apex of the dome. When the cusps retain their contour and are uniformly sclerotic or thickened, the site and size of the orifice are evident so that a rough estimate as to whether the aortic stenosis is mild, moderate, or severe is possible. In other cases, the aortic cusp calcification is heavy and irregular so that the location and dimension of the stenotic valve orifice cannot be ascertained. If the cusp morphology in systole is not very different from that in diastole, significant aortic stenosis is present. The parasternal short-axis view may in some cases reveal the valve orifice contour in sufficient detail to decide the presence and degree of stenosis, but this is generally the exception rather than rule.[35] Recently, transesophageal echocardiography (TEE) has been used to obtain optimal visualization of the aortic valve orifice for area measurement.[36]

Fluid dynamics in various regions in and around an aortic stenotic jet are important to understand (Figure 17–6). There is acceleration of velocity proximal to the stenotic orifice, peak velocity in the stenotic jet itself, and somewhat lesser (but higher than normal) velocity adjacent to this (parajet). Around that there is turbulence, sometimes dominating and obscuring other (jet) Doppler signals. Finally, downstream from the valve, the normal laminar flow pattern reasserts itself.

2D echo and continuous-wave Doppler appearances in mild, moderate, and severe aortic valvar stenosis are shown in Figures 17–7, 17–8, and 17–9, respectively. Heavy calcification in one cusp may be accompanied by only slight thickening of another cusp (Figure 17–10). The parasternal short-axis view may provide good visualization of the size and shape of the stenotic orifice and thus of the severity of the stenosis (Figures 17–11 and 17–12).

Subvalvar fixed stenosis (Figure 17–13) is much rarer than valvar aortic stenosis but may coexist with it in older patients. Continuous-wave and pulsed-wave Doppler views are very useful in localizing the site of stenosis.

Continuous-wave Doppler measurement of velocity of the aortic valve stenotic jet is now the noninvasive "gold standard" for estimation of the pressure gradient and has been universally accepted as reliable for this purpose. Good spectral Doppler recordings of the jet are usually recorded by apical window interrogation. However, the best and highest-velocity jet of aortic valve stenosis is often obtained from the right parasternal window (right first or second intercostal space; very rarely the suprasternal window provides the highest-velocity jet). The reason for the great variability among patients is a reflection of the variation in direction of the stenotic jet. In other words, the jet is very often not directed into the center of the ascending aorta but is eccentric, i.e., impinges on the aortic wall, often the anterolateral convexity of the ascending aorta.

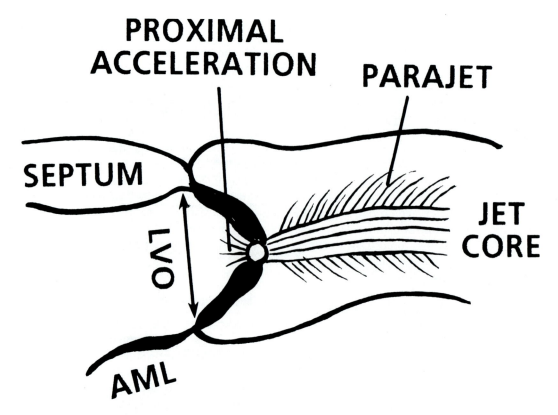

Figure 17–6. Diagram showing simplified depiction of different flow zones in patient with aortic valve stenosis. The jet core with highest velocity emerges from the stenotic orifice at the summit of the valve dome; external to the central jet a zone of increased but not as high velocity is sometimes called the *parajet.* Note zone of proximal acceleration on the ventricular side of the stenotic valve (LVO, left ventricular outflow; AML, anterior mitral leaflet).

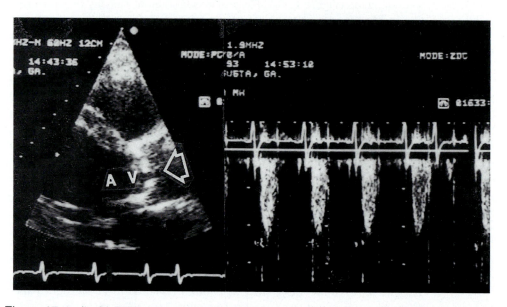

Figure 17–7. (Left) Parasternal long-axis view showing a thickened stenotic aortic valve with well-defined cusp contour and orifice (arrow). (Right) Continuous-wave Doppler shows an aortic jet peak velocity of 2.3 m/s, i.e., mild peak instantaneous valve gradient of about 20 mmHg.

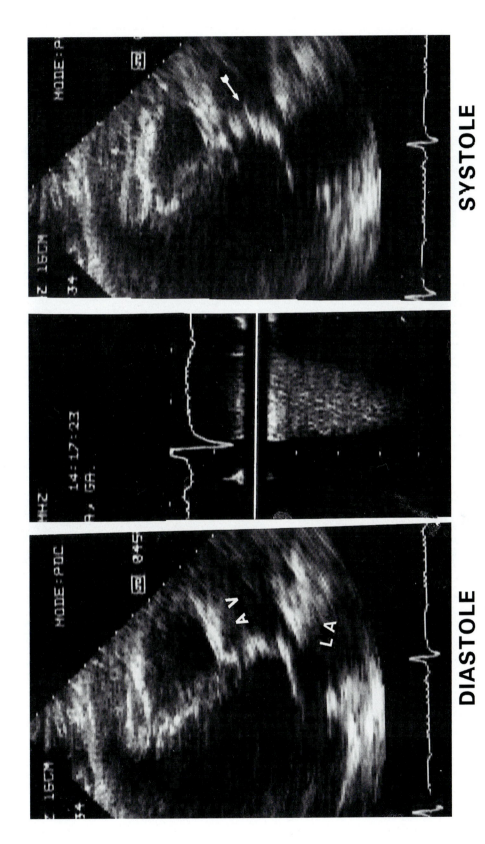

DIASTOLE   **SYSTOLE**

Figure 17–8. Long-axis view of stenotic aortic valve (AV) at end-diastole (left) and in systole (right) showing thickened cusps, systolic doming, and a stenotic orifice (arrow). Continuous-wave Doppler shows a peak instantaneous velocity of 3.6 m/s = gradient 52 mmHg (moderate aortic stenosis).

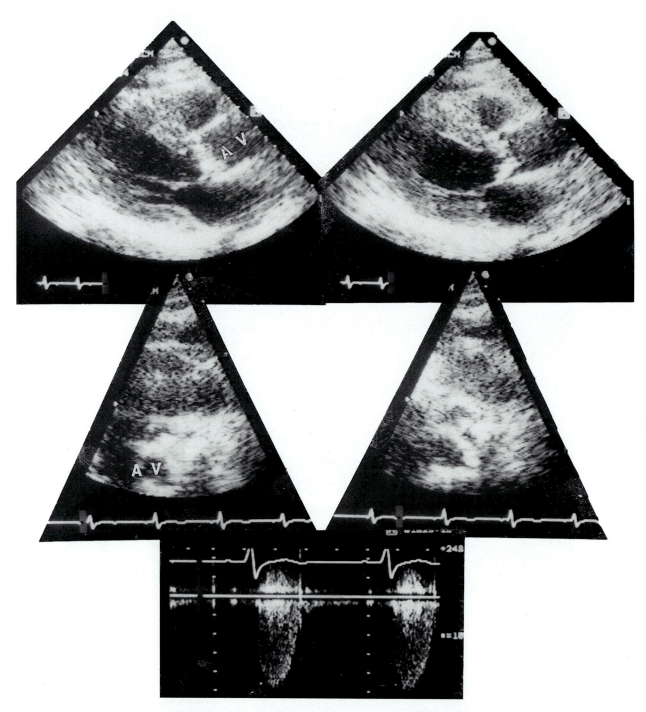

Figure 17–9. Parasternal long-axis view (above) and short-axis view (center) in a patient with severe calcific aortic valve stenosis. Comparison of the diastolic frames (left) with systolic frames (right) shows that the valve opens only slightly in systole. Continuous-wave Doppler of aortic jet velocity (below) reveals a peak velocity of about 4.8 m/s (peak instantaneous gradient of 92 mmHg).

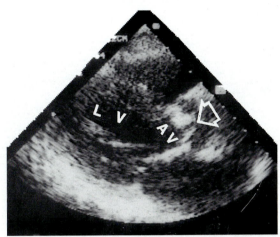

P A R A S T E R N A L
L O N G   A X I S

Figure 17–10. Parasternal long-axis view showing a stenotic aortic valve; the right coronary (anterior) cusp is heavily calcified, while the noncoronary cusp (posterior) is only mildly thickened.

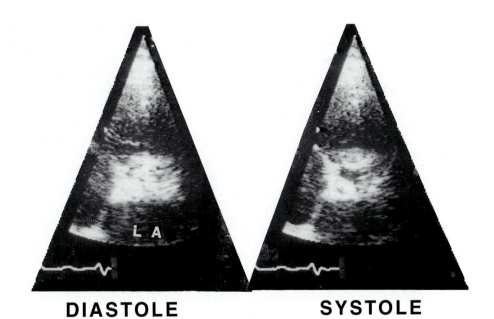

Figure 17–11. Parasternal short-axis view in diastole (left) showing heavy sclerocalcification of the aortic valve. In systole (right), the valve partly opens, but is obviously stenotic.

DIASTOLE   **SYSTOLE**

DIASTOLE   **SYSTOLE**

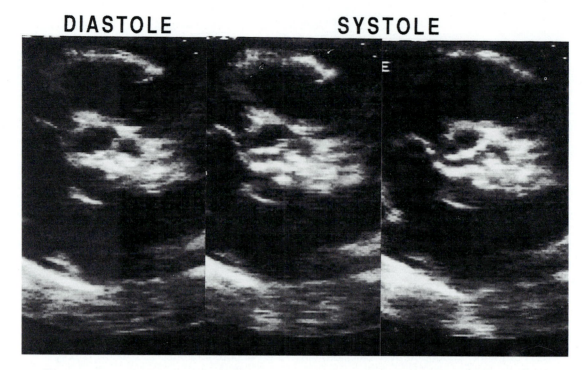

Figure 17–12. Parasternal short-axis view in a patient with aortic valve stenosis. The cusp edges are well-defined. (Left) Valve closed in diastole. (Center and right) In systole, the valve orifice can be identified as a transverse slit.

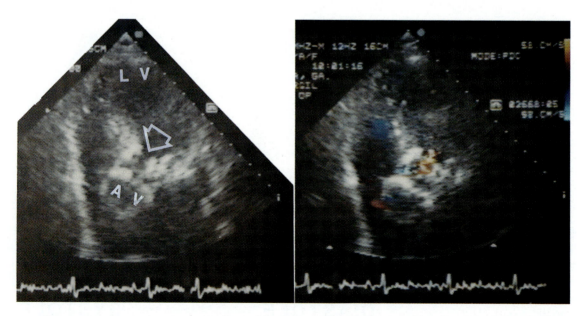

Figure 17–13. Apical four-chamber view of a patient with aortic valve (AV) stenosis. There is also subvalvar fixed (discrete) stenosis (open arrow). Colorflow Doppler shows high-velocity flow in LV outflow tract (arrow) beyond the subvalvar stenotic site.

AORTIC REGURGITATION

Aortic regurgitation is an extremely common and important valve lesion. It was formerly detectable only by auscultation and injection of radioopaque dye into the aortic root. It was possible to diagnose aortic regurgitation on M-mode echo by rapid oscillations (flutter) of the anterior mitral leaflet all through diastole, caused by the impact on it of the regurgitant jet; septal flutter was noted in a minority (Figure 17-14A).

Colorflow Doppler was a great diagnostic advance because it allowed imaging not only of the presence of the regurgitant jet but also of the direction, width, and length (i.e., penetration into the LV chamber) of the jet. Such jets may be directed anteriorly along the septum, centrally into the LV, or posteriorly along the mitral valve to the LV posterior wall (Figures 17-14 to 17-17). The width or area of the jet at its origin at the valve is a good index of the severity of regurgitation (Figure 17-18). In diastole, a mitral stenotic jet has the same general direction as an aortic incompetence jet but differs in location of origin (Figure 17-17). The colorflow Doppler appearances of an aortic incompetence jet with and without simultaneous normal mitral inflow are seen in Figure 17-19.

AORTIC VALVE ENDOCARDITIS

The main autopsy as well as echocardiographic feature of endocarditis is the presence of vegetations.[37-47] In the more acute forms of bacterial infections (more virulent organisms), the vegetations tend to be larger, more friable, and cause rapid and severe cusp destruction. In classic subacute bacterial endocarditis, on the other hand, the vegetations are smaller with slower progression of cusp damage.

Vegetations vary in size from a few millimeters to ones large enough to partly obstruct LV outflow.[43,44] They tend to fragment with resulting embolization, most importantly of the cerebral arteries. Emboli also can obstruct other arteries; notably aortic valve vegetations can pass into a coronary artery causing acute myocardial infarction.

Infection causes weakening or erosions and then rupture or perforation of one or more cusps under the pulsatile stress of high aortic diastolic pressure. A torn cusp exhibits flail motion, and severe aortic incompetence (AI) is inevitable. Alternatively, the cusp margins may remain intact, but a hole may form within the cusp (perforation or acquired fenestration), causing AI that varies in severity depending on the size of the hole.

Echocardiography of Aortic Valve Endocarditis[39-47]

A vegetation on the aortic valve presents as a mobile small mass obviously attached to the aortic valve cusp. Typically, the valve mobility is normal; i.e., even though one or more vegetations fill the aortic root in diastole, they move briskly aside in systole and do not obstruct LV outflow. By contrast, sclerocalcific nodular thickening of the aortic valve is usually (but not always) associated with limitation of the cusp motion and sometimes with actual stenosis of the valve (manifested by high velocity on continuous-wave Doppler).

Very recent vegetations may have a shaggy or fluffy texture on careful examination. However, healing or healed vegetations gradually become dense and more distinctly defined; at this stage the differentiation from degenerative sclerocalcific changes in elderly patients can be very difficult.

A torn aortic leaflet shows flail motion, characterized by abnormal motion into the LV outflow tract in diastole and forward quick motion into the aortic root in systole (Figure 17-20). When a vegetation is adherent to the flail leaflet, its very abnormal rapid to and fro motion during the cardiac cycle becomes even more conspicuous and in fact pathognomonic for flail aortic leaflet complicating bacterial endocarditis (Figure 17-21).

On the other hand, aortic cusp perforation has no typical manifestation on 2D echo. In the setting of bacterial endocarditis, the presence of severe AI without flail cusp motion should raise the suspicion of cusp perforation.

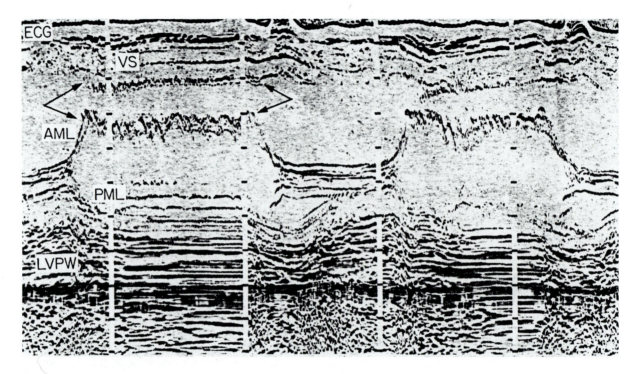

A

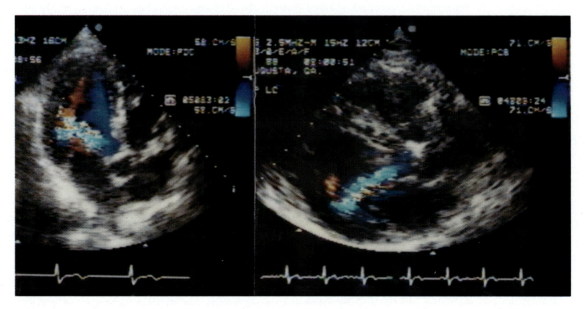

B

Figure 17–14. (A) M-mode echo in a patient with aortic regurgitation showing holodi-astolic flutter on the anterior mitral leaflet and also LV surface of ventricular septum (arrows). (B) Colorflow Doppler in parasternal long-axis view showing eccentric poste-riorly directed AI jet that impinges on anterior mitral leaflet.

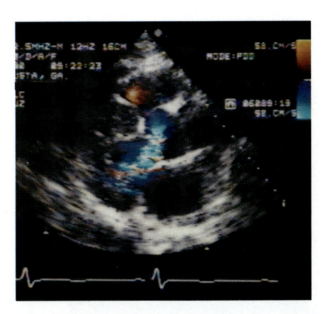

Figure 17–15. Colorflow Doppler in parasternal long-axis view showing posterior AI jet directed tangential to the anterior mitral leaflet to strike the LV posterior wall.

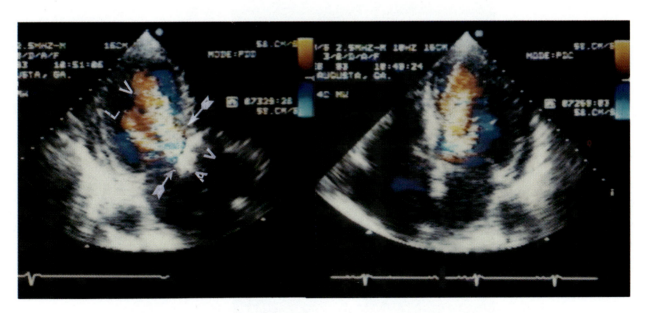

Figure 17–16. Apical long-axis (left) and four-chamber view (right) showing a large aortic regurgitant jet (arrows) that penetrates to the LV apex, signifying severe regurgitation.

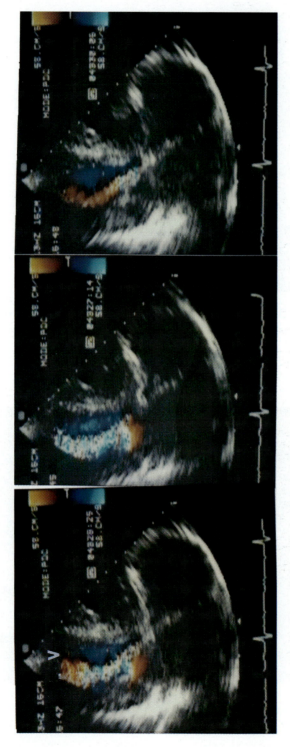

Figure 17–17. Apical long-axis view of a patient with mitral stenosis as well as aortic regurgitation. Colorflow Doppler shows merging of the two jets in the left frame, the mitral stenosis jet alone in the central frame, and the AI jet alone in the right frame.

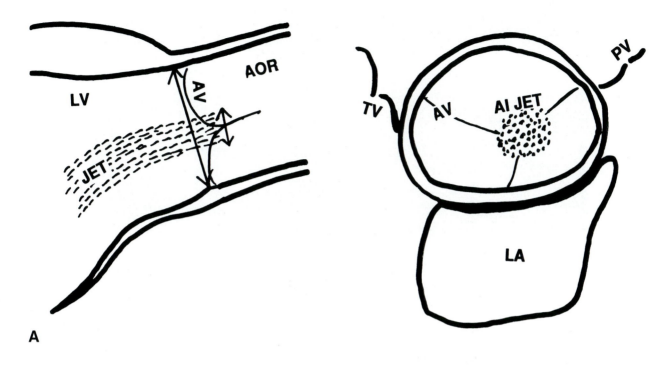

A

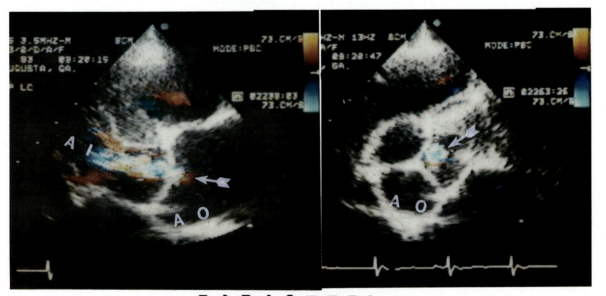

B

Figure 17–18. (A) Diagram showing width of AI jet in parasternal long-axis view (left) and area of the jet in parasternal short-axis view (right). (B) Colorflow Doppler in same views showing the AI jet, 2+ in this case.

**APICAL
LONG AXIS**

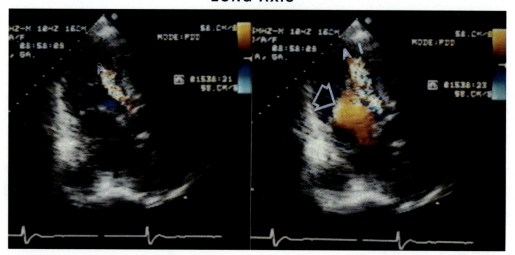

Figure 17–19. (Above) Parasternal long-axis view (left) and apical long-axis view (right) showing flail aortic cusp prolapsing into the LV outflow tract. (Below) Colorflow Doppler in parasternal long-axis view (left) and short-axis view (right) showing large, wide AI jet signifying severe AI.

Fine diastolic vibration of the aortic leaflets (diastolic flutter) is diagnostic of aortic cusp rupture or perforation. Good magnified M-mode imaging at fast speed is needed to demonstrate it well.

It has been shown in several well-documented studies that no vegetations may be detected on 2D echo (even TEE) in some proven cases of bacterial endocarditis. Valve destruction may be the only evidence in these patients; serial echocardiograms and comparison with previous ones are diagnostically very helpful if they show a striking increase in (or appearance of) significant AI that was slight (or absent) in earlier Doppler examinations.

Acute severe AI resulting from aortic valve endocarditis has several other Doppler or "pathophysiologic" manifestations such as premature mitral valve closure (best depicted on rapid-speed M-mode tracings), rapid deceleration of the AI jet velocity, etc. Though diagnostically valuable, these will not be further discussed in this chapter, which is concerned with abnormal anatomy rather than physiology.

Paraaortic (Ring or Aortic Root) Abscess

Although bacterial endocarditis has been known for a century, one of its most common and important complications—paraaortic abscess—has received the recognition it deserves only during the last two decades. These abscesses are caused by spread of infection from a cardiac valve to the vicinity of the aortic annulus. Aortic valve endocarditis is by far the most common site of the original cardiac infection, followed by mitral valve endocarditis; tricuspid and pulmonary valve endocarditis have also been known to rarely spread to the paraaortic region.

How often does paraaortic abscess complicate aortic valve endocarditis? Autopsy and surgical series reported indicate that this complication occurs in one-half to one-third of patients with native aortic valve endocarditis.[48,49] Paraaortic abscesses are found in more than half of patients with prosthetic aortic valve endocarditis who come to surgery and in virtually all fatal cases at autopsy.[50-53]

Streptococcus and *Staphylococcus* are the most common microorganisms causing aortic root abscesses. *S. aureus* is particularly notorious in causing rapid and severe de-

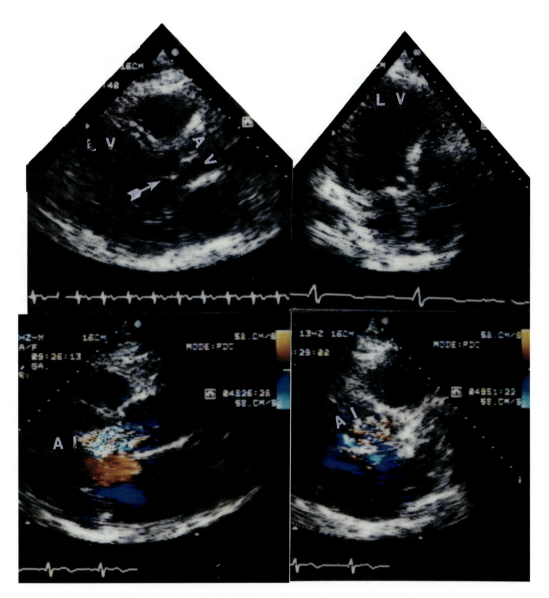

Figure 17–20. Parasternal long-axis view (left) and short-axis view (right) showing a flail aortic cusp with attached vegetation prolapsing into the LV outflow tract in diastole (arrows).

struction of valve and paravalvar tissue. Exceptionally, patients with paraaortic abscesses who have received a course of antibiotics are found to have a sterile abscess cavity at surgery or autopsy.

Vegetations on the native or prosthetic aortic valve are the rule and, when large, can actually obstruct the valve orifice. Infected thrombi within a mechanical prosthetic valve can seriously impede motion of the moving disk or disks, resulting in hemodynamically important stenosis.

The paraaortic abscess was restricted to one sinus of Valsalva in 70% of one series[54] and in 40% of another series.[55] In some cases, local destruction by the culprit organisms results in (1) a fistula between the aortic root and a right heart chamber,[55] (2) spread of infection or abscess rupture into the pericardium, causing purulent pericarditis (in other cases, a small pericardial effusion results from the contiguous abscess but is "sympathetic" rather than actually purulent), (3) first-, second-, or third-degree atrioventricular block or bundle branch block, because the central fibrous body of the cardiac skeleton through

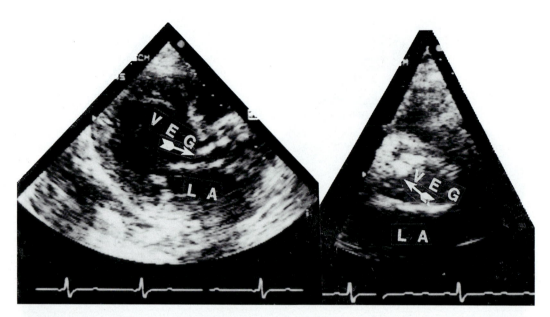

Figure 17–21. Parasternal long-axis view (left) and short-axis view (right) showing an aortic valve vegetation. In long-axis view, projection of the flail leaflet with vegetation into the LV outflow tract is seen.

which the His bundle passes is within the territory often involved by spread of paraaortic infection, and (4) tracking of the paraaortic abscess along the components of the cardiac fibrous skeleton, including the valve annuli, resulting in the dreaded situation of separation of much or most of the aortic root from the ventricle. Many of these catastrophic complications of bacterial endocarditis were described a century ago by Osler[56] in his original report on the disease.

REFERENCES

1. Friedman B, Hathaway B. Fenestrations of the semilunar cusps and "functional" aortic and pulmonary valve insufficiency. Am J Med 1958;24:549.
2. Foxe A. Fenestrations of the semilunar valves. Am J Pathol 1929;5:179.
3. Symbas PN, Walter PF, Hurst JW, et al. Fenestration of aortic cusps causing aortic regurgitation. J Thorac Cardiovasc Surg 1969;57:464.
4. Osler W. The bicuspid condition of the aortic valves. Trans Assoc Am Physicians 1886;2:185.
5. Bacon APC, Matthews MB. Congenital bicuspid aortic valves and the etiology of isolated aortic valvular stenosis. Q J Med 1959;28:545.
6. Roberts WC. The congenitally bicuspid aortic valve: A study of 85 autopsy cases. Am J Cardiol 1970;26:72.
7. Edwards JE. The congenital bicuspid aortic valve. Circulation 1961;23:485.
8. Waller F, Carter JB, Williams HJ, et al. Bicuspid aortic valve: Comparison of congenital and acquired types. Circulation 1973;48:1140.
9. Scovil JA, Nanda NC, Gross CM, et al. Echocardiographic studies of abnormalities associated with coarctation of the aorta. Circulation 1976;543:953.
10. Nanda NC, Gramiak R, Manning J, et al. Echocardiographic recognition of the congenital bicuspid aortic valve. Circulation 1974;49:870.
11. Radford DJ, Bloom KR, Izukama R, et al. Echocardiographic assessment of bicuspid aortic valves. Circulation 1976;53:80.
12. Kececioglu-Draelos Z, Goldberg SJ. Role of M-mode echocardiography in congenital aortic stenosis. Am J Cardiol 1981;47:1267.

13. Fowles RE, Martin RP, Abrams JM, et al. Two-dimensional echocardiographic features of bicuspid aortic valve. Chest 1979;75:435.

14. Brandenburg RO, Tajik AJ, Edwards WD, et al. Accuracy of two-dimensional echocardiographic diagnosis of congenitally bicuspid aortic valve. Am J Cardiol 1983;51:1469.

15. Zema MJ, Caccavano M. Two-dimensional echocardiographic assessment of aortic valve morphology: Feasibility of bicuspid valve detection. Br Heart J 1982;48:428.

16. Hurwitz LE, Roberts WC. Quadricuspid aortic valve. Am J Cardiol 1973;31:623.

17. Davia JE, Fenoglio JJ, DeCastro CM, et al. Quadricuspid semilunar valves. Chest 1977;72:186.

18. Kim HS, McBride RA, Titus JS. Quadricuspid aortic valve and single coronary ostium. Arch Pathol Lab Med 1988;112:842.

19. Chandrasekharan K, Tajik AJ, Edwards WD, et al. Two-dimensional echocardiographic diagnosis of quadricuspid aortic valve. Am J Cardiol 1984;53:1732.

20. Herman RL, Cohen IS, Glaser K, et al. Diagnosis of incompetent quadricuspid aortic valve by two-dimensional echocardiography. Am J Cardiol 1984;53:972.

21. Ellis FH, Kirklin JW. Congenital valvular aortic stenosis. J Thorac Cardiovasc Surg 1962;43:199.

22. Campbell M. Calcific aortic stenosis and congenital bicuspid aortic valves. Br Heart J 1968;30:606.

23. Roberts WC. Anatomically isolated aortic valvular disease. Am J Med 1970;49:151.

24. Roberts WC, Perloff JK, Constantino T. Severe valvular aortic stenosis in patients over 65 years of age. Am J Cardiol 1971;27:497.

25. Subramanian R, Olson LJ, Edwards WD. Surgical pathology of pure aortic stenosis. Mayo Clin Proc 1984;59:683.

26. Edwards JE. Pathologic aspects of cardiac and valvular insufficiencies. Arch Surg 1958;77:634.

27. Petersen MD. Types of aortic stenosis in surgically removed valves. Arch Pathol Lab Med 1985;109:829.

28. Selzer A. Changing aspects of the natural history of valvular aortic stenosis. N Engl J Med 1987;317:91.

29. Bulkley BH, Roberts WC. The heart in systemic lupus erythematosus and the changes induced in it by corticosteroid therapy. Am J Med 1975;48:243.

30. Larson EW, Edwards WD. Risk factors for aortic dissection. Am J Cardiol 1984;54:849.

31. Godley RW, Green D, Dillon JC, et al. Reliability of two-dimensional echocardiography in assessing the severity of valvular aortic stenosis. Chest 1981;79:657.

32. DeMaria AN, Bommer W, Joye J, et al. Value and limitations of cross-sectional echocardiography of the aortic valve in the diagnosis and quantitation of valvular aortic stenosis. Circulation 1980;62:304.

33. Vered Z, Schneeweiss A, Meltzer RS. Echocardiographic assessment of left ventricular outflow tract obstruction. Am Heart J 1983;106:177.

34. Wong M, Tei C, Sadler N, et al. Echocardiographic observations of calcium in operatively excised stenotic aortic valves. Am J Cardiol 1987;59:324.

35. Hofmann T, Kasper W, Meinertz T, et al. Determination of aortic valve orifice area in aortic valve stenosis by two-dimensional transesophageal echocardiography. Am J Cardiol 1987;59:330.

36. Stoddard MF, Arce J, Liddell NE, et al. Two-dimensional transesophageal echocardiographic determination of aortic valve area in adults with aortic stenosis. Am Heart J 1991;122:1415.

37. Conde CA, Meller J, Donoso E, et al. Bacterial endocarditis with ruptured sinus of Valsalva and aorticocardiac fistula. Am J Cardiol 1975;35:912.

38. Mills J, Utley J, Abbott J. Heart failure in infective endocarditis. Chest 1974;66:151.

39. Wray TM. Echocardiographic manifestations of flail aortic valve leaflets in bacterial endocarditis. Circulation 1975;51:832.

40. Mintz GS, Kotler MN, Segal BL, et al. Comparison of two-dimensional and M-mode echocardiography in the evaluation of patients with infective endocarditis. Am J Cardiol 1979;43:738.

41. Ramirez J, Guardiola J, Flowers NC. Echocardiographic diagnosis of ruptured aortic valve leaflet in bacterial endocarditis. Circulation 1978;57:634.

42. Chandaratna PAN, Robinson MJ, Byrd C, et al. Significance of abnormal echoes in left ventricular outflow tract. Br Heart J 1977;39:381.

43. Sternberg L, Sole MJ, Joza P, et al. Echocardiographic features of an unusual case of aortic valve endocarditis. Can Med Assoc J 1976;115:1022.

44. Pease HF, Matsumoto S, Caccione RJ, et al. Lethal obstruction by aortic valvular vegetation.

Chest 1978;73:658.

45. Krivokapich J, Child JS, Skorton DJ. Flail aortic valve leaflets: M-mode and two-dimensional echocardiographic manifestations. Am Heart J 1980;99:425.

46. Martin RP, Meltzer RS, Chia BG, et al. Clinical utility of two-dimensional echocardiography in infectious endocarditis. Am J Cardiol 1980;46:379.

47. Kinney EL, Wright RJ. Aortic valve vegetations: Examples of overestimation and underestimation of disease by two-dimensional echocardiography. Am Heart J 1987;113:1268.

48. Arnett EN, Roberts WC. Valve ring abscess in active infective endocarditis: Frequency, location, clues to clinical diagnosis from the study of 95 necropsy patients. Circulation 1976;54:140.

49. D'Agostino RS, Miller DC, Stinson EB, et al. Valve replacement in patients with native valve endocarditis. Ann Thorac Surg 1985;40:429.

50. Baumgartner WA, Miller DC, Reitz BA, et al. Surgical treatment of prosthetic valve endocarditis. Ann Thorac Surg 1983;35:87.

51. Richardson JV, Karp RB, Kirlin JW, et al. Treatment of infective endocarditis. Circulation 1978;58:589.

52. Arnett EN, Roberts WC. Prosthetic valve endocarditis. Am J Cardiol 1976;38:281.

53. Cowgill LD, Addonizio VP, Hopeman AR, et al. A practical approach to prosthetic valve endocarditis. Ann Thorac Surg 1987;43:450.

54. Fiore AC, Ivey TD, McKeown PP, et al. Patch closure of aortic annulus mycotic aneurysms. Ann Thorac Surg 1986;42:372.

55. David TE. Aortic root abscess, in RW Emery, KV Arom (eds): The Aortic Valve. St Louis: Mosby–Year Book, 1991, p 290.

56. Osler W. Gulstonian lecture on malignant endocarditis. Br Med J 1885;1:467.

18

Coronary Arteries

The right and left coronary arterial trees, though of immense importance to angiocardiographers, have seldom been of major interest to echocardiographers. The latter can image the coronaries only in their proximal extent, and it is mainly these segments that merit their attention.

The right coronary artery (RCA) arises from the right (anterior) sinus of Valsalva (Figures 18-1 and 19-4) and then emerges anteriorly and slightly rightward between the right atrial appendage and pulmonary trunk. It is this segment of RCA that can be imaged in a short-axis plane through the aortic root. Once it reaches the right atrioventricular (AV) groove or sulcus, it descends vertically to reach the acute (anteroinferior) cardiac margin and then turns posteriorly to reach the crux of the heart (area where the following four boundaries meet: right and left AV sulci and interatrial and interventricular grooves).

The left main coronary artery arises from the left sinus of Valsalva and varies tremendously in length from a few millimeters to a few centimeters. It lies on a bed of subepicardial fat between the pulmonary trunk and the left atrial appendage. On reaching the left AV sulcus, it divides into two main branches: the left anterior descending (LAD) and the circumflex arteries. Although the left main coronary artery curves leftward at this level, its entire length is approximately in the same plane and can be imaged in this plane to the left of the aortic root (Figures 18-1 and 19-4).

The LAD artery descends forward and to the left in the anterior interventricular groove as far as the apex. In one-third of cases it ends there. In the others it turns round the apex into the posterior interventricular groove. The circumflex artery continues posteriorly in the left AV groove toward the cardiac crux.

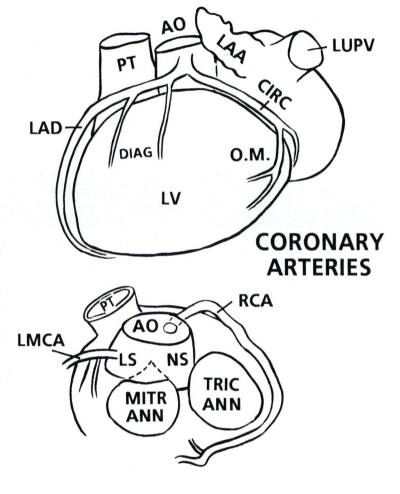

Figure 18–1. (Above) Diagram of left aspect of heart to show bifurcation of left main coronary artery into left anterior descending (LAD) artery anteriorly and circumflex artery (CIRC) posteriorly (PT, pulmonary trunk; Ao, aorta; LA, left atrial appendage; OM, obtuse marginal artery; LUPV, left upper pulmonary vein). (Below) Base of the heart, viewed from above and posteriorly, to show relationship of right coronary artery (RCA) and left main coronary artery (LMCA) to aorta, pulmonary trunk, mitral annulus (MITR ANN) and tricuspid annulus (TRIC ANN) (LS and NS, left and non-coronary sinus of Valsalva, respectively).

There is much reciprocal variation in size, length, and myocardial territory supplied by the right and left coronary arterial systems. The left main coronary artery is larger than the right in 60% of hearts, and the right is larger than the left in 17%; the two are of about the same size in 23%.

ECHOCARDIOGRAPHY OF CORONARY ARTERIES

The origin and proximal segments of the left main and right coronary artery (CA) can be visualized on short-axis view, as the aorta is imaged at sinuses of Valsalva level. The right CA emerges from the right coronary sinus of Valsalva at about the 11 o'clock position, and usually not more than 1 cm or less of it can be identified. The left main CA emerges from the left sinus of Valsalva at about the 3 or 4 o'clock position and courses leftward.

In this location the left main CA lies embedded in pericardial fat in a shallow fossa posteroinferior to the wide pulmonary trunk. The left main CA is therefore imaged by first visualizing the pulmonary valve and trunk and then shifting to a slightly inferior plane. The left main CA manifests as a narrow (few millimeters) tubular space surrounded by a dense echogenic amorphous area (mainly fatty connective tissue). The right and left main CAs are nearly, but not quite, in the same horizontal plane so that they are seldom both well depicted simultaneously.

The CAs are difficult to image well (1) because of their curved winding course in the coronary (AV) groove, and (2) because they are in constant complex motion. Because of the latter, a slow frame-by-frame sequence is usually necessary to secure the best image of the artery.

With practice and a favorable ultrasonic window, the entire left main CA may be seen from its ostium until and even beyond its bifurcation into left anterior descending (LAD) and circumflex arteries; the former turns anteriorly, and the latter continues in the same general direction as the left main.

CORONARY ARTERY STENOSIS

Feigenbaum and associates,[1-5] in a series of reports, have experienced excellent results in the visualization of the left main and LAD arteries, especially with utilization of enhanced technology of recording and digital processing. They could identify stenotic left main lesions (over 50% stenosis) in over 90% of patients and a lesser but encouraging percentage of proximal LAD lesions. However, others are not as enthusiastic about two-dimensional (2D) echo as a screening test. Block and Popp[6] studied 50 patients against the "gold standard" of angiography. The left main CA could not be properly seen in one-fourth of cases. 2D echo was correct in predicting the presence or absence of left main CA stenosis in 30 of 37 patients, but there were 6 false-positive results and 1 false-negative result.

Chandaratna and Aronow[7] found 2D echo reliable in predicting left main CA stenosis when this artery could be seen adequately, but this was possible in only about 60% of patients. Chen et al.[8] visualized the left main CA from the apical instead of parasternal window. In the apical four-chamber view, the transducer is tilted posteriorly to transect the posterior mitral annulus rather than mitral leaflets; the left main CA is detectable as a narrow tubular sonolucency embedded in the solid echogenic background of the posterior mitral annulus region. Because the left main CA is much further away from the transducer than it is in the parasternal view, resolution is inferior, and stenosis or patency of the vessel is more difficult to identify.

Arjunan et al.[9] developed normal standard values for proximal CA caliber (right as well as left main) in children and adolescents. They recommend 1 cm from the ostium as the best place to measure the width of the main CA, which is normally about 2 mm in infants and 5 mm in teenagers. Coronary artery caliber in the same patients on angiography was slightly (less than 1 mm) but consistently smaller than the 2D echo measurement.

With improved ultrasound technology, Faletra et al.[10] have succeeded in visualizing the lumen of the peripheral LAD artery in 82% of 30 patients and made a correct diagnosis of significant stenosis in 11 of 12 cases.

Superior resolution of coronary artery images by transesophageal echocardiography (TEE) (Figure 18-2) has stimulated echocardiographers to reassess the proximal coronaries from the esophageal window[11-15] using colorflow Doppler in conjunction with magnified 2D imaging. CA stenosis is considered present if hyperreflecting plaques narrowing the CA lumen are detected. The published data from several centers, using coronary angiography as the "gold standard," indicate a high specificity and sensitivity for TEE detection of stenosis of the left main, LAD, and circumflex arteries.

KAWASAKI DISEASE

This syndrome, first described only 25 years ago, is of interest to pediatric cardiologists because of CA aneurysms that occur in 15% to 20% of patients. The acute phase, known to pediatricians as the *mucocutaneous lymph node syndrome* (because of transitory inflammatory changes in the mouth, skin rash, and cervical lymph node enlargement), is followed within 10 to 30 days by CA aneurysms.[16-19] The arteries affected, in descending frequency, are the LAD, RCA, left main, and circumflex.

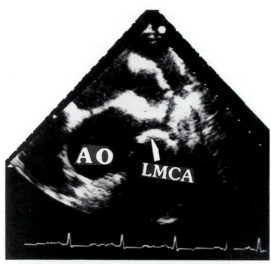

TRANSESOPHAGEAL

Figure 18–2. TEE view of left main coronary artery (LMCA) emerging from aortic root (Ao) and bifurcating into circumflex artery (directed posteriorly) and left anterior descending artery (directed anteriorly).

Aneurysms of two, three, or four arteries were found in 37%, 23%, and 13% of cases.[16] Kawasaki coronary aneurysms have been categorized by shape into saccular, fusiform, and tubular. The affected coronary arteries might develop thrombi in them, or stenosis may coexist with dilatation in different segments of the same artery. Although primarily an affliction of smaller children, it can occur in teenagers and even young adults. Although most common and most studied in Japan, it is not very rare in the United States, where it has been encountered in white, black, and Asian races. Fortunately, serial studies have shown that improvement or resolution of coronary artery aneurysms occurs in as many as two-thirds of cases.

2D echo has been proved very useful in diagnosing the presence of CA aneurysms. Aneurysms of the proximal RCA, left main, or commencement of the LAD are easy to visualize, especially if large, and thrombi may be evident within them.[19]

Since the more peripheral parts of coronary arteries are not accessible to cardiac ultrasound imaging, it might be assumed that aneurysms at these sites cannot be detected by echocardiography. However, some Japanese authors[20,21] have worked out special views or imaging planes that can reveal aneurysmal dilatation of the "peripheral" CAs as they run in the right and left atrioventricular grooves. In brief, starting from apical or subcostal windows, the transducer is tilted and rotated in unconventional planes to scan the regions of the tricuspid and mitral annuli. If present, CA aneurysms show up as small round or oval sonolucencies against a background of echogenic myocardium or pericardial fat. A potential pitfall in this regard is to mistake a narrow corner of the right atrium (RA) or right ventricle (RV) cavity for a coronary aneurysm.

CORONARY ARTERY ANOMALIES

Anomalous origin of the left main CA or (less frequently) the right CA from the pulmonary trunk is an important entity for pediatric cardiologists, though occasional instances in young adults are seen. Infants present with angina-like symptoms due to myocardial ischemia. In older children or teenagers who have survived due to adequate collateral circulation, a left-to-right shunt occurs into the pulmonary artery. At this stage, left ventricular (LV) dilatation and hypokinesis may be mistaken for dilated cardiomyopathy. On 2D echo, aided by colorflow Doppler in short-axis view, it may be possible to visualize the origin of the anomalous left main or right CA from the pulmonary trunk and also to demonstrate that the abnormal CA does not arise from its proper location on the aortic sinus of Valsalva.[22-24] Colorflow Doppler helps in showing the direction of abnormal flow, i.e., toward the pulmonary trunk, in the anomalous artery. Numerous reports documenting diagnostic use of colorflow Doppler for this purpose in early childhood have appeared, including one case in a teenager.[25] Fernandes et al.[26] have demonstrated the ability of TEE to visualize various other coronary anomalies: left main CA or LAD arising from right coronary sinus of Valsalva and RCA from left coronary sinus of Valsalva (Figure 18–3). In the former anomaly, the course of the anomalous artery between aorta and pulmonary trunk was well seen, better than by angiography. The importance of this is that this particular variant can result in sudden death.[27] Anomalous origin of the RCA from the pulmonary trunk has been identified by colorflow Doppler.[28]

Coronary artery fistula is a rare anomaly encountered in children as well as adults. The RCA is involved twice as often as the left coronary system. The RCA fistula conveys

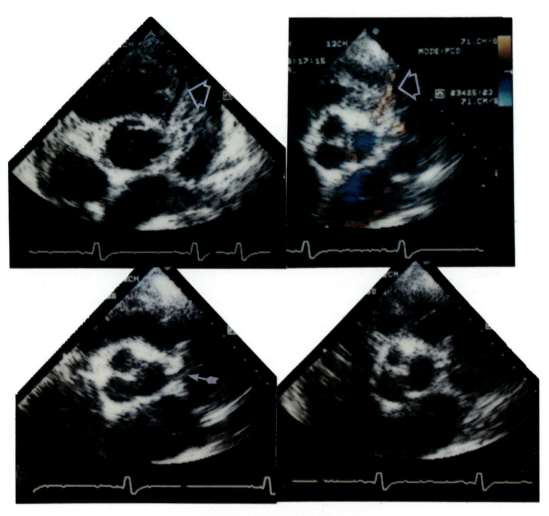

PARASTERNAL
SHORT AXIS

Figure 18–3. Parasternal short-axis views to show coronary arteries. The left main coronary artery (small thin arrows) is viewed in normal location. Also emerging from the left coronary sinus of Valsalva is an anomalous right coronary artery (open arrow) at about 2 o'clock. Colorflow Doppler (above, right) shows flow in this artery directed anteriorly.

arterial blood most frequently into the RV chamber, less often the right atrium, pulmonary artery, left heart, or superior vena cava. The affected CA is enlarged, sometimes to a huge size. 2D echo can image the abnormal fistulous track, which is dilated and tortuous.[29-32] Colorflow Doppler may permit the course of blood flow and the site of termination or emptying of the fistula to be demonstrated.[33]

REFERENCES

1. Weyman AE, Feigenbaum H, Dillon JC, et al. Noninvasive visualization of the left main coronary artery by cross-sectional echocardiography. Circulation 1976;54:169.
2. Rogers EW, Feigenbaum H, Weyman AE, et al. Possible detection of atherosclerotic calcification by two-dimensional echocardiography. Circulation 1980;62:1046.
3. Rink LW, Feigenbaum H, Godley RW, et al. Echocardiographic detection of left main coronary artery obstruction. Circulation 1982;65:719.
4. Ryan T, Armstrong WF, Feigenbaum H. Prospective evaluation of the left main coronary artery using digital two-dimensional echocardiography. J Am Coll Cardiol 1986;7:807.
5. Presti CF, Feigenbaum H, Armstrong WF, et al. Digital two-dimensional echocardiographic evaluation of the proximal left anterior descending coronary artery. Am J Cardiol 1987;60:1254.
6. Block PJ, Popp RL. Detecting and excluding significant left main coronary artery narrowing by echocardiography. Am J Cardiol 1984;55:93.
7. Chandaratna PAN, Aronow SW. Left main coronary arterial patency assessed with cross-sectional echocardiography. Am J Cardiol 1980;46:91.
8. Chen CC, Morganroth J, Ogawa S, et al. Detecting left main coronary disease by apical cross-sectional echocardiography. Circulation 1980;62:288.
9. Arjunan K, Daniels SR, Meyer RA, et al. Coronary artery caliber in normal children and patients with Kawasaki disease without aneurysms. J Am Coll Cardiol 1986;8:1119.
10. Faletra F, Cipriani M, Corono R, et al. Transthoracic high-frequency echocardiographic detection of atherosclerotic lesions in the descending portion of the left coronary artery. J Am Soc Echocardiogr 1993;6:290.
11. Yoshida K, Yoshikawa J, Hozumi T., et al. Detection of the left main coronary artery stenosis by transesophageal color Doppler and two-dimensional echocardiography. Circulation 1990;81:1271.
12. Reichert SLA, Visser CA, Koolen JJ, et al. Transesophageal examination of the left coronary artery with a 7.5-MHz annular array two-dimensional color flow Doppler transducer. J Am Soc Echocardiogr 1990;3:118.
13. Yamagishi M, Yasu T, Ohara K, et al. Detection of coronary blood flow associated with left main coronary artery stenosis by transesophageal Doppler color flow echocardiography. J Am Coll Cardiol 1991;17:87.
14. Samdarshi TE, Nanda NC, Gatewood RP, et al. Usefulness and limitation of transesophageal echocardiography in the assessment of proximal coronary artery stenosis. J Am Coll Cardiol 1991;17:87.
15. Memmola C, Iliceto S, Rizzon P. Detection of proximal stenosis of left coronary artery by digital transesophageal echocardiography. J Am Soc Echocardiogr 1993;6:149.
16. Onouchi Z, Shimazu S, Kiyosawa N, et al. Aneurysms of the coronary arteries in Kawasaki disease. Circulation 1982;66:6.
17. Capannair TE, Daniels SR, Meyer RA, et al. Sensitivity, specificity, and predictive value of two-dimensional echocardiography in detecting coronary artery aneurysms in patients with Kawasaki disease. J Am Coll Cardiol 1986;7:355.
18. Takahashi M, Mason W, Lewis AB. Regression of coronary aneurysms in patients with Kawasaki syndrome. Circulation 1987;75:387.
19. Mahoney L. Echocardiography in Kawasaki disease and other coronary abnormalities in children, in RE Kerber (ed): Echocardiography in Coronary Artery Disease. New York: Futura, 1988, pp 95–102.
20. Satomi G, Nakamura K, Narai S, et al. Systematic visualization of coronary arteries by two-dimensional echocardiography in children and infants. Am Heart J 1984;107:497.
21. Yoshida H, Maeda T, Funabashi T, et al. Subcostal two-dimensional echocardiographic imaging of peripheral right coronary artery in Kawasaki disease. Circulation 1982;65:956.

22. Fisher EA, Sephri B, Lendrum B, et al. Two-dimensional echocardiographic visualization of the left coronary artery in anomalous origin of the left coronary artery from the pulmonary artery. Circulation 1981;63:698.

23. Terai M, Nagai Y, Toba T. Cross-sectional finding of anomalous origin of left coronary artery from pulmonary artery. Br Heart J 1983;50:104.

24. Diamant S, Luber JM, Brumson SC, et al. Two-dimensional and pulsed-Doppler echocardiography in anomalous origin of the left coronary artery from the pulmonary artery. Am Heart J 1987;113:195.

25. Maire R, Gallino A, Jenni R. Initial detection in a teenager of anomalous left coronary from the pulmonary artery by color Doppler echocardiography. Am Heart J 1993;125:1802.

26. Fernandes F, Alam M, Smith S, et al. The role of transesophageal echocardiography in identifying anomalous coronary arteries. Circulation 1993;88:2532.

27. Kragel AH, Roberts WC. Anomalous origin of either the right or left main coronary artery from the aorta with subsequent coursing between aorta and pulmonary trunk. Am J Cardiol 1988;62:771.

28. Shah RM, Nanda NC, Hsuing MC, et al. Identification of anomalous origin of the right coronary artery from pulmonary trunk by Doppler color flow mapping. Am J Cardiol 1986;57:366.

29. Yoshikawa J, Katao H, Yanagihara K, et al. Noninvasive visualization of the main coronary arteries in coronary artery fistulas by cross-sectional echocardiography. Circulation 1982;65:600.

30. Kronzon I, Winer HE, Cohen B. Noninvasive diagnosis of left coronary arteriovenous fistula communicating with the right ventricle. Am J Cardiol 1982;49:1811.

31. Rogers DM, Wolf NM, Barrett MJ, et al. Two-dimensional echocardiographic features of coronary arteriovenous fistula. Am Heart J 1982;104:872.

32. Friedman DM, Rutkowski M. Coronary artery fistula: A pulsed Doppler/two-dimensional echocardiographic study. Am J Cardiol 1985;55:1652.

33. Oda H, Kawada Y, Toeda T, et al. Assessment of a coronary artery fistula to the pulmonary artery by transesophageal echocardiography. Am Heart J 1993;125:1460.

19

Aorta I: Sinuses of Valsalva

NORMAL ANATOMY (Figure 19–1)

Just above the aortic valve, the ascending aorta is dilated compared with the rest of its caliber. This dilatation takes the form of three bulges, each corresponding to a cusp of the aortic valve. These bulges are called the *sinuses of Valsalva* (SOV) after the man who described them in 1740 [but they had been discussed and illustrated earlier (1513) by Leonardo da Vinci]. The SOVs, like the corresponding cusps, are designated right coronary, left coronary, and noncoronary. Longitudinally, each SOV starts at the aortic valve cusp attachment and extends upward, where its distal extent is limited by a well-defined ridge, the supravalvar or sinus ridge, consistently demonstrable by inspection and palpation of the inner aspect of the aorta.[1] This ridge is much thicker than the adjacent aortic wall on either side and tends to be a favorite site for atheroma. On the other hand, the aortic wall is unduly thin at mid-SOV level; this fact is of interest to echocardiographers because the thin aortic wall segment often tends to drop out in the parasternal long-axis view, which the unwary may mistake for an aortic–right ventricular (RV) fistula. The artifactual nature of the apparent lack of continuity here is confirmed by the absence of any jet on colorflow Doppler.

The term *aortic root* is believed to have been introduced in 1880 by the anatomist Sibson and is commonly used at present by echocardiographers and angiographers, but is not to be found in most textbooks of anatomy, which refer only to lower and upper ascending aorta. Titus and Edwards[2] stated that the term *aortic root* should apply to that part of the ascending aorta which lies between the aortic valve attachment and the supraval-

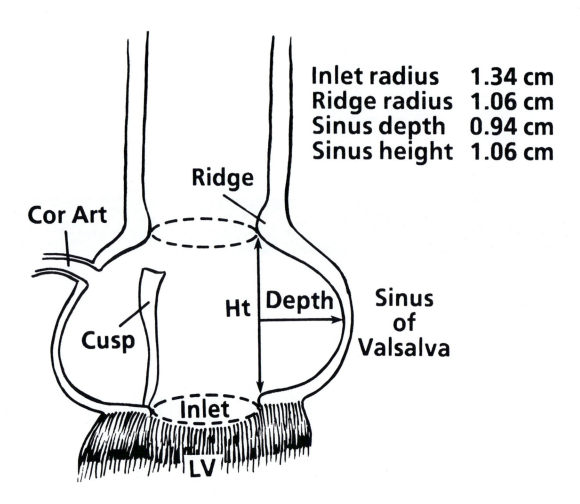

Figure 19–1. Diagram of normal aortic root showing increased caliber at sinus of Valsalva level. A ridge separates the sinus portion of the aorta from the tubular upper segment of the ascending aorta. The measurements are from the publication of Reid.[4]

var ridge, also called the *sinus portion* of the ascending aorta. The remainder of the ascending aorta above this level is sometimes called the *tubular portion.*

The degree of bulging or dilatation of the SOVs varies from one individual to another and may not affect all SOVs equally (Figure 19-2). The noncoronary SOV tends to be a little larger than the other two. The maximal diameter of the aorta at SOV level may be as much as twice the aortic caliber at or above the supravalvar ridge level; this is more obvious on aortography or echocardiography, when the aorta is distended with blood,[3] than at autopsy.

Measurements of aortic root obtained by Reid[4] are shown in Figure 19-1, slightly modified from his paper. Reid pointed out that the floor of each SOV rests to some extent on the myocardial shoulder of the summit of the ventricular septum so that the cusp is attached not only to the fibrous annulus but also to cardiac muscle at this site. This does not apply to the noncoronary SOV, which is not supported by subjacent septal myocardium.

The left and right main coronary arteries arise from their respective SOVs, virtually always within the SOV, i.e., below the supravalvar ridge. The anatomic relationship and geometry with respect to the SOV, aortic semilunar cusp, and coronary artery ostium are important. The free edges or tips of the cusps are believed to reach the supravalvar ridge, thus nearly occluding the SOV in systole; others maintain that the cusp edge falls short of the ridge.

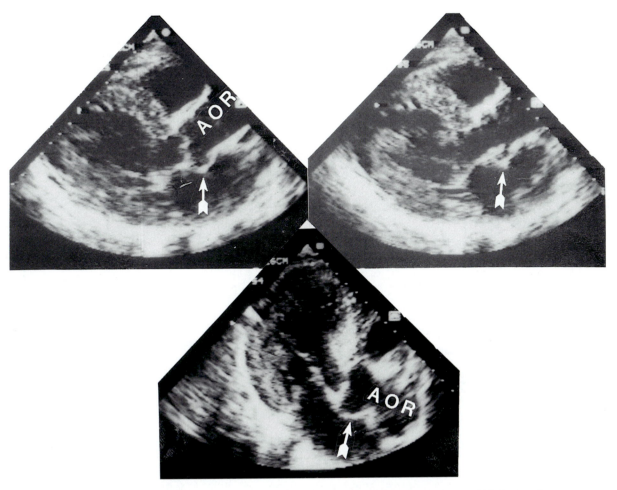

Figure 19–2. (Above) Prominence of the posterior (noncoronary) sinus of Valsalva (arrows). (Below) Bulging of the sinuses of Valsalva (arrow) with relative narrowing just above this level (supravalvar ridge) is well seen in this case.

The aortic root increases in diameter by about 10% during systole, attributable to the elastic fibers in the aortic wall. Valsalva (1740) suggested that the main function of the SOVs was to "dissipate the violence of systolic contraction by allowing blood to enter sinuses during systole."

EXTERNAL RELATIONSHIPS OF SINUSES OF VALSALVA[5] (Figures 19–3 and 19–4)

The right coronary SOV is related mainly to the RV infundibulum. The lowest part of this SOV is attached to the myocardium; above this level a wedge of epicardial fat separates the SOV from the infundibulum. The left coronary SOV is related to the pulmonary trunk anteriorly and to the proximal left main coronary artery and surrounding fat and epicardium laterally. Its most posterior third has the same relations as the noncoronary SOV.

The posterior or noncoronary SOV has several important relationships. The right one-third of this SOV is attached to the membranous part of the ventricular septum. This SOV lies above the septal leaflet of the tricuspid valve and abuts the atrial septum. It is thus closely related to both atria, but much more to the right atrium. The left two-thirds of the noncoronary SOV and the posterior one-third of the left coronary SOV have no attachment or contiguity to the left ventricular (LV) wall or ventricular septum. Instead, they

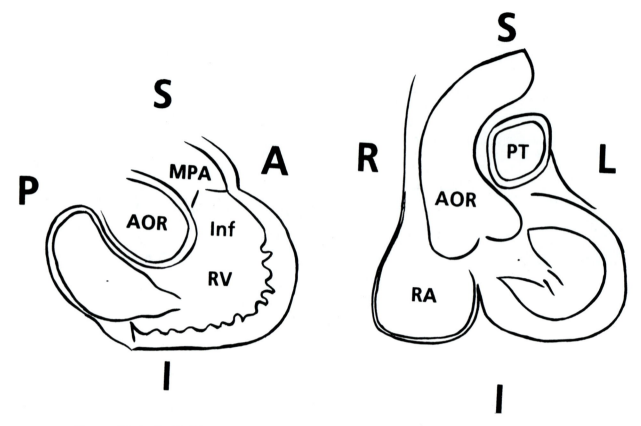

Figure 19–3. (Left) Diagram in near-sagittal plane through the right heart and aortic root to show how the former "wraps around" the latter. (Right) Coronal section through ascending aorta to show its relation to the right atrium, ventricle, and pulmonary trunk (PT) (S, superior; I, inferior; A, anterior; P, posterior; R, right; L, left).

connect or bridge over to the base of the anterior mitral leaflet by a thin fibrous sheet, the intervalvar fibrosa. This structure also has been called the *mitral-aortic intervalvular fibrosa*, the *intervalvar ligament* or *septum*, or the *fibrous trigone;* it varies in length from 2 to 10 mm.

Between the noncoronary SOV and the left atrium immediately posterior to it is a narrow wedge of pericardial fat that is limited inferiorly by the intervalvar fibrosa. This region is a favorite site for abscess formation due to spread of infection from aortic as well as mitral endocarditis.

Hemodynamics within the aortic root and coronary blood flow are determined to a large extent by anatomic factors: the geometry of the SOVs, the supravalvar ridge, the valve cusps and their position in systole and diastole, and the location of the coronary artery ostia.

Reid and Bellhouse[6] discussed vortex formation within the SOVs and balancing of forces on the SOV and the aortic sides, respectively, of the cusps in systole. These authors explained how a coronary ostium at a higher level in the SOV (at or very near the supravalvar ridge) would be fed at a higher pressure than an ostium in a lower location (closer to cusp attachment). In other words, coronary ostia located higher in the SOV result in larger coronary flow. It has been found that coronary ostia are on or almost on the supravalvar ridge in fast-moving animals such as dogs but at mid-SOV level in slow-moving animals such as the ox, sheep, and pig. In humans, coronary ostial location is intermediate between these two levels. Reid and Bellhouse[6] conclude that "it seems reasonable to assume

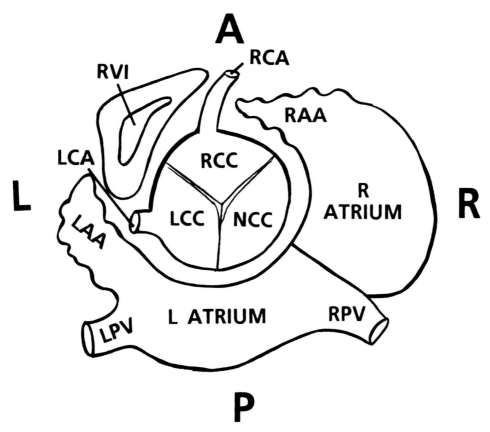

Figure 19–4. Diagram of transverse section through the aortic root and adjacent cardiac chambers, looked at from above (RCC, LCC, and NCC, right, left, and noncoronary cusps; RCA and LCA, right and left coronary arteries; RAA and LAA, right and left atrial appendages; RPV and LPV, right and left pulmonary veins; RVI, right ventricular infundibulum; L, left; R, right; A, anterior; P, posterior).

that the aortic sinuses are a means of ensuring that the coronary arteries are kept primed with blood during systole, regulate coronary flow responses during exercise, and act as pressure recovery chambers initiating valve closure during the latter part of systole." It follows that disruption of aortic root geometry by either disease or surgery would be accompanied by reduction of systolic coronary flow and defective valve closure.

CONGENITAL SINUS OF VALSALVA ANEURYSMS

First described in 1839,[7] this uncommon anomaly has been the subject of an amazing number of single case reports, as well as a few patient series.[8-10] Blackshear et al.[11] noted that by 1991 a total of 274 cases of sinus of Valsalva aneurysm (SVA) had been reported, of which 75% involved the right coronary sinus, 21% the noncoronary sinus, and 4% the left coronary sinus.

Congenital SVA begins as a small blind pouch at a weak spot in the aortic wall where the wall joins the aortic valve annulus. Whereas the local weakness is presumably congenital, the SVA enlarges and manifests in adult life, the typical patient being a young man. The SVA grows to a few centimeters in length, projecting outward from the aortic root and resembling the finger of a rubber glove. In course of time, about 80% of SVAs rupture, usually into a cardiac chamber, producing a shunt from the aorta to this chamber.

If unrepaired, death occurs in most patients within 4 to 6 weeks in refractory heart failure. Rarely, patients survive many years if the SVA perforation is small; another scenario is enlargement of a small apical rupture of an SVA causing progressive congestive failure after an initially compensated left-to-right shunt. Yet another complication is bacterial endocarditis of an SVA.

Since the aortic root is located very centrally in the heart, contiguous to all four cardiac chambers, SVAs can protrude into and then rupture into any of these chambers. Right coronary sinus SVAs rupture into the right ventricle, rarely the right atrium. Noncoronary SVAs rupture into the right atrium. Left coronary SVAs rupture into the left atrium or ventricle. Uncommon sites of SVA rupture include the pulmonary trunk and pericardial sac.

Unruptured SVAs may be discovered unexpectedly at autopsy. However, unruptured SVAs can cause serious symptoms if strategically situated. Thus, if an SVA projects into the right ventricular outflow tract, it can result in subvalvar pulmonic stenosis. If it protrudes into the right atrium, distorting the tricuspid valve, it can cause tricuspid regurgitation. If a left SVA compresses the left main coronary artery, it can result in angina or myocardial infarction. Gallet et al.[12] in 1988 found 14 cases in the literature of left coronary SVA compressing the left main coronary artery and described a new one in a 63-year-old woman. If it encroaches on the aortic valve or left ventricular outflow, aortic regurgitation or stenosis can occur. If an SVA burrows into the ventricular septum, atrioventricular (AV) block of varying degree can occur.

An association of SVA with ventricular septal defect is well known. Congenital SVA as described above is very different in morphology and natural history from aneurysms involving the SOV region in Marfan's syndrome or complicating bacterial endocarditis (mycotic aneurysm). The latter may balloon out to a large size, unlike the finger-like protrusions of congenital SVAs.

Echocardiography of Sinus of Valsalva Aneurysms

These manifest on two-dimensional (2D) echo as a rounded sonolucent space adjacent to and continuous with the aortic root lumen. The aorta itself is of normal width. The communication between the SVA and aorta is above aortic valve level; this communication or "neck" of the SVA may be obvious or may require careful imaging before the appropriate plane is obtained.

Whereas right coronary SVAs and noncoronary SVAs are well seen in the parasternal views, left coronary SVAs may be best revealed in the apical four-chamber view. Transesophageal echocardiography (TEE) has proved useful in identifying SVAs[11,13-15] when the conventional transthoracic echocardiogram (TTE) is inconclusive or the SVA coexists with aortic regurgitation or ventricular septal defect (not a rare association).

Commonly, the SVA is 1 to 2 cm in caliber, in shape as well as size resembling the distended fingers of a glove, but sometimes the SVA balloons out to large size, even occasionally wider than the aorta itself.

The majority of patients with SVAs are diagnosed after they develop congestive failure secondary to the large left-to-right shunt that ensues after the aneurysm ruptures into a cardiac chamber. Colorflow Doppler and pulsed-wave Doppler reveal a turbulent jet issuing from the aortic root into the right atrium or ventricle. Since the pressure gradient between the aorta and these chambers is high through the whole cardiac cycle, the shunt is continuous, and the turbulent jet flow is evident in diastole as well as systole.

SVAs can simulate other pathologic conditions that produce sonolucent spaces adjacent to the aortic root. These include pseudoaneurysm of the aorta, large coronary artery aneurysms, coronary arteriovenous fistulas, and congenital aortic–left ventricular tunnel.[16] Posterior (noncoronary) SVAs can mimic aortic dissection, the aortic wall being mistaken for an intimal flap.

SVAs projecting into the right atrium or ventricle present echocardiographically as an intracardiac mass, thus simulating thrombotic or neoplastic masses. Infected SVAs have been mistaken clinically and on 2D echo for tricuspid endocarditis with vegetations. Left coronary SVAs rupturing into the left ventricle can mimic regurgitation through the aortic valve.

Blackshear et al.[11] collected 14 cases of unruptured SVAs studied by 2D echo and used TEE in an additional patient. While rare, these anomalies are important to echocardiographers because they can masquerade as intracardiac masses or cause obstruction of right ventricular outflow, tricuspid regurgitation, or SVC obstruction. Yet another spectacular, though rare, variant of SVA is that of a noncoronary SVA burrowing into the ventricular septum[17,18]; a large sonolucent space distending the latter structure is seen on 2D echo. Communication with the aortic root distinguishes it from a myocardial hydatid cyst.

AORTIC ROOT FISTULA

Spread of infection from aortic valve endocarditis to the wall of the aortic root may cause its weakness and erosion, resulting eventually into a fistula between one of the aortic root sinuses and an adjacent cardiac chamber, commonly the right atrium. Such aorta-atrial fistulas have been found at autopsy, surgery, or aortography in the past, but recently, colorflow Doppler and 2D echo have made it possible to demonstrate the pathologic anatomy of such fistulas.

In some of these instances there is not only an aortic ring abscess or mycotic aortic root aneurysm but also a separation between the aorta and LV outflow tract, making surgical correction even more formidable. Prosthetic valve endocarditis tends to produce a greater circumferential extent of aortoseptal discontinuity than native valve endocarditis.

Saner et al.[19] pointed out that aortic valve endocarditis can extend in any of three directions, which conform to the three SOVs: (1) from the right coronary SOV into the membranous ventricular septum and then into the right atrium or ventricle or the muscular ventricular septum,[20,21] (2) from the left coronary SOV through the mitral-aortic intervalvar fibrosa to the base of the anterior mitral leaflet or the epicardial wedge of connective-adipose tissue between aorta and left atrium (an abscess may form here, a pseudo-aneurysm, or a rupture into the pericardial sac causing tamponade[22,23]), and (3) from the noncoronary SOV into the posterior ventricular septum and then possibly toward the RV outflow tract or anterior mitral leaflet.

Prosthetic valve endocarditis is often complicated by even more tissue destruction, i.e., separation between the prosthetic sewing ring and the aortic annulus. Severe paravalvar aortic regurgitation and valve dehiscence result.[19] The latter can be recognized by 2D echo and colorflow Doppler, even better when viewed from the TEE window, as aortic-LV discontinuity. This is of vital importance to the surgeon, who has to perform more extensive and radical surgery in such a predicament.

Several reports of rupture of a mycotic aortic root aneurysm into the right or left atrium have appeared in the echocardiographic literature recently[19,24-26] seen by either conventional echo or TEE. Mycotic fistula formation between the aortic root and the pulmonary trunk also has been reported, though more rarely.[27-30] Other known causes of an acquired aortopulmonary fistula include penetrating trauma, aortic dissection, and rupture of a syphilitic aortic aneurysm into the pulmonary artery.

In conclusion, the erosive effects of bacterial infection spreading from infected aortic valves (especially prosthetic valves) can produce a wide spectrum of anatomic and echocardiographic abnormalities (Figure 19-5) depending on (1) the virulence of the organism, (2) the circumferential extent of tissue destruction, (3) whether infection tracks above the level of the aortic valve (aortic root lesions) or below it (subvalvar lesions), and (4) whether perforation of the aortic wall or intervalvar fibrosa has occurred, thus forming a fistula or pseudoaneurysm.

SUPRAVALVAR AORTIC STENOSIS

In this uncommon variety of aortic stenosis, the stenosis affects the ascending aorta, the valve being normal. Two-thirds of cases are characterized by an "hourglass aortic deformity," with severe thickening of the media and intimal proliferation of the aortic wall

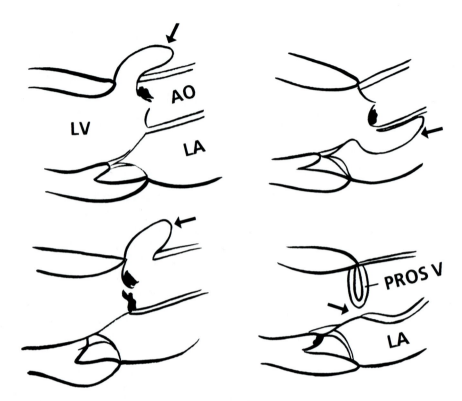

Figure 19–5. Diagram showing various complications of aortic valve endocarditis recognizable on the parasternal long-axis view: (above, left) anterior subvalvar aneurysm; (above, right) posterior subvalvar aneurysm; (below, left) sinus of Valsalva aneurysm; (below, right) prosthetic valve dehiscence.

COMPLICATIONS OF AORTIC VALVE ENDOCARDITIS MANIFESTING ON ECHO

above the SOV level.[31,32] In the remaining instances, the supravalvar aortic stenosis takes the form of a fibrous membrane with a central opening or alternatively a diffuse hypoplastic ascending aorta.

In 30% of cases the aortic valve cusps are thick and may sometimes be adherent to the adjacent aortic wall. The coronary arteries are often of large caliber, thick and tortuous, presumably because they are exposed to abnormally high pressure in the proximal obstructed aortic chamber. Mild aortic regurgitation is common.

Supravalvar aortic stenosis is frequently associated with pulmonary branch artery stenosis and less often with stenosis of the arteries arising from the aortic arch. Bacterial endaortitis has been described as a complication. Acquired supravalvar aortic stenosis has been reported as a complication of surgery on the ascending aorta. Another intriguing variety of the acquired lesion has been its development in a patient with homozygous type II hyperlipoproteinemia.

Echocardiography of Supravalvar Aortic Stenosis (SAS)

M-mode diagnosis of SAS was reported by Bolen et al.[33]; by sweeping the ultrasound beam upward through the left ventricular outflow track (LVOT), aortic root, and ascending aorta, it was possible to record aortic narrowing well above the level of the aortic valve.

2D echo can provide better imaging of the typical SAS appearance. The normal ridge at the junction of the SOVs with the upper ascending aorta appears much accentuated, dense, and thickened.[34,35] It encroaches on the aortic lumen so that aortic caliber is unduly narrow at this level but gradually widens to normal size above that level.

Vogt et al.[35] showed that the ratio of aortic diameter at SAS level to aortic diameter at nonobstructed level correlated well with corresponding aortographic measurements. In a canine model of SAS produced by aortic banding, Doppler hemodynamic correlations were made that validated estimation of the SAS area by the continuity equation method.[36]

ANNULOAORTIC ECTASIA

This awkward term was introduced in the late 1970s[37,38] to refer to symmetrical dilatation of the aortic "annulus" (site of aortic valve attachment) and of the aorta immediately above the valve (Figure 19-6). Aortic regurgitation is always present. Typically, the patient is a young adult with Marfan's syndrome. Very similar anatomic, echocardiographic, and aortographic appearances are sometimes encountered in persons who do not have the skeletal or ocular manifestations of Marfan's syndrome. Some of these have the histologic characteristics described by Erdheim six decades ago and named by him *idiopathic cystic medionecrosis* of the aorta. Other patients have less distinctive histology, but there is some degree of elastic tissue fragmentation, fibrosis, and atrophy of smooth muscle in the arterial media.

Aortographic appearances of this "syndrome" have been described.[39,40] M-mode echocardiographers recognized the condition in the 1970s.[41,42] 2D echo demonstrates the characteristic bulbous aortic root that rapidly tapers to a normal caliber in the upper ascending aorta. Aortic regurgitation is often moderate to severe in degree by colorflow Doppler and tends to increase progressively with time, as does the dilated aortic root itself.

PSEUDOANEURYSM OF THE ASCENDING AORTA

This results from perforation or rupture of the aortic wall in those cases where death did not ensue rapidly because hemorrhage was contained by the resistance of surrounding structures. A cavity is formed, often very large, containing fluid and clotted blood, which communicates with the aortic lumen through a narrow "neck." Clots get organized, and in time, fibrous capsulization of the pseudoaneurysm occurs. Unlike true aortic aneurysms, the pseudoaneurysm wall does not consist of any of the normal arterial wall components.

Most of the reported instances of pseudoaneurysm of the ascending aorta have followed surgery on the aorta.[43-48] The breach in aortic wall continuity occurs at suture sites for insertion of prosthetic valves or grafts or of vents or cannulation placement. The interval between surgery and diagnosis of aortic pseudoaneurysm usually has been less than a year but sometimes several years. Other causes of aortic pseudoaneurysm include traumatic tear (penetrating or blunt chest trauma) and erosion and perforation of the aortic wall by spread of bacterial endocarditis. The latter can complicate discrete subvalvar aortic stenosis.[49] Rarely, no obvious cause can be invoked, and the aortic perforation is presumed to be due to atherosclerotic ulceration[50] or secondary rupture of a small local aortic dissection.

The importance of diagnosis and surgical repair of an aortic pseudoaneurysm lies in its propensity to rupture. This may be preceded by expansion and increasing pain. A large pseudoaneurysm can cause stenosis of the aorta itself,[51] or it may compress the pulmonary trunk, SVC,[52] or right heart chambers.[51,52]

On 2D echo,[46-52] the aortic pseudoaneurysm manifests as a large sonolucent or partly sonolucent space adjacent to the aorta, varying from a few to 15 cm in largest diameter. The pseudoaneurysm may be anterior to the aortic root, presenting as an anterior mediastinal mass, or posterior, in which case it could simulate a left atrial mass and need TEE for better imaging.[50] The echo Doppler characteristics[46] that help to identify the mass or sonolucent space as an aortic pseudoaneurysm are (1) slow swirling "smoke" (dynamic intracavity echoes) caused by slow eddy motion of blood within the cavity, (2) a communication or gap between the aorta and the cavity, (3) permitting the passage of intracavity "smoke" from the aorta to the pseudoaneurysm or in a reversed direction, (4) pulsed-wave Doppler or colorflow Doppler appearances of turbulent flow within the cavity in systole as well as diastole, and (5) a gradient of at least 25 mm between the aorta and the cavity on continuous-wave Doppler.[46]

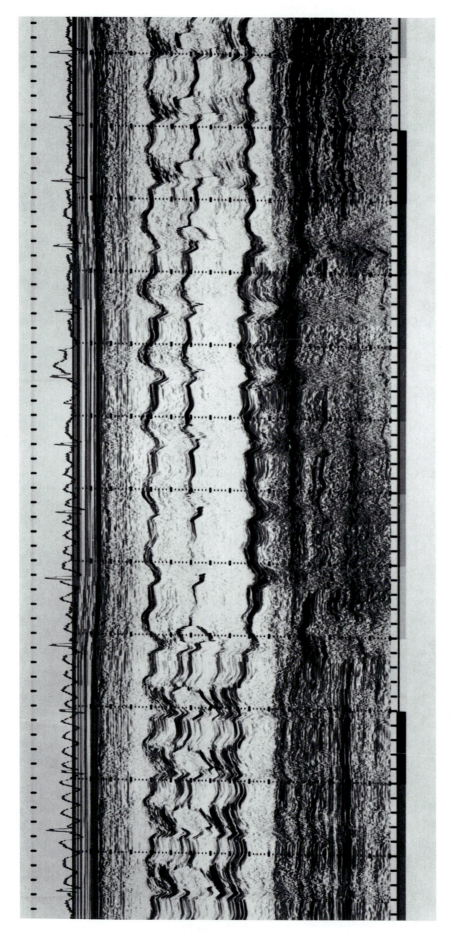

Figure 19–6. M-mode sweep of aortic root shows normal caliber (left) at aortic valve level but a wider aortic width at a higher level (center). Note abnormally small left atrial dimension due to encroachment by the dilated ascending aorta.

REFERENCES

1. Tveter KJ, Edwards JE. Calcified aortic sinotubular ridge. J Am Coll Cardiol 1988;12:1510.

2. Titus JL, Edwards JE. The aortic root and valve, in RW Emery, KV Arom (eds): The Aortic Valve. Philadelphia: Hanley & Belfus, 1991, p 3.

3. Brewer RJ, Deck JD, Cepati B, et al. The dynamic aortic root. J Thorac Cardiovasc Surg 1976;72:413.

4. Reid K. The anatomy of the sinus of Valsalva. Thorax 1970;25:79.

5. Sud A, Parker F, Magilligan DJ. Anatomy of the aortic root. Ann Thorac Surg 1984;38:76.

6. Reid KG, Bellhouse BJ. A Bio-Engineering Study of the Aortic Root. University of Oxford, Department of Engineering Science Report, 1968.

7. Hope J. A Treatise on the Diseases of the Heart and Great Vessels. London: Churchill & Sons, 1839.

8. Chiang CW, Lin FC, Fang BR, et al. Doppler and two-dimensional echocardiographic features of sinus of Valsalva aneurysm. Am Heart J 1988;116:1283.

9. Boutefeau JM, Moret PR, Hahn C, et al. Aneurysms of the sinus of Valsalva. Am J Med 1978;65:18.

10. Taguchi K, Shsaki N, Matshura Y, et al. Surgical correction of aneurysm of the sinus of Valsalva. Am J Cardiol 1969;23:180.

11. Blackshear JL, Safford RE, Lane GE, et al. Unruptured noncoronary sinus of Valsalva aneurysm. J Am Soc Echocardiogr 1991;4:485.

12. Gallet B, Combe E, Saudemonte JP, et al. Aneurysm of the left aortic sinus causing coronary compression and unstable angina. Am Heart J 1988;115:1308.

13. Katz ES, Cziner DG, Rosenzweig BP, et al. Multifaceted echocardiographic approach to the diagnosis of a ruptured sinus of Valsalva aneurysm. J Am Soc Echocardiogr 1991;4:494.

14. Rubin DC, Carliner NH, Salter DR, et al. Unruptured sinus of Valsalva aneurysm diagnosed by transesophageal echocardiography. Am Heart J 1992;124:225.

15. McKenny PA, Shemin RJ, Wiegers SE. Role of transesophageal echocardiography in sinus of Valsalva aneurysms. Am Heart J 1992;123:228.

16. D'Cruz IA, Callaghan WE, Gross CM. Imaging of the aorta: I. Two-dimensional echocardiography of nondissecting aneurysm of the aortic root and its components. Am J Cardiac Imaging 1987;1:323.

17. Raffa H, Mosieri J, Sorefan AA, et al. Sinus of Valsalva aneurysm eroding into the interventricular septum. Ann Thorac Surg 1991;51:996.

18. Dev V, Shrivastava S. Echocardiographic diagnosis of unruptured aneurysm of the sinus of Valsalva dissecting into the ventricular septum. Am J Cardiol 1990;66:502.

19. Saner HE, Asinger RW, Homans DC, et al. Two-dimensional echocardiographic identification of complicated aortic root endocarditis. J Am Coll Cardiol 1987;10:859.

20. Fox S, Kotler MN, Segal BL, et al. Echocardiographic diagnosis of acute aortic valve endocarditis and its complications. Arch Intern Med 1977;137:85.

21. Mansur AJ, Grinberg M, Lopes EZ, et al. Acquired ventricular septal defect and tricuspid valve destruction as a complication of infective endocarditis of the aortic valve. J Cardiovasc Surg 1983;24:669.

22. Pirani CL. Erosive (mycotic) aneurysm of the heart with rupture. Arch Pathol 1943;36:579.

23. Chesler E, Korns ME, Porter GE, et al. False aneurysm of the left ventricle secondary to bacterial endocarditis with perforation of the mitral-aortic intervalvar fibrosa. Circulation 1968;37:518.

24. Ontiveros MM, Calhoon JH, Garcia MA, et al. Complementary value of transthoracic and transesophageal echocardiography in detecting a mycotic aortic aneurysm ruptured into the right atrium. Am Heart J 1993;125:1447.

25. Bansal RC, Graham BM, Jutzy KR, et al. Left ventricular outflow tract to left atrial communication secondary to rupture of mitral-aortic intervalvular fibrosa in infective endocarditis. J Am Coll Cardiol 1990;15:499.

26. Thomas MR, Monaghan MJ, Michalis LR, et al. Aortoatrial fistulae diagnosed by transthoracic and transesophageal echocardiography. J Am Soc Echocardiogr 1993;6:21.

27. Thomas TV, Heilbrunn A. Prosthetic aortic valve replacement complicated by diphteroid endocarditis and aortopulmonary fistula. Chest 1971;59:679.

28. Vieneg WV, Oury JH, Tretheway DG, et al. Aortopulmonary septal defect due to *Staphyloccus* endocarditis. Chest 1974;65:101.

29. Aragam JR, Keroack MA, Kemper AJ. Doppler echocardiographic diagnosis of aortopulmonary

fistula following aortic valve replacement for endocarditis. Am Heart J 1989;117:1392.

30. Chen CH, Nanda NC, Fan P, et al. Transesophageal echocardiographic diagnosis of aortopulmonary fistula. Echocardiography 1993;10:85.

31. Edwards JE. Pathology of left ventricular outflow tract obstruction. Circulation 1965;31:586.

32. Peterson TA, Todd DB, Edwards JE. Supravalvar aortic stenosis. J Thorac Cardiovasc Surg 1965;734.

33. Bolen JL, Popp RL, French JW. Echocardiographic features of supravalvular aortic stenosis. Circulation 1975;52:817.

34. Weyman AE, Caldwell RL, Hurwitz RA, et al. Cross-sectional echocardiographic characterization of aortic obstruction: I. Supravalvular aortic stenosis and aortic hypoplasia. Circulation 1978;57:491.

35. Vogt J, Rupprath G, Grimm T, et al. Qualitative and quantitative evaluation of supravalvar aortic stenosis by cross-sectional echocardiography. Pediatr Cardiol 1982;3:13.

36. Kitabatake A, Fujii K, Tanouchi J, et al. Doppler echocardiographic quantitation of cross-sectional area under various hemodynamic conditions: An experimental validation in a canine model of supravalvar aortic stenosis. J Am Coll Cardiol 1990;15:1654.

37. Cooley DA. Annuloaortic ectasia. Ann Thorac Surg 1979;28:303.

38. Savunen T, Aho HJ. Annulo-aortic ectasia: Light and electron microscopic changes in aortic media. Virchows Arch 1985;407:279.

39. Najaki H. Aortic root aneurysm. JAMA 1966;197:173.

40. Wheat MW, Bartley TD. Aneurysms of the aortic root. Dis Chest 1965;47:430.

41. Kronzon I, Weisinger B, Glassman E. Cystic medial necrosis with severe aortic root dilatation. Chest 1974;66:79.

42. Atsuchi Y, Nagai Y, Komatsu Y, et al. Echocardiographic manifestations of annuloaortic ectasia. Am Heart J 1977;93:428.

43. Soorae AS, Cleland J, O'Kane H. Delayed nonmycotic false aneurysm of ascending aortic cannulation site. Thorax 1977;32:743.

44. Williams GD, Zimmerman SJ, Osam PN, et al. False aneurysm of aortic cannulation site occurring three years postoperatively. J Cardiovasc Surg 1976;17:266.

45. Moore EH, Farmer DW, Geller SC, et al. Computed tomography in the diagnosis of iatrogenic false aneurysms of the ascending aorta. AJR 1984;142:1117.

46. Come PC, Riley MF, Kaufman H, et al. Aortic false aneurysms: Recognition by noninvasive techniques four years after mitral valve replacement. Am J Cardiol 1986;58:1137.

47. Kong B, Ogilby JD, Poynton R. Pseudoaneurysm of a Shiley composite aortic valve and graft prosthesis. Am Heart J 1990;120:1002.

48. Lasorda DM, Power TP, Dianzumba SB, et al. Diagnosis of aortic pseudoaneurysms by echocardiography. Clin Cardiol 1992;15:773.

49. Kumar N, Prabhakar G, Kandeel M, et al. *Brucella* myocotic aneurysm of ascending aorta complicating discrete subaortic stenosis. Am Heart J 1993;125:1780.

50. Perella MA, Smith HC, Khandheria BK. Pseudoaneurysm of the aortic root diagnosed by noninvasive imaging. J Am Soc Echocardiogr 1991;4:499.

51. Wendel CH, Cornman CR, Dianzumba SB. Diagnosis of pseudoaneurysm of the ascending aorta by pulsed Doppler cross-sectional echocardiography. Br Heart J 1985;53:567.

52. McFallas EO, Palac R, Gately H, et al. Pseudoaneurysm formation with superior vena caval syndrome 7 years after aortic composite graft placement. Ann Thorac Surg 1989;48:704.

20

Aorta II: Ascending Aorta, Aortic Arch, Descending Aorta

NORMAL ANATOMY[1] (Figures 20–1, 20–2, 3–1 to 3–5, 3–8)

The aorta is a long wide tube, about 3 cm in diameter at its origin from the left ventricle (LV) and about 1.75 cm in caliber at its bifurcation in the abdomen, at the level of the fourth lumbar vertebra. For purposes of anatomic description, it is divided into (1) the ascending aorta, situated in the anterior thorax, (2) the aortic arch, situated in the superior mediastinum, crossing transversely and to the left of the trachea to the posterior mediastinum, where (3) the descending thoracic aorta courses downward just anterior to the spine and (4) is continued below the diaphragm as the abdominal aorta. See diagrams in chapter 3 (Mediastinum).

Ascending Aorta

The ascending aorta commences at the aortic valve, at the level of the lower border of the third costal cartilage, and then ascends forward and to the right in a curved oblique manner, behind the sternum, to the level of the upper border of the second costal cartilage. The ascending aorta is about 5 cm long. Its lowest segment is slightly expanded into the sinuses of Valsalva. The uppermost segment of the ascending aorta, just before it becomes the aortic arch, is approximately vertical in alignment, parallel to the adjacent chest wall.

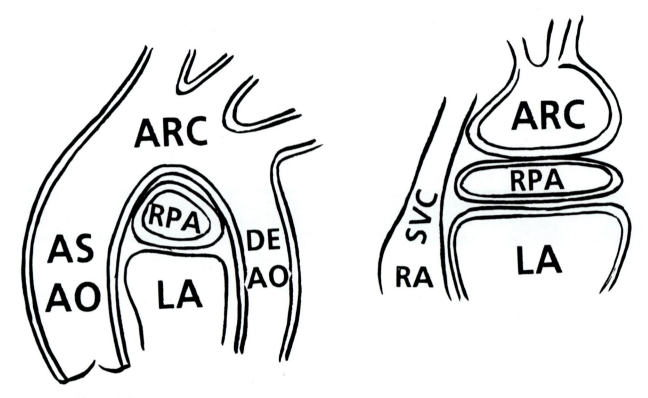

Figure 20–1. (Left) Diagram showing ascending aorta (As Ao), arch of aorta (ARC), and descending thoracic aorta (DE Ao) in long axis of aortic arch. Note right pulmonary artery located in concavity of the aortic arch and the left atrium inferior to it. (Right) Diagram of same structures in short axis (cross section) of aortic arch with superior vena cava (SVC) and right atrium (RA) alongside.

The anatomic relationships of the ascending aorta are important. At its origin (aortic valve level), it occupies a central position within the heart, as is well known to echocardiographers, in all planes that pass through the aortic root. Thus it has the right atrium to its right, and the right ventricle outflow tract and pulmonary trunk wind round the anterior and left aspect of the aortic root. The posterior aspect of the aortic root is related closely to the left atrium.

The ascending aorta is entirely enclosed in a sheath of pericardium, along with the pulmonary trunk, behind which is a pericardial recess—the transverse sinus. Anteriorly and superiorly, the ascending aorta is separated from the chest wall (sternum and second and third costal cartilages) by the right lung and pleura. Because of this fact, one is usually unable to visualize the aorta and neighboring cardiovascular structures from the right parasternal area. However, if the patient is turned to the right lateral position, it is often possible to interrogate flow across the aortic valve from the right sternal border by suitable angulation and firm pressure of the Pedoff Doppler probe, a valuable maneuver for recording aortic jet velocity in aortic valve stenosis. If the ascending aorta is dilated enough to approach the right parasternal chest wall, pushing aside the anterior border of the right lung, the ascending aorta can be visualized well from the right parasternal area.

Posterior to the ascending aorta is the right pulmonary artery as it runs across the top of the left atrium, and next to it is the right bronchus. To the right of the ascending aorta is the superior vena cava and beyond that the right lung and pleura. The superior vena cava (SVC) is partly to the right and posterior in relation to the ascending aorta. Both these structures cannot be imaged from the right parasternal view in adults but may be visualized from this site if the ascending aorta is dilated and provides a right parasternal window. They also may be well seen in some subjects from the suprasternal or right supra-clavicular window.

Aortic Arch

The aortic arch starts to the right of the midline, then runs obliquely backward and to the left across the front of the trachea and then to the left of the trachea, and ends at the fourth dorsal vertebra to the left of the midline to continue below as the descending aorta. Thus the aortic arch has two curvatures, a convexity upward as well as a convexity to the left and slightly anteriorly. Two important nerves—the phrenic and vagus—and one vein—the left superior intercostal vein—cross the convexity of the aortic arch vertically but are too small to be visualized on transthoracic echocardiography (TTE).

The anatomic relations of the aortic arch are as follows: Anteriorly and to the left, it is separated from the chest wall by a wide expanse of left lung and pleura, so the aortic arch cannot be imaged from any site on the anterior or lateral chest wall. Posteriorly and to the right of the aortic arch are the trachea, esophagus, and thoracic duct and further back the vertebral column. The proximity of the esophagus makes it possible to image the aortic arch by transesophageal echocardiography (TEE), especially by biplane or mul-tiplane techniques.

The highest point on the convexity of the aortic arch is on an average 2.5 cm below the level of the superior border of the manubrium sternum, i.e., the suprasternal notch. An ultrasound transducer placed at this site and pressed downward and posteriorly usu-ally results in adequate visualization of the aortic arch (suprasternal view). A similar view of the aortic arch also may be attained by placing the transducer just above the sternal end of the right clavicle and directing it downward, posteriorly, and to the left (right supra-clavicular view).

The aortic arch gives off three large branches from its superior convexity, the in-nominate artery (also called *brachiocephalic trunk*), the left common carotid artery, and the left subclavian artery in that order from front to back. Slightly above their origin from the arch, these arteries are crossed obliquely by a large vein, the left innominate vein, that joins the right innominate vein to form the SVC.

There is much variation in branches coming off the arch, two or even three of the usual branches occasionally arising from a common stem; on the other hand, the right carotid or subclavian artery may arise directly from the arch. Extremes of one to six branches from the aortic arch are known to occur.

Inferiorly, the aortic arch is related to the tracheal bifurcation and left bronchus, as well as a small fibrous structure, the ligamentum arteriosum. The latter structure, a rem-nant of the fetal ductus arteriosus that normally closes at birth, is attached to the inferior aspect of the aortic arch just after the origin of the left subclavian artery and at its other end to the left main pulmonary near its origin from the pulmonary trunk (see Chapter 8, Figures 8-3, 8-12, and 8-13). The right main pulmonary artery runs horizontally under the aortic arch as it extends from the pulmonary trunk bifurcation to the hilum of the right lung.

The aortic arch is, on average, 4.5 cm long and 2.5 cm in diameter in young adults, increasing to 3.5 cm or more over age 60. On its inner surface, the only normal features are the large branches arising from the arch's convexity and a dimple at the site of the ligamentum arteriosum on its concavity.

Descending Thoracic Aorta (DTA)

This segment of the aorta begins at the level of the fourth dorsal vertebra and runs verti-cally downward anterior to the spine to become the descending abdominal aorta at the level of the twelfth dorsal vertebra. At its upper end it is to the left of the midline, but it gradually approaches the midline as it descends, and at the level of the twelfth dorsal ver-tebra, it is precisely a midline structure.

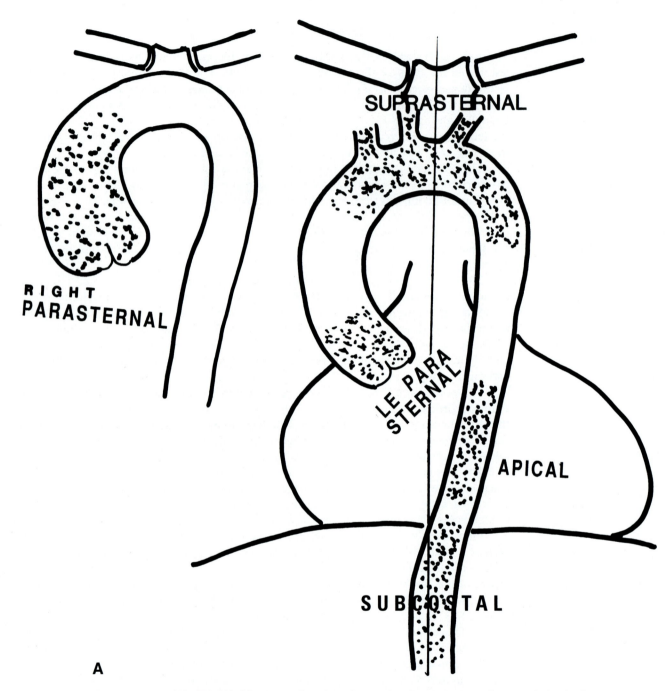

A

Figure 20–2. (A) (Right) Diagram showing the various segments of aorta (stippled) commonly visualized by 2D echo: aortic root from left parasternal window (LE PARASTERNAL), aortic arch from suprasternal window, retrocardiac descending aorta from modified apical window, and upper abdominal aorta from subcostal window. (Left) Ascending aorta from right parasternal window when it is dilated. (B) Suprasternal view of ascending aorta and aortic arch of normal caliber (above). Arch with origin of left common carotid and subclavian in same case (below).

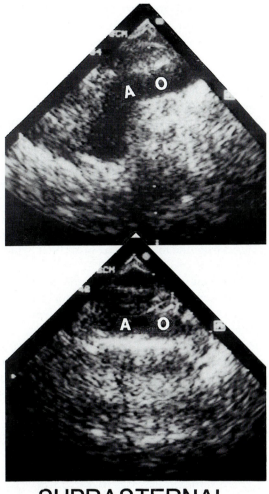

B   **SUPRASTERNAL**

Figure 20–2. *(Continued)*

Its anterior relations, from above downward, are first the hilum of the left lung, then the left atrium (separated by the oblique pericardial sinus, normally only a potential space), and finally the diaphragm.

The main posterior relationship of the DTA is the vertebral column, covered anteriorly by a thin layer of prevertebral muscles and ligaments. The hemiazygos vein is also posterior to the DTA.

To the right and anterior of the DTA are the azygos vein and thoracic duct, and lower in the thorax, the right pleura and lung. To the left of the DTA are the left pleura and lung.

The proximity of the DTA to the esophagus in the thorax has important consequences. It permits exquisite imaging of the DTA in all its extent by TEE, including aortic pathology such as intimal plaques and intimal flaps (in aortic dissection). The esophagus is to the right of the DTA in its upper third, then anterior to it in its middle (retrocardiac) third, and finally anterolateral to it at diaphragmatic level. Anatomic diagrams often depict the DTA and esophagus as two straight parallel tubes alongside each other; in fact, the two structures are mutually spiral in mild degree; i.e., each is slightly twisted around the other.

The DTA is 20 cm long on average, its diameter narrowing gradually from 2.5 cm at its upper end to 2 cm at its lower end. The abdominal aorta is 15 cm long and narrows further from 2 to 1.75 cm where it bifurcates into the common iliac arteries at the level of the fourth lumbar vertebra. The DTA gives off no large branches but has numerous small branches: paired intercostal arteries at every vertebral segment, as well as esophageal, bronchial, mediastinal, and phrenic arteries. The DTA is in contact with the left pleura in much of its extent. It can therefore be well imaged *through* a large left pleural effusion (Figure 20-3).

Abdominal Aorta

This aortic segment is a vertical midline structure located on the anterior aspect of the spine from the first to the fourth lumbar vertebrae. Although echocardiographers are not primarily involved in abdominal ultrasound, the upper abdominal aorta is of some interest because it is a feature of the subxiphoid (subcostal) view.

In long axis, the abdominal aorta appears as a tubular sonolucent space continuous with the DTA above the diaphragm. When the DTA shows evidence of pathology (dilatation or dissection), it is relevant to ascertain whether these abnormalities extend into the abdominal aorta. On either side of the upper abdominal aorta is the right and left crus of the diaphragm, the aorta descending into the abdomen under the arch formed by the crossing of these two components of the diaphragm. The right crus separates the abdominal aorta from the inferior vena cava (IVC), which lies somewhat anterior to the aorta at this level.

It is important for the echocardiographer not to mistake the aorta and IVC for each other. Both vessels appear as sonolucent tubular spaces in the sagittal or near-sagittal subcostal view. The aorta shows a strong systolic pulsation, gives off anterior branches in the upper abdomen (celiac and superior mesenteric), and lies just anterior to the spine. The IVC is in a slightly more anterior plane, normally narrows with inspiration, opens into the right atrium, receives hepatic veins coursing through the liver, and shows small-amplitude, "soft" pulsations. Colorflow Doppler further helps in identifying the aorta by demonstrating flow away from the heart, whereas flow in the IVC is mainly toward the heart.

ECHOCARDIOGRAPHY OF THE NORMAL AORTA (see Figure 20–2)

The aortic root at aortic valve level is well visualized in most standard views, perhaps best in the parasternal long-axis view. However, the upper ascending aorta normally cannot be imaged in adults from the left or right parasternal view because lung intervenes between the aorta and the chest wall. In certain special circumstances, the entire ascending aorta can be visualized:

1. If a solid mass such as a lymphoma occupies the anterior mediastinum, thereby displacing the anterior edge of the right lung, a window is created to reveal much of the mediastinum.
2. If the ascending aorta is dilated enough to impinge on the right parasternal chest wall, the dilated vessel itself provides an echocardiographic window on the aorta and adjacent structures. If this window is good enough, not only the ascending aorta but also the arch and upper DTA may be demonstrated.

In adults, the aortic arch can only be imaged from the suprasternal or right supraclavicular region. Even this may not be possible in some individuals, when the space between trachea and manubrium sternum is not large enough to insinuate the ultrasound probe.

The aortic arch manifests, by suprasternal echo (Figure 20-2B), as a curved tubular sonolucency, from the convexity of which arise three large arteries [from right to left, innominate (brachiocephalic), left common carotid, and left subclavian]. All three arteries may not be revealed in one imaging plane; the probe may have to be maneuvered at different angulations to reveal the entire arch, all three branches, and the upper DTA. One also should avoid the error of mistaking a large artery such as the innominate for the aortic arch.

The upper DTA may be visualized by suprasternal echocardiography and can be distinguished from the ascending aorta by the colorflow Doppler systolic pattern within it—

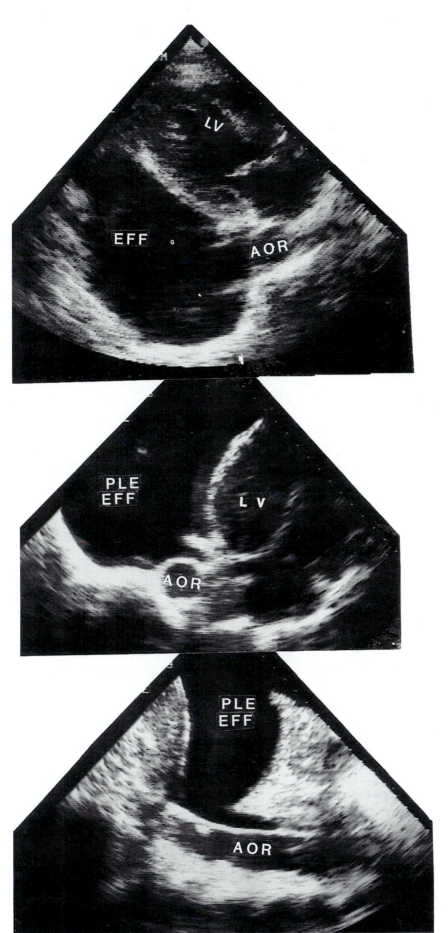

Figure 20–3. (Above) Parasternal long-axis view showing relationship of descending aorta (AOR) to left pleural effusion (PLE EFF). (Center) View of heart and descending aorta using the left pleural effusion as the echo window. (Below) View of descending thoracic aorta in its long axis, through the left pleural effusion. The large bright mass within the pleural effusion is the right lung.

toward the transducer for the ascending, aorta away from it for the DTA. All segments of the aorta are easier to visualize if they are dilated; otherwise, they are prone to partial obscuration by air in the lungs or the tracheobronchial tree.

The retrocardiac part of the DTA appears as a round or oval sonolucency in cross section, as a constant feature of the parasternal long-axis view. It is located posterior to the junction between the left atrium and ventricle; sometimes it is posterior to the left atrial chamber, the variation in precise position of DTA to the heart being attributable to tortuosity of the aorta in the elderly.

The retrocardiac DTA can be imaged in its long axis from the left anterior chest wall from a site intermediate between the parasternal border and the LV apex. The plane necessary to achieve this is also intermediate between the apical four-chamber and parasternal short-axis views. The DTA appears as a tubular sonolucency with parallel walls, with the LV chamber or atrioventricular junction anterior to it. The retrocardiac DTA can be followed inferiorly below the diaphragm as it becomes the abdominal aorta by imaging from the subxiphoid (midline epigastric) area. Its differentiation from the IVC was discussed earlier.

Computerized synthesis of two-dimensional (2D) TEE imaging has made it possible to construct very realistic three-dimensional images of the DTA (including dissecting aneurysms with division into true and false lumens). This is feasible because the DTA is a fixed structure, unaffected by respiratory or cardiac motion, and well depicted by TEE all through its extent.[2]

DILATATION OR ANEURYSM OF THE AORTA

Normal values for aortic caliber at various levels (mean and range) are shown in Table 20-1. The precise sites and modes of measurement may not have been the same in all these studies, which include one CT and one MRI paper, in addition to the 2D echo ones.

Mild dilatation of the ascending aorta is common in patients with aortic regurgitation, aortic valve stenosis (poststenotic dilatation), hypertension, and prosthetic aortic valves.

At what point does aortic dilatation justify the term *aneurysm*? The distinction is arbitrary; Mathew and Nanda[5] considered an aneurysm to be present when the aortic luminal diameter was increased to 50% or more of the maximal normal width for that aortic segment or if the increase was 50% or more of the adjacent aortic diameter.

TABLE 20–1. NORMAL VALUES FOR AORTIC CALIBER BY VARIOUS NONINVASIVE IMAGING TECHNIQUES

Aortic Level	CT (n = 102; Aronberg et al.[3])	MRI (n = 20; Kersing et al.[4])	2D Echo (n = 18; Mathew and Nanda[5])	2D Echo (n = 50; Come[6])	2D Echo (n = 25; Weyman[7])
Aortic valve	36 mm	32.9 mm	30 mm	—	29 mm
Range	24–47	30–38	26–32		24–39
Ascending aorta	35.1 mm	30.2 mm	28 mm	—	26 mm
Range	22–46	19–37	22–31		21–34
Aortic arch	—	27 mm	24 mm	—	25 mm
Range		18–37	20–29		22–27
Descending thoracic aorta	24.8 mm	27 mm	21 mm	20 mm	—
Range	16–37	18–37	15–25	13–27	

Syphilis was the dominant cause of aortic aneurysms for centuries until the middle of this century but has in recent decades been replaced by atherosclerosis and dissecting aneurysms. Rarely, the etiology is trauma or bacterial infection (mycotic aneurysm).

Syphilitic Aortitis and Aneurysm

Excellent autopsy descriptions of this entity appeared in the early 1900s,[8,9] updated more recently by the work of Heggtveit.[10-12] The primary aortic lesion is chronic inflammation and destruction of the musculoelastic structure of the medial layer, which is replaced by vascular connective tissue. These changes invariably affect the ascending aorta, frequently also the arch and/or the DTA and rarely the abdominal aorta. The intimal surface of the aorta typically has a wrinkled "tree bark" appearance. Atherosclerotic changes are the rule, superimposed on the syphilitic intimal lesions.

Syphilitic aortitis results in three main complications. *Aortic aneurysms* result from local or diffuse protrusion of the weakened aortic wall in response to the high pressure and pulsatile distension within the vessel. Saccular aneurysms are more common than fusiform ones and vary in size from outpouchings of a few centimeters to enormous aneurysms of spectacular proportions, widening and distorting mediastinal contours. Aneurysms cause symptoms and even death by (1) pressure on adjacent structures (hoarseness of voice by stretching of the left recurrent laryngeal nerve, stridor by pressure on the tracheobronchial airway, dysphagia by esophageal compression, back pain by erosion of dorsal vertebrae, anterior chest pain and even swelling by erosion of sternum, ribs, or costal cartilages) and (2) rupture of the aneurysm (in order of frequency) into left pleural cavity, mediastinum, esophagus, right pleural cavity, trachea, and externally through chest wall. TEE has been used to visualize a posterior mediastinal hematoma resulting from rupture of a nondissecting DTA aneurysm.[12a]

Mural thrombosis is very common within aortic aneurysms. Successive layers of thrombotic material cause visible stratification (lines of Zahn). In saccular aortic aneurysms, thrombus may fill almost all the aneurysmal cavity. In fusiform aneurysms, mural thrombi are not usually obstructive to aortic flow; a channel remains in it approximately equal to the nonaneurysmal aortic lumen in cross-sectional area. Aneurysmal thrombi can get infected; for unclear reasons, *Salmonella* infection is common.

Aortic regurgitation rather than aneurysm formation may dominate the clinical picture in syphilitic aortitis. Dilatation of the aortic "annulus," to which the aortic cusps are attached, is the cause of valve incompetence (valve circumference more than 8.5 cm). The commissures between the cusps may be widened. The cusps may be normal or mildly thickened, sometimes with curled edges.

Ostial stenosis of one or both main coronary arteries was found in one-fourth of cases of syphilitic aortitis in Heggtveit's series.[10] One might expect that TEE would demonstrate this finding more reliably than transthoracic echocardiography (TTE).

Atherosclerotic aortic aneurysms are caused by extension of intimal atherosclerotic lesions into the adjacent medial layer, with consequent weakening of the aortic wall and gradual dilatation under the expansile effect of intraaortic pressure. Such aneurysms are usually fusiform, rarely saccular. Abdominal aortic aneurysms are almost always atherosclerotic. The incidence of thoracic aortic aneurysms is about 6 per 100,000 per year in the United States, according to a study published in 1982.[13] The incidence of aortic aneurysms increases with age; in the autopsy series of Halpert and Williams,[14] the prevalence rose from 6% in the sixth decade to 14% in the ninth. In a recent echocardiographic study of 15 patients with ascending aortic aneurysms in California, 4 of the 5 below age 50 had Marfan's syndrome, 8 of the 10 above age 50 had atherosclerosis, and 5 had aortic dissection.[15]

Measuring the size of aortic aneurysms is important, because the risk of rupture rises with increasing aneurysmal size and hence the advisability of surgical repair. In abdominal aortic aneurysms, the risk of rupture over 5 years has been reported to be nil in aneurysms less than 5 cm but 25% in those over 5 cm by Nevitt,[16] though Crawford and

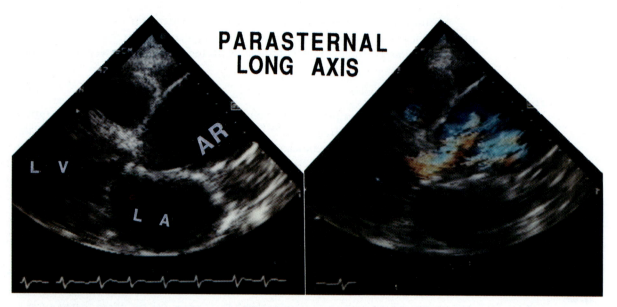

PARASTERNAL LONG AXIS

Figure 20–4. Left parasternal long-axis view showing marked dilatation of the ascending aorta (max. diameter 7 cm). The upper ascending aorta is much wider than it is just above the aortic valve. Colorflow Doppler (right) shows systolic swirling of flow.

Hess[17] believe that abdominal aortic aneurysms less than 5 cm can rupture. Nevitt estimated that the average rate of increase in aneurysmal diameter is 0.21 cm per year. For aneurysms of the thoracic aorta, surgical repair was recommended for aneurysms producing pressure symptoms and asymptomatic ones over 10 cm.[18]

Dilatation of the ascending aorta is best visualized from left and right parasternal windows (Figures 20-4 to 20-7). The latter is a much neglected echocardiographic opportunity, provided by the dilated aorta pushing the anterior edge of the right lung aside to impinge on the chest wall. The right parasternal window should be tried whenever aortic root dilatation is seen on a standard left parasternal view or when aortic valve sounds or murmurs are unusually loud on right parasternal auscultation (Figures 20-5 to 20-7). Apical views also may permit good visualization of aortic root dilatation (Figures 20-6 and 20-7).

Colorflow Doppler helps in delineating the caliber of dilated aortas; large aortic aneurysms may exhibit a swirling flow (Figure 20-4) very different from the monocolor laminar flow in normal or mildly dilated aortas. Sometimes aortic dilatation is neither saccular nor fusiform but diffuse, with uniform tubular rather than segmental ectasis (Figure 20-8).

Dilatation of one or more of the three large arteries arising from the aortic arch, especially the innominate artery, may be identified from the suprasternal window (Figure 20-9), so ultrasound imaging from this window is a useful and convenient noninvasive means for diagnosis of a pulsatile swelling at the root of the neck.

Mild dilatation of the DTA is very common in the elderly and of little clinical importance. It is relevant to echocardiography as one cause of a retrocardiac sonolucent space (Figures 20-10 and 20-11). Severe to huge dilatation of the DTA is far less common than large aneurysms of the ascending or arch segments; such enormous DTA aneurysms (Figure 20-12) can grossly distort mediastinal anatomy and may even be mistaken for a left pleural effusion or mediastinal cyst.

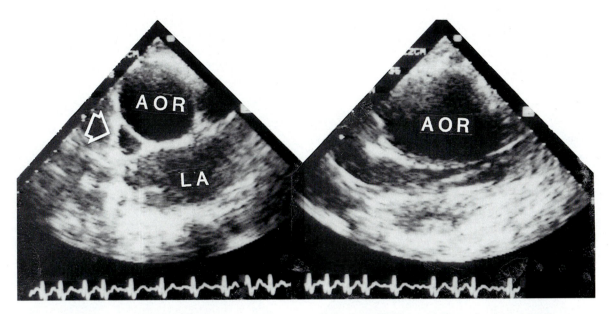

Figure 20–5. Right parasternal view in short-axis view (left) and long-axis view (right) showing dilatation of the ascending aorta (AOR). Arrow indicates SVC to the right of aorta; the left atrium (LA) is posterior to the aorta.

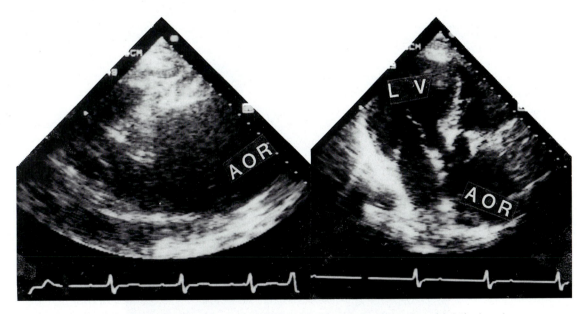

Figure 20–6. Right parasternal view (left) and apical long-axis view (right) showing severe dilatation of the ascending aorta (maximum diameter about 7 cm).

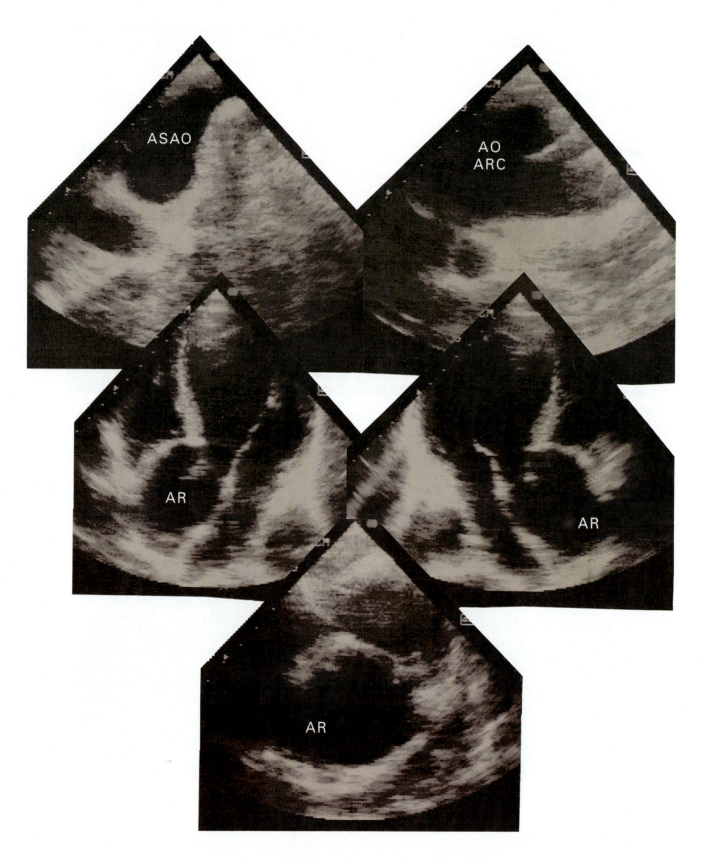

Figure 20–7. Suprasternal view (above) showing dilatation of ascending aorta (left) and aortic arch (right). (Center) Apical four-chamber view (left) and long-axis view (right) show aortic root dilatation. (Below) Subcostal view shows aneurysmal dilatation of aortic root.

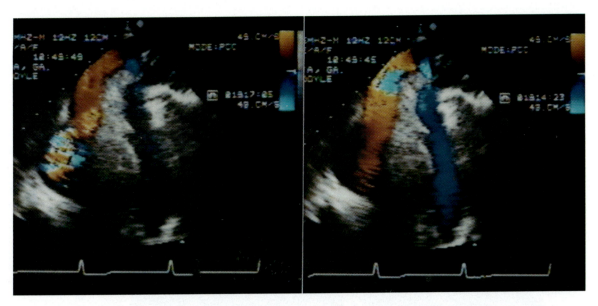

Figure 20–8. Colorflow Doppler in suprasternal view in patient with mild diffuse dilatation of entire aorta. Ascending part of aorta is red and descending part is blue in systole.

CONGENITAL ANOMALIES OF THE AORTIC ARCH (Figure 20–13)

These abnormalities, some common and others rare, are of primary interest to pediatric cardiologists; in fact, almost all the echocardiographic studies published have pertained to infants or children. They may or may not be associated with congenital cardiac defects. However, some of these aortic arch anomalies are encountered in adults, usually without congenital heart anomalies. With the exception of right aortic arch (diagnosed on a chest x-ray), these aberrancies of aortic arch development formerly could be identified only by aortography. Modern noninvasive imaging techniques (ultrasound, CT, or MRI) have made it possible to diagnose most such anomalies, sometimes aided by chest radiography, with or without barium contrast in the esophagus.

The aortic arch and its main branches, as well as the ductus arteriosus, arise from six paired branchial arches that connect ventral and dorsal aortas in early embryonic life. Normally, certain of these branchial arches, or segments thereof, disappear after a very transient appearance, whereas other arches persist. Anomalies of the system arise as a result of persistence of segments that normally reabsorb and/or disappearance of arches that normally persist. A detailed discussion of the embryologic basis of aortic arch anomalies is beyond the scope of this book, and in fact, two or more rival explanations have been advanced in some cases to account for certain abnormalities of anatomy. What is important to the echocardiographer and clinician is the actual configuration of the aortic anomalies, how they deviate from normal, and how the abnormal arch components relate spatially to other normal mediastinal structures. Adult cardiologists and echocardiographers often have only a rudimentary idea of such information.

The normal aortic arch traverses the superior mediastinum from front to back, as well as from right to left, crossing in front of the trachea and above the left bronchus. The DTA

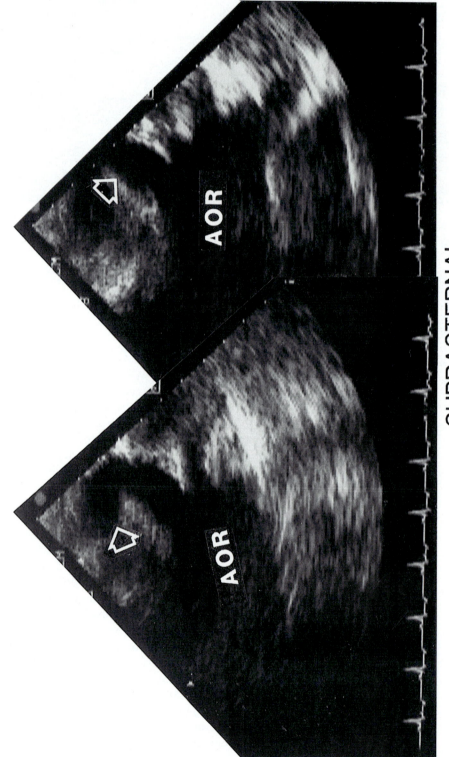

SUPRASTERNAL

Figure 20–9. Suprasternal view of aortic arch (AOR) and dilated innominate artery (arrows); the latter presented as a pulsatile swelling at the root of the neck.

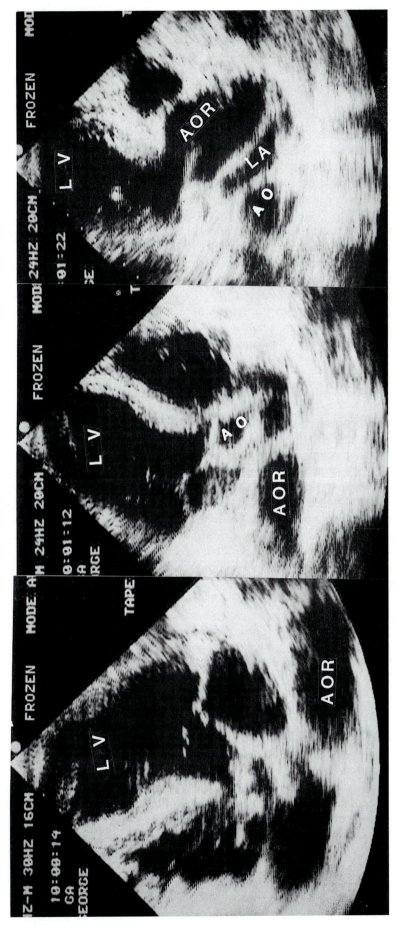

Figure 20–10. Apical four-chamber view (left) and two different apical long-axis views (center and right) showing dilatation of the descending aorta (left) and of the ascending aorta (right). The LA appears much narrowed by the aortic dilatation.

runs vertically downward, first to the left of the midline, but inclining toward the midline in the lower thorax.

Right Aortic Arch[19–23]

In this anomaly, the aortic arch crosses over the right rather than the left bronchus to reach a point to the right of the midline just anterior to the fourth dorsal vertebra. The right aortic arch can then continue in one of two ways: (1) vertically descend to the right of the midline just anterior to the spine (right DTA) or (2) cross horizontally behind the esophagus at the fourth dorsal vertebra level, and its subsequent course to the left of the midline is normal, i.e., left DTA. The retroesophageal aortic segment produces a large round impression on the barium-filled esophagus on its posterior aspect.

The ligamentum arteriosum normally connects the concavity (inferior surface) of the aortic arch to the superior aspect of the junction of the pulmonary artery and its main branch. The combination of a right aortic arch with a left ligamentum arteriosum completes one type of "vascular ring" that encircles the trachea and esophagus, causing dysphagia. The mirror image of this—left aortic arch with retroesophageal crossing of the aorta to descend on the right with a right ligamentum arteriosum—is extremely rare. Double aortic arch is obviously a complete vascular ring and commonly causes tracheoesophageal compression in infancy.

Bedford and Parkinson[24] distinguished two types of right aortic arch with (1) "mirror-image branching," in which a left innominate artery arises as the first branch and then divides into a left common carotid and left subclavian artery, and (2) with aberrant left subclavian artery, which arises as the fourth branch from the arch and then crosses the midline to reach the left upper limb. A conical diverticulum, or pouch, may occur at the origin of such an aberrant subclavian artery, which can manifest on 2D echo as a retroesophageal impression on the barium-filled esophagus.

The prevalence of right aortic arch in adult autopsies is about 1 in 1000.[22] The association of right aortic arch with tetralogy of Fallot is well known (sometimes called *Corvisart's disease*), varying from 13% to 34% in various reported series, and was at the high end of this range in 167 cases of tetralogy studied by the author and colleagues.[19] An even higher prevalence of right aortic arch is encountered in patients with persistent common truncus arteriosus.[19] A right aortic arch occurs more frequently than in the general population with various common congenital heart defects: about 8% with tricuspid atresia, 4% to 5% with complete transposition of great vessels, and 2% to 3% with ventricular septal defect (perhaps higher in the Eisenmenger syndrome). It does not occur with undue frequency in patients with congenital anomalies at the atrial level nor with pulmonary valve stenosis and intact ventricular septum. It seems likely that a right aortic arch has a developmental association with cardiac defects involving a bulboseptal malformation, as suggested by Espino-Vela and Mata.[23]

Echocardiography of Aortic Arch Anomalies

Right Aortic Arch.[25–27]   Whether the aortic arch is left- or right-sided cannot be easily ascertained in any of the standard views. It can be diagnosed from the suprasternal view as follows:

1. The aortic arch is first imaged in its long axis, and then the transducer is tilted or rocked from side to side to seek the air-filled trachea. If the trachea is found to the right of the aortic arch sonolucency, the arch is left-sided (normal location); if the tracheal air column is detected to the left of the aortic arch, the arch is right-sided.

2. Having first visualized the aortic arch, the transducer is rotated and tilted upward so as to image the first branch coming off the arch and to follow it toward the head to visualize its bifurcation, if possible. With a normal left arch, the first branch is a right innominate artery that runs upward and to the right to bifurcate into the right common carotid and right subclavian arteries. If the first aortic arch branch does not bifurcate, it

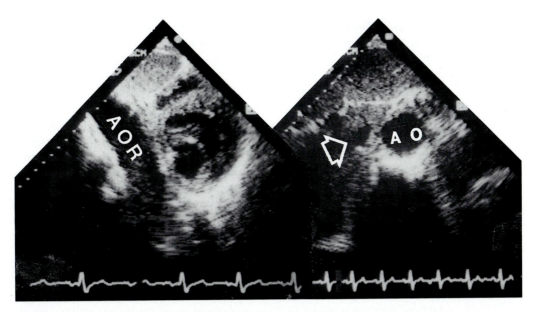

Figure 20–11. (Left) Subcostal sagittal view showing mildly dilated descending aorta (AOR). (Right) Subcostal transverse view showing the upper abdominal aorta (AO) in cross section. Arrow indicates IVC.

may be assumed that this unbranched artery is the right common carotid artery and that the right subclavian artery is aberrant such that it comes off the arch as its last branch (and then crosses behind the esophagus). If the first aortic branch crosses the midline, running upward and to the left, it is probable that a right aortic arch is present with mirror-image branching.

The rare instances of *retroesophageal aorta* (right arch crossing horizontally to descend as the left DTA or left arch continuing as right DTA) can be suspected following the aortic arch sonolucency into a posterior scanning plane. However, air in the trachea interferes with visualizing the aorta immediately behind it.

Whenever the ligamentum (or ductus) arteriosum is contralateral to the aortic arch, a vascular ring is present, a potential cause of dysphagia because of encirclement of the tracheoesophageal passages. Sometimes the site of attachment of the ductal ligament or artery to the junction of the aortic arch and DTA is expanded into an aneurysm or diverticulum opening into the aorta. This sonolucent structure (Kommerell diverticulum), when present, represents abnormal partial persistence of the fourth branchial arch.

Double aortic arch, though quite rare in adults, does occasionally occur and should be sought for in patients presenting with unexplained dysphagia. The ascending aorta bifurcates into right and left arches, the right being commonly larger while the left is hypoplastic or even atretic.[28,29] Normal vessels such as the innominate artery or vein should not be mistaken for abnormalities of aortic arch development. Colorflow Doppler can assist in identifying the branching of the ascending aorta into the two aortic arches.[30] The situs of the DTA can be ascertained by directing attention to the sonolucency of the descending aorta posterior to the left atrium in parasternal long- and short-axis views.[31]

The aortic arch can be imaged from the subcostal window in infants or children but seldom in adults. Murdison et al.[32] demonstrated how the 2D echo diagnosis of double aortic arch and other vascular rings could be facilitated by a suprasternal-view "sweep" of successive frontal plane images, sweeping from most anterior to most posterior plane including the arch and/or its vessels. The echocardiographer was in effect attempting to obtain a three-dimensional "mental" image of aortic anatomy. These authors were able to correctly diagnose the anatomy of the vascular ring in 7 of their 12 infants by this method; however, the atretic components of the vascular rings (no sonolucent lumen depicted) could not be visualized.[32]

Cervical Aortic Arch. This is a very rare yet spectacular anomaly in which the aortic arch is much elongated into a sharp loop extending above the thoracic inlet into the supraclavicular region, where it presents as a pulsatile mass. In earlier case reports, the cervical arch was right-sided, but later reports describe both left and right cervical arches. With the transducer placed on the pulsatile swelling, the long, redundant hairpin aortic loop appears as two tubular sonolucencies, one above the other. The anomalous thoracic course is visualized in appropriate suprasternal planes.[32a] The terminal segment of the long arch crosses behind the esophagus, where it cannot be imaged by suprasternal echography but can be suspected by its large, round impression on the posterior aspect of the barium-filled esophagus. In attempting noninvasive diagnosis of the anatomic variety of a vascular ring, 2D echo should be combined with barium swallow to look for site and contour of esophageal indentation by anomalous vessels, as shown by Parekh et al.[31] in 8 cases.

COARCTATION OF THE AORTA (Figure 20–14)

This well-known aortic anomaly was described by the anatomist Meckel in 1760 and later fascinated several nineteenth-century physicians.[33] In older children and adults, congenital coarctation is remarkably constant in location and anatomic configuration. The stenotic site is just beyond the origin of the left subclavian artery, near the aortic attachment of the ligamentum arteriosum.[34-36] Poststenotic dilatation is common just distal to the coarctation.

The most striking anatomic lesion in coarctation is a localized ridgelike thickening of the aortic wall at the junction of the aortic arch and descending aorta. This ridge involves the superior, posterior, and anterior aspects of the aorta at this level; the ridge projects into the aortic lumen, causing an asymmetrical (eccentric) stenosis of the latter. The outer surface of the aorta shows a sharp notch or constriction on its convexity corresponding to the site of the ridge internally.

Mitral valve anomalies are believed to occur in one-fourth to one-half of patients with aortic coarctation.[37-40] Some of these, like parachute mitral valve (fusion or near-fusion of the LV papillary muscles), cause mitral stenosis,[38] whereas other mitral abnormalities are associated with mitral regurgitation.[40] The combination of aortic coarctation, subaortic stenosis, parachute mitral valve, and supramitral valve ring[38] is well known to pediatric cardiologists, sometimes called *Shone's syndrome.*

Bicuspid aortic valve is strongly associated with coarctation of the aorta[41,42]; valvar aortic stenosis may be present on this basis. Ventricular septal defect is also known to coexist with coarctation occasionally.[43-45] Another left-to-right shunt sometimes seen in infants or young children with coarctation is patent ductus arteriosus; this goes against the theory advanced 150 years ago[33] that coarctation of the aorta is due to undue extension into the aorta of the normal phenomena of obliteration and fibrosis of the ductus arteriosus (ligamentum arteriosum) after birth.

Poststenotic aneurysms of the aorta[46] just beyond the coarctation may be an extreme form of the usual dilatation seen at this level. Ascending aortic aneurysms are also reported.

All these cardiovascular abnormalities encountered in association with coarctation can be diagnosed by 2D echo, perhaps combined with colorflow Doppler. They are mentioned here to alert the echocardiographer to seek or exclude their presence when a patient with coarctation is being studied. Suprasternal echocardiography demonstrates the coarctation at the junction of the aortic arch with the DTA.[47-49] A sharp posterior shelf projects into the aortic lumen. The left subclavian artery is larger than normal and sometimes almost appears as a lateral continuation of the aortic arch. However, a poor suprasternal echo window and great distance from the transducer often result in suboptimal visualization of aortic anatomy at and beyond the coarctation site. Pulsed-wave and continuous-wave Doppler recordings at this site are important to assess the pressure gradient.[50-53] Stern et al.[54] have used TEE to obtain high-quality imaging of aortic coarctation. It has been recently shown that the ratio of the Doppler velocity of the coarctation

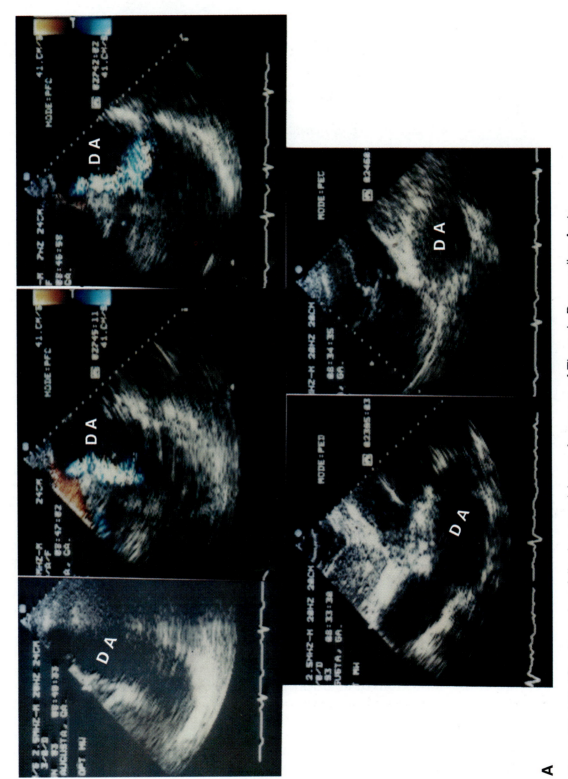

A

Figure 20–12A (*See legend on following page.*) Large Aneurysm of Thoracic Descending Aorta

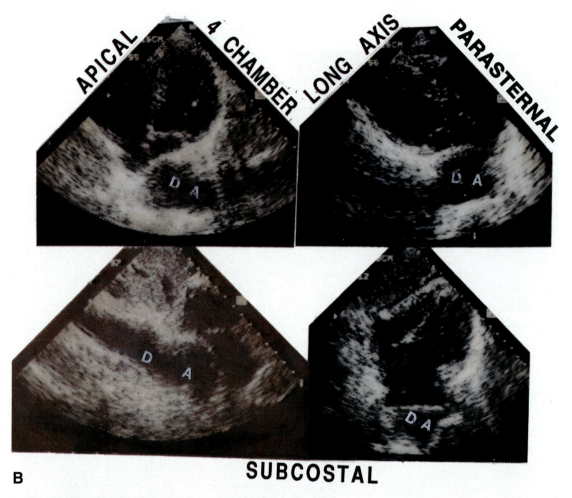

Figure 20–12. (A) Suprasternal view of thoracic descending aorta (above) showing aneurysmal dilatation with swirling of blood flow (on colorflow Doppler). Subcostal view (below, left) and parasternal long-axis view (below, right) showing aneurysmal dilatation of the thoracic descending aorta. (B) Dilatation (maximum 4 cm) of the thoracic descending aorta (DA) in four different views in a different patient. In all the dilated aorta encroaches on the left atrium.

jet to the velocity in the abdominal aorta approximates the ratio of the cross-sectional area of the latter to that of the coarctation (assessed by MRI).

Interruption of the aortic arch is almost never seen in adults but is commonly associated with various serious cardiac defects in infancy. The ascending aorta terminates after giving off both carotid arteries and (usually) one or both subclavian arteries. The DTA is continuous with a large pulmonary artery through a large persistent ductus; the pulmonary trunk—ductus—DTA vessel supplies the lower half of the body.

Pseudocoarctation of the Aorta (Kinked or Buckled Aortic Arch)

The normal aortic arch presents a smooth convex loop, making an angle of 30 degrees with the sagittal plane. In pseudocoarctation of the aorta (PCA), the distal (posterior) part of the aortic arch is acutely kinked, with an angular convexity directed forward and downward at the level of the ligamentum arteriosum, which in fact seems responsible for abnormal traction on the arch such that its shape is distorted in this manner. The aorta proximal to the kink is elongated and rises higher in the mediastinum than usual. The ascending aorta is normal. The apex of the abnormal kink is closely applied by a short ligamentum arteriosum to the posterior aspect of the left main pulmonary artery, thereby displacing the left main bronchus and the esophagus forward, downward, and to the right. The distal limb of the aortic kink may be dilated; it turns sharply backward and leftward to continue as the DTA, which is normal in the rest of its course.

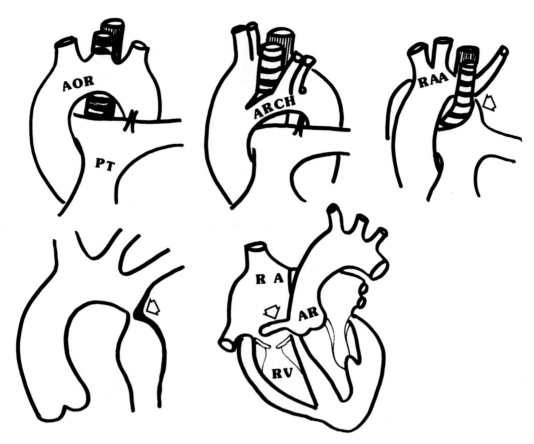

Figure 20–13. Diagram of some common aortic anomalies. (Above, left) Normal aortic anatomy. Note location of ligamentum arteriosum connecting aorta to bifurcation of pulmonary trunk (PT). (Above, center) Double aortic arch; the extra (anterior) arch is labeled ARCH. (Above, right) Right aortic arch (RAA); arrow indicates ligamentum arteriosum completing a vascular constricting ring. (Below, left) Coarctation of aorta (arrow). (Below, right) Congenital sinus of Valsalva aneurysm projecting into the right atrium.

Thus, in its radiologic, angiographic, and ultrasound morphology, PCA bears some resemblance to true aortic coarctation (even a similar systolic murmur is the rule). However, in PCA, there is no aortic obstruction, no arterial hypertension, and no pressure gradient.

The term *pseudocoarctation* was introduced 40 years ago by angiographers Dotter and Steinberg,[55] and its diagnostic features were described subsequently by several other groups correlating aortograms with radiographic and clinical findings. Its clinical significance consists of its simulation of true coarctation on one hand and left upper mediastinal masses on the other.

AORTIC DISSECTION AND RUPTURE

A tear or rupture of the aortic wall can result in a variety of clinicopathologic events.[61] (1) If the tear goes through the full thickness of the wall, it causes either (a) sudden death from massive hemorrhage or (b) false aneurysm (pseudoaneurysm), where bleeding is limited by the pressure of surrounding tissue, and a blood-filled cavity is formed that communicates with the aortic lumen. The pseudoaneurysm itself has a strong tendency to rupture sooner or later. (2) The tear may involve only the intima and inner part of the media (aortic dissection).[61-63] Under the force of pulsatile blood pressure, blood spreads through

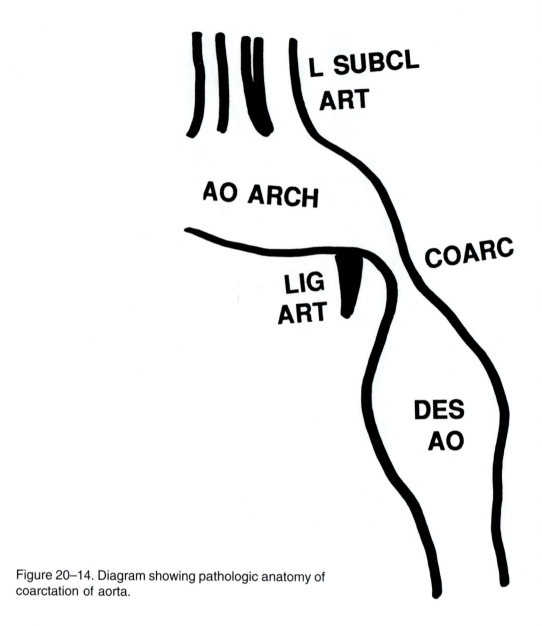

Figure 20–14. Diagram showing pathologic anatomy of coarctation of aorta.

the aortic wall longitudinally within seconds, for a varying extent, thus forming an "intimal flap" that separates the true lumen from the false lumen (Figures 20–15 and 20–16). The plane of dissection is commonly at the junction of the inner two-thirds with outer one-third of the media. Therefore, the outer wall of the false lumen is quite thin and often balloons out to a huge degree, justifying the older term *dissecting aneurysm*. Also, this aneurysm is more likely to burst externally rather than internally into the true aortic lumen. Rupture back into the true lumen causes spontaneous "healing" of the dissection with a chronic double-barreled aorta. Should aortic rupture or some other fatal complication not occur in the acute period of dissection, the patient may present months or years later with chronic aortic dissecting aneurysm, perhaps with aortic regurgitation, but with no definite history of the acute event.

The pathology of aortic dissection has been well studied in several large series.[64-67] The primary event in aortic dissection is an intimomedial tear, usually transverse, in the ascending aorta about an inch above the aortic valve. The next most frequent sites of intimal laceration are the distal aortic arch and upper DTA. Circumferentially, the tear involves one-third to one-half the circumference, only rarely being a complete annular tear.

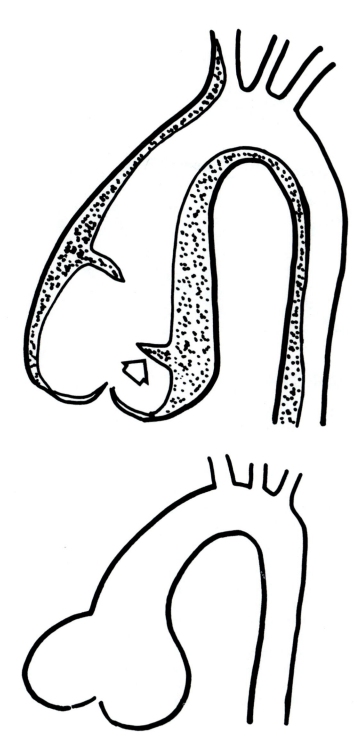

Figure 20–15. (Above) Diagram of aortic dissection showing site of intimal tear (arrow) and "double-barreled" aorta with false lumen as the stippled area. The dissection extends through the arch into the descending aorta. (Below) Diagram showing usual aortic configuration in dilatation due to Marfan's syndrome with ballooning of the sinuses of Valsalva.

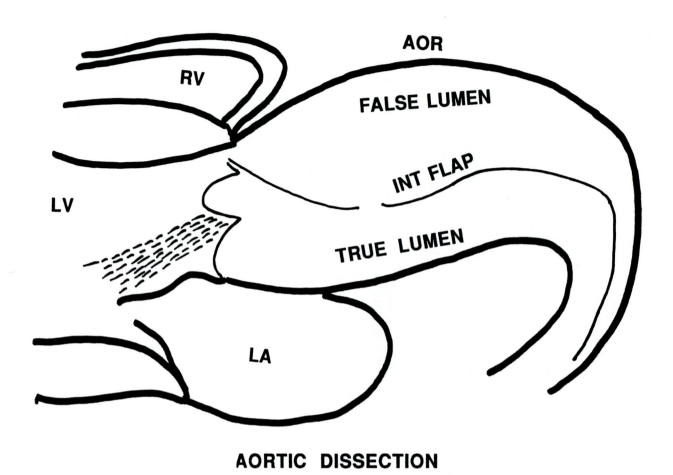

AORTIC DISSECTION

Figure 20–16. Diagram of parasternal long-axis view (including right parasternal) in patient with dissecting aortic aneurysm (AOR). The intimal flap (INT FLAP) separates the true lumen from the false lumen. Aortic regurgitation is present.

From the site of the intimomedial tear, the process of dissection spreads rapidly downward toward the aortic valve (causing aortic regurgitation), the coronary arteries, more often the right (perhaps causing myocardial infarction), and occasionally into the atrial septum (perhaps causing AV block). Distal tracking of the dissection tends to involve the convexity of the aortic arch and then part or all of the way downward to the aortic bifurcation. Dissection tends to halt at the level of atherosclerotic scarring in the aortic wall or where a major branch arises. Dissection never extends beyond the coarctation site, if coarctation is present. Major arteries supplying important viscera may be sheared off the true aortic lumen so that they are fed only from the false lumen and could be in jeopardy.

The main threat of a dissecting aneurysm is that of rupture. The most common site of rupture is the anterolateral (right) wall of the ascending aorta. This results in hemopericardium and acute tamponade within minutes or hours. The resulting intrapericardial hematoma can obstruct the aorta itself (a variety of supravalvar stenosis) or compress the pulmonary trunk.

Rupture of the dissecting aneurysm at arch or DTA level occurs into the mediastinum, left pleural cavity, or retroperitoneal space. Aortic dissection was classified by DeBakey et al.[62] in 1965 into three types: (1) involving the ascending aorta, aortic arch, and descending aorta, (2) involving the ascending aorta only, and (3) involving the DTA only. In more recent years, the simpler classification of Daily et al.[63] also has been in wide use: type A, which comprises types 1 and 2, and type B, which is type 3 of DeBakey. Type A has a grave prognosis (fatal in 90% of untreated cases) and needs emergency surgical repair. Type B has a much better prognosis and is usually managed conservatively.

Aortic dissection is more common in men than in women, in blacks, and in hypertensives. Two-thirds of all aortic dissections occur in hypertensives,[65] the risk rising with the severity of hypertension. Another uncommon though important predisposing condition is Marfan's syndrome. Dissection seldom, if ever, complicates aortitis of various etiologies, with or without mild aortic dilatation.

Echocardiography of Aortic Dissection (Figures 20–15 to 20–18)

The main 2D echo features include[68-74]

1. Aortic dilatation, which is commonly severe, often enormous, exceptionally mild or minimal. It is, of course, absent in aortic segments not involved in dissection.
2. Visualization of an intimal flap is the key diagnostic feature. This is sometimes obvious as a linear or band echo of varied contour (straight, curved, or even coiled) and varied mobility (undulating or fixed) within the dilated aorta. Spiral intimal flaps are notorious for incomplete fragments being recorded in any particular plane.
3. Spontaneous swirling echo contrast and thrombi may be detected in the false lumen, due to sluggish flow therein. Flow in the true lumen is rapid but may show swirling on colorflow Doppler secondary to gross aortic dilatation and turbulence caused by the intimal flap.
4. Colorflow Doppler reveals two distinct streams in the true and false lumina, respectively, which correspond to two channels on either side of the intimal flap. Colorflow Doppler may sometimes also reveal the site of intimal tear as a jet from the true to false lumen.
5. Important complications of aortic dissection such as aortic regurgitation and pericardial effusion (hemopericardium) can be detected and roughly quantified by colorflow Doppler or 2D echo.
6. Presence or extension of dissection into the DTA is much better visualized by TEE than transthoracic 2D echo.

In fact, TEE is extremely good at diagnosing aortic dissection, concomitantly with parasternal and suprasternal 2D echo and colorflow Doppler; the sensitivity and specificity for this purpose are very close to 100% in reported series.

Nevertheless, the echocardiographer has to beware of false-positive diagnosis of dissection caused by instrument artifacts (beam width, side lobe, or reverberatory) or by atheromatous aortic plaques. The left innominate vein crosses the left aspect of the aortic arch obliquely; the interface between the two sonolucent structures can be mistaken for an intimal flap.[68]

A large body of literature has now accumulated on the TEE manifestations of aortic dissection; from these numerous reports, only a few will be cited here.[69-74]

ATHEROMATOUS AORTIC LESIONS

The last 4 years have witnessed a surge of interest in the aorta as a possible source of emboli to systemic arteries, either of fragments of atherosclerotic plaque or of a thrombus forming on such a plaque. The impetus to such aortic endocardial disease has come from TEE, which has demonstrated that protruding atheromatous plaques, sometimes with mobile superimposed thrombus, are common in elderly patients, especially in those who have experienced embolization but do not have an obvious cardiac source.[75-80]

Amarenco et al.[81] recently reported the autopsy aortic findings in 500 patients with cerebrovascular or other neurologic diseases. Of 28 patients with unexplained stroke, ath-

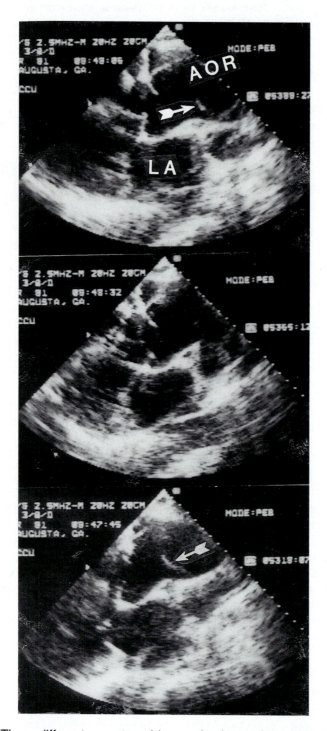

Figure 20–17. Three different parasternal long-axis views of the ascending aorta in a patient with aortic dissection (proven at surgery). The aorta is dilated and intimal flap (arrows) is seen within it.

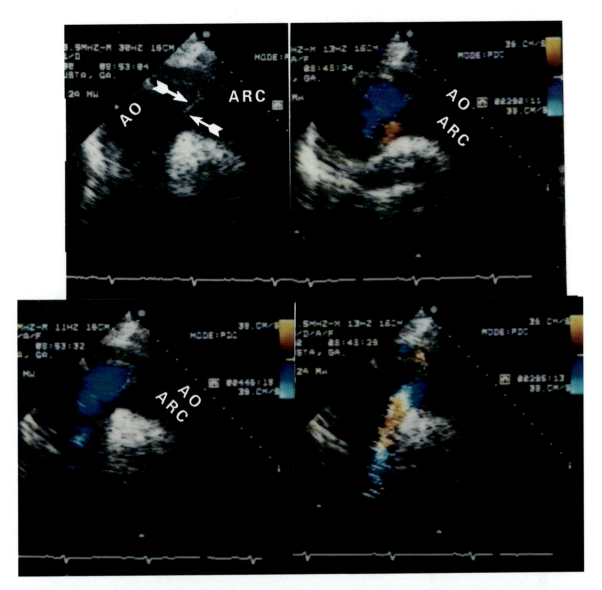

Figure 20–18. Suprasternal view in long axis of aortic arch in a patient with aortic dissection showing aortic dilatation and an intimal flap (arrows). The latter separates two streams of flow (shown by colorflow Doppler) in the true lumen (below, right) and false lumen (below, left). Both streams are seen simultaneously at top right.

erosclerotic plaques and ulcerations in the aortic arch were present in 61%. Several groups have described TEE appearances suggestive of irregular protruding atheromas, sometimes with mobile components (presumably thrombus) in the aortic arch or descending thoracic aorta (DTA). However, anatomic correlation of these intraaortic "mass" lesions were available in only a very few instances; they consisted partly of atheromatous material and partly of thrombus. Even conventional 2D echo can sometimes detect protruding aortic plaques (Figures 20–19 and 20–20).

In the experience of Tunick and Kronzon,[76] 25% of patients undergoing TEE for unexplained cerebrovascular accident (CVA), transient ischemic attack (TIA), or peripheral arterial embolization had protruding atheromas in the thoracic aorta. These authors raise the important practical issue that apart from spontaneous embolization, such patients may be at risk for iatrogenic emboli during left-sided heart catheterization or cannulation techniques at the time of cardiac surgery.

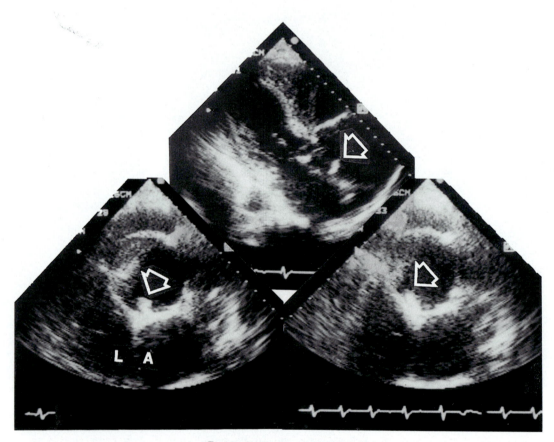

S H O R T   A X I S

Figure 20–19. Long-axis view (above) and short-axis views (below) showing small dense echo protruding from the aortic wall into its lumen, presumably an atheromatous plaque. The aortic root is dilated, but no dissection was present.

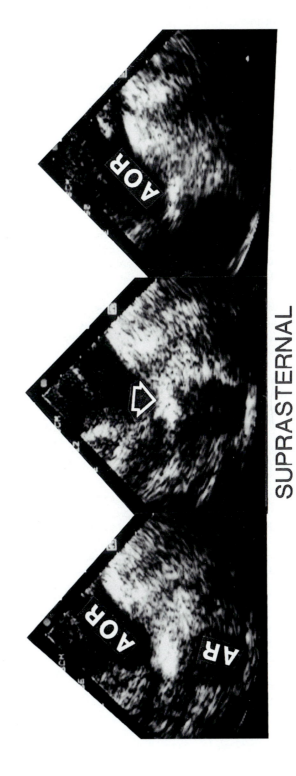

SUPRASTERNAL

Figure 20–20. Suprasternal views showing a large dense echo mass within the upper ascending aorta (arrow) presumably a calcified atheromatous plaque.

In a British series[79] of 155 patients examined for aortic lesions by TEE, 42 had had systemic emboli, and 20 of them had at least one atheromatous lesion on TEE. These authors found that patients with such atheromatous plaques had a much higher incidence of carotid, coronary, and peripheral vascular disease than those with "clean" aortas on TEE.

Penetrating atherosclerotic ulcer of the DTA has been recognized recently as a clinical simulator of aortic dissection with acute back pain. It can result not only in an intramural aortic hematoma but also in an aortic pseudoaneurysm or even fatal aortic perforation. Well established as an entity on its aortographic, CT, and MRI appearances over the last 7 years, its TEE characteristics have been reported[82]: a crater-like contour with jagged edges in the descending aorta distal to but near the origin of the left subclavian artery, and the rest of the aorta may show extensive atheromatous change. Absence of an intimal flap excludes aortic dissection.

REFERENCES

1. Gray's Anatomy, 37th ed. Edinburgh: Churchill-Livingstone, 1989, pp 727, 732.
2. Ross JJ, D'Adamo AJ, Karalis DG, et al. Three-dimensional transesophageal echo imaging of the descending thoracic aorta. Am J Cardiol 1993;71:1000.
3. Aronberg DJ, Glazer HS, Madsen K, et al. Normal thoracic aortic diameters by computed tomography. J Comput Assist Tomogr 1984;8:247.
4. Kersting-Sommerhoff BA, Sechtem UP, Schiller NB, et al. MR imaging of the thoracic aorta in Marfan patients. J Comput Assist Tomogr 1987;11:633.
5. Mathew T, Nanda NC. Two-dimensional and Doppler echocardiographic evaluation of aortic aneurysm and dissection. Am J Cardiol 1984;54:379.
6. Come PC. Improved cross-sectional echocardiographic technique for visualization of the retrocardiac descending aorta in its long axis. Am J Cardiol 1983;51:102.
7. Weyman AE. Cross-sectional Echocardiography. Philadelphia: Lea & Febiger, 1982, pp 498–504.
8. Martland HS. Syphilis of aorta and heart. Am Heart J 1930;6:1.
9. Klotz O. Some points respecting the localization of syphilis upon the aorta. Am J Med Sci 1918;155:92.
10. Heggtveit HA. Syphilitic aortitis: A clinicopathological autopsy study of 100 cases, 1950 to 1960. Circulation 1964;29:346.
11. Heggtveit HA. Syphilitic aortitis: Autopsy experience at the Ottawa General Hospital in 1950. Can Med Assoc J 1965;92:880.
12. Heggtveit HA. Nonatherosclerotic diseases of the aorta, in MD Silver (ed): Cardiovascular Pathology. New York: Churchill-Livingstone, 1991, p 310.
12a. Hust MH, Metzler B, Bickel W, et al. Transmural rupture of a nondissecting aortic aneurysm diagnosed by transesophageal echocardiography. Am Heart J 1993;125:1778.
13. Bickerstaff LK, Pairolero PC, Hollier LH, et al. Thoracic aortic aneurysms: A population-based survey. Surgery 1982;92:1103.
14. Halpert B, Williams RK. Aneurysms of the aorta: An analysis of 249 autopsies. Arch Pathol 1962;74:163.
15. Eisenberg MJ, Rice SA, Paraschos A, et al. The clinical spectrum of patients with aneurysms of the ascending aorta. Am Heart J 1993;125:1380.
16. Nevitt MP, Ballard DJ, Hallett JW. Prognosis of abdominal aortic aneurysms: A population-based study. N Engl J Med 1989;321:1009.
17. Crawford ES, Hess RR. Abdominal aortic aneurysm. N Engl J Med 1989;321:1040.
18. Morenco-Cabral C, Miller DC, Mitchell RS, et al. Degenerative and atherosclerotic aneurysms of the thoracic aorta. J Thorac Cardiovasc Surg 1984;88:1020.
19. Hastreiter AR, D'Cruz IA, Cantez T. Right-sided aorta: I. Occurrence of right aortic arch in various types of congenital heart disease. Br Heart J 1966;28:722.
20. D'Cruz IA, Cantez T, Namin EP, et al. Right-sided aorta: II. Right aortic arch, right descending aorta, and associated anomalies. Br Heart J 1966;28:725.
21. Shuford WH, Sybers RG, Edwards FK. The three types of right aortic arch. AJR 1970;109:78.
22. Anson BJ. The aortic arch and its branches, in AA Luisada (ed): Development and Structure of the Cardiovascular System. New York: McGraw-Hill, 1961, p 119.

23. Espino-Vela J, Mata LA. Eisenmenger's complex. Am Heart J 1956;51:284.

24. Bedford DE, Parkinson J. Right-sided aortic arch. Br J Radiol 1936;9:776.

25. Celano V, Pieroni DR, Gingell RL, et al. Two-dimensional echocardiographic recognition of the right aortic arch. Am J Cardiol 1983;51:1507.

26. Shrivastava S, Berry JM, Einzig S, et al. Parasternal cross-sectional echocardiographic determination of aortic arch situs. Am J Cardiol 1985;55:1236.

27. Kveselis DA, Snider AR, Dick M, et al. Echocardiographic diagnosis of right aortic arch with a retroesophageal segment and left descending aorta. Am J Cardiol 1986;57:1198.

28. Sahn DJ, Valdes-Cruz LM, Ovitt TW, et al. Two-dimensional echocardiography and intravenous digital video subtraction angiography for diagnosis and evaluation of double aortic arch. Am J Cardiol 1982;50:342.

29. Enderlein MA, Silverman NH, Stanger P, et al. Usefulness of suprasternal notch echocardiography for diagnosis of double aortic arch. Am J Cardiol 1986;57:359.

30. Kan M, Nanda NC, Stopa AR. Diagnosis of double aortic arch by cross-sectional echocardiography with Doppler colour flow mapping. Br Heart J 1987;58:284.

31. Parekh SR, Ensuing GJ, Darragh RK, et al. Rings, slings and such things: Diagnosis and management with special emphasis on the role of echocardiography. J Am Soc Echocardiogr 1993;6:1.

32. Murdison KA, Andrews BAA, Chin AJ. Ultrasonic display of complex vascular rings. J Am Coll Cardiol 1990;15:1645.

32a. D'Cruz IA, Stanley A, Vitullo D et al. Non invasive diagnosis of right cervical aortic arch. Chest 1983; 83:820.

33. Craigie D. Instance of obliteration of the aorta beyond the arch, illustrated by similar cases and observation. Edin Med Surg J 1841;56:427.

34. Abbott ME. Coarctation of the aorta of adult type. Am Heart J 1928;3:574.

35. Edwards JE, Christensen DA, Clagett OT, et al. Pathological considerations in coarctation of the aorta. Proc Mayo Clin 1948;23:324.

36. Elzenga NJ, Gittenbirger-deGroot AC. Localized coarctation of the aorta. Br Heart J 1983;49:317.

37. Becker AE, Becker MJ, Edwards JE. Anomalies associated with coarctation of the aorta. Circulation 1970;41:1067.

38. Carey LS, Sellers RD, Shone JD. Radiologic findings in the developmental complex of parachute mitral valve, supravalvular ring of left atrium, subaortic stenosis and coarctation of aorta. Radiology 1964;69:924.

39. Celand V, Pieroni DR, Morera JA, et al. Two-dimensional echocardiographic examination of mitral valve abnormalities associated with coarctation of the aorta. Circulation 1984;69:924.

40. Freed MD, Kean JF, Von Praagh R, et al. Coarctation of the aorta with congenital mitral regurgitation. Circulation 1974;49:1175.

41. Edwards JE. The congenital bicuspid aortic valve. Circulation 1961;23:485.

42. Tawes RL, Berry CL, Aberdeen E. Congenital bicuspid aortic valves associated with coarctation of the aorta in children. Br Heart J 1969;31:127.

43. Newcombe CP, Ongley PA, Edwards JE, et al. Clinical, pathological and hemodynamic considerations in coarctation of the aorta associated with ventricular septal defect. Circulation 1961;24:1356.

44. Neches WH, Park SC, Lenox CC. Coarctation of the aorta with ventricular septal defect. Circulation 1977;55:189.

45. Anderson RH, Lennox CC. Morphology of ventricular septal defect associated with coarctation of aorta. Br Heart J 1983;50:176.

46. Edwards JE. Aneurysms of the thoracic aorta complicating coarctation. Circulation 1973;48:195.

47. Huhta JC, Gutgesell HP, Latson LA, et al. Two-dimensional echocardiographic assessment of the aorta in infants and children with congenital heart disease. Circulation 1984;70:417.

48. Sahn DJ, Allen HD, McDonald G, et al. Real-time cross-sectional echocardiographic diagnosis of coarctation of the aorta. Circulation 1977;56:762.

49. Weyman AE, Caldwell RL, Hurwitz RA, et al. Cross-sectional echocardiographic detection of aortic obstruction. Circulation 1978;57:498.

50. Shaddy RE, Snider AR, Silverman NH, et al. Pulsed Doppler findings in patients with coarctation of the aorta. Circulation 1986;73:82.

51. Marx GR, Allen HD. Accuracy and pitfalls of Doppler evaluation of the pressure gradient in aortic coarctation. J Am Coll Cardiol 1986;7:1379.

52. Anders SD, MacPherson D, Yeager SB. Temporal flow velocity profile in the descending aorta in coarctation. J Am Coll Cardiol 1986;7:603.

53. Simpson IA, Sahn DJ, Valdez-Cruz LM, et al. Doppler flow mapping in patients with coarctation of the aorta. Circulation 1988;77:736.

54. Stern H, Erbel R, Schreiner G, et al. Coarctation of the aorta: Quantitative analysis by transesophageal echocardiography. Echocardiography 1987;4:387.

55. Dotter CT, Steinberg I. Angiography in congenital heart disease. Am J Med 1952;12:219.

56. Stevens GM. Buckling of the aortic arch (pseudocoarctation, kinking). Radiology 1958;70:67.

57. Pattison JN, Grainger RC. Congenital kinking of the aortic arch. Br Heart J 1959;21:555.

58. Griffin JF. Congenital kinking of aorta. N Engl J Med 1964;271:726.

59. Nasser WK, Helman C. Kinking of the aortic arch (pseudocoarctation). Ann Intern Med 1966;64:971.

60. Smyth PT, Edwards JE. Pseudocoarctation kinking or buckling of the aorta. Circulation 1972;46:1027.

61. Murray CA, Edwards JE. Spontaneous laceration of ascending aorta. Circulation 1973;47:848.

62. DeBakey ME, Henley WS, Cooley DA, et al. Surgical management of dissecting aneurysm of the aorta. J Thorac Cardiovasc Surg 1965;49:130.

63. Daily PO, Trueblood HW, Stinson ER, et al. Management of acute aortic dissections. Ann Thorac Surg 1970;10:237.

64. Hirst AE, Johns VJ, Klime SW. Dissection aneurysm of the aorta: A review of 505 cases. Medicine 1958;37:217.

65. Hume DM, Porter RR. Acute dissecting aortic aneurysms. Surgery 1963;53:122.

66. Leonard JC, Haselton PS. Dissecting aortic aneurysms: A clinicopathological study. Q J Med 1979;189:55.

67. Larson EW, Edwards WD. Risk factors for aortic dissection: A necropsy study of 161 cases. Am J Cardiol 1984;53:849.

68. Applebe AF, Olson S, Biby LD, et al. Left branchiocephalic vein mimicking an aortic dissection on transesophageal echocardiography. Echocardiography 1993;10:67.

69. Mathew T, Nanda NC. Two-dimensional and Doppler echocardiographic evaluation of aortic aneurysm and dissection. Am J Cardiol 1984;54:379.

70. Erbel R, Engberding R, Daniel W, et al. Echocardiography in diagnosis of aortic dissection. Lancet 1989;1:457.

71. Hashimoto S, Toshiaki K, Osakada G, et al. Assessment of transesophageal Doppler echocardiography in dissecting aortic aneurysm. J Am Coll Cardiol 1989;14:1253.

72. Roudaut R, Chevalier JM, Barbeau P, et al. Mobility of the intimal flap and thrombus formation in aortic dissection. Echocardiography 1993;10:279.

73. Iliceto S, Nanda NC, Rizzon P, et al. Color Doppler evaluation of aortic dissection. Circulation 1987;75:748.

74. Khanderia BK, Tajik AJ, Taylor CL, et al. Aortic dissection: Review of value and limitations of two-dimensional echocardiography in a six-year experience. J Am Soc Echocardiogr 1989;2:17.

75. Tunick PA, Kronzon I. Protruding atherosclerotic plaque in the aortic arch of patients with systemic embolization. Am Heart J 1990;120:658.

76. Tunick PA, Kronzon I. Protruding atheromas in the thoracic aorta. Echocardiography 1993;10:419.

77. Karalis DG, Chandrasekharan K, Victor MF, et al. Recognition and embolic potential of intraaortic atherosclerotic debris. J Am Coll Cardiol 1991;17:73.

78. Amarenco P, Cohen A, Baudrimont M, et al. Transesophageal echocardiographic detection of aortic arch disease in patients with cerebral infarction. Stroke 1992;23:1005.

79. Nihoyannopoulos P, Joshi J, Athanasopoulos G, et al. Detection of atherosclerotic lesions in the aorta by transesophageal echocardiography. Am J Cardiol 1993;71:1208.

80. Dee W, Geibel A, Kasper W, et al. Mobile thrombi in atherosclerotic lesions of the thoracic aorta. Am Heart J 1993;126:707.

81. Amarenco P, Duyckaerts C, Yzourio C, et al. The prevalence of ulcerated plaques in the aortic arch in patients with stroke. N Engl J Med 1992;326:221.

82. Mosvovitz HD, David M, Mosvovitz C, et al. Penetrating atherosclerotic aortic ulcers: The role of transesophageal echocardiography in diagnosis and clinical management. Am Heart J 1993;126:745.

21

Prosthetic Valves

MECHANICAL VALVES

A large number of different mechanical heart valves have been devised over the last three decades. Most of these are no longer marketed; only a few that have stood the test of experience have continued in vogue among surgeons in recent years (Figures 21-1 to 21-4). However, an occasional patient who had one of the earlier models installed 10 to 15 years ago or even longer still shows up in the echocardiography laboratory; the valve may be obsolete, but the patient is still extant.

Ideally, a prosthetic valve should be efficient mechanically (i.e., open well when flow normally occurs and close perfectly or almost so when regurgitation is to be prevented). It should not get thrombosed or infected nor interfere with function of adjacent structures. It should stay securely in place and last indefinitely with no adverse effects of wear. No such ideal valve exists, but changes in valve design to minimize complications have led to obsolescence of many earlier models.

Mechanical valves consist of a prosthetic fixed valve ring and a poppet (movable ball or disk) that opens and closes the valve within a metal cage. The valve ring is surrounded by a cloth sewing ring that is stitched by the surgeon to the valve annulus after removal of the diseased native valve. The sewing-ring cuff has two surfaces exposed to blood (inflow and outflow aspects). The inner rim of the sewing ring forms the edge of the prosthetic valve orifice.

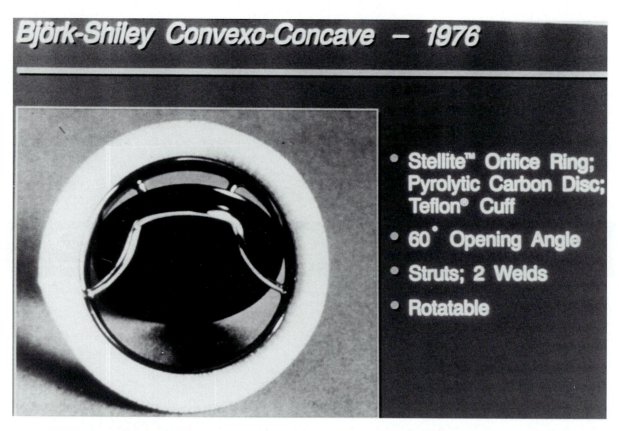

Figure 21–1. Bjork-Shiley Convexo-Concave Valve (Tilting disc).

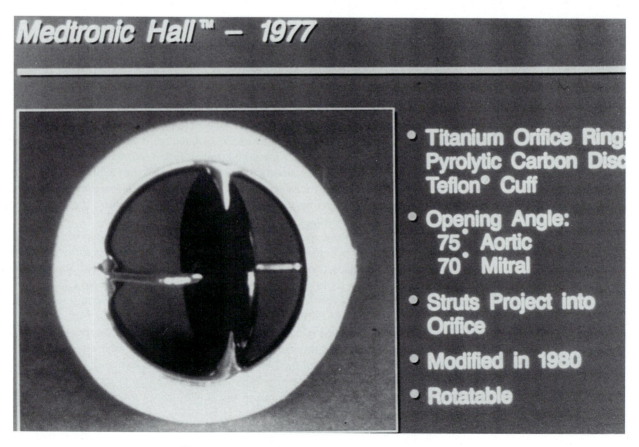

Figure 21–2. Medtronic-Hall valve—Tilting disc.

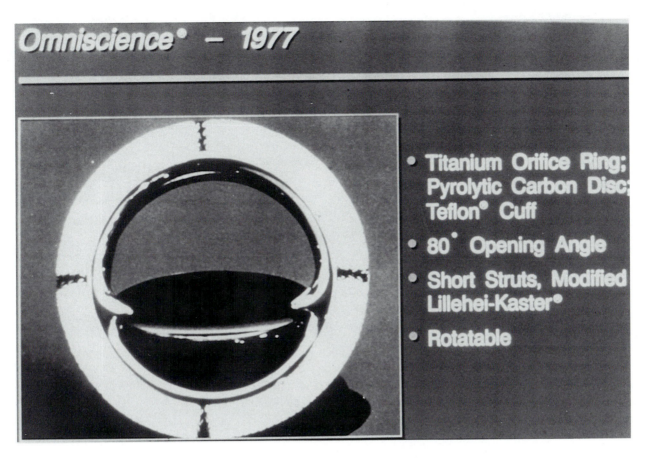

Figure 21–3. Ominscience Valve—Tilting disc.

Motion of the poppet (ball or disk) is confined within a cage formed by the metal ring and by metal struts of varying shape and size. The most popular valve currently, the St. Jude Medical, has neither ball, disk, nor cage but consists of two leaflets that pivot on an axis between open and closed positions (see Figure 21–4). Mechanical prosthetic valves thus have metal and cloth plus perhaps other synthetic material components. In recent years, surfaces of the valve that come into contact with blood have been covered by black pyrolitic carbon, which is very durable and resistant to thrombus formation. A systematic description of all known varieties of prosthetic valves can be found in the publications of Mehlman[1] and Silver.[2]

Complications of Mechanical Valves

Thrombosis and infection are the main complications. Certain other adverse mechanical consequences, including dehiscence, valve-chamber disproportion, and sequels of turbulence, are either less common or less serious.

Thrombosis.[2–6] A thin layer of thrombus on the sewing-ring surface is probably beneficial, because it is presumed that host tissue grows along and into it, gradually covering the sewing-ring cloth and rendering it smooth and less prone to thrombosis. But thrombus formation in excess on the sewing ring or at any other valve site is undesirable and dangerous inasmuch as it can lead to thromboemboli, valve obstruction, or valve infection.

Thrombi tend to form at cloth-metal interfaces and where valve shape allows relative stasis to occur. Thus thrombosis is common where the cloth sewing ring meets the metal

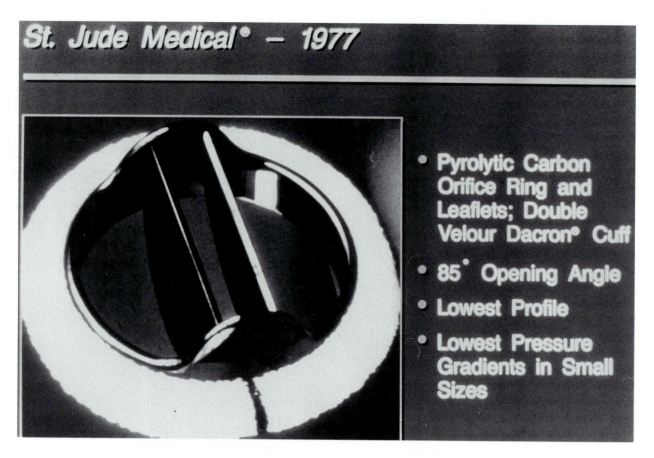

Figure 21–4. St. Jude Medical—Bileaflet valve.

ring (in ball and disk valves), where the struts meet the inner metal ring, and rarely at the summit of the metal cage. Atrial fibrillation and discontinuation of anticoagulant therapy predispose to prosthetic valve thrombosis.

A dangerous form of thrombus is that which encroaches or grows across the valve orifice, because it directly obstructs flow or because it restricts disk or ball motion and therefore proper valve opening or closure. Such poppet "sticking" or "freezing" is ominous, heralding a fatal outcome. Valve thrombus itself causes more stasis and further thrombus formation, a vicious cycle.

Thromboembolic phenomena commonly manifest as cerebral emboli, less often as coronary or other embolization. Extensive prosthetic valve thrombosis also can be responsible for the appearance or aggravation of heart failure. Poppet sticking or entrapment can cause syncope or near-syncope. It has been estimated that thromboembolic phenomena are more frequent with mitral than aortic prosthetic valves (4% versus 2% per 100 patient-years).[4]

Better valve design to eliminate or reduce stasis and coating of valve surfaces with pyrolitic carbon have reduced the thrombotic risk.

Bacterial Endocarditis of Prosthetic Valves.[2–7] Two types of this dreaded complication are distinguished: (1) *early*, in the postoperative period, is presumed to be due to inadvertent introduction of infection during surgery or to flaring up of the original infection if valve replacement was done for bacterial endocarditis, and (2) *late*, occurring months or years after valve replacement, estimated as 0.2% to 0.5% per year, afflicting 3% of patients with prosthetic valves. Bacteremia following dental or other manipulations or from a pyogenic focus results in bacteria lodging on an area of thrombosis or roughened endocardium.

Apart from the systemic effects of refractory septicemia and of embolization of infected thrombi, an extremely common complication of prosthetic valve endocarditis is a ring or annular abscess (see Chapter 17). Infection spreads to the valve annulus and its vicinity, over part or all of its circumference. Such ring abscesses may lead to fistulas or pseudoaneurysms leading from the left ventricular (LV) chamber or aortic root to the paraaortic or paramitral extracardiac space.

Prosthetic valve endocarditis does not usually cause mobile pedunculated or projecting vegetations (as seen in native valve endocarditis). At surgery or autopsy, a variable amount of amorphous infected thrombus is found in and around the prosthesis. Valve thrombosis is thought to predispose to endocarditis by providing a nidus on which blood-borne bacteria settle; conversely, valve infections engender new thrombus, further stasis, and an ominous cycle leading to certain death if untreated.

Dehiscence of Prosthetic Valve.
Small local separation of the sewing ring from the adjacent annulus (less than 5 mm) is not rare (Figure 21-5) and not serious. It is attributable to tissue retraction during postoperative healing or "giving way" of one or two stitches. On the other hand, valve dehiscence over a large segment of its circumference is serious not only because of its mechanical effect (severe regurgitation) but also because it usually signifies valve infection. The untethered part of the valve has an abnormal "loose" or rocking motion.

Other Prosthetic Valve Adverse Effects.
Unlike normal native valves, all prosthetic valves have some built-in stenosis[8]; a pressure gradient is present varying from small to moderate, its degree depending on valve type and size (orifice diameter). Trivial valve regurgitation is not only harmless but may be beneficial by preventing stasis.

Turbulence.
In contrast to smooth laminar flow through normal native valves, *turbulent flow* is the rule through prosthetic mechanical valves. However, turbulence is greater with lateral or eccentric valve flow patterns than with central flow as in St. Jude valves. Turbulence causes endocardial thickening, sometimes extensive, thought by some to impair LV function[9] by splinting subjacent myocardium or by interfering with subendocardial myocardial nutrition. Intimal thickening in the aortic root associated with prosthetic valve turbulence rarely can cause coronary ostial stenosis.

Valve-Chamber Disproportion.
This complication sometimes occurred with "high-profile" mechanical valves with long struts as a result of shrinkage in size of preoperatively dilated ventricles.[10] Impingement of the projecting struts of the valve on the adjacent LV wall or septum may cause endocardial thickening or grooving. Rare instances of such contact provoking ventricular arrhythmias have been reported. Free strut ends in open-cage valves can "hook" trabeculations and impair poppet motion.[11]

Ball variance was important two decades ago when silicone-rubber balls were used in Starr-Edwards ball valves. Such balls swelled up by absorbing lipids from the blood.[12,13] Thus the ball got too big for the cage, impairing normal motion or even resulting in impaction and death. Such a poppet could fracture and a fragment embolize.[14]

Strut fracture is a catastrophic event[15-17] notoriously associated with a particular model of Bjork-Shiley valve[16,17] manufactured during a specific period by welding the struts to the ring. Strut breakage results in release of the disk into the aorta and massive overwhelming regurgitation. Such potentially breakable valves are no longer installed, but a fairly large number of patients still exist with such possibly hazardous devices within their hearts. Isolated examples of other valve models having similar fractures have been reported.[15,18]

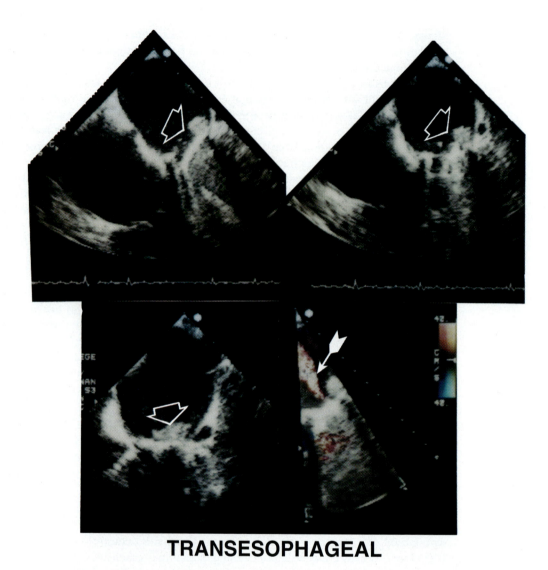

TRANSESOPHAGEAL

Figure 21–5. *TEE* views prosthetic tilting-disc mitral valve, showing disk (open arrow) and small paravalvar leak (small white arrow), in right lower panel.

Echocardiography of Mechanical Valves[18–20]

M-mode and two-dimensional (2D) echo are usually limited in their ability to detect abnormalities of mechanical prostheses. This is due to the following:

1. Very strong ultrasound reflections from prosthetic materials produce artefactual echoes and reverberations obscuring valve details and pathology (Figure 21-6). However, abrupt change in disk position from systole to diastole and back is usually noted (Figure 21-7).
2. Motion of prosthetic ball, disk, or leaflet may not be well visualized because it occurs in a plane or axis very different from that of the ultrasound probe.
3. Thrombi or vegetation, in or on mechanical valves, cannot be imaged separately from dense valve echoes.

Extensive thrombosis causing gross restriction of poppet motion may be appreciated on M-mode or 2D echo if poppet "sticking" is present, i.e., failure to move when expected, in some beats at least. Significant valve dehiscence manifests as a typical rocking motion

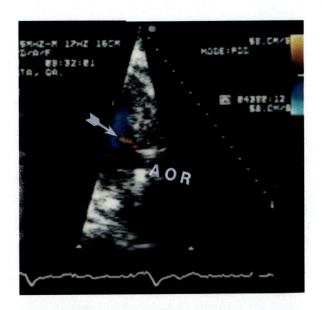

PARASTERNAL LONG AXIS

Figure 21–6. Long-axis view showing small perivalvar leak (arrow) between the prosthetic valve and septum.

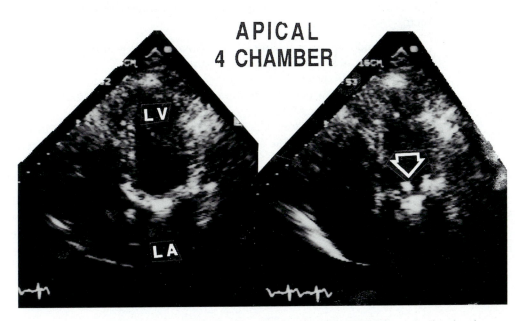

Figure 21–7. Apical four-chamber view of patient with Bjork-Shiley mitral valve in systole (left) and early diastole (right). In the latter the edge of the tilting disc shows up on the ventricular aspect of the valve (arrow).

independent from the normal annulus motion. Endocardial thickening is common with high-profile Starr-Edwards valves. The severed stumps of mitral chordae may present as multiple mobile echoes near the prosthetic valve and should not be mistaken for vegetations.

Fortunately, Doppler and especially colorflow Doppler are informative in assessing the presence and severity of prosthetic valve stenosis or regurgitation, though they are not quite as accurate in this respect as with native valves. A large number of Doppler studies of normal and abnormal prosthetic function appeared during the 1980s.

Colorflow Doppler [transesophageal echo (TEE) or transthoracic echo (TTE)] is useful in distinguishing regurgitation *through* a prosthetic valve from regurgitation at its outer edge (paravalvar leak). Colorflow Doppler also can demonstrate rare instances of fistulas from the LV or aortic root into adjoining cardiac chambers or vessels.

Doppler signals in the left atrium due to mitral regurgitation are difficult or impossible to interpret with mechanical mitral prostheses because of obscuration by valve artefacts (see Figure 21-6). This technical obstacle sometimes can be overcome by right parasternal scanning in the right lateral position and even better by TEE; both techniques interrogate the left atrial (LA) chamber without intervening valve artefacts.

Ring (annular) abscesses should be sought in every patient with suspected prosthetic valve endocarditis because they are very common and because their presence influences prognosis and management. The usual echo appearance is that of a sonolucent or partly sonolucent space around a variable part of the circumference of the prosthetic aortic valve in the parasternal short-axis view. A common location is posterior to the aortic root, between it and the left atrium; the sonolucent abscess space is evident in parasternal long- as well as short-axis views. An abscess in this location also can result from mitral valve endocarditis spreading through the intervalvar fibrosa (between aortic and mitral valve fibrous rings). Rarely, infection might burrow *into* a mitral leaflet, the ventricular septum, or the LV wall, causing intramural abscesses. Certain uncommon prosthetic valve complications are worth mentioning because echocardiography has been used to diagnose them:

1. Pseudoaneurysm (Figure 21-8) following local wall rupture at the annulus region below the site of the prosthesis[21-23]
2. Fistulas between the LV chamber and the right atrium or coronary artery[24]
3. Protrusion or deep impaction of the prosthetic valve (Starr-Edwards) into the ventricular septum[25]
4. Atrial wall aneurysm secondary to malattachment of a mitral prosthesis[26]
5. Thin, delicate, mobile strands attached to the periphery of a mechanical prosthesis[27]
6. Dehiscence of a Carpentier mitral ring causing severe mitral regurgitation[28]

In some of the unusual types of prosthetic valve disorders mentioned above, as well as in more common complications, including valve thrombosis, ring abscess, and perivalvar leaks, colorflow Doppler assessment of valve regurgitation, i.e., TEE, has proved invaluable, as documented by a plethora of recent reports.[29-36] Comparisons between TTE and TEE in the same patients have amply established the superiority of TEE for the diagnosis of all aspects of prosthetic valve dysfunction.[30,31]

BIOPROSTHETIC VALVES

These prosthetic valves are made of animal or human tissue, usually chemically treated and mounted on a prosthetic stent. Those commonly used are *heterografts* (tissue of another species), e.g., the pig aortic valve or (used less often) bovine pericardium. The stent supports are of plastic or metal wiring with a sewing ring of Dacron. Stents are coronet-shaped, with rounded projections called *struts*.

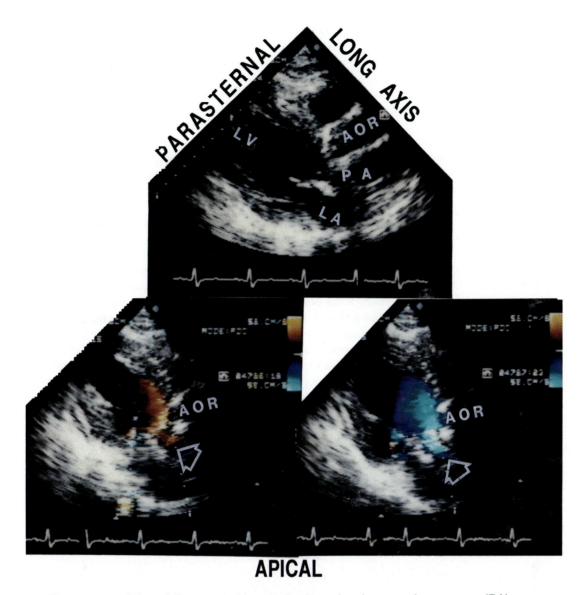

Figure 21–8. (Above) Parasternal long-axis view, showing pseudoaneurysm (PA) opening into the LV through a perforation in the fibrosa between aortic and mitral valve rings (prosthetic aortic valve). (Below) Colorflow Doppler shows flow (arrows) from pseudoaneurysm to LV chamber in diastole (left), and in the reverse direction in systole (right).

Homografts are bioprostheses containing valve tissue from the same species, e.g., a human cadaver. *Autografts* are valves transplanted from one site to another in the same patient (pulmonic valve excised and placed in aortic valve location) or fashioned out of tissue (pericardium or fascia lata) from the same individual.

The Ionescu-Shiley valve consists of bovine pericardium treated with glutaraldehyde and mounted on a Dacron-covered titanium frame. It was in vogue in some centers several years ago. However, almost all bioprosthetic valves recently installed are porcine aortic valves, which include the aortic wall adjacent to the valve cusps. The two popular models, the Hancock and the Carpentier-Edwards valves (Figures 21–9 and 21–10), are very similar in gross appearance and also in durability and complication rates. They differ in minor details such as concentration of glutaraldehyde used for preservation and stent composition. The pig aortic valve resembles the human one except for a muscular shelf within the right coronary cusp that slightly narrows the valve inlet. Encroachment of this shelf, present in Hancock and Carpentier-Edwards valves, is minimized by ingenious techniques of mounting on the stent. Pericardial bioprostheses are prepared from selected areas of the cow parietal pericardium that are cut to the desired shape and size. Pericardial valve cusps are 0.3 to 0.5 mm thick; porcine cusps, about 0.2 mm thick. The collagen components provide strength to these very thin cusps.

Alignment of bioprosthetic mitral valves with the LV chamber can vary. Accordingly, colorflow Doppler shows the mitral inflow stream directed into the central LV (Figure 21–11) or more often toward the ventricular septum (Figure 21–12).

Once implanted, the porcine valve cusps undergo certain changes over time that are relevant to eventual valve functioning as well as to the echocardiographer. Within a few days, the cusps are covered by a layer of fibrin, platelets, and inflammatory cells. The basal areas of the cusps (up to 1 cm from attachment) get covered by a thick fibrous sheath, of variable thickness and extent, growing inward from the adjacent host tissues. When excessive, this fibrous layer (pannus) stiffens the cusp and can affect function adversely. Pericardial valve tissue also may undergo deleterious changes in course of time, becoming granular, thick, and stiff, or may get progressively stretched ("creep").

Complications of Bioprosthetic Valves[37–44]

The overall incidence of porcine bioprosthetic failure (death or reoperation due to valve-related complications) is quoted as 35% to 50% at 10 years and 50% to 75% at 15 years. *Structural deterioration* is by far the most common cause of bioprosthetic failure (74%). Bacterial endocarditis and noninfective paravalvar leak each account for about 10% to 12% and thrombosis for 4%. The latter is four or five times more frequent with mechanical prostheses. Degenerative porcine cusp changes include calcification, which occurs progressively more rapidly and extensively the younger the patient, especially below age 35. However, cusp deterioration also can occur without calcification, due to collagen degradation. Clinically significant structural deterioration is strongly time-dependent, the rate accelerating after 5 years. Regurgitation is the usual manifestation, due to cusp tears. Stenosis due to calcific cusp rigidity is less common (10% to 15%), as is cusp perforation.

Two types of cusp calcification are recognized by pathologists: (1) *intrinsic,* calcium being deposited in the original implanted cusp tissue, and (2) *extrinsic,* calcification occurring in material added later to the valve, such as thrombus, host tissue overgrowth, or old vegetations.

Cusp tears have been divided into four types:

- Type I involves the free edge and is more common in pericardial than in porcine valves. Large tears can result in flail cusp motion.
- Type II involves arclike linear tears along the base of the cusp and occurs parallel to the line of cusp attachment. Disruption is thought to occur at this site because it is subjected to undue stress as the cusp opens by "hinging" here.
- Type III involves large, round perforations in the cusp center, often resulting from bacterial endocarditis with severe focal full-thickness destruction.
- Type IV involves small pinhole openings in the cusp, commonly multiple, which if confluent may eventually progress to type III.

Endocarditis is said to occur in 4% to 6% of prosthetic valve replacements, not strikingly different in bioprostheses from mechanical prostheses. Valve infection may be lo-

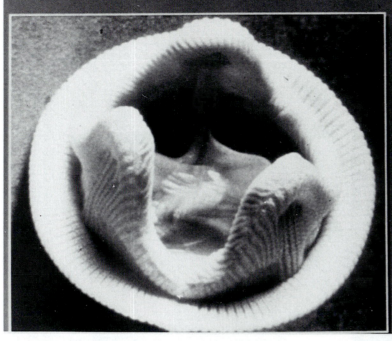

Figure 21–9. Hancock bioprosthetic (porcine) valve.

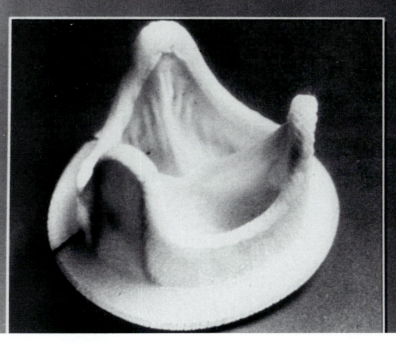

Figure 21–10. Carpentier-Edwards bioprosthetic (porcine) valve.

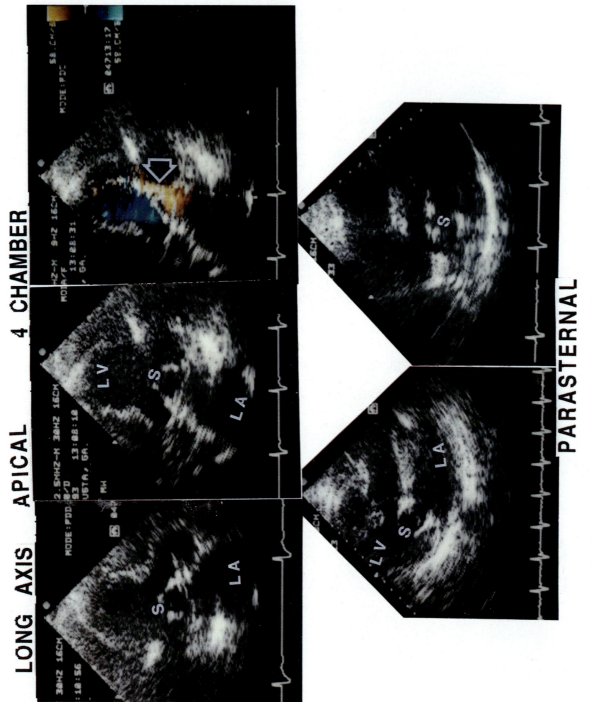

Figure 21–11. Apical long-axis view (above, left) and apical four-chamber view (above, center and right) of a patient with a normal porcine mitral valve. Colorflow Doppler (above, right) shows mitral inflow stream passing through the valve. The contour of the stents (S) is seen in the apical views as well as the parasternal long- and short-axis views (below).

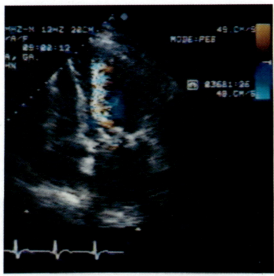

APICAL 4 CHAMBER

Figure 21–12. Colorflow Doppler in apical four-chamber view, in a patient with a porcine mitral valve. The alignment of the prosthetic valve with the LV chamber is such that flow into the ventricle is directed toward the ventricular septum.

calized to the sewing ring, from which it frequently spreads to the vicinity of the annulus (ring abscess). Vegetations also may occur on the prosthetic cusps and, when large, have been known to cause valve stenosis. Cusp tears or perforations are more common, causing severe regurgitation. Such obvious disruption of cusp continuity is presumptive evidence of extensive full-thickness cusp destruction.

Thrombosis is uncommon with bioprostheses, but not if atrial fibrillation and/or a low-output-failure state is present. Early postoperative thrombus formation usually occurs in the sewing-ring vicinity, but within a few months this area gets endothelialized, and the risk of thrombosis decreases. Late valve thrombosis has a predilection for the outflow aspect of the cusps, in the concavity of the porcine sinus of Valsalva.

Rarely, the stent of a bioprosthetic valve may impinge on the septal or ventricular wall, in which case ventricular ectopy may be provoked, and even perforation of myocardium or aortic wall has been reported. Abnormal angulation or malalignment of a bioprosthesis may cause the valve and its stents to be directed against the septum (for mitral) or the aortic wall (for aortic prosthesis) rather than into the LV chamber or aortic lumen. This has been attributed to asymmetrical annular scarring or gross calcification. Rare examples of LV outflow obstruction or coronary ostial obstruction can ensue.

Echocardiography of Bioprosthetic Valves[45–54]

The stents with the characteristic three rounded strut projections are easily identified in all views (Figure 21-13). Ultrasound artefacts shadowing adjacent structures or the left atrium are not as obscuring of these structures as with mechanical valves. They rarely show any echo abnormality, except for the rare instances of valve dehiscence. Ring abscesses are common with endocarditis and have the 2D echo features mentioned above with respect to mechanical prosthetic valves.

The important parts of the bioprosthetic valve to image are the cusps. Very thin and delicate, they may be difficult to visualize and may manifest as no more than a barely visible small linear flickering. As the valve thickens with time, the cusps are easily identified, and when calcified, cusps are good evidence of advanced structural deterioration. Cusp tears (Figure 21-14) and perforations may not be diagnosed except indirectly by color-

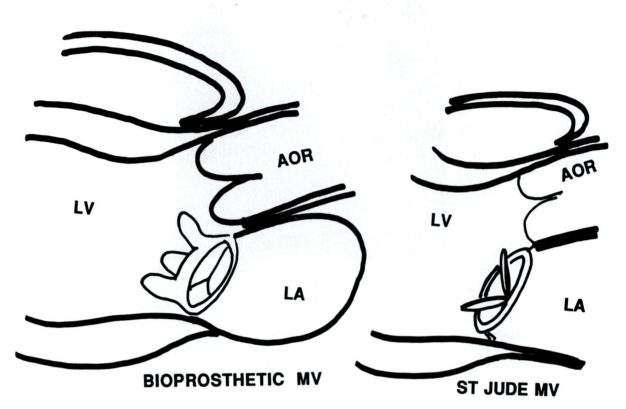

Figure 21–13. Diagram of parasternal long-axis view, with bioprosthetic mitral valve (left) and St. Jude mitral prosthesis (right).

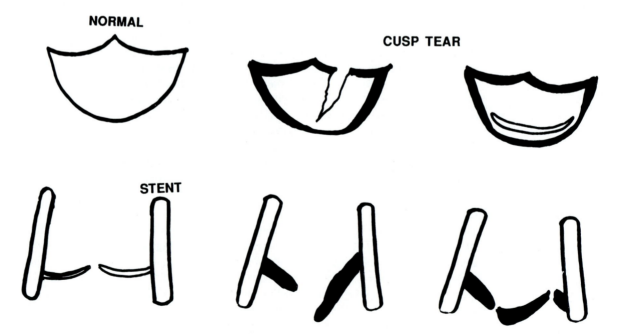

Figure 21–14. Diagram showing different types of prosthetic porcine cusp tear.

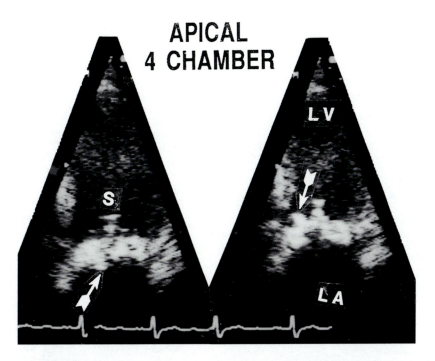

APICAL
4 CHAMBER

Figure 21–15. Apical four-chamber view of porcine mitral valve with flail mitral cusp (proven at surgery). In systole the flail thickened cusp prolapses into the left atrium (left); in diastole it moves into the LV chamber (right), as shown by arrows.

flow Doppler recognition of moderate to severe mitral regurgitation with a few exceptions:

1. Flail motion of a torn leaflet, especially if calcified or with an attached vegetation, presents a very abnormal motion pattern, whipping forward and backward with every cardiac cycle (Figure 21–15).
2. Tears at the base of the cusps in mitral prostheses, a common site, may cause the cusp to sag or prolapse toward the LA without flail motion (Figure 21–16).
3. Rapid flutter or vibration of a prosthetic valve leaflet is diagnostic of a leaflet tear and best depicted on M-mode imaging (Figure 21–17).
4. Paravalvar regurgitation can be recognized on colorflow Doppler as with mechanical valves (Figures 21–18 and 21–19).
5. Endocarditis and vegetations can be better diagnosed by 2D echo on bioprosthetic valves (Figures 21–20 and 21–21) than they can on mechanical valves.
6. Abnormal valve alignment is well appreciated in long-axis parasternal and apical views. It is not unusual to see the mitral valve stent impinge or almost impinge on the septum, apparently causing LV outflow obstruction; however, continuous-wave or pulsed-wave Doppler rarely demonstrates significant obstruction.

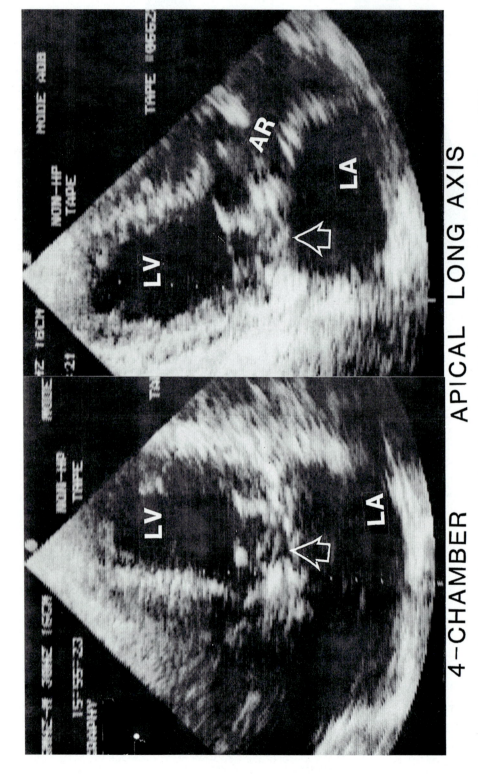

4-CHAMBER   APICAL LONG AXIS

Figure 21–16. Apical four-chamber view of a porcine mitral valve. The prosthetic valve leaflets are thickened and tend to sag into the left atrium (right), evidence of cusp degradation. A basal cusp tear was found at surgery.

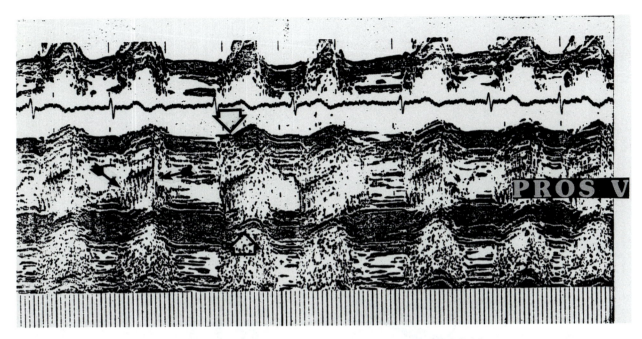

Figure 21–17. M-mode of a porcine mitral prosthetic valve (PROS V), open arrows. Systolic flutter of its leaflets (small thin arrows) indicates torn leaflet, confirmed at surgery,

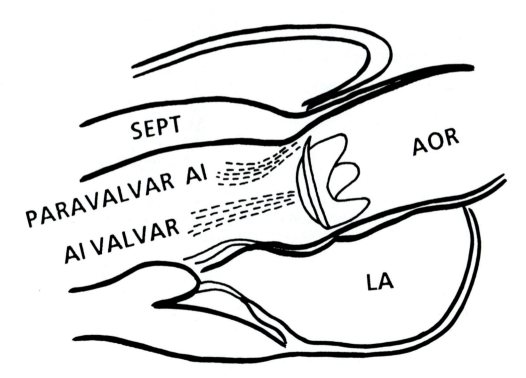

Figure 21–18 Diagram showing a bioprosthetic mitral valve, and sites of regurgitation, either through the valve center (VALVAR) or between the prosthetic valve and posterior aortic root, as seen on Colorflow Doppler (PARAVALVAR).

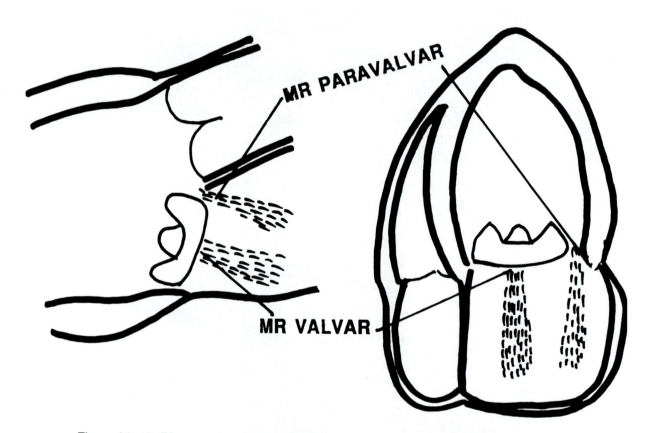

Figure 21–19. Diagram showing a bioprosthetic aortic valve and the sites of regurgitation, either through the valve center (AI VALVAR) or between the valve and aortic annukus (PARAVALVAR AI), as seen on Colorflow Doppler.

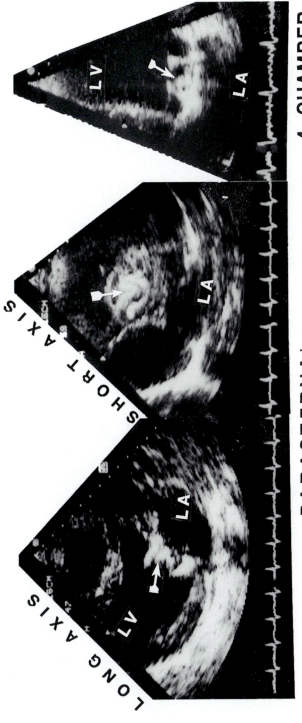

Figure 21–20. Parasternal long-axis (left), short-axis view (center) and apical four-chamber view (right) of a patient with a bioprosthetic mitral valve. Arrows indicate a vegetation on a prosthetic valve cusp, confirmed at surgery.

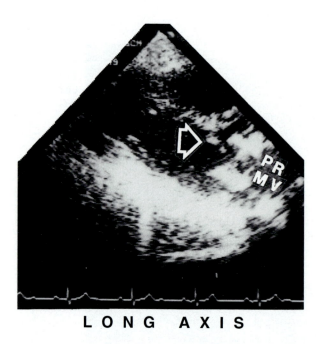

LONG AXIS

Figure 21–21. Parasternal long-axis view of patient with endocarditis of a porcine mitral valve (PRMV). Arrow indicates a long mobile vegetation.

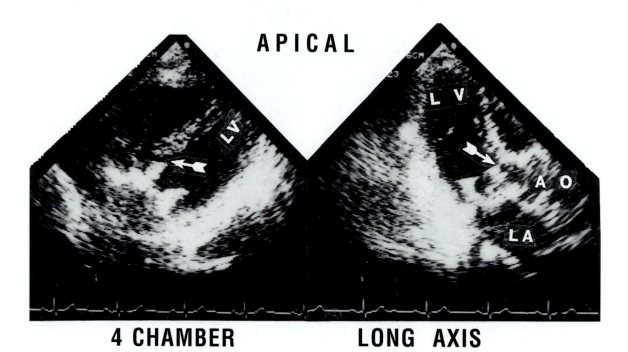

APICAL

4 CHAMBER   **LONG AXIS**

Figure 21–22. Apical long-axis view (right) and modified apical four-chamber view (left) in a patient with bioprosthetic mitral valve. Note that a stent of the porcine valve abuts the ventricular septum and apparently obstructs the LV outflow tract.

REFERENCES

1. Mehlman DJ. A pictorial and radiographic guide for identification of prosthetic heart devices. Progr Cardiovasc Dis 1988;30:441.
2. Silver MD. Cardiovascular Pathology, 2d ed. New York: Churchill-Livingstone, 1991, p 1487.
3. Yoganathan AP, Corcoran WH, Harrison EC, et al. The Bjork-Shiley aortic prosthesis: Flow characteristics, thrombus formation and tissue. Circulation 1978;58:70.
4. Edmonds LH. Thromboembolic complications of current cardiac valvular prostheses. Ann Thorac Surg 1982;34:96.
5. Akbarian M, Austen WG, Yurchak PM, et al. Thromboembolic complications of prosthetic cardiac valves. Circulation 1968;37:826.
6. Boskovic D, Elezovic I, Boskovic D, et al. Late thrombosis of the Bjork-Shiley tilting disc valve prosthesis. J Thorac Cardiovasc Surg 1986;91:1.
7. Watanakunakorn C. Prosthetic valve endocarditis. Prog Cardiovasc Dis 1979;23:181.
8. Rahimtoola SH. The problem of valve prosthesis-patient mismatch. Circulation 1978;58:20.
9. Roberts WC, Morrow AG. Secondary left ventricular fibroelastasis following mitral valve replacement. Circulation 1968;38(suppl II):101.
10. Kennedy JW, Doces J, Steward DR. Left ventricular function before and following aortic valve replacement. Circulation 1977;56:944.
11. Kalke B, Korns ME, Goot B, et al. Engagement of ventricular myocardium by open-cage atrioventricular valvular prostheses. J Thorac Cardiovasc Surg 1969;58:92.
12. McHenry MM, Smeloff EA, Fong WY, et al. Critical obstruction of prosthetic heart valves due to lipid absorption by Silastic. J Thorac Cardiovasc Surg 1970;59:413.
13. Grunkmeier GL, Starr A. Late ball variance with the model 1000 Starr-Edwards aortic valve prosthesis. J Thorac Cardiovasc Surg 1986;91:918.
14. Hameed K, Ashfaq S, Waugh DOW. Ball fracture and extrusion in Starr-Edwards aortic valve prosthesis with dissemination of ball material. Arch Pathol 1968;86:520.
15. Dillelo F, Flemma RJ, Mullen DC, et al. Strut fracture of the Starr-Edwards cloth covered metallic ball prosthesis. J Thorac Cardiovasc Surg 1988;95:1020.
16. Lindblom D, Rodriquez L, Bjork VO. Mechanical failure of the Bjork-Shiley valve. J Thorac Cardiovasc Surg 1989;87:95.
17. Vilacosta I, Sanroman JA, Camino A, et al. Disc escape after minor strut fracture in a Bjork-Shiley mitral valve prosthesis. Echocardiography 1992;9:265.
18. Silver MD, Torok PR, Slinger RP, et al. Late strut fracture of the Beall model 105 disc valve prosthesis. J Thorac Cardiovasc Surg 1988;96:448.
19. Kotler MN, Mintz GS, Panidis I, et al. Noninvasive evaluation of normal and abnormal prosthesis valve function. J Am Coll Cardiol 1983;2:151.
20. Panidis IP, Ren JF, Kotler MN, et al. Clinical and echocardiographic evaluation of the St Jude cardiac valve prosthesis. J Am Coll Cardiol 1984;4:454.
21. Comess KA, Baron SB, Cossgrove NA, et al. Doppler ultrasound diagnosis of aortic subvalvular pseudoaneurysm with left ventricular fistula. J Am Soc Echocardiogr 1988;1:226.
22. Ascah KJ, Patrick E, Chilton C, et al. Atypical pseudoaneurysm after mitral valve replacement. J Am Soc Echocardiogr 1991;4:625.
23. Sakai K, Nakamura K, Ishizuka N, et al. Echocardiographic findings and clinical features of left ventricular pseudoaneurysm after mitral valve replacement. Am Heart J 1992;124:975.
24. Yee GW, Naasz C, Hatle L, et al. Doppler diagnosis of left ventricle to coronary sinus fistula: An unusual complication of mitral valve replacement. J Am Soc Echocardiogr 1988;1:458.
25. Rosenzweig MS, Nanda NC. Two-dimensional echocardiographic detection of left ventricular wall impaction by mitral prosthesis. Am Heart J 1983;106:1069.
26. Garcia-Fernandez MA, SanRoman D, Torrecilla E, et al. Transesophageal echocardiographic detection of atrial wall aneurysm as a result of abnormal attachment of mitral prosthesis. Am Heart J 1992;124:1650.
27. Stoddard MF, Dawkins PR, Longsaker RA. Mobile strands are frequently attached to the St Jude Medical mitral valve prosthesis as assessed by two-dimensional transesophageal echocardiography. Am Heart J 1992;124:671.
28. Gindea AJ, Schwinger M, Freedberg RS, et al. Dehiscence of a Carpentier mitral ring: Diagnosis by transesophageal echocardiography. Am Heart J 1989;118:841.
29. Taams MA, Gussenhoven EJ, Cahalan MK, et al. Transesophageal Doppler color flow imaging in the detection of native and Bjork-Shiley mitral valve regurgitation. J Am Coll Cardiol 1989;13:95.

30. Hixson CS, Smith MD, Mattson MD, et al. Comparison of transesophageal color flow Doppler imaging of normal mitral regurgitant jets in St Jude Medical and Medtronic Hall cardiac prostheses. J Am Soc Echocardiogr 1992;5:57.

31. VandenBrink RBA, Visser CA, Basart DCG, et al. Comparison of transthoracic and transesophageal color Doppler flow imaging in patients with mechanical prostheses in the mitral position. Am J Cardiol 1989;63:1471.

32. Alam M, Serwin JB, Rosman HS, et al. Transesophageal color flow Doppler and echocardiographic features of normal and regurgitant St Jude Medical prostheses in the mitral valve position. Am J Cardiol 1990;66:871.

33. Khanderia BK, Seward JB, Oh JK, et al. Value and limitations of transesophageal echocardiography in assessment of mitral valve prostheses. Circulation 1991;83:1956.

34. Chaudhry FA, Herrera C, DeFrino PF, et al. Pathologic and angiographic correlations of transesophageal echocardiography in prosthetic heart valve dysfunction. Am Heart J 1991;122:1057.

35. Dittrich HC, McCann HA, Walsh TP, et al. Transesophageal echocardiography in the evaluation of prosthetic and native aortic valves. Am J Cardiol 1990;66:758.

36. Karalis DG, Chandrasekharan K, Ross JJ, et al. Single-plane transesophageal echocardiography for assessing function of mechanical or bioprosthetic valves in the aortic valve position. Am J Cardiol 1992;69:1310.

37. Foster AH, Greenberg GJ, Underhill DJ, et al. Intrinsic failure of Hancock mitral bioprostheses. Ann Thorac Surg 1987;44:568.

38. Magilligan DJ, Lewis JW, Tilley B, et al. The porcine bioprosthetic valve. J Thorac Cardiovasc Surg 1985;89:499.

39. Milano A, Botolotti U, Talenti E, et al. Calcific degeneration as the main cause of porcine bioprosthetic valve failure. Am J Cardiol 1984;53:1066.

40. Nistal F, Garcia-Martinez V, Fernandez D, et al. Degenerative pathologic findings after long-term implantation of bovine pericardial bioprosthetic heart valves. J Thorac Cardiovasc Surg 1988;96:642.

41. Schoen FJ, Hobson CE. Anatomic analysis of removed prosthetic heart valves. Hum Pathol 1985;16:549.

42. Wheatley DJ, Fisher J, Reee IJ, et al. Primary tissue failure in pericardial heart valves. J Thorac Cardiovasc Surg 1987;94:367.

43. Walley WM, Keon WJ. Patterns of failure in Ionescu-Shiley bovine pericardial bioprosthetic valves. J Thorac Cardiovasc Surg 1987;95:925.

44. Fernicola DJ, Roberts WC. Frequency of ring abscess and cuspal infection in active infective endocarditis involving bioprosthetic valves. Am J Cardiol 1993;72:314.

45. Simpson IA, Reece IJ, Houston AB, et al. Noninvasive assessment by Doppler ultrasound of 155 patients with bioprosthetic valves. Br Heart J 1986;56:83.

46. Melacini P, Villanova C, Thiene G, et al. Long-term echocardiographic Doppler monitoring of Hancock bioprosthesis in the mitral valve position. Am J Cardiol 1992;70:1157.

47. Grenadier E, Sahn D, Roche AHG, et al. Detection of deterioration or infection of homograft and porcine xenograft bioprosthetic valves in mitral and aortic positions by two-dimensional echocardiographic examination. J Am Coll Cardiol 1983;2:452.

48. Daniel WG, Murge A, Grote J, et al. Comparison of transthoracic and transesophageal echocardiography for detection of abnormalities of prosthetic and bioprosthetic valves in the mitral and aortic positions. Am J Cardiol 1993;71:210.

49. Vandeberg BF, Dellsperger KC, Chandran KB, et al. Detection, localization and quantitation of bioprosthetic mitral valve regurgitation. Circulation 1988;78:529.

50. Chambers JB, Monoghan MJ, Jackson G, et al. Doppler echocardiographic appearance of cusp tears in tissue valve prostheses. J Am Coll Cardiol 1987;10:462.

51. Adamick RD, Glekel LC, Graver LM. Acute thrombosis of an aortic bioprosthetic valve. Am Heart J 1991;122:241.

52. Alam M, Rosman HS, Polanco GA, et al. Transesophageal echocardiographic features of stenotic bioprosthetic valves in the mitral and tricuspid valve positions. Am J Cardiol 1991;68:689.

53. Rothbart RM, Castriz JL, Harding LV, et al. Determination of aortic valve area by two-dimensional and Doppler echocardiography in patients with normal and stenotic bioprosthetic valves. J Am Coll Cardiol 1990;15:817.

54. Pinto FJ, Wranne B, Schnittger I. Transesophageal echocardiography for study of bioprostheses in the aortic valve position. Am J Cardiol 1992;69:274.

22

Transesophageal Views

The rapidly increasing application of transesophageal echocardiography (TEE) over the last decade has occurred because of greatly enhanced quality of imaging of posterior cardiac and posterior mediastinal structures by this technique. However, the new diagnostic potential provided by TEE can be fully implemented only if the anatomy of this previously unfamiliar perspective on the heart and great vessels is well understood.

Thus the echocardiographer embarking on TEE must acquire not only the expertise of passing and then manipulating the TEE probe but also of becoming familiar with the topography of all the TEE views. This includes the sizes, shapes, and anatomic relationships of cardiac chambers and vessels in numerous horizontal and longitudinal planes. In other words, cardiothoracic anatomy must be mastered before one can proceed with the application of TEE to clinical diagnosis. The various biplane TEE views have been categorized by Bansal et al.,[1] Seward et al.,[2,3] and Nanda et al.[4] As with conventional transthoracic echo (TTE) views, these views should not be regarded each as rigid and standard, but rather as a family or range of imaging planes with some variation secondary to individual differences in cardiac chamber size, shape, and alignment with the thorax and direction of the TEE probe.

Most higher TEE views show some part of the left atrium, nearest to the transducer; this chamber is directly subjacent to the TEE probe and thus constitutes a convenient "window" on the rest of the heart.

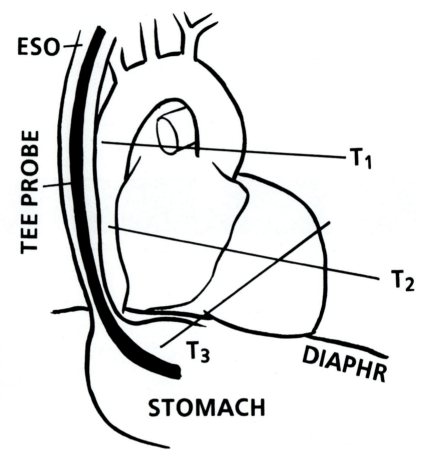

Figure 22–1. Diagram showing position of TEE probe in esophagus (ESO) and stomach. T₁ and T₂ represent transverse TEE planes, T₃ a transverse transgastric plane. These three planes are only a few of numerous TEE planes. DIAPHR, diaphragm.

HORIZONTAL (TRANSVERSE) TEE VIEWS (Figures 22–1 and 22–2)

Short-axis views of the base of the heart reveal the aortic valve, proximal coronary arteries, left atrial appendage, superior vena cava (SVC), right ventricular (RV) outflow tract, pulmonary veins, and pulmonary arteries.

Midesophageal four-chamber views image the aortic root, aortic valve, and left ventricular (LV) outflow tract and are therefore ideal for demonstrating the abnormal anatomy of fixed (discrete) or dynamic subvalvar obstruction. Aortic valve vegetations and paravalvar ring abscesses are also well seen. On colorflow Doppler, the presence, severity, and direction of aortic regurgitation are very obvious. In a different orientation, the atrial septum and its defects, including abnormalities of the fossa ovalis region, are clearly seen; colorflow Doppler is likewise exquisitely sensitive in depicting shunts at this level. Mitral and tricuspid leaflets and their abnormalities of structure and motion are also imaged well in this four-chamber view. Other structures visualized include the ventricular septum and defects in it, the RV inflow tract, and papillary muscles of mitral as well as tricuspid valves.

Transgastric views are helpful for obtaining short-axis views of the LV chamber, the ultrasound beam being directed upward through the diaphragm. The LV is seen as a circular structure, either at papillary muscle or mitral valve level. LV chamber size and contractile performance are easily appreciated and can be monitored during anesthesia or surgical procedures. Longitudinal and apical transgastric views are also possible.

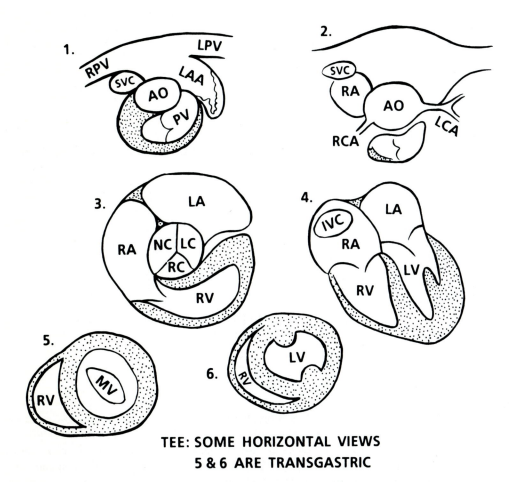

TEE: SOME HORIZONTAL VIEWS
5 & 6 ARE TRANSGASTRIC

Figure 22–2. Diagram showing some common transverse TEE views (No.1 to No.4) through the base of the heart. No.1 is at the level of the upper pulmonary veins (RPV and LPV) and the left atrial appendage (LAA). No.2 is at the level of the coronary arteries (RCA and LCA) from the aortic root. No.3 is at the level of the aortic valve and atrial septum. No.4 is a four-chamber view through the crux of the heart. SVC, superior vena cava; Ao, aortic root; RA, right atrium; RV, right ventricle; RC, LC, and NC, right, left, and noncoronary aortic cusps; LA, left atrium; LV, left ventricle; IVC, inferior vena cava. No.5 and No.6 are transgastric views of the left ventricle at mitral valve and papillary muscle levels respectively.

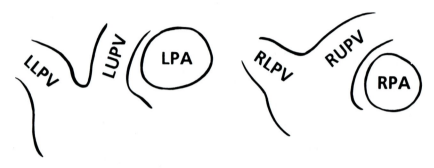

Figure 22–3. Diagram showing longitudinal TEE views through left and right pulmonary veins: LLPV and LUPV, left lower and left upper pulmonary veins; RLPV and RUPV, right lower and right upper pulmonary veins. The left and right pulmonary arteries are seen in cross-section, superior to the pulmonary veins.

TEE: SOME LONGITUDINAL VIEWS

Continuous-wave Doppler interrogation of a stenotic aortic valve jet can sometimes prove more successful from this apical gastric site than from TTE windows.

LONGITUDINAL TEE VIEWS (Figures 22–3 to 22–5)

As the ultrasound beam sweeps from far right to far left across the mediastinum, numerous basal cardiac longitudinal planes can be obtained from extreme right to extreme left. However, five basic planes are usually described: extreme right, near right, central, near left, and extreme left. In all, the left atrium appears at the apex of the sector image and is in fact the window through which all other cardiac structures are visualized.

Extreme Right. The right upper pulmonary vein, entering the left atrium, is the main feature; the right pulmonary artery, in cross section, is seen above it. The right lower pulmonary vein also may be brought into view.

Near Right. The SVC and atrial septum are the main features in this plane. Thus fossa ovalis and sinus venosus atrial septal defects are clearly depicted and their size measured. The valve-flap anatomy of a patent foramen ovale is also well demonstrated. Slight manipulation can bring into view the inferior vena cava (IVC) and eustachian valve. Anteriorly, the RA chamber leads into its appendage; posterosuperiorly, the right pulmonary artery is seen in cross section.

Central. The ascending aorta (aortic root) is the central feature. The aortic valve cusps are transected obliquely and may therefore appear somewhat different than in transthoracic views, in which they are in strict longitudinal or transverse orientation. Posterior to the ascending aorta is the left atrium; anterior to the aorta is the RV outflow tract; in a

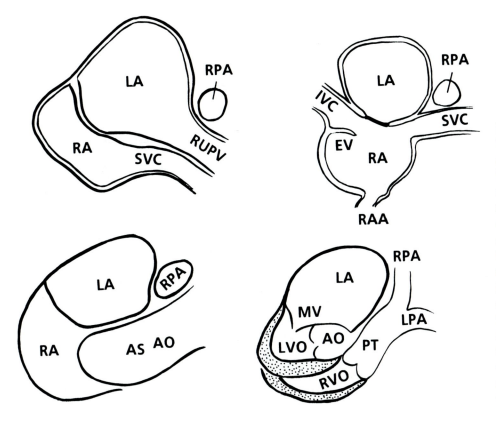

Figure 22–4. Longitudinal TEE views through the base of the heart. (Top left) Through SVC and interatrial septum. (Top right) Through same structures at fossa ovalis level, also showing right atrial structures such as Eustachian valve and right atrial appendage. (Bottom left) Through long axis of ascending aorta and cross-section of right pulmonary artery. (Bottom right) Through outflow tracts of LV as well as RV (LVO and RVO); the pulmonary trunk (PT) and its bifurcation are also seen.

LONGITUDINAL VIEWS OF THE LEFT VENTRICLE

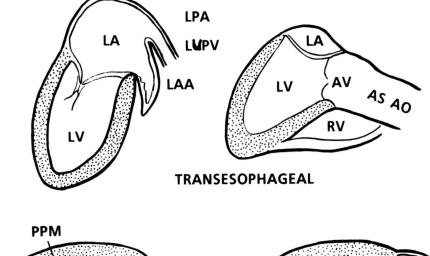

TRANSESOPHAGEAL

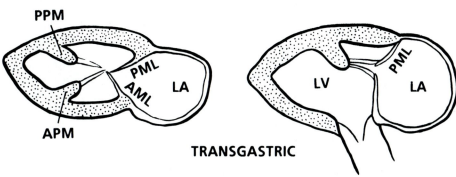

TRANSGASTRIC

Figure 22–5. Longitudinal TEE views of LV chamber. (Top left) Through left atrial appendage (LAA) and left upper pulmonary vein (LUPV). (Top right) Through aortic valve (AV) and ascending aorta (AsAo). (Bottom) Views are transgastric: The left is a two-chamber view of LV and LA chambers; the right includes the aortic valve and root.

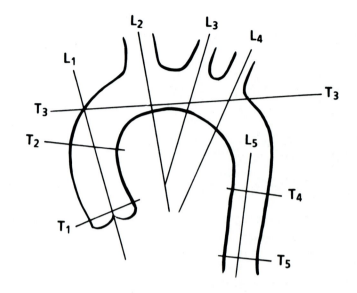

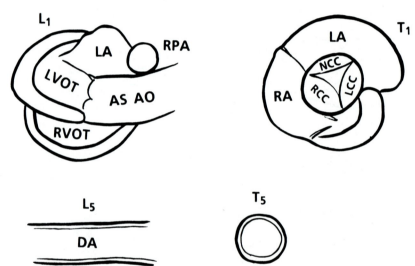

Figure 22–6. (Above) TEE views of the aorta. Transverse planes T_1 and T_2 are short axis views of the ascending aorta; T_4 and T_5 are of the descending aorta; T_3 transects the aortic arch. L_1 is a long axis view of the ascending aorta, L_5 of the descending aorta. L_2, L_3, and L_4 pass through the aortic arch in the long axes of the innominate, left common carotid, and left subclavian arteries respectively. (Center) The ascending aorta occupies a central position in the heart, in long axis (L_1, left) and in short-axis (T_1, right). NCC, LCC, RCC, non-, left, and right coronary cusp of aortic valve. (Bottom) Descending thoracic aorta in long-axis (L_5, left) and short axis (T_5, right).

posterosuperior corner is the right pulmonary artery. The echocardiographer is already familiar with these anatomic relationships in the parasternal and apical long-axis views. The atrial septum also appears in this plane, rightward of the aorta.

Near Left. The RV outflow tract, pulmonary valve, and pulmonary trunk are the main features. The latter's bifurcation into left and right pulmonary arteries can be brought into view. Posterior to the RV outflow is the LV outflow tract; even more posteriorly is the LA chamber.

Extreme Left. The main features are the left upper pulmonary vein and left atrial appendage, both opening into the LA. These two orifices are very close together, forming an acute ridge or spur at the junction. Superiorly is seen the left pulmonary artery and inferiorly the inflow part of the LV chamber.

The aorta, especially the descending aorta, can be imaged in much finer detail by TEE than by TTE (Figure 22–6). Much of the ascending aorta cannot be visualized by (horizontal) TEE views because of the intervening air-filled trachea; however, it can be better imaged by biplane TEE. The anatomic relationship of the descending aorta to the esophagus and the spine is also relevant to TEE (Figure 22–7).

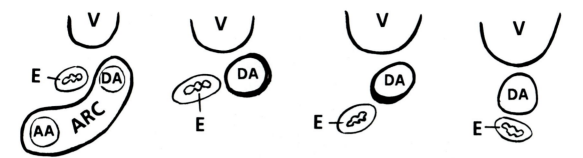

RELATION OF ESOPHAGUS TO AORTA

Figure 22–7. Diagram to show relationship of aorta to esophagus at different levels: Aortic arch level (far left); lowest thoracic level where descending aorta (DA) passes through the diaphragm, (far right). The central two sections are in the upper and lower mid thorax respectively. As the esophagus descends, it gradually moves from right of the aorta to directly anterior to it. AA, ascending aorta; ARC, aortic arch V, vertebra; E, esophogus.

PITFALLS IN TEE DIAGNOSIS[5]

A sound knowledge of cardiac anatomy is important to avoid pitfalls in echocardiographic interpretation, in TEE as well as in conventional TTE. In other words, the inexperienced or untutored often commit the blunder of mistaking normal variants or even constant normal structures for tumors, thrombi, or vegetations. Some of such common fallacies are briefly mentioned below.

Right Atrium

The eustachian valve is situated at the anterior rim of the IVC orifice, thus projecting into the lower right atrium. This is a vestigial structure in adults, with a tremendous range of persistence varying from virtual absence to a long, large flap stretching from the crista terminalis laterally to the atrial septum medially. It can be misdiagnosed as an atrial "mass," especially when transected obliquely by the ultrasound beam. A fenestrated eustachian valve or an attached Chiari network (which looks somewhat similar) may be misinterpreted as a fungating neoplasm or vegetation.

Another false "mass" on TEE can appear at the junction of the SVC and right atrium. Normally, there is a ridge at this site, corresponding to a sulcus on the atrial exterior. Incidentally, the sinus node is located at this site.

The crista terminalis is a narrow ridge on the inside of the lateral right atrial wall that runs vertically from the SVC to the IVC orifice. It corresponds to the sulcus terminalis on the right atrial exterior, which separates the posterior smooth sinus venosus portion of this chamber from the corrugated anterior portion. The latter shows a pattern of ridges that resemble the teeth of a comb and which are continuous with the ridges in the right atrial appendage. The pectinate ridges and crista terminalis form small endocardial elevations that should not be mistaken for mural thrombi. The former have a recognizable regular size and shape and move with the atrial wall as it contracts. In contrast, atrial mural thrombi are larger, and while they may be adherent to the underlying atrial wall, they do not participate so closely in the atrial wall motion.

Left Atrium

The left atrial appendage, like its right counterpart, presents a corrugated inner surface that needs to be differentiated from thrombi in this location. Thrombi are larger than the endocardial ridges, often round, sometimes quite dense (if calcified), and obviously separate from the atrial wall, though partly contiguous with it.

The left atrial appendage is usually roughly tubular or cylindrical in shape and could therefore be mistaken for the left upper pulmonary vein in a transverse TEE plane. One

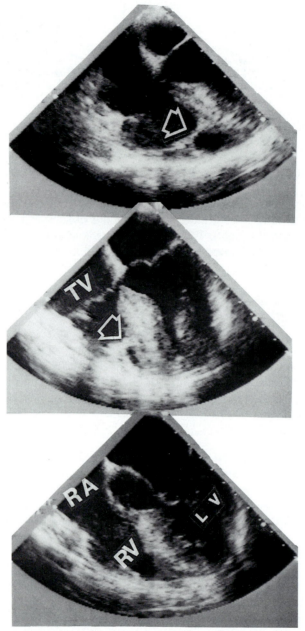

TRANSESOPHAGEAL

Figure 22–8. Four-chamber TEE view. The moderator band (arrow) is clearly visible in the RV chamber. TV, tricuspid valve.

is less prone to make this error in the longitudinal TEE plane. The left upper pulmonary vein is smooth, whereas the inner aspect of the atrial appendage shows multiple small ridges or folds.

A conspicuous ridge at the junction of the orifice of the left upper pulmonary vein and that of the left atrial appendage is a normal finding in TEE as well as TTE (apical four-chamber view). This sharp angular echogenic spur can project as much as 1 cm into the LA chamber and is often mistaken for an LA "mass" by the unwary. Anecdotal accounts of such patients being sent for CT, MRI, or angiocardiography or being placed on long-term anticoagulants are numerous.

TRANSESOPHAGEAL

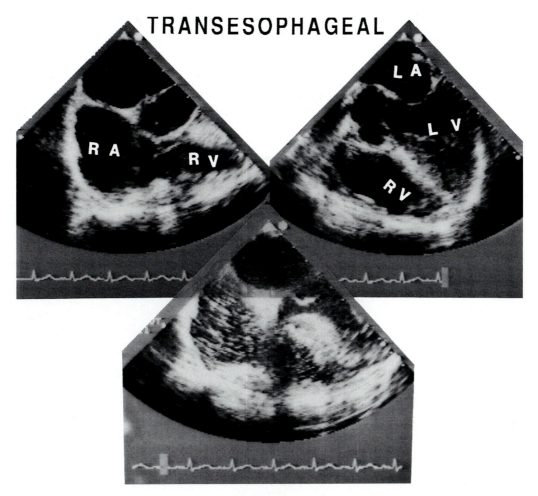

Figure 22–9. (Above) TEE views showing right as well as left heart chambers. (Below) Injection of agitated saline into an arm vein opacifies the right heart chambers. Absence of microbubble contrast in left heart chambers rules out right to left atrial shunt.

TRANSESOPHAGEAL

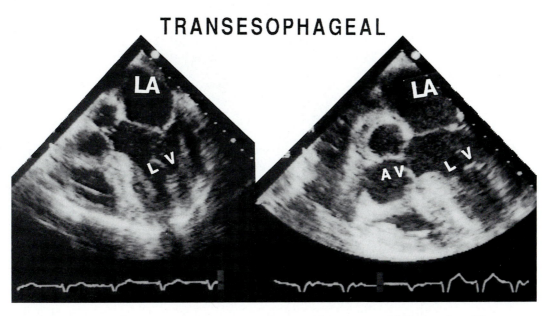

Figure 22–10. TEE showing inflow as well as outflow tracts of LV chamber. The aortic valve (AV) as well as mitral valve. LA, left atrium; LV, left ventricle.

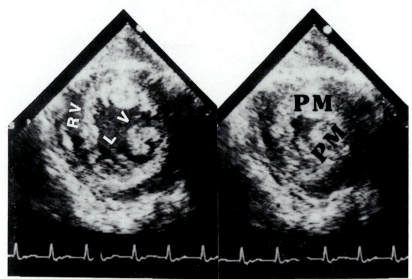

Figure 22–11. TEE view of LV at papillary muscle (PM) level, in diastole (left) and in systole (right).

TRANSESOPHAGEAL

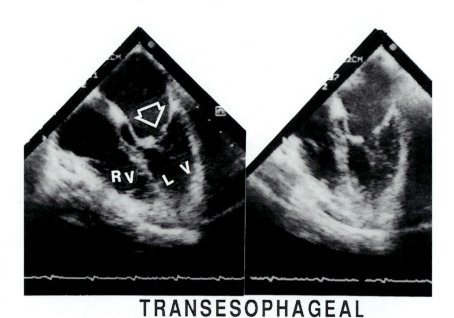

Figure 22–12. TEE view of mitral stenosis. The mitral leaflets are only slightly thickened and show diastolic doming.

TRANSESOPHAGEAL

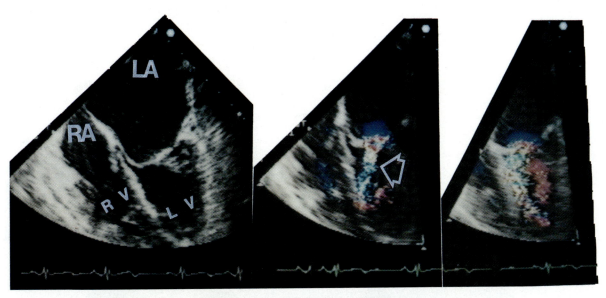

TRANSESOPHAGEAL

Figure 22–13. TEE in a patient with mitral stenosis showing LA dilatation and diastolic doming of pliable mitral leaflets. Color-flow Doppler shows a high velocity turbulent jet (arrow) through the stenotic mitral valve into the left ventricle.

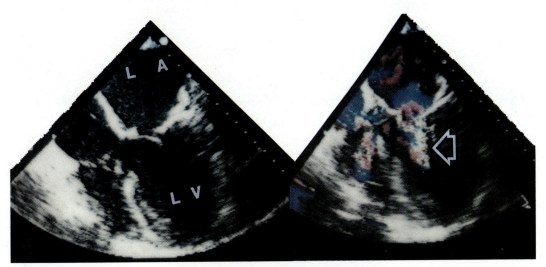

TRANSESOPHAGEAL

Figure 22–14. TEE with Color-flow Doppler in a patient with mitral stenosis showing a turbulent narrow stream entering the LV chamber in diastole.

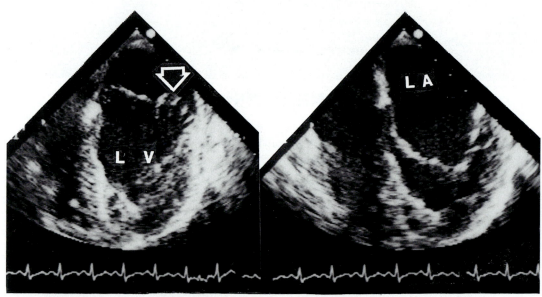

TRANSESOPHAGEAL

Figure 22–15. TEE showing prolapse of the mitral leaflets (arrow) in systole (left). In diastole (right) the long redundant mitral leaflets fall deep into the LV chamber.

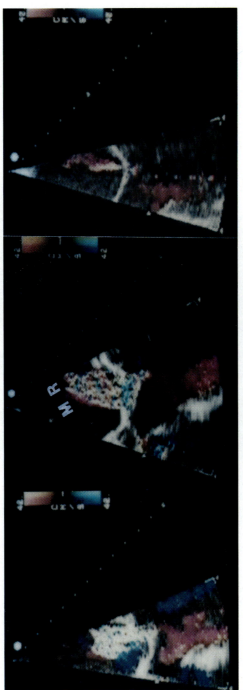

TRANSESOPHAGEAL

Figure 22–16. TEE in Color-flow Doppler mode, showing a turbulent MR jet entering the LA chamber (left and center). At a different phase of the cardiac cycle the MR jet is very small (right).

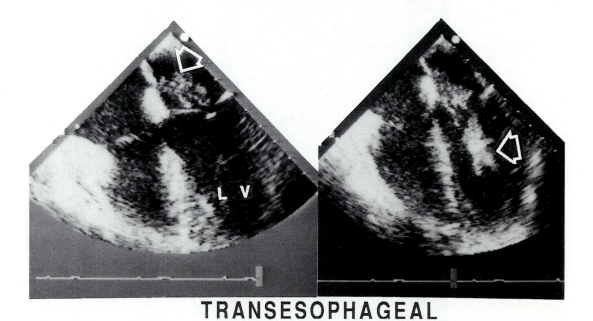

TRANSESOPHAGEAL

Figure 22–17. TEE four-chamber view showing LA myxoma (arrows), which is located in the left atrium in systole (left), but moves into the left ventricle in diastole (right).

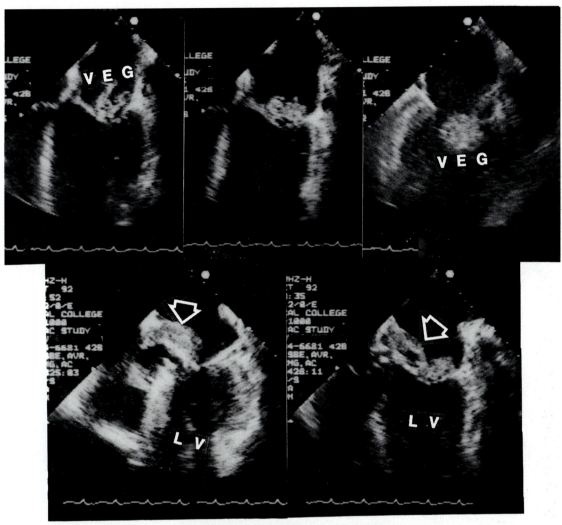

TRANSESOPHAGEAL

Figure 22–18. (Above) TEE showing large vegetations (VEG) on the mitral valve in a patient with staphylococcal endocarditis. (Below) TEE views in a slightly different plane show a paravalvar ring absess (arrow).

A small pericardial recess between the pulmonary trunk and the left atrial appendage is little known to cardiologists. Echocardiographers should be aware of it, because if pericardial fluid accumulates at this site, the small sonolucent space could be mistaken for the left atrial appendage, in which case the actual appendage floating in it might be taken for an atrial thrombus. Such a sonolucent space has even been mistaken for an aneurysm of the left main coronary artery, which is located in this vicinity.

Spontaneous echo contrast in the left atrium is not uncommon in TEE, especially in patients with mitral stenosis or prosthetic mitral valves. These nebulous echoes could be confused with intraatrial thrombi, which are frequent in the same patients. Spontaneous echo contrast attributable to clumping of red blood cells in slow-moving blood can be diagnosed from thrombi because of its fine powdery echo "texture," ill-defined borders, and slow swirling motion pattern.

Valves

Echocardiographers are accustomed to seeing the aorta and mitral valve cusps as thin linear echoes in parasternal and apical views. However, in certain commonly used TEE planes,

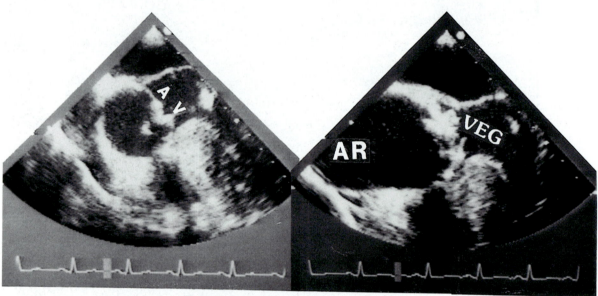

TRANSESOPHAGEAL

Figure 22–19. TEE showing vegetation (VEG) on the aortic valve (AV).

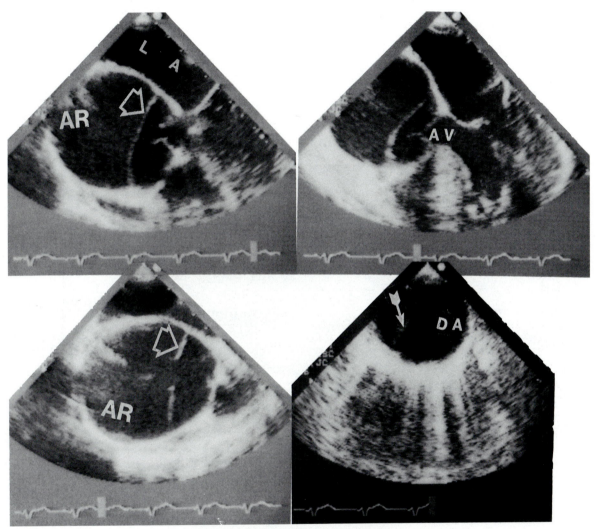

TRANSESOPHAGEAL

Figure 22–20. TEE showing aortic dissection. The aortic root (AR) is very dilated and contains an intimal flap (arrow). The false lumen is less sonolucent because of spontaneous echo-contrast (signifying stasis) in it. AV, aortic valve. Aortic dissection extends into the descending aorta (DA) which is dilated and contains a faint echo representing an intimal flap (small arrow).

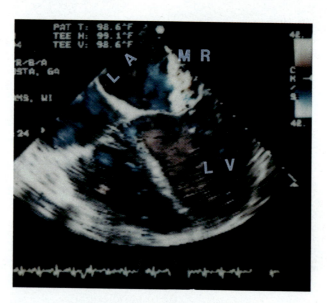

TRANSESOPHAGEAL

Figure 22–21. TEE view showing all four cardiac chambers. A mitral regurgitant (MR) jet is seen entering the LA from the LV.

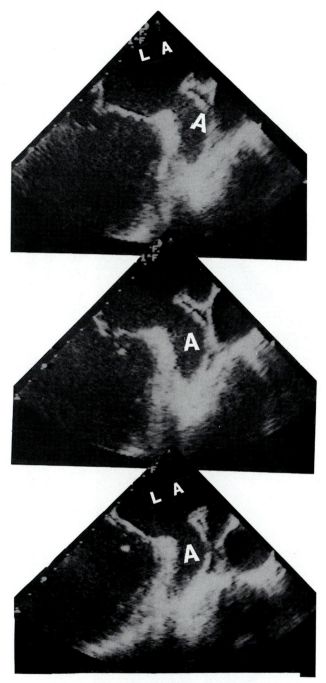

TRANSESOPHAGEAL

Figure 22–22. TEE view in slightly different planes to show the LA with its appendage (A). Note the narrow tubular shape with conical tip of the appendage.

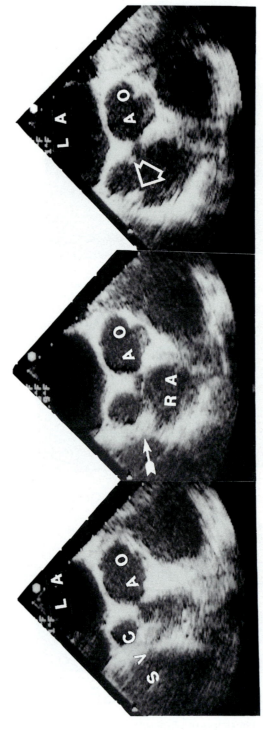

TRANSESOPHAGEAL

Figure 22-23. TEE views in three transverse planes. In the highest (left) the superior vena cava (SVC) is seen to the right of the ascending aorta (Ao). In a slightly lower plane (center) at SVC-RA junction, a normal ridge or indentation (small arrow) can simulate a mass. At a slightly lower level, a small ridge on the inner aspect of the lateral RA wall represents the crista terminalis (open arrows).

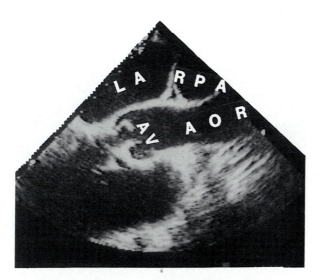

TRANSESOPHAGEAL

Figure 22–24. TEE showing long-axis plane of the ascending aorta (AOR). The aortic valve (AV) is clearly visible. The LA and right pulmonary artery (RPA) are visualized posterior to the aorta.

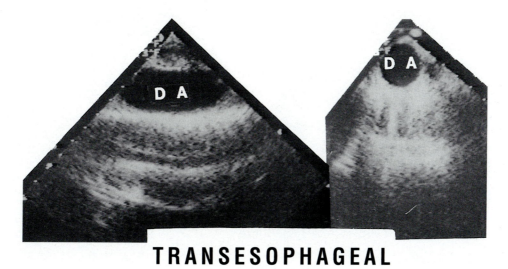

TRANSESOPHAGEAL

Figure 22–25. TEE views showing the descending aorta (DA) in long-axis (left), and in short-axis (right).

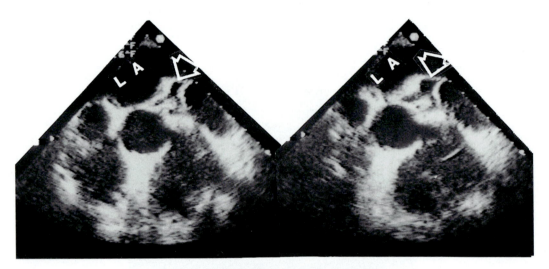

TRANSESOPHAGEAL

Figure 22–26. TEE in a patient with a pericardial effusion. Fluid in a small pericardial recess (open arrows) forms a sonolucent space which is wider during atrial contraction (right) than during atrial relaxation (left).

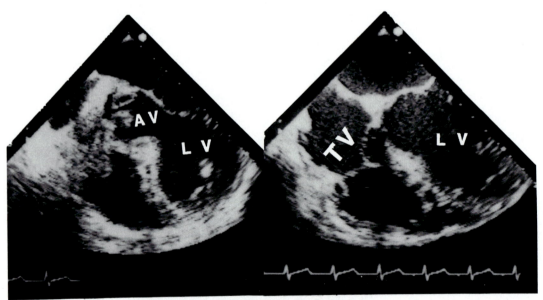

TRANSESOPHAGEAL

Figure 22–27. TEE views in the same patient transecting the LV outflow tract (left); the tricuspid valve is clearly visible at right. The appearance of the aortic valve (AV) simulates vegetations because of the oblique cut.

the ultrasound beam transects the aortic valve cusps obliquely so that the cusps appear artefactually thick, perhaps simulating a vegetation. A similar effect may be obtained with oblique imaging of the mitral or tricuspid leaflets.

Lambl's excrescences are harmless "normal" fine small strands or tags on the aortic cusps, not evident on TTE but visible with the much higher resolution of TEE.

Aorta

On TTE, the aorta commonly has sharply defined smooth walls. Atheromatous plaques are not evident unless particularly large and dense. On TEE, however, the aortic arch and descending aorta are visualized in such fine detail that it is common to encounter atheromatous plaques projecting into the aortic lumen. These are of varying size and contour and may exhibit a mobile component representing superimposed thrombi or atheromatous debris. Such intraaortic objects should not be mistaken for the intimal flap of aortic dissection. Some TEE illustrations are scattered through the preceding 21 chapters. A few more examples of commonly encountered cardiac lesions are shown in Figures 22-8 to 22-17.

REFERENCES

1. Bansal RC, Sakudo M, Shah PM. Biplane transesophageal echocardiography: Technique, image orientation, and preliminary experience in 131 patients. J Am Soc Echocardiogr 1990;3:348.
2. Seward JB, Khandheria BK, Oh JK, et al. Transesophageal echocardiography: Technique, anatomic correlations, implementation and clinical applications. Mayo Clin Proc 1988;63:649.
3. Seward JB, Khandheria BK, Edwards WB, et al. Biplanar transesophageal echocardiography: Anatomic correlations, image orientation, and clinical applications. Mayo Clin Proc 1990;65:1193.
4. Nanda NC, Pinheiro L, Sanyal RS, et al. Transesophageal biplane echocardiographic imaging: Technique, planes and clinical usefulness. Echocardiography 1990;7:771.
5. Blanchard DG, Dittrich HC. Problems and pitfalls, in HC Dittrich (ed): Clinical Transesophageal Echocardiography. St Louis: Mosby-Year Book, 1992, pp 39-47.

INDEX

page numbers in *italics* indicate figures
page numbers followed by t indicate tables

A